KU-997-116

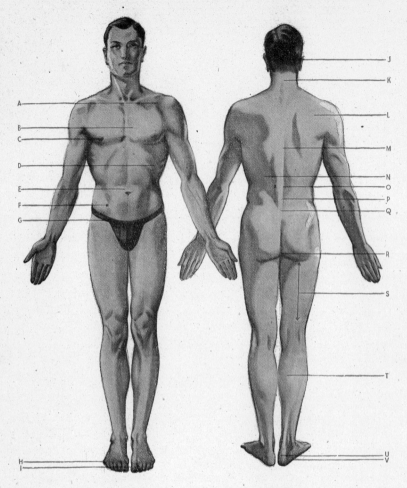

Letters indicate the centre of the areas where warning pains may occur

A, Rheumatism, neuritis, neuralgia, dyspepsia, pleurisy.

B, Anæmia, heart disorders, angina pectoris, dyspepsia.

C, Pleurisy, pneumonia, muscular rheumatism, shingles, pericarditis, phthisis, aneurysm (left side only), dyspepsia (left side only).

D, Dyspepsia, gastric ulcer, acute gastritis, enlarged spleen, colitis, floating kidney, renal colic.

E, Appendicitis (early stages), colic, peritonitis, gastroenteritis, obstruction of bowels, spinal disease.

F, Appendicitis (later stages), *McBurney's Point.*

G, Renal colic, hernia, varicocele, bubo.

H, Corns, neuralgia.

I, Bunion, gout.

J, Neurasthenia, eye-strain, meningitis, rheumatism.

K, Meningitis, spinal disease.

L, Gall-stones, liver disease (right side only), rheumatism, affections of stomach (right side only), neuritis, neuralgia.

M, Dyspepsia, gastric ulcer, spinal disease, rheumatism.

N, Affections of spleen.

O, Constipation, gastric ulcer (often specially tender at x).

P, Lumbago, kidney disease, influenza.

Q, Affections of bladder, prostate, testicles, piles, disease of rectum, sciatica.

R, Piles, anal fistula or fissure, ischio-rectal abscess, coccygeal neuralgia, pruritus ani.

S, Sciatica, affections of rectum.

T, Cramp, phlebitis, varicose veins.

U, Teno-synovitis, neurasthenia.

V, Neuralgia, flat foot.

See also Diagnosis Diagram: The Female Anatomy, Plate I

EVERYBODY'S
FAMILY
DOCTOR

✵

ODHAMS PRESS LTD.
LONG ACRE, LONDON, W.C.2

Copyright

S1244 3RS.
Printed by Wm. Collins Sons and Co. Ltd. Glasgow

INTRODUCTION

THE purpose of this book is a practical one. By consulting it readers will be able to recognize and understand warning symptoms and summon medical assistance in good time, where ignorance might cause delay and aggravate the complaint. To apply correctly these general facts to each individual case, medical training is, of course, necessary; and the importance of the doctor's personal diagnosis and skilled treatment of disease cannot be too much emphasized.

Moreover, medical research has made such strides in the last ten years that the possession of a really up-to-date book of medical knowledge is essential to every home. Treatments given only a few years ago have been superseded to-day by directly opposite methods, and scientific research is continually making new discoveries that show former knowledge to be insufficient and misleading. In this new and revised edition, many new facts are included which have not yet had time to find their way into the standard medical textbooks.* To assist the reader and to ensure immediate and accurate reference, this volume has been arranged alphabetically, with cross-references to other subjects associated with each entry.

It is hoped that this work will not only prove of great practical value and interest in times of sickness, but will also serve as a helpful guide to the best ways of maintaining the health of the individual and the home. Prevention is always better than cure, and it is a matter of supreme importance to us to be able to turn our attention from disease and to concentrate it instead on the creation of sound and lasting health.

THE EDITOR

Harley Street, London, W.1.

---

* See under the following sections: Agranulocytosis, Anæsthetics, Angina Pectoris, Appendicitis, Avertin, Barbiturates, Bronchiectasis, Calciferol, Chiropractic, Coeliac Disease, Deficiency Diseases, Diabetes, Embolectomy, Epilepsy, Lupus, Measles, Menière's Disease, Myasthenia gravis, Obesity, Pernicious Anæmia, Raynaud's Disease, Spondylitis, Undulant Fever, Vitamins, etc.

LIST OF PLATES IN MONOCHROME

The following is the list of plates contained in the inset facing page 128.

EVERYBODY'S FAMILY DOCTOR

A.B.C. LINIMENT. A liniment or rubbing mixture made up of equal parts of the drugs aconite, belladonna and chloroform. It is very good for relieving pain caused by lumbago, sciatica, neuralgia, rheumatism, stiffness after exercise, etc.

ABDOMEN. The abdomen is the main part of the trunk of the body and consists of a large cavity containing the various abdominal organs. It is popularly known as the belly or stomach, but the stomach proper is merely one of the organs contained in the abdomen.

Abdomen, Contents of. The organs of *viscera* which lie in the abdomen are contained in a cavity which is lined by a smooth membrane called the *peritoneum*. This membrane is attached to the wall of the abdomen on its outer side, and on its inner side stretches over the organs beneath it. It is lubricated by a small amount of *serous fluid* and thus the organs are protected from friction with the peritoneum and each other.

The organs contained in the abdomen are described from the diaphragm downwards : The *liver* is to the right and is situated mostly under the right ribs, but it also extends partly across the body and under the left ribs. Underneath the liver is the *gallbladder*, which is a small bag in which the bile or juice produced by the liver is stored and concentrated before it is poured into the duodenum. In front of the liver and to the middle and left

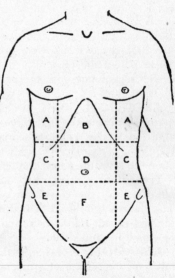

Abdomen : Divisions of

A. Hypochondriac;　　B. Epigastric;
C. Lumbra; D. Umbilical; E. Iliac;
F. Hypogastric Regions.

of the abdomen lies the *stomach*, which joins, on the right side of the body, on to the duodenum. Below the stomach and to the left of it is the *spleen*, and a long body called the *pancreas* (called sweetbread in animals), which lies behind the stomach between the spleen and

7

the duodenum. In front of the liver and below it, but behind and below the stomach, are the *kidneys*, one on the right and one on the left of the abdomen. Attached to them above are the *suprarenal glands* or *adrenals*. The rest of the abdomen proper is taken up with the coils of the small bowel or *intestine*, and the *large intestine* which is divided into the *cæcum* and *appendix* and the ascending, transverse and descending *colon*. The whole of this *intestinal tract* is popularly known as the bowels. In the pelvis or lower part of the abdomen are the *bladder*, which acts as a reservoir for the urine until it is ready to be voided, part of the colon, the whole of the *rectum*, which is the lower end of the intestinal tract, and most of the organs of reproduction.

ABDOMINAL TUMOURS IN WOMEN. Tumours of one sort or another are fairly common in women. They can be present at all ages and whether the woman is married or single. In a great many cases they are either cystic tumours of the ovary, which are commonly called ovarian cysts, or they are solid fibroid tumours of the womb, known as fibroids. These tumours may remain small and be quite harmless, but sometimes they grow to an enormous size and cause trouble by pressing on the surrounding organs. There is also the possibility that they may turn malignant, which in fact means turn into cancer. It is safer, therefore, to have such tumours removed. (*See also* FIBROIDS ; FLOODING.)

ABORTION. When the contents of the womb are lost prematurely during the first three months of pregnancy, this is called abortion. The word miscarriage is usually applied when this expulsion takes place between the fourth and seventh months, and after the seventh month the term premature delivery is used.

Treatment. Pains, of the same character as labour pains, and bleeding, are the two main symptoms of a threatened abortion. The patient should go to bed immediately and the bottom end of the bed raised. If the pain and bleeding continue, a doctor should be called in immediately.

ABRASION. Abrasion is the term generally applied to a slight injury of the skin or of a mucous membrane. The most important thing is to keep the wound clean, and this may be done by applying a simple antiseptic lotion, such as boracic lotion, or iodine, and covering with a dressing in order to prevent germs from entering.

ABSCESS. An abscess is a collection of pus, or matter, which comes to a head in any part of the body. The centre of the abscess where the pus collects has a yellowish appearance, and is surrounded by a hot and painful area of hard, reddened flesh which is called the abscess wall, and which serves to keep the pus away from the healthy flesh. There is usually quite a definite swelling and the pain is a throbbing one. Plenty of nourishing food, rest, fresh air and a tonic should therefore be taken by anyone who is inclined to have abscesses.

Abscesses which are described under separate headings are Gumboil, Whitlow, Breast Abscess, Iliac Abscess (Appendicitis), Ischio-rectal Abscess, Lung Abscess, Psoas Abscess, and Retro-

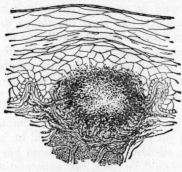

Abscess

pharyngeal Abscess. (*See also* DISEASES OF THE BRAIN, BONE, RECTUM AND ANUS, LUNG, LIVER, SPINE, EAR, GLANDS *and* JOINTS.)

ABSCESS, COLD. There is a form of chronic abscess which is due to the tubercle bacillus, and which is called a " cold abscess." It is of slow development and in the early stages may give rise to few or no symptoms. The usual signs of festering are not often present, but pus is slowly gathering under the skin and its presence may be recognized from the fact that the skin pits on pressure, i.e. remains white for a short time after it is pressed. The parts most often attacked are the spine, hips, joints, genito-urinary organs and the glands.

Treatment. In the very early stages non-operative treatment may be tried, and a cure is sometimes obtained. The first essential of such treatment is absolute rest of the affected part for a very long period, even for several years. This rest is secured by means of splints and plaster of Paris bandages or jackets. The patient in the meantime should live almost entirely in the open air on a generous diet which includes eggs, milk and butter in abundance. Cod-liver oil, or halibut-liver oil, should be taken daily.

ABSCESS, EXTERNAL. An external abscess is one which forms in the fleshy parts of the body, or in glands or the cellular tissue just under the skin.

Treatment. The treatment of an external abscess should be

directed towards maintaining the strength, and therefore the
resisting powers, of the patient, and assisting the pus to come to
the surface or to point as it is called. The patient should therefore
rest and especially should keep the affected part at rest. If the
temperature is raised, the resting should be done in bed. Hot
fomentations or poultices should be used continuously and as hot
as the patient can bear comfortably, until the abscess begins to
point, when it should be opened. Antiphlogistine is a very convenient form of poultice. To leave the abscess to burst of its own
accord only means a longer period of suffering for the patient, and
the additional risk of septicæmia or blood-poisoning. After the
abscess has been opened with a carefully sterilized instrument—
and this operation should be carried out by a doctor—special care
should be taken to keep the wound clean. The wound should be
squeezed to expel as much pus as possible, and then the surrounding
skin should be cleaned with a mild disinfectant. A dressing of
boracic lint, rung out in warm water, should be laid on the wound
and covered with oil-skin. After the abscess has been opened no
further poultices should be used, but antiseptic dressings applied.
(*See also* BOIL ; CARBUNCLE.)

ABSCESS, INTERNAL. An internal abscess is one which
forms in one of the internal organs of the body, such as the liver,
kidneys or lungs, or in one of the passages through the body such
as the bowels, the œsophagus, the bladder, etc. These internal
abscesses are always a matter for the doctor and are often a very
serious affair.

ABSORPTION. This means that one substance takes up or
absorbs another. The absorbent most often used in medicine is
wood charcoal which is given as a powder, or in the form of lozenges
or biscuits to absorb gases in the stomach or bowels, thus relieving
flatulence. Charcoal has also been recommended as a means of
removing the odour from foul ulcers.

ACARUS. This is the name applied to a tick, or mite, which
takes up its abode in the skin, and is responsible for the skin disease
known as the itch or scabies.

ACCIDENTAL HÆMORRHAGE *See* BLEEDING.

ACCOMMODATION (OF EYE). The eye in health has a
changing refractive power ; this is known as *accommodation*. If the eye
is directed towards a distant object the rays of light entering it
should be focused exactly on the retina ; and if the eye is turned
towards an object a few inches off, as in reading, the elastic circular
ligament, in the centre of which the lens is suspended, is drawn
together by the muscle, which allows the lens to become more
globular. The lens therefore becomes a lens of higher power, and

the diverging rays from a near object are still brought to a focus on the retina. The amount of power possessed by the eye of thus suiting itself for far and near objects is known as its range of accommodation.

At the age of 45, the lens has lost much of its elasticity, though this change has been slowly going on through life, owing to the gradual sclerosis or hardening of the lens. By the age of 60, though the lens may be quite clear, it is incapable of this accommodative change in shape. That is, it has now a constant refractive power such as a glass lens has, and its focus is for distant objects only. Consequently, a natural change with advancing years is that persons become unable to read, sew, or do other fine work without glasses, though for distant vision no such aid is necessary. This natural change is known as presbyopia (old-sightedness).

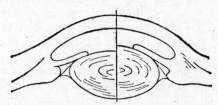

Accommodation of Eye : Showing Change in the lens

In addition to this, there are three errors in the refractive power of the eye, which may be present at birth, or come on early in life, or in the course of some disease, and persist through life. In these conditions the movements of the lens are not always sufficient to focus rays of light accurately on the retina. They are known as astigmatism, hypermetropia, and myopia. (*See also* VISION, ERRORS OF.)

ACCOUCHEMENT. The French term for child-birth. A professional male attendant at child-birth is called an accoucheur and a professional female attendant an accoucheuse, but this term should not be applied to the ordinary midwife.

A.C.E. MIXTURE. This is a mixture of alcohol, chloroform and ether, and is often used as an anæsthetic.

ACETABULUM. A cup-shaped depression on each side of the pelvis, into which the head of the thigh bone (femur) fits.

ACETIC ACID. Acetic acid is the acid contained in vinegar. It is a colourless liquid and must not be taken internally. Acetic acid or vinegar is very often taken internally as a means of reducing stoutness. Whether it has the desired effect it would be difficult to say, but it would certainly be at the expense of good health. It is often applied to warts and corns, but great care should be taken when using it for this purpose, as, owing to its burning action, it may cause irritation to the surrounding skin.

In cases of poisoning by strong acetic acid, the mouth is burnt, and the breath has an odour of vinegar. The treatment is to give chalk or whitewash in water immediately, and later white of egg or olive-oil. No emetic should be given.

ACHE. This term is applied to any continuous or throbbing pain. It may occur owing to a variety of conditions. For instance, in rheumatism, it is not unusual for people to describe their symptoms as a " dull ache." In cases of abscess the pain may be of the throbbing variety.

ACHILLES TENDON. The Achilles tendon is the tendon at the back of the heel. It is so called after Achilles, one of

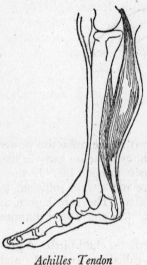

Achilles Tendon

the Greek leaders against the Trojans, about whom the story is told that his mother dipped him in the river Styx as a baby in order to make him invulnerable. Unfortunately she had to hold him by some part of his body while she dipped him into the river. She therefore held him by the smallest possible place she could grip him by, which was the narrow part of the back of his heel. When he grew to manhood no spear or arrow could harm him, until one day his enemy, Paris, shot him in the back of the heel and thus killed him. The muscles of the calf of the leg are attached to the heel bone by this tendon. It is the strongest tendon in the body and is not easily put out of order. If torn, it may require an operation to heal it. *(See also* FOOT.)

ACHONDROPLASIA is a condition met with most often in one child of a large family. The bones grow hard at too early an age, so that the skeleton becomes dwarfed. The face and skull are the normal size, with the result that the head appears too large for the stunted body. The nose is usually depressed at the bridge and is described as " saddle-shaped." The child develops normally and is healthy and intelligent. A peculiarity of these children is the extraordinary way they rise from the sitting to the standing position without bending the knees. Pairs or troupes of achondroplasiacs may be seen appearing as professional comedians. There is no known cure for the condition and no treatment is needed.

ACHYLIA. Deficiency of the normal gastric juice in the stomach.

ACID. This is a term generally applied to any substance which has a sour taste. It should be noted that many acids are poisonous and some are corrosive.

Treatment of Acid Poisoning. If strong corrosive acid is taken internally it produces a burning sensation in the mouth, throat and stomach, and this is followed by severe pain. The patient should be given liberal doses of chalk, magnesia, baking soda or whiting in water. The doctor should be called at once, but in the meantime *no* emetic should be given to the patient to cause vomiting. Demulcents may be given, such as white of egg, olive-oil, or arrowroot. As the patient may have difficulty in breathing owing to irritation of the throat, cloths wrung out in hot water may be applied to relieve the pain.

ACIDITY. Commonly called "heartburn," this is a condition in which there is a sour or burning taste in the throat and at the back of the tongue, due to sourness of the stomach and the welling up of acid fluid from the stomach into the mouth, together with an increased flow of saliva. (*See also* HYPERCHLORHYDRIA, HYPER-SECRETION, HYPOCHLORHYDRIA.)

ACIDOSIS. This means a condition in which there is not enough alkali in the blood, with the result that the acids are present in too great a proportion. In children, acidosis often accounts for the long continued slight feverishness to which some children are prone and for which no obvious reason is visible to the parents. Care should be taken that such children are not described as "nervous" and left without any attempt at remedying their deficiency of alkalis. A still worse fault is to consider the condition to be due to rheumatism and to give acid in the form of salicylic acid, which makes matters worse. In grown-up persons acidosis may cause feverishness, headache, neuralgia, faintness, dyspepsia and the form of difficulty in breathing in which the patient suffers from "air hunger." A striking result of acidosis is extreme drowsiness amounting almost to a state of coma.

In order to prevent acidosis it is necessary to see that there is a sufficient supply of carbohydrate in the diet, and in the case of diabetes, insulin. Bicarbonate of soda should be taken several times a day, and glucose up to 2 oz. a day.

ACNE (Acne vulgaris). Acne, or "Blackheads," is probably the most common form of chronic skin disease, and is most usual between the ages of sixteen and twenty-six. It attacks certain definite areas of skin : the forehead, nose, and cheeks ; the ear ; the back of the neck ; and the upper part of the body, both back and front. In rare cases, it covers the whole of the trunk and the limbs.

The essence of the disease is hyperkeratosis or overgrowth of the horny layer of the skin. In the mouths of the sweat glands of the skin this overgrowth forms a *comedo*, which is a tiny black speck shaped like an elongated onion, and with its horny scales arranged in a similar way. The yellow material which can be squeezed out below this black speck is not really part of the comedo, but is oil which has been unable to get away. In this will be found the roots of a hair, a germ known as the *Bacillus acnes*, and several varieties of other germs, which add to the trouble. The comedo or " blackhead " as it is commonly called, does not get its colour from dirt, but from the upper layers of the blackheads becoming dry and horny, and changing in colour as they do so.

Acne, causes of. The cause of acne is now generally considered to be the *Bacillus acnes*, which is always found in the comedones. Among other causes are the increased activity of the skin and hair at the age of puberty, and the changes in the glands which occur at that time. Seborrhœa (dandruff) of the hair and skin (*See* SEBORRHŒA) is very frequently found with acne, and many specialists believe that there is a definite connection between the two diseases. The treatment of acne should therefore always include that of seborrhœa. Other contributory causes are defective general nutrition, constipation, anæmia, and menstrual irregularities.

Treatment. The main factors in the cure of acne are time, attention to the general health, and perseverance with local treatment. Most cases, even if untreated, slowly clear up in the twenties ; but few patients are willing to endure an unpleasant disease for years without some attempt at curing it. Also the scars left are as disfiguring as the disease, and one may act as a starting-point for worse trouble.

With regard to general treatment, the patient should attend most carefully to the rules of hygiene. He should take regular exercise in the open air, and eat plain but sufficient food, avoiding the rich, " fried-fat " type of diet, and having instead plenty of vegetables and fruit. A cold morning bath, followed by a brisk rub-down with a rough towel, helps to promote a healthy reaction of the skin. A general tonic is often useful ; constipation, anæmia, and menstrual irregularities, if present, should be treated. The first, especially, is often to blame for a continued unhealthiness of the skin which, though not actually causing the disease, renders it unfit to combat infection.

Internal remedies for acne proper are of little or no use ; several have been advocated from time to time, but have invariably proved disappointing.

With regard to local treatment, one has always to remember the local symptoms of tough skin, greasiness, anæmia, and flabbiness. One treatment, luckily, has an influence on all four, and that is the vigorous washing with plenty of soap accompanied by rubbing, which not only removes the grease and thickened horny layer, but by means of the friction with which it is applied, invigorates the blood-supply and the muscles. Sulphur soap is generally recommended.

ACNE ROSACEA. This is a skin disease which appears only on the face. It starts as a slight flush or congestion of the nose and cheeks, sometimes of the chin and the middle part of the forehead. This redness, which is due to over fullness of the surface blood-vessels, is apt to become chronic. Accompanying this, there is often an oily appearance of the skin, with red pimples and spots ; the appearance is rather like that in ordinary acne, though comedones (blackheads) are absent, and the nose becomes coarsened and enlarged.

Treatment. General health treatment is of special importance in this disease. Particular attention should be paid to regularity of the bowels, opening medicine being taken at least twice weekly whether the patient needs it or not. As to diet, the patient should avoid anything which he notices causes flushing of the face, especially alcohol, tea, coffee, highly-flavoured dishes such as curry, condiments and tobacco. Vegetarianism has been suggested in obstinate cases. Extremes of temperature should be avoided as far as possible, even to taking warm baths in preference to hot or cold.

ACONITE. Aconite, aconitine, and their preparations are obtained from roots collected from *Aconitum Napellus* or monk's-hood. The root, which is dark brown outside and white inside, is dried in the process of extracting the aconite. It has often been mistaken for horseradish and, as aconite is a powerful poison, the results have sometimes been fatal.

Aconite produces local anæsthesia on the skin and it is frequently used in cases of neuralgia. Care should be taken that it does not come in contact with any mucous membrane or broken skin. It is used a great deal in the form of an ointment, but much more frequently as a liniment. This drug was, at one time, used internally in cases of fever, with the object of decreasing the force and tension of the pulse.

Poisoning by Aconite. The symptoms come on very quickly when this most powerful poison has been taken internally. In a few minutes there is a severe tingling sensation and burning in the mouth, followed by numbness. Vomiting usually takes place after an hour or two and is very severe in character. The burning sensation is usually felt in the stomach also, and the skin may feel very cold and clammy. The pupils of the eyes are usually enlarged and the eyes may become fixed and staring. The muscles become weak and the pulse is very irregular. Death takes place from suffocation and the patient is often conscious to the end.

Treatment consists of washing out the stomach as promptly as possible. Emetics should be given ; one to two tablespoonsful of mustard in half a glass of warm water is a very common one. Artificial respiration should be administered early. Strychnine and digitalis may be given hypodermically, and brandy or strong coffee should be given per rectum. Hot blankets and hot-water bottles should be placed around the patient's abdomen and extremities. Artificial respiration should be kept up unceasingly. (*See also* ARTIFICIAL RESPIRATION.)

ACOUSTICS. The science of sounds, on which hearing depends.

ACQUIRED CHARACTERISTICS. The changes in one or more organs of the body which have occurred during the lifetime of the individual.

ACRIFLAVINE. This is also termed flavine, and is a new antiseptic which is powerful in character, but quite harmless. It is bright yellow when mixed with water.

ACRODYNIA. The name of this disease, derived from the Greek, means " pain in the extremities," and this describes its most troublesome symptom. It is a comparatively rare disease, but sometimes breaks out in epidemic form. It is probably toxic in origin, i.e. is due to poisons in the blood, though there are no symptoms of fever. It is found amongst uncleanly people.

The symptoms are those of a severe " bilious attack," nausea, vomiting and diarrhœa ; pains in the extremities, followed by loss of feeling ; and a rash which varies in character, from red spots to small or larger blisters. It usually clears up entirely in a month to eight weeks.

The treatment is to treat the symptoms. Counter-irritation over the spine is generally advised.

ACROMEGALY. This is a strange disease affecting certain bones of the body, especially the bones of the head, hands, and feet. The bones become enlarged and other tissues may become affected. It is due to some alteration in the working of the pituitary gland, the little gland which lies at the base of the brain and manufactures a substance which is necessary for the growth of the body. In some cases a change in the pituitary gland causes growth of the whole body, especially if it occurs early in life, but if it occurs later, the over-development is more local. Sometimes there may be a serious loss of sight owing to the pressure of the pituitary growth on the nerves of the eye. Pituitary extract and thyroid extract have proved of some benefit in a good many cases, and surgical operation may be tried. (*See also* BRAIN ; DUCTLESS GLANDS.)

ACROMION. The acromion is a bony projection at the summit of the shoulder-blade or scapula.

ACTINO - THERAPY. This is the medical name for treatment by artificial sunlight, and by the different rays that go to make up sunlight, such as ultra-violet rays, etc. (*See also* LIGHT TREATMENT.)

ACUTE. If an illness begins suddenly and gets quickly worse with pronounced symptoms, which in a few days or even hours are at their height, the illness is called *acute*. Diseases are described as acute, sub-acute or more gradual than acute, and chronic where the condition settles down and remains for a long period of weeks or months in a stationary condition without becoming either acute or cured. (*See also* DISEASE.)

ADAM'S APPLE. The lump seen under the skin in the front of the throat is commonly known as the Adam's apple. It is really the most prominent cartilage of the larynx, and is much larger in men than in women. (*See also* LARYNX.)

ADDER BITE. For treatment *see* BITE ; BITES AND STINGS.

ADDISON'S DISEASE. This disease was named after the physician, Thomas Addison, who was on the staff of Guy's Hospital in the early part of the nineteenth century. It is usually due to tuberculosis of the suprarenal capsules, two glands which are situated just above the kidneys. The symptoms are the bronze colour of the skin, extreme muscular weakness, vomiting, and enfeebled heart action. The blood-pressure is low and the temperature is usually subnormal. Secondary anæmia may be present. Recovery has been recorded in some cases, but the disease is a very serious one and death may occur in a few weeks or be delayed for several years. The introduction of injections of cortical extract (eucortone) has undoubtedly brightened the outlook for recovery, but at present this remedy is very expensive. (*See also* DUCTLESS GLANDS.)

ADDUCTOR. Muscles which move the structures to which they are attached towards the middle line of the body are called adductor muscles.

ADENITIS. This term means inflammation of a gland. Inflammation of the lymph glands of the neck is common and often due to unhealthy tonsils. (*See also* LYMPHADENITIS.)

ADENOIDS. This is common among young children, and is due to inflammation and swelling of the mass of tissue that lies between the nose and the throat, up behind the uvula. The uvula is the flap of tissue that can be seen hanging down at the back of the mouth guarding the entrance to the throat. Behind the uvula and higher up, quite out of sight except when looked for with a special mirror on the end of a long handle, lies a mass of tissue which is called the naso-pharyngeal tonsil. A swollen condition of this is known as adenoids. It is composed of the same sort of tissue as the ordinary tonsils, and is always normally present in young children, but it should not be so large and swollen that it blocks the back of the nose and interferes with the child's breathing. Catarrh in the nose and infectious fevers are common causes of the inflammation and swelling which cause adenoids. Infected adenoids are a common cause of deafness and of inflammations of the ear in children. A child with adenoids usually has a characteristically " stupid " look, with open mouth, long face, narrow nose, prominent front teeth, high arched roof of the mouth and flat chest. But in the early stages of the condition, all or at least some of these symptoms may not be present, and the adenoids may only be detected on examination by a doctor.

Treatment. There is no doubt that the best treatment for adenoids is removal by operation, which is only a slight affair, and the child's health nearly always improves at once. Whether the tonsils should always be removed at the same time is another matter : under the age of five it is not usually advised nowadays, unless there are enlarged glands in the neck.

ADENOMA SEBACEUM. This disease is characterized by an overgrowth of the sebaceous glands of the face, forming tumours. They are whitish or reddish-yellow in colour, and cover the whole face, being most numerous on the nose, cheeks, and chin. Enlargement of the small veins of the face also takes place, which adds to the mottled appearance of the patient.

ADHESIONS. By adhesions are meant the undesirable attachments that occur in a joint or organ after injury or inflammation. Any joint which has been injured is very apt to become stiff and limited in its range of movement. To prevent adhesions, massage and movements of the joint are begun at an early stage in the treatment. If the joint does become set it may be a very troublesome business to get back its range of movement, and the adhesions may have to be forcibly broken down under an anæsthetic.

ADHESIVE PLASTER. This is better known as sticking plaster and is chiefly used for holding dressings in position over a wound.

ADIPOSE TISSUE. Fatty tissue distributed throughout the body, the cells of which contain fat-globules. (*See also* OBESITY.)

ADIPOSIS DOLOROSA. Adiposis dolorosa, or Dercum's disease, is characterized by the formation of soft nodules or swellings throughout the flesh of the body, accompanied by neuralgic pains. This usually occurs in women after middle age. Treatment is not very satisfactory, but injections of pituitrin and adrenaline may prove helpful.

ADOLESCENCE, IN BOYS. Adolescence or " growing up " in boys usually lasts about ten years, from the age of fifteen to about twenty-five. This is the most critical time in the life of a man, as it is during these years that his character is formed and the basis for his conduct during the rest of his life usually takes shape. It is a stage which is full of difficulties, and one which should interest the parents or guardians to the fullest extent.

ADOLESCENCE, IN GIRLS. Just as the age of puberty and adolescence plays an important part in the life of a boy, so it is of no less importance in that of a girl. The age at which puberty commences varies between the eleventh and seventeenth year. Adolescence, by which we mean the time in which the girl is growing into the adult type, usually ends about the twenty-first year, but may go on until the twenty-fifth.

The periods of menstruation should commence about this time, and should normally occur about once a month. There is a wide variation in the amount and duration, but it should not be accompanied by much pain or distress. It is true that most authorities say that no pain should accompany the menstrual period, but in the majority of cases there is to be found a certain amount of distress with a marked lowering of the vitality. Any cessation or abnormality of the menstrual period should be looked upon as serious, and medical advice should be sought.

The mental and moral outlook during the period of adolescence is usually developing rapidly in the growing girl. Her doubts and anxieties are numerous, and it is at this time that a mother should show her greatest sympathy and understanding and prepare her for the important part she may be called upon to play later on in life.

ADRENAL. The word adrenal means " near to the kidney," and is commonly used to denote the suprarenal capsules or adrenals, which are two small bodies placed at the upper end of the kidneys. The juices which they produce, and which are released into the blood as it passes through them, are of great importance to health.

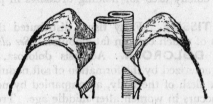

Adrenals or Suprarenal Gland

ADRENALIN. The trade name for a preparation containing the chemical produced by adrenals (the suprarenal glands). It is of great use in arresting bleeding and can be applied locally to the sockets of teeth after extraction, to the bleeding-point in the nose for nose-bleeding, and internally to arrest hæmorrhage from the stomach, intestines, bladder or womb.

ADSORPTION. The process whereby one substance becomes a part of another without becoming chemically combined with it.

ADULT. A person of mature or legal age. The age of legal responsibility in this country is 21, though a person is allowed to drive a motor-car at the age of 17, and the age of legal marriage is 16.

AEROBIC. Aerobic means requiring oxygen or air to live. This term is applied to microbes which require oxygen.

AEROPHAGY. "Air-swallowing," the taking in and swallowing of air. This is a bad habit usually found in hysterical patients. (*See also* FLATULENCE.)

AFEBRILE. Without fever.

AFFERENT. This term means carrying towards the centre. Nerves which convey impulses towards the central nervous system are afferent nerves. The same term is applied to blood-vessels, such as the arteries, which convey blood to the tissues.

AFFUSION. The pouring of water upon the body, or a part of the body, is known as affusion. This method is used to reduce the temperature in fevers.

AFTER-BIRTH. This is the popular name for the placenta, cord, and membranes by which the unborn child is attached to the womb. The placenta comes away a little time after the birth of the child, and it is of the greatest importance that the whole of these membranes should be expelled from the womb. In cases where a portion has been left behind, there is the possibility of decomposition taking place and blood-poisoning arising. (*See also* CHILDBIRTH ; LABOUR.)

AFTER-PAINS. A short time after a child has been born, pains set in again ; these are due to the contractions of the womb expelling the after-birth (placenta, etc.), and pass off again when the placenta has successfully come away.

AGITATION. Mental disturbance or excitement. Restlessness. From the Latin *agito*, I stir.

AGITOGRAPHIA. A condition in which the handwriting is defective owing to omission, slurring or distortion of letters or words, occurring in some nervous diseases.

AGITOPHASIA. A condition of excessive rapidity of speech with sounds or syllables slurred, omitted or distorted.

AGLANDULAR. The state of being without glands.

AGONY. Persons may say they are " in agony " when they are suffering violent pain or extreme anguish. The phrase " the agony of the death-struggle " is often used.

AGORAPHOBIA. This term is applied to an exaggerated and unhealthy fear of open places or spaces. The word literally means " fear of a market place." (*See also* CLAUSTROPHOBIA.)

AGRANULOCYTOSIS. This is a disease only recently recognized, which usually begins with a sore throat and mouth and feeling of general weakness, and progresses rapidly to severe ulceration and necrosis involving the lips, mouth, tongue and throat. It is not usually diagnosed at an early stage unless a blood examination is made, which reveals a peculiar condition of the blood cells. Agranulocytosis has been found to follow the use of certain drugs, especially pyramidon, which is frequently found in patent medicines and compound tablets. The treatment is as for pernicious anæmia, using liver extract ; injections of pentnucleotide are also used successfully.

AGRAPHIA. This is a condition in which the patient is unable to express ideas in writing. In certain forms of this trouble, the patient may be able to write, but what he has written conveys no meaning whatever. Sometimes the patient may be quite unable to copy writing, but be perfectly able to write from dictation, while another form is loss of capacity to write from dictation.

AGUE. An old-fashioned name for Malarial fever, in which there are always severe chills and sweatings and which recurs at regular intervals. Three hundred years ago England was full of " ague." (*See also* MALARIA.)

AILMENT. A disease, sickness, or complaint.

AILUROPHOBIA. An unnatural fear of cats. This is different from the easily understandable dislike of the domestic cat found in people who get asthma when they are in the same room as a cat.

AINHUM. This is a disease of the dark-skinned races who live in warm countries ; it is limited to the toes, and characterized by their becoming diseased and dropping off of their own accord. The treatment consists in amputation of the affected part.

AIR. The air or atmosphere consists of a mixture of gases : 77 parts of nitrogen, 21 parts of oxygen and a trace of carbon dioxide. It also contains traces of ammonia, argon, nitrites and organic matter, as well as a varying amount of water vapour. The purest air is to be found on the tops of mountains or far out at sea. In towns the air is always polluted by gases given off from factories, drains, coal-heated houses, etc., and bad ventilation encourages the growth and spread of germs which produce disease.

AIR HUNGER. Difficulty of breathing or dyspnœa when a person gasps for breath is referred to as air hunger. The condition is usually due to heart disease. (*See also* DYSPNŒA.)

AIR-SWALLOWING. *See* AEROPHAGY.

ALBINISM. Albinism is a condition in which a person or animal is born without the usual colouring matter in the skin. The hair is quite white and the eyes are pink. Every person who has to do with the breeding of small animals will probably be familiar with albinos, which turn up from time to time in litters of rabbits, rats, mice, etc. But there are also human albinos as well. In most cases of albinism, however, it will be found that the parents or other ancestors have shown a similar absence of colouring matter. The condition lasts throughout the lifetime. Usually the eyes of an albino are very weak and they have to wear glasses of a special kind.

ALBUMIN. Albumin is the chief substance found in the tissues of human beings. It contains carbon, hydrogen, nitrogen, oxygen and sulphur. The white of an egg (called albumen) is largely composed of albumin.

ALBUMINURIA. When albumin, which is an important substance present in the human tissues, appears in excess in the urine, the patient is said to have albuminuria. Its appearance may mean very little if it is temporary and due to faults of the diet or to a feverish condition, but it is also a symptom of disease of the kidneys, and its presence should always lead to a thorough investigation. In pregnant women especially, the presence of albuminuria should always be looked upon as a warning that there may be a danger of the serious condition known as eclampsia or " fits " arising, and for this reason the urine should be regularly examined during pregnancy.

Albuminuria occurs without any apparent reason in children, but they usually grow out of it. There may also be a considerable amount of albumin present in the urine of athletes directly after strenuous exercise. This has no significance.

Many cases of albuminuria are first discovered when the patient submits to examination for life insurance, to which it is usually a bar, owing to the serious outlook regarding a long life for the person with a chronic kidney disease such as Bright's disease.

ALCOHOL. The " alcohol " which is commonly referred to, is one of a large group of chemical substances known as the alcohol group. Many of these are produced by the fermentation of sugary fluids, ethyl alcohol (alcohol) being much the most important. A simpler member of the same series is methyl alcohol, which is obtained by distilling wood, and is called wood alcohol or wood spirit. It has similar actions to alcohol, but in human beings is apt to produce fatal and serious results from a single dose. Blindness is not infrequently caused thus.

When it is pure, alcohol is a colourless liquid with a faint and fleeting odour.

ALCOHOL. ACTION ON MAN. In dealing with the action of any drug on living tissues, its strength at the point at which it acts is very important. Strong alcohol used locally on any particular spot is capable of producing great irritation and damage. This property may, however, be used for hardening the skin, and also as an antiseptic since it will kill bacteria. The drinking of strong liquors is liable to lead to damage of the delicate lining of the stomach unless this be protected by the presence within it of other liquids or solid food. It is also associated with a violent burning sensation both in the mouth and in the gullet, as well as in the stomach. This may vary from the pleasant warming sensation which makes for good fellowship, to a severe pain. Different individuals vary considerably in the way they are affected by strong liquors, and many suffer from a severe inflammation of the stomach after small amounts of alcohol which do not affect others. This ability to tolerate alcohol or " hold one's liquor " may be lost during or after an illness.

The local irritation caused by drinking strong liquor leads to changes in the body which may not appear to have any connection with it, such as the raising of the blood-pressure, or the quickening of the rate of breathing. The administration of alcoholic stimulants is thus frequently useful in attacks of fainting, where both the blood-pressure and the breathing are impaired. Other irritants, such as smelling-salts (sal volatile), serve equally well.

Drinking dilute alcohol induces a feeling of warmth and well-being, and a marked flushing of the face. Not infrequently gas contained in the stomach is also released and allowed to escape by the mouth. These combined actions are known as a carminative effect, and are due to a combination of factors. The most quickly acting cause is the expansion of the blood-vessels, which expansion is directly produced by the alcohol. It may be caused indirectly by the irritation to the nerves of the stomach. The " hiccough " is caused by the local effect on the muscles of the stomach causing them to relax. As the upper opening, or sphincter of the stomach, is normally closed, alcohol, by relaxing them, causes them to open and allows the gas to escape. This latter action is used in medicine, and also to relieve the feeling of excessive fullness after a heavy meal by the taking of a small amount of concentrated liquor such as port or liqueur.

Alcohol in the stomach also causes an abundant production of the gastric, or digestive juices, which property is valuable in cases where these juices are scanty and poor owing to fatigue, exhaustion, general weakness or excitement. Strong solutions, however, may themselves diminish the juices and should not be taken on an empty stomach.

ALCOHOLIC NEURITIS. *See* MULTIPLE NEURITIS.

ALE. An alcoholic beverage brewed from hops and malt. It contains from 3 to 7 per cent. of alcohol.

ALEPPO BUTTON. Also known as Oriental sore, Oriental boil, Delhi boil, Baghdad sore, and by other names, according to places in which it is found. It begins as a pimple which spreads and breaks down into an ulcer. This heals very slowly, usually taking from six months to two years to clear up. As a rule a few sores make their appearance, often leaving unsightly scars, so that if the disease occurs on the face there may be much disfigurement.

It is caused by infection with a parasite, and the disease is probably spread by a special sort of sand-fly. One attack of Aleppo Button usually gives lifelong protection against any subsequent attack. Treatment is usually successfully carried out by injections of sodium antimony tartrate.

ALEUKEMIA. Deficiency in the proportion of white cells in the blood.

ALIMENTARY CANAL. The passage through which food passes from the mouth to the anus or lower opening of the bowel. Its parts are called, in the order in which they occur, the mouth, pharynx, œsophagus (or gullet), the stomach and pylorus, duodenum, jejunum, ileum (small intestine), cæcum and appendix, colon (large intestine), the rectum and anus.

ALIMENTARY SYSTEM. The digestive tube which extends

from the mouth to the anus is known as the alimentary canal or tract ; but the accessory glands such as the salivary glands, the pancreas and the liver are also included in the alimentary system. (*See also* Digestion.)

ALKALI. This term is derived from an Arabic word meaning soda-ash. Chemical substances which are alkalis include bicarbonate of soda, which is one of the most frequently used medicines in cases of acidity. When an alkali comes in contact with an acid substance, the two unite and neutralize each other ; in other words, they form a salt substance which is neither alkaline nor acid.

ALKALINE POISONING. Strong alkalis such as caustic soda, strong ammonia, etc., act as very corrosive poisons. Emetics should not be given, as the act of vomiting would only increase the irritation of the throat. While the doctor is being called, the patient may be given a small quantity of lemon juice or vinegar, in about half a glass of water. This may be followed by milk, white of egg beaten up with a little water, barley water, arrowroot or olive-oil. To relieve pain in the abdomen and throat, hot fomentations should be administered and the patient should be kept as warm as possible.

ALKALOID. Alkaloids are substances extracted from plants, which have a powerful action in one way or another. They are alkalis and are nearly all bitter to the taste. Some of our most powerful and useful drugs are alkaloids. A few of the more common ones are aconite, obtained from monk's-hood, atropine from deadly nightshade, cocaine from coca leaves, digitalin from foxglove, ergotin from rye, morphia, heroin and codeine from poppies, nicotine from tobacco, quinine from cinchona bark and strychnine from nux vomica seeds.

ALKALOSIS. The chemicals in the body are either acids or alkalis and to keep the body in perfect health a definite amount of each sort is required. Alkalosis is simply the disordered state of the body in which there is too much alkali for the amount of acid in the blood. The condition is usually the result of taking large amounts of alkalis, such as bicarbonate of soda or magnesia, which are prescribed in large amounts in certain diseases of the stomach such as stomach ulcer, but it may also be the result of severe vomiting. It is found also in mountain sickness and heart failure, when it is due to lack of oxygen in the blood.

The chief symptoms are a feeling of uneasiness, headache, giddiness, loss of appetite, vomiting, twitching limbs, and coma. As soon as alkalosis is discovered to be present, all alkalis should be stopped at once, and sugar in the form of glucose should be given ; at least 1 oz. in water three times a day. Glucose is very sickly to the taste, so if the patient is unable to keep down the glucose taken by mouth, it may be given by injection into the bowel. Calcium may also be prescribed.

ALLERGY. This is a condition present in certain individuals which is best described as a chemical " idiosyncrasy." Its manifestations, such as swelling and itching, and bodily discomfort, are often brought about by a particular article of food, the most common being fish, eggs, milk and wheat. If, for example, after a meal all of the participants become ill, something was probably wrong with the food ; but if only one person becomes ill, with all eating the same food, something was probably wrong with that individual. In the first case, the condition is food poisoning ; in the second case, food *allergy*. But allergy is not necessarily associated only with a disposition to being upset by certain foods. *Hay-fever*, in which the person is upset by the irritation of certain pollens—timothy grass being the most common—is a form of allergy ; and so is *asthma*, which, however, may often be brought on by certain articles of food ; one person may get an attack of asthma from the same article of food, that another allergic person may get an attack of nettle-rash (urticaria). The real cause of allergy is still obscure, but it can be controlled by the avoidance of the upsetting articles of food, and by injections of adrenaline, ephedrine or peptone. (*See also* ANAPHYLAXIS.)

ALOES. Aloes is one of the most popular drugs used for the purpose of purging the bowels. It is included in many patent medicines and pills, acts chiefly on the lower bowel and is very useful in the treatment of chronic constipation.

ALOPECIA AREATA. This is the term given to the development of small rounded areas on the scalp, which have become completely bald. These sometimes increase in size and run together until the whole scalp appears absolutely hairless. The cause of this disease is not definitely known. The recovery from this condition is usually slow, and if occurring in elderly persons, will probably take longer.

All forms of treatment aim at stimulating the scalp in some way or another. The scalp should be kept thoroughly clean and sulphur ointment should be rubbed in every night. Other remedies are turpentine, vinegar, paraffin oil, etc. It should be remembered that the rubbing necessary for the application of these remedies is probably the most important part of the cure. Applications of ultra-violet rays have sometimes proved of great benefit in the treatment of Alopecia Areata.

ALUM. Alum is an astringent formerly used in a throat paint. Powdered alum applied to a cut will often stop bleeding. One or two teaspoonsful dissolved in a pint of hot water may be used as a vaginal douche in cases of leucorrhœa or " whites." A solution of alum is useful to destroy slugs, snails, and their eggs without harming the plants.

ALVEOLAR ABSCESS. *See* GUMBOIL.

ALVEOLUS. The bony socket in which the tooth is fixed is known as an alveolus. A gumboil is known as an alveolar abscess and is usually due to a decayed tooth.

AMAUROSIS. The technical name for part or total blindness. (*See* BLINDNESS.)

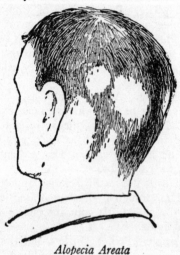

Alopecia Areata

AMAUROTIC CAT'S EYE. This is the name given to a condition of the pupil of the eye in which it glows like a cat's eye in the dark. It occurs when the eye is pushed forward as, for instance, by a tumour.

AMBIDEXTROUS. A person who is able to use both hands equally well is said to be ambidextrous.

AMBLYOPIA, or AMAUROSIS; blindness with no ophthalmoscopic changes. The causes suggested are very numerous, the most important being (excluding diseases of the eye and neighbouring parts) toxins such as tobacco and lead ; functional or reflex ; and defective development. In toxic amblyopia, the poison may be introduced from without, or manufactured in the body. Tobacco and lead are by far the most important in the first group, though quinine, sodium salicylate, morphia, and other drugs are sometimes the cause. Body toxins, which cause more passing and less characteristic symptoms, are chiefly uræmia ; megrim, caused by digestive disorders ; and, more rarely, fevers, such as malaria. (*See also* BLINDNESS AND DEFECTIVE SIGHT.)

AMBRINE. A dressing for burns and wounds. It is composed of a mixture of paraffin and resin.

AMBULANCE. A vehicle for conveying injured or ill persons.

AMENORRHŒA. This means the absence of the " courses " or menstrual flow during the period of life in which they should be present. (*See also* MENSTRUATION.)

AMMONIA. A strong, colourless, pungent gas which is very easily dissolved in water. Preparations of ammonia are used extensively in medicine as heart stimulants, gastric stimulants, and also in cases of headache and hysteria, etc. It is also useful in bronchitis. Aromatic spirit of ammonia or *sal volatile* is used in many forms of smelling-salts. Ammonia is a very good application in cases of insect bites or stings.

Ammonia Poisoning. Ammonia acts as a corrosive poisoning and breathing its vapour has been know to cause death. No emetic should be given. Lime juice or vinegar in half a glass of water followed by bland substances such as milk, egg white, arrowroot, or olive-oil may be administered. The patient should be kept warm and the doctor called for.

AMNESIA. This is the medical name for loss of memory.

AMNION. The amnion is the bag or sac in which the fœtus or unborn child is enclosed. It contains one or two pints of fluid in which the child floats.

AMŒBA. A single-celled, colourless, jelly-like germ found in the sea and in fresh waters. The form of inflammation of the bowels called dysentery is due to an amœba.

AMPOULE. An ampoule is a small, sealed glass capsule. Ampoules are used for holding small measured quantities of drugs, vaccines or serums sterile and ready for use.

AMPUTATIONS. By amputation is meant the cutting off of a limb or other part of the body. Amputations are never carried out nowadays unless the surgeon has found himself unable to cure the disease which makes the amputation necessary, or unless to prevent serious and possibly fatal complications arising from the disease which is present. In performing an amputation a surgeon always preserves as much of the limb as he can, but at the same time he must consider how to make the stump which results as suitable as possible for having an artificial limb fitted on to it. (*See also* ARTIFICIAL LIMBS.)

AMYL ALCOHOL. A form of alcohol known as fusel oil or potato-starch alcohol.

AMYL NITRITE. A clear, yellowish liquid, with a penetrating odour. It is a very important drug in the treatment of heart disease as it has a stimulating effect on the heart's action. Amyl nitrite is usually supplied in small capsules which can conveniently be carried and used by crushing in a handkerchief when necessary. (*See also* ANGINA PECTORIS.)

AMYLOID DISEASE. This name is given to a condition in which a starch-like substance is found in the tissues owing to disease.

The process affects the tissues of the blood-vessels of various organs, especially the liver, spleen, kidneys and bowels, and is connected with chronic suppuration in the body. Another name for this condition is lardaceous disease. (*See also* BRIGHT'S DISEASE.)

ANACIDITY. The lack of normal acidity; subacidity. (*See also* ALKALOSIS.)

ANAL. Anything to do with the anus, or lower opening of the bowel, is described as anal.

ANALGESIA. By analgesia is meant insensibility to pain. (For a description of various analgesics *see also* ANÆSTHESIA.)

ANÆMIA or BLOODLESSNESS. Anæmia may mean a deficiency of blood as a whole in the body, or it may be a deficiency of the number of red cells in the blood, or of the red-colouring matter (hæmoglobin) of the blood. About one-twentieth of the whole weight of the body should be blood.

Anæmia may be local, e.g. affecting a small portion of the body only, when it is known as *ischæmia*, or it may be general throughout the whole system when it is divided into two main types—*primary anæmia* and *secondary anæmia*. A primary anæmia is one in which there is no obvious cause, while a secondary anæmia is one which follows some obvious reason such as excessive bleeding from an accident, or prolonged loss of blood in small quantities such as occurs from piles, stomach, ulcer, etc. The anæmia may be due to a failure to manufacture enough blood, to increased use of it in the body, or to loss by bleeding.

Causes of Anæmia. It is most common in girls, just after puberty. It seems to be associated with the beginning of the menstrual periods in women. It is more common among those who work under poor conditions and have insufficient food. Lack of exercise causes the waste products to be retained in the blood. These act as a poison to the red corpuscles and reduce their power of taking in oxygen.

Sometimes atmospheric conditions, such as living at high altitudes, may produce an anæmia due to the fact that the oxygen leaves the blood-cells too readily. After a time the red cells increase enormously in number ; and whereas the average number of red cells in a cubic millimetre of blood is five millions ; under these special conditions the number may increase to ten millions ; but the hæmoglobin in each cell is much diminished. (A cubic millimetre is the size of an ordinary pin's head.)

Treatment. General hygiene is important ; proper ventilation of the bedroom at night, so that the air breathed out is not allowed to accumulate. Damp should be avoided as it favours rheumatism. Clothing should be sufficient for warmth, but should not be excessive. Porous clothes which provide sufficient warmth are the best as they allow the skin to work freely and to regulate its own temperature. Diet must be non-irritating so as not to increase the indigestion which is usually present. Meals must be regular and no food must be taken between meals. Fluids should not be taken with meals, but a bland fluid such as water should be drunk half an hour before a meal. Tender meat rather underdone and finely minced is very useful. Later on exercises, which must be graduated and should always stop before producing fatigue, are very useful, since they assist the circulation generally. The exercises increase the activity of the skin and tone up the whole body generally.

Drug Treatment of Anæmia. Iron is the most important remedy in this disease, but it must be given in large quantities. An excellent form is as Blaud's pills, which are not a patent medicine, but an old and valuable formula. They are given in large doses, up to 45 grains a day. Iron and ammonium citrate is also valuable, up to 90 grains a day being given. It is most important to go on taking the iron for at least three months, and if necessary to resume it afterwards in smaller doses as recurrences are so common.

Arsenic, in the form of Fowler's solution, can be combined with the iron with advantage. It should be given in small doses, as large ones may have a destructive effect on red blood-cells.

Hæmoglobin extracted from bullock's blood is a valuable form of iron. The chlorophyll (green colouring matter) of plants is also a form of iron which can now be obtained in tablet form and has produced some very good results.

In the case of children it is necessary to accustom them to the iron gradually, giving iron and ammonium citrate in small increasing doses ; it can be given in milk. Infants are said to be better with traces of copper and manganese with the iron.

ANÆMIA, PERNICIOUS. *See* PERNICIOUS ANÆMIA.

ANÆSTHESIA. By anæsthesia is meant the state of unconsciousness or insensibility to pain to which patients are reduced before a surgeon performs an operation on them. Anæsthetics are divided into the two classes, *general* and *local*, according to whether the whole body is to be rendered insensible or only a small part.

In 1847 Sir James Simpson discovered the anæsthetic use of chloroform at Edinburgh. It was not, however, until Simpson administered chloroform to Queen Victoria at one of her confinements that general anæsthesia received the approval that made it so universal as it is to-day.

The drugs chiefly used to-day for general anæsthetics by the vapour method are nitrous oxide, commonly called " gas," chloroform, ether, and ethyl chloride. Avertin, nembutal and evipan are newer anæsthetics used by injection or other methods and have proved satisfactory. Whatever the anæsthetic drug used the effects and method of giving it are much the same. There is first a semi-conscious state in which the patient feels the world swirling around him and in which he may talk, sing or laugh. With a skilled anæsthetist this only lasts a very short time, perhaps only seconds. In the matter of taking an anæsthetic well the patient can help the doctor considerably by overcoming his dread beforehand and going to the operation with a quiet mind.

Local Anæsthesia. In local anæsthesia or analgesia only a portion of the body is rendered insensitive to pain, and the patient remains conscious. Large operations can be performed under a local anæsthetic, and this is sometimes done when the patient's heart is in a bad condition.

Drugs used. Of the drugs used for local anæsthetics, cocaine is the best known. Several new preparations have been introduced which are used in the same way as cocaine, but have not its disadvantages. It is sufficient merely to give the names of some of them, as for example, novocain, novutox, stovain, eucain, borocain, pantocain, and percain. Quinine-and-urea-hydrochloride is found useful in some conditions when a prolonged anæsthesia is desired, as its effects may last several days.

Dental Anæsthesia. For general work on the teeth the stand-by is nitrous oxide gas, commonly referred to as gas, or laughing gas. In the early days of anæsthetics nitrous oxide sometimes had the effect of making the patient laugh hysterically as the anæsthetic wore off, so it gained the popular name of laughing gas. This rarely happens nowadays, and very little discomfort is felt afterwards.

Anæsthesia and Analgesia in Childbirth. Birth is always looked upon as a natural function, but the pain which now accompanies it is probably one of the penalties of civilization and the mixture of races.

Suffering, such as is often felt during child-birth, will cause exhaustion which is the chief cause of delay in the birth and the most frequent cause for forceps having to be used. The results of exhaustion may be shock, faintness, bleeding, and perhaps even blood-poisoning. The main difficulties to be met are that the pains of labour are prolonged for several hours, and that there are two lives to be considered, while the effects of drugs upon the unborn child are practically unknown.

Twilight Sleep. As soon as the mother begins to feel that labour pains are beginning, small doses of scopolamine should be given. In order to carry out the proper procedure for twilight sleep, the patient should be put to bed in a darkened and sound-proof room. Small doses of scopolamine should be given as long as the patient is still able to recognize familiar objects handed to her, and repeated until a state of amnesia, or loss of memory is reached. The object of this treatment is that the patient shall have no recollection of anything that takes place while she is in labour or while the child is being born.

Chloroform. Chloroform is a very satisfactory anæsthetic and can be used as soon as the patient feels the labour pains beginning. Small doses of chloroform are now being put up into ampoules so that anyone can use it without fear of taking an overdose.

Ether is used a great deal and is safer than chloroform ; it seems to have less effect on the child and does not in any way interfere with the normal processes of childbirth.

Treatment of Vomiting after an Anæsthetic. The patient should be turned over to the right side. Strong black coffee or chloretone may be given by mouth. Counter-irritation, such as a mustard leaf over the pit of the stomach, may help.

The " pernicious " type of vomiting, characteristic of delayed chloroform poisoning, is very serious ; but the condition is treated by means of injections of glucose and insulin.

ANALYSIS. By analysis is meant the separation of anything that is made up of several different things into those different substances which compose it. Clinical analysis of a disease means a thorough examination of the symptoms and course a disease is running. A chemical analysis is the splitting up of a mixture into the different drugs that compose it. In the new treatment, called psycho-analysis, which is sometimes used for certain mental conditions, the contents of the mind as represented by thoughts, dreams, etc., are analysed, and this process is called the "analysis" of the patient.

ANAPHRODISIAC. This is a drug which diminishes the sexual desires. Bromides are anaphrodisiacs if taken for a long time.

ANAPHYLAXIS. Anaphylaxis is a state in which an individual is so sensitive to certain substances that they constitute a poison for him, whereas they are harmless for other persons. Everyone knows someone who cannot touch fish, must not eat eggs, gets a rash when he eats strawberries, etc. Sometimes these people are born anaphylactic to the particular thing which disagrees with them, but sometimes the condition comes on after the nervous system has been subjected to some severe shock or strain. In women, anaphylaxis may develop after the birth of a child, for instance. It is often found that the things to which a person becomes anaphylactic are things for which he or she has had a great liking. A common beginning of anaphylaxis is when a serum or vaccine is being taken in continually increasing doses and suddenly one dose makes the patient violently ill for a short period, and any further dose would cause a similar or worse attack ; the patient has become anaphylactic to the serum. Anaphylaxis is part of the condition known as allergy, and the article on allergy should be read by anyone interested in the subject. (*See also* ALLERGY.)

ANASARCA. Dropsy, or the accumulation of fluid in the tissues of the body. To tell whether the condition is present press firmly with the finger on the skin. If the depression made by the finger takes some time to fill up dropsy is present.

ANASTOMOSIS. The junction between two blood-vessels is called the anastomosis of the vessels when the circulation is established by communicating branches when the main channel is

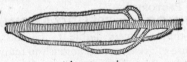

Anastomosis

blocked. Sometimes it is necessary to establish a new channel of communication between two organs or two distinct parts of the same organ. This also is an anastomosis.

ANATOMY. By the term anatomy is meant the study of the various structures which make up the human body. The knowledge of anatomy which we have to-day has been gained during hundreds of years of painstaking dissection of the human body, and the amount of knowledge that has been thus acquired is indeed vast.

ANDROPHOBIA. Fear or dislike of the male sex.

ANEURYSM. An aneurysm is a swelling caused by an abnormal swelling of an artery. The most serious form of aneurysm is that of the aorta, or large artery, into which the blood from the heart is pumped. The most common cause of aneurysm is syphilis ; but chronic alcoholism, rheumatism, Bright's disease and other diseases may cause it. It usually occurs in persons over the age of thirty, and men are more frequently attacked than women. Occupations involving strain predispose towards it.

The symptoms of aneurysm are very variable, but there will be pain, faintness, swelling of the face, neck, arms or hands, breathlessness on exertion and often coughing and bringing up of blood. The throbbing of the artery may be visible on inspection of the chest. The veins of the chest may stand out or the aneurysm itself may be seen as a throbbing lump. In some cases there is a distinctive thickening or clubbing, as it is called, of the fingers of the left hand. The left arm may also be considerably swollen.

Treatment. The treatment of aneurysm is always a matter for a doctor. The treatment should begin with some months in bed with treatment of the various symptoms, and when the patient is allowed up again, he must be careful to avoid all violent exertion.

ANGINA. Angina is a term meaning literally choking, and is used for conditions where there is a sense of choking or of suffocation, especially diseases of the throat or chest which have such symptoms. Vincent's angina is a non-infectious disease of the throat closely resembling diphtheria, in that the throat becomes ulcerated and has a foul-smelling membrane, but it is not dangerous to life like diphtheria. Angina pectoris or cardiac angina is a heart disease in which a characteristic symptom is the sudden feeling of suffocation. (*See also* ANGINA PECTORIS.)

ANGINA MINOR, or PSEUDO-ANGINA. A condition with symptoms that are very liable to be mistaken for angina pectoris is the cause of great mental anguish to many men, especially youngish men, who think they have got the true angina. This " false angina " is a nervous complaint brought on by over-smoking, too much tea-drinking, or coffee-drinking.

ANGINA PECTORIS. Angina pectoris (breast pang) is a disease affecting the heart and sometimes leading to sudden death. It is most common in those whose life is one of stress and strain. Worry seems to be an active factor in causing it, and it has been called the doctor's disease because it is very common in the medical profession. The typical sufferers from angina pectoris are business men or shopkeepers, leading lives of strain, eating, drinking and smoking to excess. It is to some extent hereditary, and has been found in members of the same family for several generations.

Symptoms. The symptoms depend upon the severity of the attack. In the mildest form there may be only a feeling of tension or discomfort, which may grow to positive pain, deep in the region of the breast-bone. This discomfort often follows emotion and sometimes exertion. It may be present on rising to speak in public, but this soon passes off. Muscular effort, such as climbing a hill or going upstairs, may bring on the sensation. In a " high pressure " life a man may feel this tension in the breast for weeks without any pain, or without being able to pin it down to any one spot. It disappears after a night's rest and may disappear entirely when the " harness " is taken off.

Severe Angina. In severe angina there is definite disease of the heart or blood-vessels leading to the heart, as well as the nervous condition which causes the anginal attacks, and it is in this form that there is a liability to sudden death. Mental emotion or muscular effort are the usual causes which bring on attacks.

An attack of Angina Pectoris. As stated previously an attack is usually brought on by emotion or exertion, an angry scene at a meeting, or a " late for the train " rush to the station and the person is seized with a violent pain in the region of the heart and a feeling of tightness as if the heart had been seized in a vice. He either falls to the ground or remains doubled up and motionless on a bench or against some such support as a wall. Pains shoot down his left arm and there may be numbness of the fingers and round about the heart. His face grows pale and ashy and often a profuse sweat breaks out. It has been described by a sufferer as though the " icy hand of death had clutched the heart." The attack may occur when he is crossing the road and even though there may be cars bearing down upon him he will be powerless to move. The attack lasts from a few seconds to a minute or two, and during the attack the sufferer feels that he is going to die. This feeling of approaching death is typical of angina pectoris.

The attack, though so severe, is mercifully short. It is all over in a few seconds or minutes. The patient may pass into a faint, he may drop dead at the height of the attack, or he may be suddenly relieved of his pain, straighten himself up and proceed on his way. He will feel exhausted and shaken for some time.

Treatment. When a man has had an attack of true angina he must realize that the time has come to " go slow." If he can retire from business he should do so, keeping a small interest in it if he would be happier that way, but not an interest which would involve him in any responsibility.

There is a wonderful drug called nitrite of amyl which gives instant relief when inhaled. Sufferers from angina pectoris carry this around with them in their pockets and use it when they feel an attack coming on. It is put up in little capsules for this purpose.

These are crushed in the fingers in a handkerchief and held to the nose. When a doctor can be on the scene quickly enough he may give morphia.

Angina pectoris is a warning by Nature that life must be slackened down, because the machinery is wearing thin. Recently removal of the thyroid gland by operation has been performed successfully for angina pectoris in a number of cases, because this had the effect of slowing down the metabolism or working of the body. The question of diet has become one of great importance to the sufferer. He must, if he is to continue living, give up heavy meals, smoking and alcohol in any quantity. If he takes care of himself he will probably live comfortably for years.

ANGIOLOGY. The science of the blood-vessels and lymphatic vessels and lymph glands.

ANGIOMA. A tumour or swelling which consists of a mass of any kind of blood-vessel. The form of angioma which is most common is a birthmark or nævus.

ANGIONEUROTIC ŒDEMA, or GIANT URTICARIA. *See* URTICARIA.

ANGOSTURA (Cusparia Bark) is a bitter and stimulating tonic. (*See also* BITTERS.)

ANILINE. A colourless liquid with a faint, peculiar odour. Combined with chlorine, the chlorates and hypochlorites, it yields the various aniline dyes known as aniline blue, aniline green, etc.

Poisoning by Aniline. In cases of poisoning, an emetic should be given as soon as possible.

ANIMAL HEAT. The temperature—the heat of the body —is one of several guides to a person's condition, and it is taken with a thermometer.

ANISOCORIA. This is a condition in which the pupils of the eyes differ in size. (*See also* EYE.)

ANKLE. The ankle is the joint where the bones of the leg meet the bones of the foot. It is a joint of the hinge variety, and allows two movements. The movement of raising the foot is called dorsiflexion, and the movement of lowering the foot plantarflexion.

The ankle-joint is formed by the lower ends of the bones of the leg, which are called the tibia and fibula, and the ankle bone, or astralagus, as it is called. Underneath the ankle-bone lies the heel-bone, or os calcis, and in front of it the five tarsal bones which form the instep or tarsus.

The ankle is surrounded by ligaments which connect the surface of the lower end of the tibia to the ankle bone. Other ligaments bind the ankle bone to the heel and bones of the foot.

The ankle joint is a very powerful joint, and is not often dislocated, but it is the most frequently sprained joint in the body, and is very often the site of synovitis or watery swelling, and disease or injury may lead to ankylosis or severe stiffening of the ankle joint. (*See also* ANKLE, INJURIES TO.)

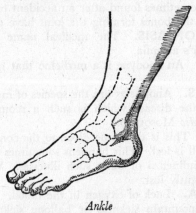

Ankle

ANKLE, INJURIES TO. The ankle joint, which has to support the entire weight of the body, is necessarily a very strong joint and is strongly supported by ligaments. It is not therefore easy to dislocate it, though dislocation sometimes does occur, most often in cases where there is a smashed bone as well. A less severe form of dislocation and fracture at the ankle is that known as Pott's fracture, where the fibula is fractured at its lower end, the ligaments of the ankle joint are torn, and the foot is bent in an outward and backward direction. This may happen by some such accident as slipping off the sidewalk, or landing after a jump with the feet turned out. It may not incapacitate the individual at the time, but may be regarded as only a severe sprain until X-ray examination shows the true situation. In another fracture of the ankle called Dupuytren's fracture, the two leg bones, the tibia and fibula, may be separated and the ankle bone may be pushed up between them.

Sprained Ankle. There is no joint which is so easily and so frequently sprained. A sudden turning of the foot may be enough to cause a sprain, which is a tear of a whole or part of the ligament at the side of the ankle. The symptoms are intense pain, marked swelling and discolouration, but the joint can still be freely moved. A firm bandage should be applied and kept on for forty-eight hours, after which massage may be started and the joint kept strapped in the intervals. In a slight case the patient may begin to put weight on the foot after a few days, provided that the ankle is well strapped and a strong boot is worn. Slippers should not be worn again for a considerable time.

ANKYLOSIS. This is the name given to the stiffness of the joints which is sometimes found after an accident or some diseased condition when the bones forming the joint have grown together.

ANKYLOSTOMIASIS. The medical name for Hookworm Disease or miner's anæmia.

ANODYNE. An anodyne is a medicine that gives relief from pain.

ANOPHELES. Anopheles are the species of mosquitoes which carry malaria, the disease which is such a scourge in tropical countries. (*See also* Mosquito.)

ANOSMIA. This is the name given to the condition in which the sense of smell is lost. This happens sometimes for a few days, or weeks, after influenza or other such illnesses. Very rarely the sense is permanently lost.

ANOXÆMIA. Lack of oxygen in the blood. The condition is then called mountain sickness or balloon sickness. (*See also* Mountain Sickness.)

ANT BITES. These should be treated by bathing with some alkaline solution such as bicarbonate of soda, and otherwise treated as like midge or mosquito bites. (*See also* Bites and Stings.)

ANTACID. Any substance which counteracts or neutralizes acidity. Any alkali substance is an antacid. (*See also* Acidosis ; Alkalosis.)

ANTE-NATAL CARE. For the normal and healthy woman the months before her baby is born should be a time of physical well-being and happy preparation ; but in some cases she drifts into serious conditions, which may even cause her to lose her own or her baby's life at the time of birth or in the first few months after. Thirty years ago, at the beginning of the present century, more than 150 babies out of every 1,000 were doomed to be born dead or die shortly afterwards, and 4 or 5 mothers out of every 1,000 died in childbirth. To-day the situation with regard to infant life has improved by half, but the death-rate amongst mothers remains almost as great and more than 3,000 women in England and Wales die each year giving birth to children. Being a mother is still the most dangerous profession in the world, even more dangerous than coal mining.

Every woman should have herself examined as soon as she knows that she is going to have a baby. Any abnormality or deformity will then be discovered, and she will be told how to conduct her life and look after her health in the way best suited to her condition ; and it must not be forgotten that for the nine months before birth the mother's health is the baby's health. (*See also* CHILDBIRTH ; PREGNANCY.)

ANTERIOR POLIOMYELITIS. *See* INFANTILE PARALYSIS.

ANTHELMINTIC. Any drug which is used to kill intestinal worms is called an anthelmintic. In many cases the parasites are not killed in the intestines, but are so violently stimulated or stupefied by the drug that they are swept away by the usual castor-oil purge, which is administered after an anthelmintic is given. Some examples of anthelmintics are Thymol and Male Fern.

ANTHRACOSIS. Anthracosis (or Silicosis), commonly called *black lung*, or coal-miner's lung, is a disease of the lungs arising from the continuous breathing of air containing particles of coal dust. The disease is growing less prevalent, and with still better ventilation of our coal mines, the adoption of wet drilling or direct exhausts to the drills, and, if the circumstances require it, the use of respirators, the disease would become a rarity. The lung becomes black in appearance and tough in texture. The chief symptoms are breathlessness, and cough with black expectoration. The patient must be removed from mine dust permanently, and should take particular care to avoid chills or anything which would lead to catarrhal colds and bronchitis. Diet should be light and any exertion which causes breathlessness should be avoided.

ANTHRAX. An acute infectious disease due to a germ called the Bacillus anthracis. It is common amongst animals, such as sheep, cattle and horses, which become infected with it after eating infected grass. Human beings become infected on the skin by handling the infected hides of animals, or by using infected shaving-brushes which are usually made from horse-hair. The lung variety of anthrax results from inhaling bacilli in the handling of wool (wool-sorter's disease).

The first thing that may be noticed may be itching on the skin of the face, arm or neck, and a small red pimple may appear at the site of the itching, which quickly becomes inflamed and angry-looking. This may at first be mistaken for an ordinary boil or septic spot, but the appearances quickly become very characteristic in anthrax. The pimple becomes encircled by small whitish blisters, and in a day or two, black slough or dead matter may appear in the centre. The neighbouring glands are usually enlarged and the temperature may be anything from normal to about 103° F. If the case is treated efficiently within a day or so of its onset the hope of recovery is very good, but in severe cases death may occur within a week. The sore should not be opened, as this increases the risk of blood-poisoning.

Treatment consists in cutting out or cauterizing the pustule and giving injections of special serum. (*See also* ANTIBODIES ; SERUM.)

ANTHROPOLOGY. The science of the nature of man and mankind, both from bodily and mental points of view.

ANTIBODIES. The body has the power to produce substances in the blood and tissues which destroy bacteria and neutralize the poisons which they manufacture in the blood. These other substances are called antibodies and antitoxins. When a sufficient number of antibodies have been produced in the blood to deal with the bacteria and get the upper hand of them the person will recover from the disease, or will become immune to it. This is the principle at the root of vaccination and inoculation against disease.

ANTIDOTE. An antidote is any substance which prevents or counteracts the action of a poison.

ANTIFEBRILE. Anything used for bringing down the temperature and reducing fever.

ANTIMONY. Antimony is a metal possessing a bluish-white shiny appearance. In medicine it is used in the treatment of syphilis and malaria, and in certain diseases caused by parasites such as bilharziasis.

Poisoning by Antimony. Give an emetic of a tablespoonful of mustard, or salt, in half a tumblerful of warm water. Strong tea should then be given, and the patient should be fed on milk and white of egg. He should be kept warm by putting hot-water bottles at his feet and sides.

ANTIPARASITIC. Any drug which is used to kill parasites.

ANTIPHLOGISTINE. *Antiphlogistine* is the name of an antiseptic paste which is used a great deal instead of poultices.

ANTIPYRETIC. A drug which is used for lowering the temperature. The most important antipyretics are phenacetin and phenazonum. Cold, such as a cold bath, or sponging, or the application of ice packs, is the method which is used a great deal for lowering the temperature in cases of fever. Quinine and salicylic acid are necessary drugs in cases of malaria and rheumatic fever.

ANTISCORBUTIC. Substances which are necessary to prevent or cure scurvy. Scurvy arises through lack of certain vitamins, chiefly the vitamin known as " water-soluble C." The best-known antiscorbutics are orange and lemon juice, fresh green vegetables, and fresh milk.

ANTISEPTICS. An antiseptic is a substance which is used to prevent the growth of germs.

Antiseptic surgery was first introduced by Lord Lister when he was professor of surgery at Glasgow in the year 1868, and since then the method has developed into aseptic surgery, germs being *prevented* and not merely killed off when present. (*See also* DIS-INFECTION.)

ANTISPASMODIC. Antispasmodics are drugs which relieve colic or spasms, sudden convulsions, or contraction of muscles. These drugs include the narcotic drugs such as belladonna and opium, and carminative drugs such as sal volatile, etc. In severe colic, the spasmodic pains may be relieved by the application of a hot-water bag or a hot fomentation over the abdomen.

ANTITOXIN. An antitoxin is a substance formed in the blood to protect the body against an invasion of germs. It neutralizes or combats the poisons produced by the germ, but the antitoxin for any particular disease will only neutralize the toxin or poison of that disease. For example, the antitoxin for diphtheria will have no effect against the toxin for lock-jaw, and vice versa.

ANTRUM. The antrum is the largest of the sinuses or spaces filled with air in connection with the nose, and lies within the upper jaw. The opening into the nose is situated high up in the antrum, and is thus badly placed for drainage. When, therefore, the antrum becomes infected, either from the nose through influenza or a similar cause, or from an abscess at the root of a tooth in the upper jaw, it is difficult for the infection to clear up naturally, and the antrum usually has to be drained surgically, either by having a small cannula passed into it, or by an operation under local or general anæsthetic. A one-sided nasal discharge makes a doctor suspicious that the antrum is infected, and sometimes there is an unpleasant smell in the nose. (*See also* SINUS.)

ANUS. The opening at the lower end of the rectum, or lowest part of the large bowel, is known as the anus. In certain cases an opening may have to be made from the lower bowel to the outside at some point above the normal anus ; this is termed an artificial anus. Imperforate anus is the term applied to complete absence of the natural opening which is found sometimes in new-born babies ; in such cases a surgical operation is necessary. Fissure, fistula, piles, abscess, pruritus, prolapse and stricture, are conditions which occur in the region of the anus.

AORTA. The aorta is the largest artery of the body. It begins at the left side of the heart and extends downwards and backwards, keeping to the left of the backbone until it enters the abdominal cavity.

The main artery of the lower body is the *abdominal aorta*, which supplies the abdomen and the organs contained in it with blood. It is a continuation of the artery called the *aorta* through the dia-

2 *

phragm into the abdomen, where it lies in front of the backbone, and behind the duodenum and coils of the small intestine.

APERIENT. Drugs or substances which produce a mildly purgative action on the intestine and lead to two or three soft motions of the bowels daily are called aperients or laxatives. The most useful drug in this class is cascara in some form. Various forms of health salts taken in a tumbler of water last thing at night or before breakfast make a very pleasant aperient. Where the bowel needs a lubricant, liquid paraffin is of great benefit and is obtainable in a great variety of forms.

APEX. The summit or top of anything. When applied to the lungs, the apex of the lung is the top part behind the border of the first rib. The apex beat of the heart is the beat of the heart felt between the fifth and sixth ribs, about $3\frac{1}{2}$ in. from the middle of the breast-bone. The apex beat may alter its situation in cases of enlargement of the heart and other conditions.

APHASIA is a defect in, or loss of, the power of expressing ideas by speech, writing, or signs, or of understanding what is spoken or written. It is due to injury or disease of certain parts of the brain. (*See also* APOPLEXY ; BRAIN ; NERVOUS SYSTEM.)

APHONIA. Aphonia means loss of the power of speaking. The most usual cause of loss of voice is inflammation of the vocal cords, due to over-use or misuse of the voice. Teachers and public speakers are very prone to lose their voices for these reasons. The voicelessness may also be due to paralysis and sometimes to hysteria. (*See also* CLERGYMAN'S SORE THROAT ; HYSTERIA.)

APOMORPHINE. Apomorphine is made from morphine. It is the most powerful emetic known, and is largely used in the treatment of cases of poisoning. It is usually given by injection under the skin, and is almost certain to produce rapid and violent vomiting.

APONEUROSIS. A particular sort of tough, membraneous tendon which is attached to muscles, or encloses and binds down muscles.

APOPLEXY or STROKE. A loss of consciousness with some paralysis, which is due to a sudden interference with the blood supply of part of the brain. It occurs most commonly in elderly people, in whom the arteries of the brain are inelastic, so that the blood tends to clot in them, thus cutting off the supply of blood from certain areas of the brain ; or the walls of the arteries may be so weakened that they become fragile, and if any strain is put upon them they burst, giving rise to hæmorrhage. In younger people, in middle life, syphilis plays an important part in producing apoplexy.

Apoplexy in people under forty is rare, but it may occur.

A few unfortunate people have arteries inside their skulls with thinner walls than usual, and some day, when the unfortunate person is making a bigger effort than usual, for example, running, or coughing hard, or indulging in a violent fit of temper, an artery will give way and the person has a stroke. This type of stroke may occur at any age, and the person who has had such a stroke, although he may survive one or two even, may be said to be living on the edge of a volcano, since no one can prophesy when the next one will occur.

It must, however, be emphasized that this type of stroke in young people is rare, compared with the type seen in the elderly from blood clotting in an artery, or from bursting of a weakened vessel. The common type, that due to clotting of the blood, most frequently occurs when the apoplexy happens during sleep or under conditions of quiet. The history is often that the patient went to bed feeling extra tired, and next morning woke up and found that he was paralysed down one or other side. If the left side of the brain is damaged, then most probably speech will be lost, at least temporarily, as this side of the brain controls speech, but if the right side of the brain has suffered, then speech will be preserved.

On the side of the paralysis, that is, on the side opposite to the hæmorrhage, the pupil of the eye is very large, and does not get smaller when a bright light is thrown into that eye. Although the patient is breathing noisily and hurriedly and puffing out his cheeks, it can readily be seen that on the side of the paralysis the cheek is less puffed out at each breath than it is on the sound side. And even though a patient be deeply unconscious it is possible to show that the limbs on the paralysed side when raised, and allowed to fall again, do so " all of a piece," in a more lifeless manner than upon the sound side.

The outlook for complete recovery depends on many factors, especially on the condition of the blood-vessels and heart. *Re-education* of the paralysed limbs as regards movements is of the utmost importance, and the patient should be urged to try to move his paralysed limbs as much as possible, as soon as he is completely conscious. There is no fear that by moving the limbs he will bring on another stroke. Many patients who have had one stroke caused by clotting of the blood in a vessel go for many years without another and finally succumb to a hæmorrhage that is rapidly fatal. The best preventive measure against a stroke in those who are known to have bad arteries is moderation in all things : in diet, alcohol, physical, and mental exercise.

APOTHECARIES' WEIGHTS AND MEASURES.

Apothecaries' Weight.

Grains.	Scruples.	Drachms.	Troy Oz.	Pound.
20 =	1			
60 =	3 =	1		
480 =	24 =	8 =	1	
5,760 =	288 =	96 =	12 =	1

Apothecaries' Measure.

Minims.	Fluid Drms.	Fluid Oz.	Pints.	Gallon.
60 =	.			
480 =	8 =	1		
7,680 =	128 =	16 =	1	
61,440 =	1,024 =	128 =	8 =	1

For domestic use the measures given below may prove a valuable help.

A teaspoonful is rather over a fluid drachm.

A dessertspoonful is about two fluid drachms.

A tablespoonful is about half a fluid ounce.

A wineglassful is about one and a half to two fluid ounces.

A teacupful is about five fluid ounces.

A breakfastcupful is about eight fluid ounces.

A tumblerful is about eleven fluid ounces.

APPENDICITIS. Inflammation of the appendix, a small worm-like projection from the cæcum, or blind end of the commencement of the large intestine. The cause of appendicitis is not definitely known. In most cases it appears to be due to invasion of germs, such as streptococci, etc., which enter the appendix from the intestine, or in other cases it may be due to germs from a distant source of infection such as the tonsils, or teeth. These latter are blood-borne, i.e. they travel in the blood-stream from some distant part of the body to the appendix. Some cases are said to be due to internal obstruction of the appendix by lumps of hardened fæces, pips and skins of fruit, thread worms in masses, and swallowed foreign bodies. External obstruction from adhesions and bands may also cause appendicitis. It is on the whole a disease of youth and middle-age ; males are attacked slightly oftener than women, and it is more common amongst civilized races.

Appendicitis is a disease which comes on in definite attacks with, usually, a pain-free interval between them. There may be vomiting, constipation or diarrhœa. The temperature rises and the pulse is rapid. There is a well-marked tenderness in the region known as

McBurney's point. An appendix which is causing symptoms should always be removed, as the condition rarely cures itself, and the results of neglect are so serious. After repeated attacks the appendix may become gangrenous, and each attack will add to the number of adhesions in the abdomen and the severity of the operation for the removal of the appendix. Appendicitis is often the original cause of diseased conditions higher up the alimentary track such as gastric or duodenal ulcer, inflammation of the gall-bladder, etc.

In an acute attack of appendicitis the patient is obviously very ill and in great pain, and no time should be lost in sending for the

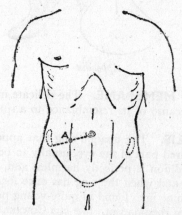

Appendicitis. A : McBurney's Point

doctor. *No aperient should be given* as is sometimes done under the impression that the case is one of colic due to constipation.

Nowadays immediate operation is advised when the condition has been present for less than forty-eight hours, but when it has been present for several days operation is usually deferred, to allow an appendix abscess to form before operating.

APPENDIX. The vermiform appendix, or appendix as it is more usually called, is a relic which probably has no definite use in modern human beings. In animals such as the rabbit or horse, which feed entirely upon vegetarian matter, it is large and appears to be of some importance, whereas in meat-eating animals like the lion and tiger, it is even more minute and shrivelled up than in human beings who live on a mixed diet of flesh and vegetables. In shape it is tubular, attached at one end to the cæcum, into which it has a small opening which is protected by a valve. The other end swings free, but is usually adherent to the cæcum or some part of the lining of the abdomen. In length appendices vary from 1 to 10 in., the average being 3 or 4 in. in length. (*See also* APPENDICITIS ; INTESTINES.)

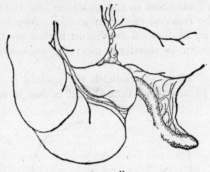

Appendix

ARACHNOID MEMBRANE. The delicate membrane of the brain, so called because of its resemblance to a spider's web. (*See also* BRAIN.)

ARCUS SENILIS. The opaque ring that appears at the edge of the iris or coloured part of the eye, usually to be seen in elderly persons. The condition is perfectly harmless and, indeed, normal to advancing age, and when the ring has once formed it proceeds no further. It is sometimes found in quite young people, especially those suffering from rheumatism. (*See also* CORNEA ; EYE.)

AREOLA. The brownish space surrounding the nipple of the breast. During pregnancy a second areola occurs, surrounding this. Areolar tissue is the medical name for any loose tissue that lies beneath the skin, and which goes to fill up all the odd corners of the body. (*See also* BREAST ; NIPPLE.)

ARGYROL. Argyrol is a silver proteinate containing 20 to 25 per cent. of silver. It is used a great deal in the treatment of eye and nose and throat affections, and is especially useful in gonorrhœal conditions.

ARM. The arm is properly the upper extremity from the shoulder to the wrist, but the part from the elbow to the wrist is sometimes called the forearm. The bones of the arm are the humerus, the large bone in the upper arm, and the ulna and radius in the forearm. The scapula or shoulder-blade does not belong to the arm. The arm is moved by muscles coming from the shoulder-blade, the collar-bone and the main trunk of the body. They are the coraco-brachialis, the biceps, the brachialis anticus and the triceps. The blood-supply is conveyed to the arm by the brachial, radial and ulnar arteries. (*See also* ELBOW ; WRIST.)

ARMPIT. The armpit or axilla is the space between the upper part of the wall of the chest and the upper part of the arm. The important nerves and blood-vessels going to the arm are near the surface in the armpit, so it is a dangerous part in which to have a cut. Care must be taken, too, that where crutches are worn they are well padded and do not press unduly in the armpit, or paralysis of the nerves of the arm may occur, a condition which is known as *crutch palsy*. The glands of the armpit are liable to abscesses (axillary abscess) which may be very troublesome to heal. It must not be forgotten, too, that the glands of the armpit enlarge in cases of chronic inflammation or cancer of the breast, and should they be found to be enlarged should be seen by a doctor.

ARNICA. Tincture of arnica is often used for bruises and injuries, but it may produce dangerous rashes and should never be used if the skin is broken.

ARRHYTHMIA. Absence of rhythm, irregularity of the heart's beat. This irregularity may be due to serious heart disease, but may also be constitutional and of no importance. It is fairly common in young adults and may cause no symptoms and only be discovered accidentally. This form requires no treatment.

ARSENIC. Arsenic is a highly poisonous substance; it should never be taken internally except under medical supervision. This drug is contained in many preparations sold for agricultural purposes, such as sheep-dip, weed killers, and insect destroyers, and many deaths have occurred through the careless handling of these preparations.

In medicine it is given internally as a general tonic and nerve tonic, and it is used in the treatment of anæmia, diabetes, malaria, and for chronic skin diseases. One peculiarity of arsenic is that it may be found many years after death in the bodies of those who have taken it during life.

Poisoning by Arsenic. Cases sometimes occur in which a patient who has been given arsenic as a medicine may show slight symptoms of poisoning. These symptoms often occur in workers who handle arsenic in the manufacture of various articles, especially wallpapers and fabrics. Long-continued use of arsenic may cause peripheral neuritis, the chief symptoms of which are paralysis of the muscles of the limbs accompanied by darting pains, herpes zoster, and rapid muscular atrophy.

In cases of acute poisoning, the onset of symptoms is very rapid.

Treatment consists of washing out the stomach thoroughly and emetics should be given. Large amounts of magnesia should be administered or large doses of castor-oil and water. The patient should be kept as warm as possible with hot blankets, and hot-water bottles to the feet and abdomen ; hot coffee may be given.

ARTERIO-SCLEROSIS. The term means hardening of the arteries, but the name is now commonly applied to the general condition of a patient in whom this hardening of arteries has occurred. In late middle life, or early old age, the elastic walls of the arteries, which are chiefly composed of muscle, begin to stretch as elastic does when it begins to wear out. In order to repair the elastic, as it were, fresh muscle is formed in the walls of the arteries, but this muscle is of an inferior quality to that which the individual was born with, and it soon breaks down (or degenerates, as it is termed), leaving the walls of the arteries weaker than before. Most of the symptoms of arterio-sclerosis are due either to this weakening of the walls of the arteries in the various organs of the body, or to bursting of a blood-vessel, the final result in many cases of the weakened wall. It is in this condition that the blood-pressure becomes very high, and kidney disease is liable to occur. One of the early symptoms is having to pass water more than once during the night. Dyspepsia and constant, though not severe, diarrhœa are also early symptoms which are often disregarded. Headache, of a throbbing and bursting character, generally felt in the back of the head, is constantly complained of, whilst giddiness, a full feeling in the head and noises in the ears are very common symptoms. In many cases patients complain that they are unable to walk more than a few steps in comfort, not because their legs have no power, but on account of the severe cramps in the legs they get after taking a few steps.

More severe symptoms may show themselves in the form of diminution of vision, shortness of breath on very slight exertion, vomiting and very intense headaches. The desire to pass water frequently at night increases, but little is passed at a time. In the worst cases, death results either from bursting of a blood-vessel in the brain, giving rise to one form of apoplexy, or from failure of the kidneys to carry out their proper functions.

Treatment. The treatment of the condition, while it obviously cannot restore the lost elasticity of the arteries, can do much to rid the patient of his troublesome symptoms. Moderation in food and drink is essential and a meatless diet is recommended. Spirits and heavy wines are not allowable and heavy beers are decidedly bad for such patients, but light wines and ales are permissible. Regular exercise of not too strenuous a nature is advisable, walking being one which is often neglected. It is of the greatest importance to ensure regular action of the bowels, and in cases with a high blood pressure, the use of a brisk purgative pill once a week and a dose of health salts each morning. This " mild dose of salts " has much to recommend it. Patients with arterio-sclerosis should be kept as free from worry as possible, and in bad cases should be urged to " take things easily " as there is always the risk of worry or anger bringing on the dreaded final hæmorrhage into the brain.

ARTERY. The arteries are the tubular vessels which convey the blood from the heart to the tissues. The arterial system of the body has been compared to a tree, the trunk of which is the main artery called the aorta, whilst the smaller arteries branch off at intervals to the different limbs and organs of the body. They, in their turn, have smaller arteries branching off them. The joining together of two arteries is called an anastomosis. The aorta and

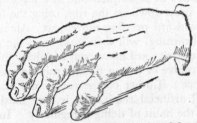

Arthritis, showing arthritic joints of fingers

its dependent arteries convey the blood from the lungs to the tissues of the body and are called the arteries of the systemic circulation. The pulmonary artery conveys the bad blood to the lungs to be mixed with oxygen, and is the main artery of the pulmonary system. The main arteries of the body are the aorta, the pulmonary, the innominate, right and left subclavian, common carotid, axillary, brachial, radial, ulnar, iliac, femoral, anterior and posterior tibial.

ARTHRITIS. Inflammation of a joint is called arthritis. A fuller description will be given under the titles Rheumatoid arthritis, Osteoarthritis, Spondylitis deformans, and Still's disease.

ARTIFICIAL RESPIRATION. Artificial respiration means artificial breathing and has to be used in cases where the heart is strong and undiseased, but the breathing has been stopped by some such reason as an accident, or drowning. In these cases the heart goes on beating for a short time after the actual breathing has stopped, and it happens in the majority of cases that if artificial respiration can be employed at once, the heart will continue beating and the breathing will be restored. For this reason it is very desirable that all able-bodied adults who mix much amongst their fellow-people should have a working knowledge of one or other of the means of performing artificial respiration. The heart, as has been said above, continues to beat after breathing has stopped and artificial respiration, therefore, tries to imitate as far as possible the movements of breathing.

Schafer's Method. This is the method in most general use. If practised a few times on healthy normal people its movements will return readily to the mind when an emergency arises and something has to be done in a hurry.

Place the patient on the ground, face downwards, with a coat or cushion under the lower half of the chest. Turn the patient's face sidewards in such a way that the nose and mouth are clear of any obstruction such as sand if it is on the beach. Kneel astride of the patient or to one side facing his head. Place the hands on the lower part of the patient's back on each side at a level of the lowest ribs. In this position press down on the ribs, using the full weight of the body in the downward pressing movement. Air and water (if the case is one of drowning) will then gush from the patient's mouth. At the end of the downward movement withdraw the hands. Repeat this movement twelve or fifteen times a minute and continue for at least half an hour ; if other competent people come up they may take turns. All artificial respiration is very hard work for those who are not in the habit of doing it regularly. In this method no attempt is made to imitate the indrawing movements of breath-taking, only those of expelling air, the lungs themselves do the rest by expanding again naturally and of their own accord. Schafer's method is the system most generally used nowadays when there is only one person available to render first-aid.

Marshall Hall's Method used to be much more used than it is now, but a knowledge of it is still valuable because, as in other conditions, one method may succeed where another fails. It is a very simple method. A prop at least six inches high is placed under the patient's chest while he is lying face downwards on the ground. This prop may be made of a roll of coat or even stone or wood in the absence of anything else. The position of the operator is the same as in Schafer's. With the same movements as in Schafer's method, press on to the back to expel air, then take the patient by the shoulders and firmly roll him over on one side in order to allow the lung to expand. Replace on the face again and repeat the pressing movement to expel air. Take care that the patient is turned on the same side each time and keep the support under his chest. Repeat both movements alternately about fifteen times a minute. The value of this method is that one lung will clear and recommence breathing sooner than two, and as soon as any measure of natural breathing is re-established the battle may be said to be almost won.

Sylvester's Method. Where helpers are available Sylvester's method is a useful one. The patient lies on his back in this method. With the patient on his face, first repeat a few minutes of Schafer's method to free the lungs of air and water. Then turn the patient on his back with a support under his shoulders, a roll of clothing being sufficient. If a slight incline, with the patient's head higher than his feet, can be arranged, so much the better. To keep the throat clear the tongue must be pulled forward out of the mouth, and it may be necessary for someone to hold it there by means of a cloth or forceps if they are at hand.

Kneel at the patient's head, and grasp his arms just above the elbows. Draw them upwards to the side of the head, keeping them there while two can be counted ; this represents " breathing in." Next bend the patient's elbows, let them down and press them into the patient's chest while two can be counted. This imitates " breathing out." Repeat the two movements alternately at the rate of fifteen series to the minute. The patient's feet are better to be held steady by another helper, and the tongue must be kept from falling back in the mouth and thus blocking the throat.

These three methods are the recognized ways of applying artificial respiration, which can be undertaken by amateurs.

In some hospitals there is a machine designed for cases where artificial respiration must be kept up for long stretches at a time.

It may be necessary to practise artificial respiration on a new-born baby, in order to start it breathing for the first time. The way to do this is described under the heading ASPHYXIA.

ARTIFICIAL SUNLIGHT. *See* LIGHT TREATMENT.

ARYTENOID. This term is used to refer to two small pieces of cartilage or gristle, which are placed at the back of the larynx or voice box, and to which the vocal cords are attached.

ASAFŒTIDA. A very disagreeably smelling gum-resin obtained from the root of a plant called Ferula fœtida. It is used in cases of hysteria and other mental disturbances, and it is extremely nasty to the taste.

ASCARIS. A species of parasitic worm which inhabits the intestines of most animals. (*See* WORMS.)

ASCITES. The name given to the collection of fluid in the abdomen in dropsy. This fluid is non-purulent, that is, it does not contain pus. It is generally the result of heart or kidney failure or cirrhosis of the liver, but may also be found in diseases which cause pressure such as tuberculosis, cancer, aneurysm or thrombosis.

ASPHYXIA, or SUFFOCATION. General asphyxia is a state produced when air is prevented by any reason from entering the lungs.

The condition may be accidental, as occurs in drowning ; when objects such as food, tin whistles, etc., are accidentally drawn into the larynx ; or it may be due to disease. The most common cause here is diphtheria, which causes a membrane to grow at the back of the roof of the mouth. This membrane may extend downwards to the vocal cords where the airway is narrowest, and restrict the passage of air still further till cyanosis or intense blueness occurs, and finally asphyxia. A large goitre or swelling in the neck may press on the windpipe and narrow it ; in fact any tumour growing outside the windpipe or bronchial tubes may narrow them and finally cause suffocation.

Drowning. Complete and prolonged immersion in water causes death, which is called death by drowning. But always try to resuscitate persons who are rescued, for breathing can often be started again by artificial respiration.

Choking. Loosen the collar, if any, lean the affected person forward and thump between the shoulders. A child may be held upside down and thumped. If this fails, introduce a finger into the mouth and try to reach the obstruction.

Swelling of the throat. Apply hot fomentations (a piece of flannel or other cloth wrung out of boiling water) to the throat. If the patient is breathing give ice to suck or cold water to drink. Also a few spoonfuls of a vegetable oil if available.

Strangulation. In a case of hanging, act promptly. Grasp the lower limbs and lift so as to reduce the tension on the rope. If alone do not go for help, but try to cut the rope and get the body down. Then free the neck, loosen any tight clothing and perform artificial respiration.

Suffocation by smoke, gases or fumes. The would-be rescuer must protect himself by tying a wet handkerchief, folded diagonally, across the bridge of his nose so that it hangs down over his mouth. Crawl swiftly along the floor and drag the affected person out. Once in a safe place loosen the clothing and, if breathing has ceased, perform artificial respiration.

" Blue Asphyxia " in the New-born. This is characterized by the blue colour and a strongly beating heart. It is usually due to an obstructed air-way, or it may be due to a narcotic drug previously administered to the mother, e.g. chloroform, morphia, etc.

The treatment is first to clear the air passages with a suction pump and then to start artificial respiration, being careful not to injure the infant's chest. If possible a mixture of carbon dioxide and oxygen should be given by a tube down the throat. If the lungs are healthy, normal breathing is rapidly established again.

" White Asphyxia " in the New-born. Corresponds to the stage described above which occurs when the heart is failing. It is characterized by pallor, muscular weakness and a feeble circulation. It is really a condition of heart failure and the treatment must be gentle. The infant must be kept warm and should be given the carbon dioxide oxygen mixture as above. Failure to respond to this usually denotes severe damage in the brain of the child.

Asphyxia, Local. A condition where the fingers, toes, ears, and sometimes patches of skin on the arms and legs, become intensely congested and livid, the circulation of blood to the part being almost stopped. This state of affairs is liable to occur in Raynaud's disease, or when a too tight bandage has been wound round the part.

ASPIRATION. This term is applied to the act of sucking up or sucking in. It is a method used for withdrawing fluid from a cavity such as the chest, etc.

ASPIRIN. Acetyl-salicylic acid is more commonly known as aspirin. It is one of our most useful drugs and is used extensively by the public. It is very beneficial in cases of rheumatism in order to relieve pain and promote sweating.

ASTHENOPIA. This mean " weak sight " and is described under the heading VISION, ERRORS OF.

ASTHMA. Asthma is one of the most distressing complaints that a person can suffer from, and it is often almost worse for the onlooker than for the actual patient. It is an affection of the bronchial tubes characterized by spasmodic attacks of breathlessness and coughing, and a feeling of suffocation and tightness in the chest and throat. Although its symptoms are referred to the lungs and bronchial tubes it is really a nerve disease and is one of the small group of allergic diseases. Allergic diseases run in families. One member of the family may have asthma, another hay-fever, another urticaria (nettle-rash), and another certain types of eczema, all of which are different manifestations of various forms of allergy, which is a kind of poisoning peculiar to these individuals. For instance, in asthmatic patients certain things which would not affect another person act as irritants to them and bring on an attack of asthma ; one man may get asthma at the seaside and another among the mountains ; the breathing of grass pollen or the dust of feathers ; the eating of shell-fish, fish, strawberries, eggs, milk, aspirin tablets, etc., are all examples of the diversity of things that may cause asthma. It is interesting to note, too, that the proximity of certain domestic animals may cause attacks. The cat and horse are fairly common examples. The late Field-Marshal Lord Roberts was well-known to be a cat asthmatic. Horse-hair mattresses, down pillows and eiderdowns are also frequent unsuspected causes. Some cases of asthma are due to reflex causes, that is, they arise from disorders in distant parts of the body. The most frequent of these causes are to be found in affections of the nose and throat such as nasal polypi, but the condition may also arise from trouble in the stomach, intestines, bladder, kidneys, etc. Eye strain has also been known to cause attacks. Mental influences such as emotion, fatigue, or even the picture of some article which causes asthma such as flowers, a cat, etc., may be sufficient to start an attack.

The attacks very often come on in the middle of the night after the patient has been sound asleep and wakes to find himself struggling for breath. He is in great distress and may get up and go to an open window in search of air, an action that has occasionally led to a fatal accident. A bad attack of asthma is always very distressing to the onlookers. The patient's face becomes pale and drawn with an anxious expression. His lips may be blue, his breathing is short and jerky, and he may look as if he were going to die, but, fortunately, he never does. Asthma is not a fatal disease, however troublesome it may be.

Attacks may last for two hours or even longer, and usually finish with a fit of coughing and the bringing up of sputum. The patient will probably be so exhausted that he will drop asleep, and for the next two or three days he may continue to breathe in a wheezy, laboured fashion.

Treatment. At the first symptom of the attack an adrenaline, ephedrine or peptone injection under the skin may stop the attack at once. As skilled attention is not usually at hand when an attack begins, it is as well for an asthmatic to find out between times what drugs agree with him and have something always within reach in tablet form, such as tablets of ephedrine sulphate or even aspirins, which in some people give relief. A strong cup of coffee helps some people. Inhaling amyl nitrite, stramonium cigarettes or stramonium burnt in a saucer are other things that may help ; sometimes an operation on the nose may be desirable. (*See also* ALLERGY.)

ASTIGMATISM. This means " short sight," and is described under the heading VISION, ERRORS OF.

ASTRINGENT. Any drug or substance which produces contraction of the tissues is called an astringent. An astringent is also used to arrest bleeding, diarrhœa, etc. The number of astringents is fairly large, and among the more well-known ones are vinegar or acetic acid, alum, tannic acid, silver nitrate, copper sulphate and adrenalin.

ATAVISM. This term is applied to a peculiar trait of heredity in which the child is a " throw-back " to a distant ancestor. He does not develop the characteristics of his immediate parents, but of his grandparents or of an ancestor still more remote. This inherited characteristic may take the form of a disease such as hæmophilia or gout.

ATAXIA. Ataxia or ataxy is a nervous condition in which the patient is unable to walk without staggering or swaying. In some forms of ataxia there is a hereditary tendency which may occur in several members of a family, and sometimes in several generations of the same family. Friedreich's ataxia is a form which generally appears between the ages of 5 and 15 years, and both sexes are equally affected. The spinal cord may appear smaller than normal, and there may be wasting of certain of the nerves of the body. The disease usually begins very slowly, and the mother may not notice very much beyond a gradual deformity of the child's feet and a definite clumsiness and difficulty in walking, especially in the dark. The eyesight may become poor, and there may be twitching of the muscles of the face and tremors of the tongue. The disease usually gets slowly worse, until the patient eventually is confined to bed. There is no known cure, but in some cases the disease may be stopped. The limbs should be carefully massaged, and special walking exercises should be encouraged.

Ataxia is a very common symptom of many nervous diseases which may be quite temporary and unimportant, as in cases of hysteria, etc. The ataxic walk is very characteristic, and although it is often confused with the walk of a drunken man it should not be described as the latter. The patient walks with his legs rather wide apart, and the feet are thrown out in rather an aimless fashion. There is usually difficulty and stumbling in the effort to lift the feet up steps, and when the patient is standing still he places his feet wide apart in order to balance himself better. Much can be done to re-educate and train a patient in the way of using his limbs, but it takes a long time, and patience and perseverance would be required. (*See also* LOCOMOTOR ATAXIA.)

ATHEROMA. Hardening of the arteries, due to inflammatory or degenerative changes in their coverings. It is associated with many diseases such as scarlet fever, rheumatic fever, syphilis and tuberculosis and is usually associated with high blood-pressure. (*See also* ARTERIO-SCLEROSIS.)

ATHLETE'S HEART. A slight incompetency of the aortic valve, one of the large valves of the heart. This is a condition sometimes found in athletes.

ATOMIZER. An atomizer is an instrument for transforming a liquid into a fine spray and for projecting the spray as required.

ATROPHY. When there is a wasting of the tissues of the body or when the tissues diminish in bulk, this process is termed atrophy. It is inevitable in old age, where the reparative capacity of the tissues is greatly diminished, and general atrophy or wasting takes place. Muscular atrophy may set in by the inability of a patient to move his limbs for himself. This may be lessened by massage or stimulation by electricity.

General wasting often occurs in children who are being starved from insufficient or improper feeding. Rickets, syphilis and tuberculosis, as well as many other serious diseases, generally give rise to wasting, especially in young children. (*See also* MARASMUS.)

ATROPHY (SENILE) OF THE SKIN. The skin, like all other parts of the body, undergoes changes as we pass from middle to old age. It not only receives less nourishment, but can deal with less. Its glands become inactive, and the skin itself becomes dry, thin and " poor." Its elasticity also goes and with it the power of accommodating itself to the size and shape of the parts underneath, so that it becomes loose and wrinkled.

In a great many old people, however, the real complaint is itching of the skin called pruritus. This may be limited to certain parts —commonly the anal region and the middle of the back—or may be more or less all over the body. It is not usually very severe, but is a constant annoyance. Many people complain that it is most troublesome for the first half-hour or so after going to bed.

The general health must be carefully regulated. If the itching occurs, the doctor should make a thorough examination to be sure that no general disease is present. A mild form of diabetes or Bright's disease may show itself in this way, or various other diseases, which would probably be missed if the skin were acting healthily. Anal itching is frequently associated with hæmorrhoids (piles), which again may give rise to no trouble in themselves. Grease in some form is the best treatment ; it not only relieves the itching, but counteracts the dryness and scurfiness of the skin. A hot bath at night is often very helpful, followed by the ointment. For use in the daytime, a lotion is more convenient.

Medicated baths, and many varieties of lotions and ointments, are also in use. The itching is often alleviated by the wearing of cotton or silk next the skin, in preference to wool.

ATROPINE. A drug obtained from the plant, Atropa belladonna, more commonly known as the deadly nightshade. The actions of belladonna and atropine on the body are the same. If atropine is placed by itself upon the unbroken skin it does not become absorbed ; but if it is placed with substances which are absorbed, such as alcohol, glycerine, or camphor, or applied to a broken surface, it produces local anæsthesia.

Given internally or by hypodermic injection, atropine lessens the perspiration and stops the flow of saliva in the mouth. It is often injected to relieve bronchial spasm, whooping cough and asthma, and also in cases of sciatica and cystitis. Atropine acts on the nerve endings in the muscles of the eye. If it is dropped into the eye, or given by mouth, the pupil of the eye dilates to a very marked degree ; this fact is made use of when examining the eyes. Belladonna is one of the favourite remedies for bed-wetting, as children do not suffer from any ill-effects from this drug. Injections of atropine given at bedtime will often check the excessive sweatings which occur in diseases such as tuberculosis, etc.

Poisoning by Atropine. Poisoning often occurs as the result of eating the leaves of the deadly nightshade plant or through having an overdose of the drug. The mouth and throat will become dry and difficulty will be experienced in swallowing ; the pulse may be a little slow. The pupil will be dilated and the vision may become confused ; the skin will feel very dry. Later, the patient may become delirious and death may take place from failure of the breathing. Treatment consists of emetics or washing out the stomach. Artificial respiration should be employed if necessary and the patient should be kept warm with hot-water bottles. Strong coffee may be given later.

AUDITORY or ACOUSTIC NERVE. Is the eighth cranial nerve and is the nerve of hearing. It comes out from underneath the brain and goes through a little opening in the skull to the internal ear. This analyses the sounds brought to it by the external ear and sends on the messages to the brain by the auditory nerve.

AURA. This word is applied to the slight warning symptoms which go before an attack of epilepsy. The " aura " may appear in various ways. Sometimes the patient is warned by a peculiar taste in the mouth, or an itching on some part of the body, or the warning may be a mental one. (*See also* EPILEPSY.)

AURICLE. This name is applied to the expanded portion or pinna of the ear. It is also the term given to two very important parts of the heart which are rather ear-like in shape. One is the upper chamber of the heart which receives the arterial blood from the lungs and is called the left auricle, and the chamber which receives the venous blood from the general circulation is the right auricle.

AUSCULTATION. This is a method of finding out the conditions and functions of various organs of the body by the sounds they themselves give out. Much can be learned about the heart by listening to its movements and the same applies to the lungs and other organs.

AUTOGENOUS VACCINE. An autogenous vaccine is one made from the patient's own germs. Stock vaccines are usually made from germs grown in the laboratory. (*See also* GERMS ; VACCINES.)

AUTO-INTOXICATION. By auto-intoxication is meant the poisoning of the body by products which, owing to faulty working of the various organs, are manufactured within the body. It is therefore self-poisoning by the body's own products.

The symptoms of auto-intoxication are very varied and the condition may lead to prolonged ill-health. There may be headache, giddiness, flatulence and dyspepsia, anæmia, muscular pains, skin troubles, physical and mental deterioration, nervousness and depression.

AUTOMATISM. This is the term applied to that state in which persons go through various actions without the mind controlling them. Automatic actions occur in some hysterical patients or in cases of epilepsy, and also in certain mental conditions. Somnambulism or sleep-walking may be regarded as a form of automatism.

AUTOPSY. The post-mortem examination or examination of a body after death. (*See also* POST-MORTEM.)

AUTO - SUGGESTION. Means to suggest to one's self, and as a method of treatment in illness which exists only in the patient's imagination, it is of great value. Auto-suggestion has received much attention recently from the propaganda work of Coué, a French psychologist, and has proved of a certain value, when used in the way Coué recommended, in sleeplessness, where the cause is mental anxiety or stress. The patient repeats, quite mechanically, the words " I'm going to sleep," in a soft monotonous whisper, until he falls asleep. After a few nights it becomes a habit to repeat this phrase and often sleeplessness can be completely cured by this means.

BACILLURIA. The presence of any kind of bacillus or germ in the urine is called bacilluria.

BACILLUS. Certain types of germs or microbes which are shaped like little rods, are termed bacilli, which is the plural for bacillus. A great number of diseases owe their origin to bacilli in some form or another. For instance, tuberculosis, meningitis, anthrax, diphtheria, typhoid fever, dysentery, and very many more diseases, are all caused by bacilli. (*See also* GERMS.)

BACK. The back consists of the spinal column or backbone with the back parts of the ribs and of the haunch bones and sacrum, with the muscular tissue which binds these bones together. The muscles of the back are very strong and powerful and have to support the head, as well as move the upper and lower limbs. A well-developed muscular back can be bent almost to the floor backwards and forwards and sidewards, but because of its great supply of muscular tissue it is very frequently the seat of muscular rheumatism, and is apt to become stiff. Strains and twists are of frequent occurrence also. Diseases and injuries of the spinal column are usually of a serious nature. A theory is held by people who call themselves *chiropractors* that most disease is due to pressure on the nerves of the spinal column owing to displacements of the *vertebræ* or small bones of the spinal column. There is, however, no truth in the theory, as the openings between the vertebræ are very large and pressure could only take place if there were some very noticeable deformity of the spine. (*See also* BACKBONE.)

BACK-ACHE. Pain, stiffness or tenderness in the back is a symptom to be met with in a number of different diseases. An early symptom of smallpox is severe aching in the back, and there is always a certain amount of back-ache in fevers. In meningitis, or brain-fever, any pressure along the whole spine usually causes pain and tenderness ; this is often accompanied by great stiffness at the back of the neck. In rheumatism, chronic or acute, there may be much pain and stiffness. Pain in the back about the level of the waist is very often due to spinal disease, or it may be due to kidney trouble. Lumbago is a very common form of back-ache which is always made worse by stooping.

In women, pain in the back is very common. In some cases the pain may be due to a disorder of the reproductive organs. In such cases the pain is usually felt low down in the back and relief may sometimes be had from surgical operation. There are, however, many women who suffer from pain in the small of the back without any sign of disease and who are otherwise perfectly well. It is usually worse when the woman is tired, and before and during the courses. Rest, especially lying down, is the only way of relieving the pain, but it does not cure it.

Muscular overstrain, constipation, neuralgia, hysteria and anæmia are among a few other causes of back-ache, and in order to treat this complaint, the patient would be advised to undergo a medical examination to find out the real cause of the pain.

BACKBONE. The backbone is the popular name for the spinal column or vertebral column, the strong supporting column of bone which stretches from the head to the bottom of the back and has the shoulder bones, the ribs and the haunch bones attached to it. In the normal adult who is standing erect, the spinal column curves slightly in four parts. Beginning at the head it curves slightly out, then in a sweeping curve inwards under the shoulders, out over the haunches and in at the end of the spine. Abnormal curvatures are called *lordosis*, *kyphosis* and *scoliosis*. The spinal column is composed of thirty-three small bones, called *vertebræ*, which are joined together by cartilage and ligaments. Each vertebra has a hole through it, through which the spinal cord runs for the whole length of the spine.

The spaces between the vertebræ are filled with elastic tissue which acts as a buffer from shock, so that a severe blow on either end of the spine such as would be caused by sitting down suddenly on something hard or being hit violently on the top of the head, does not fracture the spine, as it certainly would if the spine were composed of solid bone. The spinal cord inside the backbone is very strongly protected from injury, and dislocations of vertebræ are very rare. (*See also* SPINAL CURVATURE.)

BACTERIA. The modern medical name for germs. Other names for germs are microbes or micro-organisms. These will be described under the heading GERMS.

BACTERIOPHAGE. Anything which destroys bacteria and prevents them from growing is called a bacteriophage.

BALANITIS. This is the name given to inflammation of the head of the penis, or organ of reproduction in the male. Lack of cleanliness is often the cause of the complaint. The foreskin should be drawn back and the part washed carefully. In some cases it might be better if the operation of circumcision or cutting short of a too long foreskin, were performed, thus allowing the part to be kept clean more easily.

BALDNESS. The question of the relation between the general health and baldness is a much discussed one, but there can be no doubt that there is a close relationship between the two. The loss of hair in old age shows that this is so. Loss of colour and thinning of the individual hairs almost always start about the age of forty, when the health and physical strength are about to begin their journey on the downward path to old age.

Scurf usually makes its appearance long before it becomes troublesome enough to attract attention. It attacks the scalp gradually and may go on for years. The condition is caused by a germ which is infectious, and is usually spread by hair-brushes, combs, hats, towels, etc.

Premature baldness is much more common in men than in women. In men, thinning of the hair generally begins on the crown of the head, but in some cases the hair recedes from the temples, leaving the crown of the head well covered.

Temporary loss of hair often occurs owing to certain diseases, and a change of climate, especially if it is to a warm one, will sometimes account for this condition. During the summer months many people find that their hair becomes noticeably thinner. This is of course a natural process.

Complete baldness. In cases of typhoid fever and scarlet fever or severe measles, people have been known to become completely bald, and in some wasting diseases, such as tuberculosis, the hair also falls out. In any form of illness it is usual to find the hair losing its glossiness and becoming thin and easily broken. It is generally the rule that the hair will return to its normal state once the blood has been freed of the poisons which have been causing the temporary illness.

Treatment. To increase the growth of the hair the general health must be carefully attended to. Once the body is in perfect health, the hair will naturally improve in glossiness and growth. To treat a diseased condition of the scalp, absolute cleanliness is the first and most important step. Dandruff is a condition which may take a long time to get rid of. The head should be washed with a pure soap, such as the ordinary liquid green soap which is obtainable in bottles quite cheaply from any chemist. It should be rinsed thoroughly with repeated fresh waters. This should be done every other day in the case of a man or short-haired woman, and at least twice a week even if the hair is long and difficult to wash and dry. After washing, rub in and repeat daily, an ointment made up of 25 grains of salicylic acid to 1 ounce of vaseline. Stimulating the scalp by the use of electricity is also very helpful, and most hairdressers have the apparatus for carrying out this treatment. Treatment by mercury vapour lamps has had some wonderful results in baldness. These special treatments may be worth the expense in cases where baldness makes a person look so much older than his years that he finds himself being passed over for jobs in favour of men whose hair is younger than his, although they themselves are not.

Baldness which occurs in patches is medically termed *alopecia areata*, and will be found under its own heading.

Baldness may be due to an abnormal state of the roots of the hair which is present from birth, and is usually found in other members of the same family. Nothing much can be done for them and they usually have to wear wigs.

BALNEOLOGY. Balneology is the science of the treatment of disease by baths of various sorts, and by mineral waters. There are many forms of treatment of this sort which will be described fully in the article on BATHS. (*See also* BATHS AND BATHING.)

BALSAM. Balsams are oily, pleasant - smelling substances which are obtained from the stems of certain trees and plants. A balsam, generally speaking, is a mixture of oils, resins, and acids.

Friars' Balsam, which was discovered by the friars many hundreds of years ago, is the balsam which is best known. Its medical name is compound tincture of benzoin. Benzoin or Gum Benjamin is a resin obtained from a plant which grows in tropical countries, and to make Friars' Balsam it is mixed with other ingredients. It is almost a cure-all, being used as a dressing for wounds and sores of all sorts, and as an antiseptic. It is used in the making of sticking plaster. As well as these uses it is very popular in cases of bronchitis and sore throat, or severe cold in the head. It may be swallowed in doses of a teaspoonful to loosen a cough and help to bring up expectoration, but more often it is used as an inhalant.

Balsam of Peru comes from the bark of a tree which grows in South America. It is used as a disinfectant in skin diseases such as itch or ring-worm.

Balsam of Tolu is chiefly used as a syrup in cough mixtures for children.

Storax and **Copaiba** are two other balsams which are in general use. Storax has the same effect as balsams of Tolu and Peru and benzoin, and may be used for the same purposes, but is only given internally as one of the ingredients in Friars' Balsam. Copaiba is another South American balsam. Its use is as a disinfectant in cases of diseases of the bladder, kidneys, or in gonorrhœa. It gives the breath a very disagreeable odour, however, and so is not often used except in gonorrhœa.

BANDAGES AND BANDAGING. There are two chief varieties of bandage, the *triangular* and the *roller*. They are generally made of calico, bleached or unbleached, or of white cotton sheeting. Linen is an excellent material for the purpose, but too costly.

In first-aid work the triangular bandage is far the more commonly used. It is made by cutting diagonally across a piece of material from 36 to 42 inches square. Two triangular bandages are thus formed, measuring 36 to 42 inches along the sides and 50 to 60 inches along the base.

The parts of a triangular bandage are the point or apex, the base, the two sides and the two ends.

Always tie the ends of a triangular bandage with a reef knot. A granny knot is not safe and should never be used.

Place the knot so that it does not press into or chafe the patient. If it is likely to be uncomfortable, place a pad between it and the patient's skin. When a knot is completed the ends should be tucked out of sight. If tying a knot is not practicable, large safety-pins are used to secure the ends of the bandage.

Triangular Bandages

(a) **Large Arm Sling.** This is used to support the forearm. Pass one end of the bandage over the shoulder on the normal side and round the back of the neck. Bring it down nearly to the level of the breast on the injured side. Slip the apex of the bandage across the front of the body and behind the elbow of the injured arm. Bend the elbow and lay the forearm over the middle of the bandage. Bring up the lower end and tie just below the collarbone. Now bring forward the apex from behind the elbow and fix with two safety-pins.

(b) **Narrow Arm Sling.** This bandage supports the wrist, leaving the elbow free. It is used for (a) a fracture of the upper arm, and (b) minor injuries to the hand or shoulder.

Pass a broad-fold bandage over the sound shoulder, behind the neck and down nearly to breast-level on the injured side. Bend the elbow so that the forearm is at right angles to the upper arm. Place the wrist over the middle of the bandage so that half the little finger extends beyond the edge of the bandage. Carry the second end up to the first and tie just below the collar-bone on the injured side.

(c) **St. John's Sling.** This bandage supports the arm and keeps it close to the side. For an injury on the *right* side proceed as follows. If the injury is on the *left* side, substitute " left " for " right " and vice versa.

1. Fold the patient's right forearm flat across his chest, fingers pointing to his left shoulder.

2. Take an unfolded triangular bandage with its apex in your left hand and one end in your right. Lay it over the patient's forearm, the end on his left shoulder, the apex well beyond his right elbow.

3. Tuck the base of the bandage well in under the hand and forearm, supporting the elbow meanwhile. Bring the lower end across the patient's back, up over the left shoulder to the front and tie the ends.

4. Hold away the side of the bandage lying on the forearm and tuck the apex well in between the forearm and the side you hold. This produces a fold which you bring round behind the arm and pin securely to the bandage where it runs up the back.

There are many simple ways of improvising a sling. Take two handkerchiefs. Tie one loosely round the neck. With the other make a sling, the ends being tied in the loop formed by the first handkerchief. This will give a sling of the necessary length. Or simply support the hand well inside the buttoned coat. This is more effective if the sleeve be pinned to the coat as well. A third method is to turn up the lower edge of the coat and pin it near the lapel.

Bandage for Hand. Spread out a triangular bandage on a flat surface and fold a hem along its base. Place the open hand on the bandage, palm downwards, the wrist on the hem. Fold back the apex over the back of the hand and wrist. Cross over the ends and pass them round and round the wrist, finally tying them over the back of the wrist. Now fold back the apex over the knot towards the fingers and pin it.

Bandage for the Wrist. Place the hand palm downwards over the centre of a narrow-fold bandage. Pick up the ends and bring them round the hand, leaving the thumb clear. Cross them over the back of the hand and round and round the wrist and lower forearm. Tie off on the back of the forearm.

Bandage for the Elbow. Fold a 3-inch hem along the base of a bandage. Bend the injured elbow and lay the middle of the hem on the back of the forearm, folded side inwards, and the point of the bandage reaching up the back of the upper arm. Cross the ends in front of the elbow, then round and round the back of the arm above the elbow. Tie them behind, turn down the point to hide the knot, and pin it to the bandage.

Bandage for the Shoulder. To keep a dressing on top of the shoulder, two bandages are needed. Fold a 3-inch hem along the base of the first bandage. Place its centre, hem inwards, against the upper arm, the apex running up the side of the neck to the ear. Pass the ends round and round the arm and tie. With the other bandage apply a narrow arm sling with the knot on top of the apex of the first bandage. Draw up the apex and fold it down neatly over the knot and pin securely to keep the whole thing in place.

Bandage for the whole Foot. To keep a dressing on the foot. Fold a 2-inch hem along the base of a triangular bandage. Place the foot in the centre of the bandage, the toes pointing to the apex. Fold back the apex over the toes and instep and leave it pointing up the front of the ankle. Gather up the ends so that the heel is covered and cross them over the instep. Take them round behind the ankle, cross them and bring them forward again. Tie them in front. (If the bandage is too long, pass the ends once round the sole of the foot before tying off.) Draw up the apex, fold it over and pin it to the bandage above the instep.

Bandage for the Ankle. When treating an injured ankle

place the centre of a narrow-fold bandage against the sole of the foot. Bring up the ends and cross them over the top of the foot. Pass them round behind the ankle, cross them and bring them forward. Cross them again and down round the sole of the foot. Continue until the ends are short and tie them off where convenient.

Bandage for the Knee. Fold a 2-inch hem along the base of the bandage. Place the apex in front of the middle of the thigh and the centre of the base just below the knee-cap. Cross the ends behind the knee. Then bring them round to the front and tie above the knee. Pull up the apex to smooth out the bandage. Fold it over the knot and pin.

Bandage for the Hip. To keep a dressing in position on the hip, two bandages are needed. With the first make a narrow-fold bandage and tie it round the patient just below the rim of the haunch-bone (pelvis), with the knot on the outer side of the affected hip. Lay the second bandage on the hip and pass the apex under the knot of the first bandage. Draw it up for about 4 inches. Fold the base of the second bandage inwards in a 2-inch hem and pass the ends horizontally in and round the thigh, and round and out again. Tie them on the outside. Pull up the apex to smooth out the bandage. Turn it down over the knot and pin in position.

Bandage for the front of the Chest and Abdomen. Spread an open triangular bandage over the chest and abdomen, the base lying across the chest and the apex pointing down. Pass the ends under the armpits, behind the body and tie. Spread a second bandage similarly, but with the base lying across the lower abdomen and the apex pointing to the chin. Tuck the apex in under the first bandage and pin it there. Pass the ends round the patient and tie behind. Turn up the apex of the first bandage and pin it. *N.B.*—The foregoing is an emergency bandage to be replaced later by the orthodox " many tailed " bandage.

Bandage for the Chest. Used to keep a dressing on the chest. Stand in front of the patient and place an open triangular bandage on his chest. Push the apex well over the shoulder on the dressed side. Fold the base over inwards in a 3-inch hem. Bring the ends round behind the back and tie them vertically below the apex. One end will be longer than the other. Carry it up and tie to the apex on top of the shoulder.

Bandage for the Back. This is applied in the same way as the bandage for the chest, except that the patient stands with his back, not his front, towards the dresser.

Bandage for the Scalp. Used to keep a dressing on top of the head. Lay an open triangular bandage on top of the patient's

E.F.D.

head, so that the apex hangs down over the nape of the neck.
Fold a hem about 2 inches wide in the base, so that it lies above
the eyebrows.   Go behind the patient and draw back the ends,
so that they pass just above the ears.   Cross them over and pass
them to the front again.   Tie neatly in the centre of the forehead.
Gently pull down the apex until the bandage is smooth, then turn
it up and pin on top of the head.

Bandage for the Eye.   Place the centre of a narrow-fold
bandage over the dressing on the eye.   Carry one end round below
the ear on the injured side and the other end over the top of the
head on the uninjured side.   Cross the ends at the back of the head,
bring them forward again and tie off over the injured eye.

Roller Bandages

Roller bandages are strips of material rolled into firm cylinders
for easy application.   They are usually some yards in length and
of various widths suitable for different parts of the body.

Bandages $\frac{3}{4}$–1-inch wide are used for fingers and toes, $2\frac{1}{2}$-inch
for the head and arms, 3-inch for the legs, and 4-inch for the trunk.

When a roller bandage is ready for use, the roll is called the
" head " and the loose end the " tail."

These bandages may be rolled by hand, but can be more quickly
and efficiently rolled by machine.

When rolled up, the free end should always be secured by a safety-
pin, this ensures a pin being to hand to fasten the bandage when
needed.

The principal uses of a Roller Bandage are :

1. To retain dressings or splints in position.
2. To support a sprained or dislocated joint, when the patient
   begins to use it again, and to prevent swelling.
3. To treat or prevent varicose veins.
4. To drive the blood to a different part of the body, as is done
   by bandaging limbs in extreme collapse from hæmorrhage.
5. To prevent hæmorrhage after operations.

Rules for applying Roller Bandages :

1. Apply the outer surface to the skin.
2. Bandage from below upwards, and from within outwards.
3. Bandage the chest from below upwards ; but the abdomen
   from above downwards.
4. When bandaging to retain a dressing or splint, leave the
   tips of fingers or toes exposed.   The colour of the nails indi-

cates the state of the circulation of the blood in the limb. If congested, numb, or swollen the bandage is too tight, and the splint or dressings need to be readjusted.

5. Each fresh layer of the bandage should cover two-thirds of the preceding layer.
6. Fix the finished bandage securely.
7. Whenever possible place a layer of wool under the bandage. This permits the bandage to be drawn tighter, without constricting the veins.
8. Use a bandage of appropriate size.

Methods of applying Bandages. The four principal methods of applying roller bandages are :

1. The Simple Spiral. Adopt this method when the part to be bandaged is of uniform thickness, e.g. the finger or wrist.
2. The Reverse Spiral. The bandage is twisted upon itself at each circuit of the injured part. Adopt this method for parts of varying thickness, e.g. the forearm or leg.
3. The Figure of Eight. This is used for a joint or its vicinity. It is made by passing the bandage obliquely round the limb upwards and downwards, so that the loops look like the figure 8.
4. The Spica. This is a modified figure of 8, and is so called because when completed, the crossings of the bandage resemble in their relative positions, the grains in a head or " spike " of barley. It is described in detail under the appropriate headings.

Bandages for various parts of the body. *To Bandage a Finger* (¾- or 1-inch bandage). Turn the hand palm downwards and separate the injured finger. To dress the right hand, hold the bandage in your left, and vice versa. Make two or three fixing turns by passing the bandage round the wrist from within outwards. Lead the bandage from the root of the thumb to the injured finger and up to its tip in a long spiral. Cover the finger in a series of spirals down to its root. Thence lead the bandage across the back of the hand to the wrist, on the little-finger side. Fix with a couple of turns round the wrist.

Any or all of the fingers may be bandaged thus, but between each two a fixing turn must be taken round the wrist.

Finger-tip. If this is injured, proceed as above, but pass the bandage over the centre of the finger-tip down the upper aspect of the finger to its middle joint. Fold the bandage back upon itself and carry it over the tip again to the underside of the middle

finger joint.   Make three such folds, the second and third overlapping the first on either side.   Fix these folds in place by bandaging from tip to root of the finger in a simple spiral and finish
off as above.

To Bandage the Thumb (1-inch bandage).   Lay the tail of
the bandage across the front of the wrist.   Pass the head across
the back of the thumb between the thumb and forefinger.   Make
a simple turn round the top of the thumb and come down diagonally
across the back of the hand to the wrist.   Carry on across the palm,
round the thumb again and so on until the thumb is covered.
Finally take a turn round the wrist and secure.   This is a " spica "
bandage.

To Bandage the Hand (2-inch bandage).   Stand opposite the
injured hand, which should be extended palm downwards.   Place
cotton-wool pads between the fingers.   Lay the tail of the bandage
on the inner surface of the wrist and bring the roll obliquely over
the back of the hand.   Bandage the left hand in a clockwise, and
the right in an anti-clockwise direction.   Pass the roll round the
little finger edge of the hand, across the palm, round the forefinger side of the hand and horizontally across the back of the fingers,
so that the little finger-nail is just exposed.   The bandage circles
the fingers again and passes obliquely over the back of the hand
and round the wrist and obliquely up over the back of the hand
again.   Continue this process three or four times until the figure of
8 loops quite cover the hand and wrist.

To Bandage the Closed Fist (2-inch bandage).   Place a pad
in the palm of the hand and cotton-wool between the fingers.
Start with two fixing turns round the wrist from within outwards.
Carry the bandage over the back of the hand, round over the
little finger and on to the front of the wrist at the root of the thumb.
Circle the wrist and pass again over the back of the hand, the third
finger, the front of the wrist, and so on five or six times.   The last
loop will project 1 inch beyond the margin of the forefinger.   Now
pass the bandage twice or thrice round the bent fingers enclosed in
the loops and finish off at the wrist.

To Bandage the Forearm (2–2½-inch bandage).   Make a
few fixing turns at the wrist, from within outwards.   Bandage the
lower forearm with a simple spiral.   When the muscular part is
reached, the bandage will no longer fit snugly ; the lower edge
will be loose.   To overcome this difficulty make a reverse spiral
for the upper part of the limb.   Support the forearm with your
free hand and bring the bandage round the back of the limb in
such a way that it lies flat.   While in this position place your free
thumb on the bandage and bring the head downwards.   Turn

it over in such a way that its upper edge folds' over the thumb. A " reverse " has now been made and the *inner* surface of the roll is next the skin. Pass the bandage round the forearm again and make another reverse. (The outer surface of the bandage will now be next skin again.) Continue in this manner. When the bandage nears the elbow bend the forearm at right angles to the arm, the palm facing inwards. Carry the bandage over the elbow by four figure of 8 turns. Of each, one loop encircles the top of the forearm, the other the lower part of the arm. The four crossings are in front of the elbow.

To Bandage the tip of the Elbow ($2\frac{1}{2}$-inch bandage). Lay the tail of the bandage on the inner side of the bent elbow, and pass the roll round the limb over the elbow tip. Circle the arm with a second turn and the forearm with a third, so that each overlaps the margin of the first turn. Continue these figure of 8 turns round the arm and forearm alternately until half a dozen or so are made.

To Bandage the Arm ($2\frac{1}{2}$-inch bandage). Make two fixing turns just above the bent elbow. Carry on with simple spirals. If the limb is exceptionally muscular, reverses may be needed. If so, make them high up on the outer aspect of the arm.

Recapitulation. To bandage the whole arm : Begin with a simple spiral at the wrist and change to reversed spiral over the forearm. Use a figure of 8 to negotiate the elbow. Complete the upper arm with a simple spiral, with perhaps a few reverses.

To Bandage the Shoulder (4-inch bandage). Place a pad of cotton-wool in the *uninjured* armpit to prevent chafing. Make two fixing turns, with reverses if necessary, round the upper arm. Carry the bandage across the back to the opposite armpit, across the chest, and round the shoulder. Continue these figure of 8 turns four or five times until the whole of the shoulder is covered.

To Bandage the Chest (4-inch bandage). A spiral bandage on the chest tends to slip down. To overcome this split a $1\frac{1}{2}$-yard length of 4-inch bandage along its centre so as to make a hole $2\frac{1}{2}$-feet long. Pass this over the patient's head so that one end reaches to the small of the back, the other to well below the navel. Now take a 4-inch bandage and make two fixing turns round the lower chest and on top of the first piece of bandage. Proceed with reversed spirals well up the chest. Finish off with two fixing turns and pin the bandage in front. Turn up the free ends of the brace over the bandage and fix with safety-pins in front and behind.

If preferred, use two braces, one passing over each shoulder and finish off in the same way.

The Many-tailed Bandage. After surgical treatment a many-tailed bandage is used to retain dressings on the chest and abdomen. It has the merit of enabling the wound to be examined and the dressings changed without moving the patient. It can be made by laying several strips of roller bandage of the right length parallel to and overlapping each other. The strips are then sewn to another strip laid across their centres.

A many-tailed bandage should be long enough to go once and a quarter times round the part and deep enough amply to cover the area involved. For the chest and abdomen the tails are $3\frac{1}{2}$ to 4 inches in width.

To apply a many-tailed bandage to the chest spread the bandage underneath the patient. Then cross the right and left lower ends over each other in front. Then the second lowest pair, the third lowest, and so on, each successive pair securing the preceding pair. Fix the last tail with a safety-pin.

To Bandage the Breast. To support one breast. Take a 3-inch bandage and make two fixing turns round the body below the breasts from the sound to the affected side. Carry the third turn under the affected breast, up and over the shoulder, down the back, and round the body again. Continue until five or six turns have been made. Safety-pins may be used at intervals to fix the crossing loops in position.

To support both breasts. Proceed as for one breast, but take the bandage up and over the right and left shoulders alternately until each breast is covered by four or five turns.

To Bandage the Heel (3-inch bandage). Support the leg so that the foot projects. Stand opposite the injured foot and place the tail of the bandage on the front of the ankle. Pass the roll round the tip of the heel from within outwards. Make a second round passing the bandage slightly above the first turn. Make a third round just below the first turn on the sole of the foot. Continue like this, the fourth round passing just above the second and the fifth just below the third. But when the fifth turn reaches the inner side of the foot, do not pass it over the instep. Bring it back diagonally over the inner side of the heel across the previous turns and pass it round the back of the ankle and down over the top of the foot from without inwards. Take the top of the foot from without inwards. Take the sixth turn under the foot and back diagonally across the *outer* side of the heel and round the back of the ankle. It is the same as the fifth turn, but in the opposite direction. Finish off with a turn or two round the ankle.

To Bandage the Foot — leaving the heel exposed (3-inch bandage). Place the tail of the bandage beneath the sole of the foot. Make a figure of 8 by bringing the roll from within outwards

over the top of the foot, round the ankle, across the top of the foot
to the root of the little toe, and round under the foot to the starting-
point. Now bandage up the foot in spiral turns, with reverses, if
necessary, over the instep. Finish off with two figure of 8 turns
round the ankle and foot, pinning behind the ankle.

To Bandage the Knee (3-inch bandage). There are two
methods.

(*a*) *Permits movement of the joint.* Slightly bend the knee and
make a fixing turn from within outwards over the knee-cap. Make
a second turn *below* and half overlapping the first, and a third *above*
and half overlapping it. The fourth turn overlaps the upper two-
thirds of the third turn. Continue in this way until the knee is
covered. Finish with a turn or two round the upper leg.

(*b*) *Restricts movement of the joint.* Raise the knee so that the roll
can be passed beneath it. Make a fixing turn just below the knee-
cap. Bring the bandage round the back of the knee and out to
the front on the inner surface of the bottom of the thigh. Encircle
the thigh and carry the bandage down over the knee-cap. Pass it
round the leg just below the knee and then upwards round the lower
thigh just above the knee. Carry it round the thigh and then down
in a descending loop, which overlaps the last one. Continue until
the knee is covered.

To Bandage the Leg (3-inch bandage). Fix the bandage
with a figure of 8 turn round the foot and ankle. Carry on up the
leg with simple spirals until the bulge of the calf muscles call for
reverses. Make them on the outside of the leg. Finish off with two
simple spirals just below the knee.

To Bandage the Thigh. Apply a 3-inch bandage to the
thigh in an ascending spiral with reverses. Sometimes a many-
tailed bandage is used. (*See also* CHEST AND ABDOMEN.)

To Bandage the Groin. If the patient cannot stand, the
pelvis must be firmly supported.

(*a*) *The St. Andrew's Cross* (3-inch bandage). Make two fixing
turns round the waist from left to right. Pass the bandage down
the left groin and up behind the right buttock. Come round the
waist from left to right and down the right groin ; up behind the
left buttock, round the waist from left to right and down the left
groin again. Continue until the desired support is achieved.

(*b*) *Single Spica*—To cover one groin. Take a long 4-inch bandage and stand on the side to be bandaged. Make a fixing turn
round the upper thigh, from within outwards. Carry the bandage
up along the groin and round the back. Bring it forwards and
downwards to cross the first turn directly over the dressing in the
groin. Pass it round the thigh and up over the groin again, making

a figure of 8. Continue these turns until the dressing is covered and secure.

(c) *Double Spica*—To cover both groins. Stand on the patient's right side, or facing him if he is on his feet. Begin as for a single spica on the right side, but bring the bandage forwards and downwards over the *left* groin and round the *left* thigh. Then take it up across the abdomen to the right groin and over the first turn of the bandage. Carry it round the right thigh, behind the waist and down to the inner side of the left thigh. This completes one turn. Continue a series of such turns.

To keep a Dressing between the Legs. Make a ⊤ bandage by stitching a piece of 4-inch bandage one yard long at right angles to the centre of another piece one and a half yards long. Tear the first piece up its centre for half its length. To apply, tie the second piece round the waist like a girdle with the knot in front. Pass the first piece between the legs from behind and tie the tails to the girdle on either side of the knot. Alternatively, use the St. Andrew's Cross. (*See also* GROIN.)

To Bandage the Chin (four-tailed bandage). Cut off a yard from the widest bandage available. Tear from both ends down the middle. Stop when 3 inches from the centre. This will leave an undivided central portion 6 inches long.

To apply. Place the centre of the bandage on the patient's chin. Carry the lower tails upwards in front of the ears and tie them on top of the head. Bring the upper pair of tails along the line of the jaw and tie behind the neck. As the bandage is 1 yard long, four ends are left over. Tie the two right ends and the two left ends together.

To Bandage the Head. The triangular bandage is undoubtedly the most useful, but a modified roller bandage is sometimes used.

Roll up a 2-inch bandage from each end, or stitch the tails of two bandages together so as to form one long, double-headed, or capelline bandage.

To apply. Stand behind the seated patient with one roll in either hand. Place the centre of the bandage on the forehead, just above the eyebrows. Bring round the two ends and cross them well down at the base of the skull. Carry the upper end round to the front again. Turn up the other end, which lays underneath, and bring it over the crown of the head and down to the centre of the forehead. Let the horizontal portion pass over it and round to the back of the head again. Turn up the hanging portion and take it back over the crown, so that it overlaps one-third of the first strip. Cross the two portions at the back and bring the hanging portion forwards again so that it overlaps the *other* side of the centre strip. Carry the horizontal portion on round the head as before. In front, secure the hanging portion once again and carry on backwards and forwards on alternate sides until the whole scalp is covered. Finish off by taking both ends round the head and pinning them.

To Bandage the Eye (2-inch bandage). Make a fixing turn round the head, starting on the uninjured side just above the ear. When the starting-point is reached, bring the bandage over the affected eye, below the ear on that side, round the back of the head to the forehead again. Make as many turns as may be necessary and fix with a safety-pin. Both eyes can be bandaged by passing every other turn of the bandage below the other ear and up over the other eye, to form a crossed bandage.

BANTING. This is the name given to a slimming diet for over-fat people, which was made popular by William Banting, a London undertaker of enormous size who lived in the earlier part of the nineteenth century. (*See* OBESITY.)

BANTING, SIR FREDERICK GRANT. Born in Canada in 1892, the discoverer of the method of treating diabetes by insulin (in association with Dr. Best, Dr. Collip and Professor MacLeod) in 1922. A research institute in Toronto has been named after him.

BARBER'S ITCH. Barber's itch or " foul shave " is the popular name for a skin disease, the medical names of which are sycosis, tinea sycosis, or tinea barbæ. Many little yellow pimples are to be seen, each surrounding a hair, and the skin between is swollen and red. In bad cases the upper lip and eyebrows may be affected. The cause of barber's itch is mainly a germ of the staphylo-coccus group, but other germs have been found to be present. Barber's itch must not be confused with other diseases which at first sight look like it, such as impetigo, ringworm of the beard, and dermatitis.

Barber's itch is a very chronic disease and very difficult to cure.

Treatment. The hair of the beard should be clipped as short as possible. An antiseptic soap should be used, and if possible the hair in the centre of each pimple should be pulled out before shaving. An antiseptic ointment must then be rubbed in, and·it is very important to rub the ointment thoroughly into the skin. Even a weak ointment, thoroughly rubbed in, is better than a strong ointment if it is only smeared on. Rub the ointment in twice a day for ten minutes at a time. This treatment, if continued long enough, should cure simple cases.

Vaccines may be tried for more severe cases, and are often very useful—especially if they can be made of the patient's own germs (autogenous vaccines). Injections of the vaccine are usually given

3 *

once a fortnight. In severe cases X-ray treatment is also used and is generally very successful.

A useful ointment for rubbing in is white mercurial ointment.

BARBITONE. This drug is better known as veronal, and although looked upon generally as a harmless hypnotic, it is sometimes uncertain in its action and should be used with care.

Cases of acute fatal poisoning have occurred owing to an overdose of barbitone, but fatalities rarely follow unless the dose has been as large as 50 grains or so. Deep coma may result lasting for two or three days, and paralysis of the organs used in breathing may develop. In cases of poisoning, the stomach should be washed out with warm water, and hot strong coffee and about one ounce of castor-oil should be given through a stomach tube. If the pulse is feeble oxygen may have to be administered.

BARBITURATES. The name given to veronal (barbitone) and its derivatives, such as luminal, dial, medinal, etc. They have become very popular as sedatives and hypnotics, but care should be exercised in taking them, as their action is rather uncertain. (*See* BARBITONE, VERONAL.)

BARIUM MEAL TEST. Barium is a heavy, white, odourless powder which is insoluble in water and, being mineral, can be seen by the X-rays. It is used therefore to obtain photographs of the working of the digestive system. A bowl of barium powder is made into a porridge and is swallowed by the patient, who is then photographed under the X-rays at intervals of a few hours during the next twenty-four hours.

BARKING COUGH. This is a dry, hoarse cough which sounds exactly like the bark of a dog. It may be due to laryngitis or to food crumbs which " have gone down the wrong way," but is more usually met with in cases of hysteria.

BARLOW'S DISEASE. (*See also* SCURVY.)

BARRENNESS. The state of being unable to bear children. The reasons for this are discussed under the heading STERILITY.

BASEDOW'S DISEASE. (*See* EXOPHTHALMIC GOITRE.)

BATHS AND HEALTH. Baths have an effect on the system by improving the action of the skin. The nerves of the skin control the temperature of the body by distributing heat over the surface of the body and by evaporating moisture from it.

Baths, given at different temperatures, also have a powerful effect on the circulation of the blood, and can be used to improve it to a great extent. The same applies to the nervous system, which can be affected by heat and other influences which are employed in electrical, chemical and mechanical baths.

BAY RUM. Bay rum is a hair-oil obtained from the oil of

the bay. It is used a great deal in the treatment of greasy scalps and other conditions, and also to impart an agreeable smell to many toilet preparations.

BAZIN'S DISEASE or "SHOPGIRL'S DISEASE." Under this name two diseases are grouped. The first occurs in girls and young women whose occupation involves a great deal of standing. These girls frequently have a family history of tuberculosis, and they themselves may show symptoms of tuberculosis, such as enlarged glands, and the germ of tuberculosis has been found in the ulcers that appear on the legs. The girl is frequently delicate and anæmic. In these cases the skin at the back of the legs between the knee and ankle is affected usually on both legs. The condition begins by the formation in the skin and soft tissues beneath the skin of livid, bluish, hard lumps or nodules, as they are called. These nodules grow larger, then soften and turn into ulcers. The skin over them " sloughs " or comes away, leaving a small open sore with ragged edges. Fresh crops appear near by, and they in turn become ulcers. In the nodular or lumpy stage of the disease there is pain, but not in the ulcerated stage.

The second variety of Bazin's disease is found most often in fat women with inflamed varicose veins, " bad legs " as they would call them. In appearance this form is the same as the other, but it is not tuberculosis in origin. The treatment of both forms is much the same.

Treatment. If it is left untreated, the disease may spread widely over the calves of the legs and may last for months and years. In these neglected cases the affected tissues are better removed by operation and skin from some other part of the body grafted over the area. If seen early, the condition will improve rapidly under treatment, though relapses are common unless the general condition of the patient is improved. The treatment consists chiefly of rest in bed and generous diet. The legs should be raised on pillows. For the tubercular type, cod-liver oil and tonics are advised ; where the varicose veins are the real cause of the trouble, these may be suitably treated. The use of strapping, with or without Ichthyol paste, often promotes healing of the ulcers. (*See also* TUBERCULOSIS ; VARICOSE VEINS.)

BEAT HAND. Beat hand, beat elbow, and beat knee are terms applied to an inflamed condition which arises through constant pressure and friction caused by handling tools. It is a very common complaint among miners, but occurs in other trades also. The condition is a painful one, and unless it is treated early by the application of suitable antiseptics, surgical measures may have to be taken. (*See also* BURSITIS ; TENNIS ELBOW.)

BED-BUGS. These insects may develop into a source of great danger and annoyance if measures are not promptly taken to destroy the eggs as well as the insects themselves. The bed-bug gives forth a disagreeable smell which seems to fill the whole room, and is quite characteristic.

Not only is the bed-bug an unpleasant visitor to have in one's house, but as a carrier of disease it must be looked upon as extremely dangerous. After it has been feeding on the blood of a person suffering from fever or any other infectious disease, it will spread the germs in the most indiscriminate way to other persons whom it may bite.

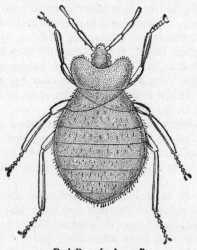

Bed-Bug (enlarged)

Drastic measures may have to be taken in order to rid a house of this pest. Mere simple cleaning will not be found enough, as these little creatures lurk in the skirting-boards and flooring. The premises which are to be cleaned must be thoroughly dismantled and all possible breeding-places must be treated with crude creosote of tar. All furniture, especially if made of wood, should be washed with soap and, after it is thoroughly dry, turpentine should be applied to all holes and cracks. Sulphur fumigation is also an excellent way of disposing of bed-bugs, or kerosene may be used. Should clothing require treatment, this may be carried out by soaking the garments in a Lysol solution. In order to relieve the intense irritation caused by the bites of these insects, the parts may be bathed with dilute ammonia or toilet vinegar. (*See also* BITES.)

BED-CRADLE. In certain cases, such as fracture of the limbs or painful abdominal conditions, it is necessary that the bed-clothes should be lifted from off these particular parts of the body. A bed-cradle is used for this purpose. It is a cage-like arrangement, made of wooden or metal struts. In cases of emergency, an ordinary foot-stool with legs can be used for this purpose.

BED-SORE. Bed-sores can develop into a very serious condition, especially in a patient who requires all his energy and strength to cope with the condition which has caused him to be bed-ridden. Any sign of redness on the skin of a person who has to stay in bed for some time should be attended to immediately, as once a bed-sore commences, it is very difficult to get rid of.

The prevention of bed-sores depends very largely on good and efficient nursing, but there are certain conditions, such as complete paralysis, etc., in which they may make their appearance towards the end of the illness. When the circulation becomes poor and the vitality of the patient is low, bed-sores will undoubtedly make their appearance unless the greatest precautions are taken.

All prominent parts, such as the spine, shoulder-blades, hips, heels, elbows, etc., are especially likely to become sore, and these parts should be given attention. The patient should be washed, and before the skin is dried, the nurse should soap her hands well and gently massage the back and hips. The movement should be round and round in order to encourage the circulation of the blood where it has been hindered by constant pressure on the bed. In order to harden the patient's skin, the soap should be left on unless it creates irritation. It will be found better to dry the skin by dabbing it with a towel instead of rubbing, as the rough towel is apt to crack the skin, and a bed-sore may be the result. When the skin is thoroughly dried, it should again be thoroughly rubbed with methylated spirits, or eau-de-Cologne. Finally, the body should be dusted with some fine powder, such as zinc, white fuller's earth, or talc.

If in spite of all precautions a bed-sore appears, the slough should be removed by warm boracic lint or eusol dressings until the surface is clean. After this a return should be made to dry dressings, such as boracic acid or aristol powder, with a large cotton-wool pad over the sore.

BED-WETTING (ENURESIS). This condition may occur in children after the age when they should have control over their own bladders. It appears to be more common among boys than girls. In some cases it is difficult to cure and the greatest care and tact are necessary in the handling of the child. It is extremely unwise to punish hastily when bed-wetting occurs, as it is very often a matter beyond the child's control.

Treatment. Proper attention to the bowels during the day and regular emptying of the bladder is the first important step in treatment. The diet should be nourishing but not irritating, and fluids should not be taken for a few hours before bedtime. The child should be made to empty the bladder before going to bed and should be waked to do so after a few hours' sleep. It is wrong to make the child feel that it is doing something unpleasant, as this often increases the child's nervousness and makes the complaint worse. The co-operation of the little patient may be gained by kindliness, and his own eagerness to obey his mother's wishes will do much to bring about a cure. Many drugs are used to try and cure children of bed-wetting. Amongst the ones generally used are belladonna, hexamine, alkalies and thyroid extract. Treatment by suggestion and hypnotism have been tried with quite good results. If the child is a boy with a tight foreskin, the simple operation of circumcision will probably cure him of the habit. Sometimes removal of adenoids will bring about a cure, by the good effect on the nerves. (*See also* BLADDER, DISEASES OF.)

BEEF. In various forms beef juice is a very valuable addition to the diet of ill people and convalescents.

BELLADONNA. This powerful drug is obtained from the belladonna plant, which is more popularly known as the deadly nightshade and is a well-known inhabitant of our hedges and woods. It can be readily recognized by its clusters of small purple flowers with orange centres, rather like lilac in appearance, which climbs about amongst a tangle of other plants in the hedges. Later on the flowers turn into bunches of bright scarlet berries and as they ripen about the same time as the blackberries and often grow amongst them, a summer never passes without some children being poisoned by eating them in mistake.

Belladonna is one of the most useful drugs we have, and atropine —the alkaloid which comes from the same plant—is also of the greatest use. Its chief use is in treating diseases where there are painful " spasms." A spasm is a tightening of the muscles in any part of the body so that that part cannot continue its work and the tightened muscles cause great pain. Such spasms occur in a large variety of diseases such as asthma, bronchitis, stomach troubles, gall-stones, inflammation of the bladder. Belladonna or atropine will usually cause the muscles to relax, thus relieving the spasm. It is sometimes prescribed for troublesome cases of bed-wetting. In whooping cough it is of the greatest use, and will often be successful where other remedies fail.

Belladonna plasters are still very comforting remedies in lumbago, phlebitis and painful rheumatic conditions, or in cases where the

liver is congested and painful. It used to be thought that a belladonna plaster applied to the breast of a nursing mother would
stop the flow of milk, but now it is considered that it is the pressure
that affects the flow and that a tight bandage will do as well.

Belladonna liniment is useful to rub in in order to ease the pain
of such conditions as rheumatism and neuralgia and lumbago.
Care must be taken, however, that poisoning is not caused by too
much being absorbed through the skin, as sometimes happens.

Poisoning by Belladonna. If the berries have been eaten or
too much of the drug taken and there is poisoning, an emetic
should be given at once and after the vomiting has stopped large
drinks of water with sal volatile or alcohol as a stimulant. Artificial
respiration may have to be performed if the breathing becomes very
feeble.

The symptoms of belladonna poisoning are great dryness of the
mouth and throat, enlarged pupils or dark centres of the eyes,
rapid beating of the heart, sickness, excitement and delirium with
great bodily weakness.

BELL'S PALSY. This is paralysis of the facial nerve. It
is called after a famous Scottish physician, Sir Charles Bell, 1774–
1842. It is described under the heading FACIAL PARALYSIS.

BENGER'S FOOD. This is a food in which the process of
digestion is begun before the patient swallows it. For this reason
it is very suitable for infants who find it difficult to digest cow's
milk ; it is also a very useful food for persons suffering from severe
illness or stomach conditions such as gastric ulcer, where no solid
food can be taken. The food being partly digested before it is
taken into the stomach by the patient, the stomach is thus relieved
of much of its work. Full directions for making it are given on
each tin and these should be carefully followed in order to obtain
the fullest benefit from the food.

BENIGN. This term is applied to certain tumours which are
not dangerous to life and health. If tumours are dangerous to life
they are called " malignant."

BENZOIC ACID. Obtained from the gum benzoin. Benzoic acid is a powerful antiseptic, and lint soaked in a preparation
of it is a very favourite dressing for wounds and sores of all sorts.
Benzoated lard is a common basis for ointments. Benzoin, benzoic
acid and its compounds are very often used in the treatment of
bronchitis.

BENZOL. Benzol or benzene is a light colourless fluid obtained from coal-tar oil. It has a very strong characteristic odour.
Applied externally, one liberal application will destroy lice. It
is a highly inflammable substance and should never be used near

a naked light. In cases of poisoning by benzol, an emetic should be given followed by stimulants.

BERGONIÉ TREATMENT OF OBESITY. One of the most effective treatments for fatness or obesity, as it is called, is by means of the special chair invented by the French physician after whom it is called. The patient reclines in this specially built chair, which is attached to a battery of faradic electricity.

The Bergonié treatment is specially useful for cases where the muscles have become weak, and where the patient is, for some reason such as a diseased heart, unable to take enough exercise. In order to obtain exercise for the debilitated muscles without fatiguing the heart, the patient is connected up with weak electricity all over the body in the manner described above, sandbags are placed over the electrodes, and the electricity is turned on. All the muscles of the body are stimulated and forced to contract painlessly and rhythmically ; thus the patient obtains general exercise of the muscles without strain or the using up of nervous energy. As much as a pound may be lost in weight at one sitting, and the loss is likely to be permanent. The patient improves in general health and feels buoyant and exhilarated. If it is not desired to exercise the whole body, any given part can be exercised by simply changing the position of the electrodes and sandbags. The sandbags serve to keep the electrodes in place and also to give the muscles more work to do by forcing them to push against their weight.

BERI-BERI. Beri-beri is a disease caused by the absence from the diet of vitamin B1 (which is described in the article on VITAMINS) and is therefore known as a " deficiency " disease. The disease is usually found in countries where rice is the chief article of food (Japan, China, India, Malay Peninsula). It is due to the eating of rice which has been polished in order to remove the husk. The vitamin is in the husk. This vitamin is found in various other foods, such as eggs, vegetables, cereals, pulses, meat and milk, and although the disease is more common in rice-eating countries, it has been known to break out in ships, jails, and institutions, wherever the diet has a deficiency in this vitamin.

Symptoms usually begin to develop after there has been a shortage of vitamin B1 for about three months. There are two main types of beri-beri : " dry " and " wet." In the " dry " type, there is much weakness and wasting of the leg muscles, loss of feeling in various parts of the skin, and pain in the limbs and joints. Tender swellings may appear in the calf of the leg, and the skin may feel dry. In the " wet " variety, there may be acute dropsy commencing in the legs and spreading upwards to the belly and lungs. The heart is usually affected and becomes very much enlarged, also the veins become too full and there is enlargement of the liver. The temperature remains normal and the mind remains quite clear.

Treatment consists of an ordinary mixed diet with the addition of the substances which contain vitamin B1. This can be quickly supplied in the form of yeast, Marmite, rice husks, wholemeal bread and milk. If the disease has become serious the patient must be kept in bed. Bleeding may be carried out to give relief in cases where the veins have become swollen, and massage may be useful for the legs. Heart stimulants do not have much effect since the main treatment lies in correcting the diet.

BICARBONATE OF SODA. A white powder, which is alkaline, used in the treatment of acid dyspepsia, for nasal douches, and for soothing irritable skin troubles. (*See also* SODIUM.)

BICEPS. Biceps, which means two-headed, is commonly used to denote the well-known muscle in the upper arm, but is also the name of another muscle in the upper leg. The two muscles are alike in that they each begin in two different places and join

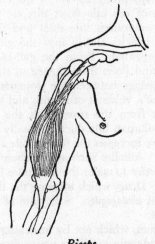

Biceps

together to form one muscle, thus earning their name. The biceps in the arm is the muscle responsible for bending the forearm on the upper arm and is thus used in weight-lifting. It comes into play in most athletic pursuits such as rowing, boxing and swimming. The biceps in the leg is a muscle at the back of the thigh.

BIDET. A bidet is a small hip bath used for administering douches and enemas. It may be raised on legs and be fixed in a special chair.

BILE. Bile or gall is the substance which is produced by the liver. It plays an important part in the process of the digestion of food. In appearance bile is a slightly sticky fluid, varying in colour from deep golden yellow to greenish yellow, according to whether it is collected from the liver itself or from the gall-bladder, and how concentrated it is. It has a very bitter taste and is composed of a mixture of substances known as *mucin* and *cholesterol*, together with certain salts and two colouring matters, one of which is green and the other is red. The liver also abstracts certain poisons, or toxins as they are called, from the blood for the purpose of turning them out of the body by way of the stream of bile which carries them to the intestines. It will be seen, therefore, that if the liver is sluggish and the bile not flowing properly, these poisons get taken back into the system and cause the toxic state known as " liverishness " or " biliousness." Calomel and Epsom salts are the two remedies which are specially useful in increasing the flow of bile and relieving this state of sluggishness.

The amount of bile produced varies from one to two pints a day. A large part of the bile flows directly from the liver into the tube called the common bile duct and from there into the duodenum. Some trickles slowly into the gall-bladder where it is stored and concentrated. From the gall-bladder it enters the common bile duct and flows from thence to the duodenum. The duodenum is the passage between the stomach and the intestines. It works by means of a valve at each end, and the entrance of food into the duodenum from the stomach is the signal for the bile to flow out of the common bile duct in greatly increased amounts. Active bodily exercise increases the flow of bile and will often relieve liverishness at once. Alkalies such as bicarbonate of soda in large doses are given in order to make the bile more liquid and enable it to flow more easily. Drugs which increase the flow or manufacture of bile are known as *cholagogues*. Salicylate of soda and aloes are useful in this respect.

Indirect cholagogues, which act by hastening the passage of the bile through the duodenum and thus preventing waste matter from having time to get back into the blood, are calomel, magnesium sulphate, podophyllin, etc. The action of olive-oil on the bile is being studied nowadays. It undoubtedly has a beneficial action in some cases of gall-bladder disease, probably by hastening the flow of the bile.

BILE DUCTS. Bile is collected in numerous small vessels in the liver, called the bile-capillaries, and flows into two large ducts or tubes called the right and left *hepatic ducts*. These two ducts join together to form the *hepatic duct*, and about ¾ in. farther on the hepatic duct is joined by the *cystic duct*, which is the duct leading from the gall-bladder. The joint hepatic ducts and cystic duct form the *common bile duct*, and as such carry the bile into the duodenum.

As these ducts are narrow tubes less than a ¼ in. wide, it will be seen that they can be easily blocked by stones from the gall-bladder or by bands and adhesions outside, in which case the gall-bladder

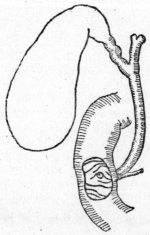

Bile Duct: Coming from Gall-bladder joining Liver and opening into Duodenum

may become over-full and distended and the patient suffers from stomach troubles as a result of the insufficient supply of bile to the intestine.

BILHARZIASIS or LIVER-FLUKE DISEASE. Bilharziasis is a disease not found in England, but which is very common in Africa, especially Egypt, the West Indies, South America, China and Japan. It is caused by the entrance into the body of certain parasites known as fluke-worms.

BILIARY COLIC. Biliary colic is the intense pain caused by the contractions of the bile ducts in their efforts to expel a stone or gravel which has entered the duct and is blocking it. The onset of the pain is usually very sudden and it is so severe that it is usually described as " excruciating." It is felt sometimes round and above the navel and sometimes all over the abdomen and it may shoot up to the right shoulder region. A pain at the point of the right shoulder is often described but in practice the pain is generally not so localized. It comes on in sharp paroxysms and the patient rolls about in agony and doubles up to obtain relief. There may be vomiting and sweating.

Treatment. During the attack morphia must be given to ease the pain, and if this is not successful, it may be necessary to give whiffs of chloroform. In less severe attacks a hot bath and tincture of belladonna or atropine given by the mouth may be sufficient. After the pain has been dealt with the condition which caused it must be attended to.

BILIOUSNESS. The word biliousness is popularly applied to states where there is a feeling of nausea or an inclination to sickness, dirty tongue, headache, discomfort in the stomach and constipation. The term " liverish " is also used. Strictly speaking this state has nothing to do with the bile itself except in so far as the fact that the liver is not working very well may cause the system to be overloaded with toxins which it is the liver's job to remove from the blood. In children an attack of " biliousness " follows very often after eating too much rich food at a party. This type of bilious attack is really acute gastritis or upset of the stomach and is easily dealt with by a couple of days on starvation diet and some simple alkaline medicine such as magnesia. Should the condition continue, however, or return from time to time, especially in middle-aged or older people, a thorough overhaul by the family doctor or at hospital should be arranged for, as it may be the beginning of more serious trouble.

BINDERS. After her confinement it is usual for a woman to wear a binder round the abdomen for a week or more until the muscles of the abdominal wall have regained their elasticity and tone. This binder is made of strong linen and is 12–16 inches in breadth and wide enough to fold well over the abdomen. It is better not to hem the edges as they may press into the delicate skin of the abdomen and cause discomfort.

A similar binder in narrower flannel is wrapped round the abdomen of the new-born baby until the cord has dropped off and the navel is quite healed. (*See also* CHILDBIRTH ; CLOTHES.)

BINOCULAR. This means the ability to use both eyes at once. Each eye has its own power of vision, which is obvious if one closes one eye at a time and looks at an object. The object will be seen by each eye separately, but by using the two eyes together, the object will appear much clearer. (*See also* EYES ; VISION.)

BIOCHEMISTRY. Biochemistry is the name for the science dealing with the chemistry of the body. It is physiological chemistry.

or the chemistry of living tissues and organs, and is a science in which a great deal of research work is now being done. Discoveries such as insulin come into the sphere of the biochemist.

BIOLOGY. This term is applied to the science of life and living things. The structure and function of all living things are studied in this science so that it forms a very wide field of medical knowledge.

BIPP. This is a preparation of bismuth, iodoform, and paraffin which was used extensively during the Great War as a dressing for wounds. Wounds of all sorts did very well with this treatment, but to-day it is used chiefly in treating abscesses in bone, such as mastoid abscess. (*See also* BISMUTH.)

BIRTH. The birth of a child normally takes place nine months after the date at which the mother had her last menstrual period or " courses." If the child arrives after only seven months it is said to be *premature*. It may still live and in time become strong, but will require very careful attention in its early years. Birth earlier than six and a half months but later than three months, is called a *miscarriage*. Before three months it is an *abortion*. The birth of all babies born after twenty-eight weeks of pregnancy, whether alive or dead, must be notified to the Medical Officer of Health of the district within thirty-six hours. This must be done by the father or any person in attendance on the mother at the time of the birth. In addition the birth must be registered with the Registrar of Births, Marriages and Deaths. It is a criminal offence to conceal a birth. A *stillborn* child is one that is born dead. (*See also* CHILDBIRTH ; LABOUR ; PREGNANCY.)

BIRTHMARKS. Birthmarks or nævi (which is the plural of the word nævus, meaning present at birth) are blemishes on the skin which are present at birth. They are of many different sorts and the term should, strictly speaking, include moles and warts as well. In general, however, when we talk of birthmarks we mean the red or purplish stains or swellings on the skin with which some children are born, and which do not fade away in the first few weeks of life but remain stationary or in many cases grow larger as the child grows.

The two most usual sorts are the " spider " and the " port-wine stain." In the case of the spider or arachnoid nævus, the dilated blood-vessels spread out from a centre with a spider's-web appearance. These birthmarks may be very small or may grow to a large size. The port-wine stain is the birthmark most commonly found on the face. It is called port-wine stain from its dark purple colour, and it is unfortunately very disfiguring. In some cases the whole of one cheek may be covered, or the stain may be no larger than the size of a small coin. Often moles are present as well and there may be a heavy growth of hair to add to the disfigurement.

Treatment. In the treatment of all varieties of birthmark the chief aim is to remove the birthmark with as little scarring as possible. This is naturally a difficult task. Of course if the birthmarks are of some size on the covered parts of the body, where the presence of a scar does not matter, and removal is desired, by far the most useful method of treating such cases is that of removal by surgery. A single operation is sufficient, and the cure is speedy and certain. Skin may be brought from another part of the body and be grafted on if necessary.

" Spider " nævi are treated by applying an electric needle to the central point, or by using a cauterizing needle. Birthmarks are also treated by freezing with carbon dioxide snow (liquid air), or by burning with a caustic such as acid nitrate of mercury, nitric acid, or carbolic acid ; but in the latter case the treatment is found to be not altogether satisfactory, as traces of the tumour frequently remain, and a new growth may appear. If advised, treatment by radium is very good, as it does not disturb the patient at all and it is especially good for young children, which cannot be said of the other methods. It is also better for birthmarks about the size of a shilling or larger, as these are difficult to destroy by the cautery.

The very extensive " port-wine stains " are so difficult to treat satisfactorily that many authorities advise leaving them alone entirely. The blood-vessels of this type are, unlike the other varieties, embedded in firm, solid tissue, and cannot be destroyed without running the risk of damaging the surrounding tissues as well. As these birthmarks on the face cause a great deal of mental suffering to their unfortunate possessors, expert advice should be sought at an early stage, and one or other of the treatments mentioned above may be tried. If an adult with a large port-wine mark is anxious for treatment, several small areas may be treated at each sitting and the mark gradually reduced, or at least made paler. It is, however, a process that may literally take years to complete, so that none but the most persevering should be encouraged to try it.

BISMUTH. Bismuth and its preparations are included in the class of heavy metals used in medicine. Used externally, salts of bismuth may be dusted on sores and wounds as a protective and mild drying agent, but the antiseptic action is very slight.

In the treatment of stomach ulcers, either gastric or duodenal, bismuth mixtures are greatly used in combination with alkalies such as magnesium carbonate. In cases of diarrhœa large doses can be given without any ill effects.

BITES AND STINGS. Insect Bites. It is sometimes difficult to distinguish between a rash and a crop of insect bites, when a child or person has been badly bitten without the insect being seen that did the damage. An insect bite has always a small red puncture in the middle of each spot where the sting of the insect broke through the skin, and the spots due to a rash have no such central point. Unless one is looking for insect bites, however, it is quite easy to overlook this central puncture and it is not uncommon for a baby to be covered with what its mother calls " teething rash," which if more closely looked at would be seen to be a fine crop of flea or other bites!

The insects which most often bite human beings are fleas, bed-bugs, lice, mosquitoes, harvest-bugs, sand-fleas (also called jigger) and wood-ticks. Ticks generally remain under the skin at the point where they made the wound ; so do sand-fleas.

Treatment. Insect bites are always very itchy, and dilute ammonia water, or a strong solution of bicarbonate of soda or baking-powder, dabbed on to the bites at intervals or bound over them on a pad of cotton-wool will help the irritation. The common blue-bag which is to be found in most kitchens and wash-houses is also useful. It should be wet and held over the spot. An onion may be rubbed on. These are easily obtained domestic remedies, but they are often as useful as the more expensive preparations sold for the purpose in shops. If the skin is very much irritated, however, simple calamine lotion may be spread on and allowed to dry on the skin.

Sand-fleas and ticks must be killed before they are removed. Kerosene, turpentine or tobacco juice, which is the most likely thing to be handy, will all kill the insects if the wound is bathed in them. The dead insects must then be picked out with a blunt needle which has been put into a flame for a moment to sterilize it, and afterwards calamine lotion may be put on.

Dog Bite, etc. Mad dogs, fortunately, are rare in England nowadays, so that unless there is any evidence to the contrary, a dog bite should be treated as an ordinary torn wound. That is to say, wash the wound thoroughly, pour in some iodine or methylated spirits, and apply a dressing of clean lint. The bites of other large animals should be treated in the same way as those of dogs. A cat more often scratches than bites, but cat bites are not unknown. A pig can give a very nasty bite, and any other animal is liable to snap at a human being, especially if it is alarmed, or if it is accompanied by its young.

But if there is any reason for suspecting that the dog was mad, there is a danger of hydrophobia and prompt treatment is of the utmost importance. The poison in this case comes from the dog's saliva and passes rapidly from the wound into the system of the bitten person.

Treatment. Emergency treatment must be given with the object of removing as much as possible of the poison from the wound, and of stopping it from getting into the blood stream. (*See* HYDROPHOBIA.)

Snake or Poisonous Adder Bites. The poison in these cases acts quickly, so immediately suck the bite hard, spitting out at once and being careful not to swallow any of the matter sucked out. Apply a tight bandage above the wound and try to make the wound bleed freely, opening it with a knife if necessary. Hold it under a tap if there happens to be one handy. If any crystals of potassium permanganate are available, rub a few well into the wound, otherwise use iodine or methylated spirits freely. Give the bitten person stimulants and get him to the doctor as soon as possible.

Wasp and Bee Stings. Wasp and bee stings are extremely painful and happen to everybody sometime during their life. A bee which has once stung becomes harmless because it leaves its sting in the wound and cannot sting again ; but a wasp keeps its sting and may return to the attack again and again. If the sting has been caused by a bee, therefore, the first thing to do is to find the sting and gently pull it out. Rub the area with a blue-bag, dab on dilute ammonia, methylated spirits, iodine, or whisky, or any specially prepared remedy for insect bites. If the bitten person is suffering from shock, make him lie down, loosen his clothing, but keep him warm. Give stimulants such as whisky or brandy or sal volatile in water, and if necessary send for the doctor. If a person gets stung by a bee, wasp or mosquito about the mouth or throat or on the upper lip, he must be taken at once to a doctor or hospital as stings on these parts swell very rapidly and may have fatal results. It sometimes happens that there is a wasp or bee in a piece of fruit or other food that a person puts in his mouth. If he is stung like that, it is not a matter to treat lightly, as the bite may easily have fatal results if it is not attended to at once.

Other Stings. Under this title are included those domestic accidents caused by jellyfish, hairy caterpillars, and nettles, and commonly spoken of as " stings."

Jellyfish (some varieties only) cause an itchy red rash at the site of contact, by the discharge of small threads which are intensely irritating or " poisonous " to the skin. Hairy caterpillars often cause a similar rash through puncturing of the skin by their brittle poisonous hairs. In both cases an application of vinegar or olive-oil relieves the condition.

Nettles " sting " because their hairs, when broken by contact, discharge formic acid into the skin. They are therefore relieved by a mild alkaline solution, such as dock leaves moistened by the saliva, or the blue-bag. Most children know that, by a merciful act of Nature, dock leaves always grow where nettles are found, and when stung they run of their own accord to rub on a dock leaf.

BITTER ALMOND POISONING. (*See* PRUSSIC ACID.)

BITTERS. In medical language the group of " bitters " contains substances which possess the common property of very bitter taste. These bitter drugs are usually given to increase the appetite and thus aid the digestion.

The action of bitters is to stimulate and increase the amount of digestive fluid produced by the salivary glands and also by the stomach. This greatly increases the appetite and aids the digestion of food. Bitters should never be used by persons who suffer from gastric ulcer or any form of inflammation of the stomach. In cases where dyspepsia is due to a general weakness of all the organs of the body, such as occurs in anæmia, starvation, tuberculosis, and convalescence from acute diseases, calumba is especially valuable in stimulating the working of the digestion and thereby improving the appetite.

Bitters must not be given in too strong a form, nor be given for too long, as they are likely to over-irritate the stomach. (*See also* APPETITE ; DIGESTION.)

BLACK DEATH. This awesome term used to be applied to the plague which at one time was the scourge of Europe. In 1664–1665 the greatest epidemic occurred in London. (*See also* PLAGUE ; EPIDEMICS.)

BLACK EYE. A black eye is generally the result of a bruise in the neighbourhood of the eye, often caused by a direct blow on the eye. The condition is too well known to need description. Owing to the fact that the skin of the eyelids and that about the eyes is very loose, blood is able to gather very easily under the eye, so the bruise may often look as if the blow had been much more violent than it was. A curious effect is sometimes seen when some of the blood flows under the conjunctiva (the thin membrane covering the eye) ; this may remain bright red, while the blood in the eyelids is nearly black.

After operations on the nose and the hollow cavities round the nose,

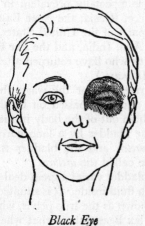

Black Eye

there are very often black eyes caused by blood which has come from the point of the operation. This disappears in a few days of its own accord.

Treatment. If the black eye is seen immediately after the blow has been struck, cold wet cloths should be applied to the eye, or pads of cotton-wool wet with lead lotion. This will do as well as the slab of raw beef-steak, which is still used sometimes, and is cheaper too. Later on, when the " black eye " has become quite evident, hot compresses may be used, also gentle pressure and massage with pure olive oil. If the eye continues to be painful, however, this should be discontinued and an oculist should be consulted, as there may be some other injury to the eye itself.

The discoloration may be concealed during the day by means of a flesh-coloured (water-colour) paint, which is quite harmless to the skin, or by a little theatrical grease-paint.

BLACKHEAD. A blackhead is a dark plug about the size of a pinhead, which appears in the sweat glands in the skin. They are found usually on the face, back of the neck, chest, and back, and are a symptom of acne. They are found, as a rule, in young people. (*See also* ACNE VULGARIS.)

BLACK MOTIONS. (*See* MELÆNA.)

BLACK VOMIT. Black or dark-coloured vomit is usually due to the presence of blood in the stomach when there is an ulcer. It is vomited up as a dark sediment, usually described as resembling coffee grounds. (*See also* STOMACH, ULCER OF.)

BLACKWATER FEVER. This disease is a complication of malaria. Its chief symptom is *hæmoglobinuria* or the presence of hæmoglobin—the colouring matter of the red blood cells—in the urine. The disease is especially prevalent in Africa, certain parts of Spain, Italy, Greece, Russia, the Near East and Palestine ; it is also found in some parts of the United States, South America, the West Indies, and in Asia, India, and the Far East. It is only found in England in patients who have returned after contracting malaria abroad. (*See also* MALARIA.)

BLADDER. A reservoir for the waste fluid of the body. It stores up the water and salts passed on by the kidneys until it is convenient to pass them out of the body in the urine. Each kidney is connected with the bladder by a long narrow tube of muscular tissue known as a *ureter*, and the bladder is connected with the exterior by a passage called the *urethra*.

The shape of the bladder varies a great deal according to whether there is little or much fluid inside. It is situated in the lower portion of the bony girdle known as the true pelvis, where it is kept in place by means of rather lax ligaments so that when empty it is so con-

tracted that there is practically no cavity, whereas when filled
it expands until it holds from 8–12 ounces of urine. In abnormal
conditions it will hold well over 40 ounces.

When the urine has collected in the bladder sufficiently to raise
the pressure above a certain point, slow rhythmical contractions
take place in the muscle walls. These get stronger and stronger
until they become powerful enough to overcome the circular
muscle fibres which guard the exit of the bladder into the urethra.
The urine is then expelled. This action is known as a " reflex "
action, and occurs in the lower animals and in man until it comes
under the control of the " will " which has the power of regulating
the reflex mechanism.

The bladder is lined on the inside by mucous membrane which
is loosely attached to the muscular coat so that it is thrown into folds
when the cavity is small, and smoothed out when it is distended.

Diseases of the Bladder. The bladder is not afflicted with
very many diseases, perhaps because it lies buried so deeply in
the abdomen and access to it is not very easy for poisons and infections. The commonest disease of the bladder is cystitis or inflammation of the bladder. This will be discussed under its own
heading. The two commonest disabilities of the bladder, which
may be due to disease of the bladder itself or to disease in some
other part such as the nervous system which affects the working
of the bladder, are incontinence of urine and retention of
urine. These conditions will be discussed below. Besides these
the bladder is subject to rupture due to accidental crushing, foreign
bodies inserted into it, tumours, stone or calculus, and such conditions as fistula and diverticula.

Incontinence of Urine. Incontinence of urine is present when
a person is unable to hold back the contents of the bladder until
he wishes to evacuate them. The urine may escape in a sudden
rush without his having the power to stop it, or it may continually
dribble away. In both these cases incontinence is present. In the
case where a full flow of urine is suddenly passed without the
will of the individual the condition is more likely to be due to
trouble in the nervous system than to actual disease in the bladder.
This condition is known as *enuresis* and is very well known in its
most common form as " bed-wetting " amongst children.

Incontinence due to mechanical causes. Incontinence due
to mechanical causes such as outside pressure on the bladder
are more frequent in women than in men. In the latter stages
of pregnancy the pressure of the enlarged womb almost always
causes a certain amount of dribbling, and some women have the
same experience in the last few days of each month just before the

period begins ; here, again, the swollen womb is the cause. The condition called prolapse which is common amongst women who have had children is also frequently a cause of incontinence. In these cases the incontinence is usually slight and may follow on some sudden exertion. In men this form of incontinence is usually found in connection with an enlarged prostate gland, and is in fact the most obvious symptom of that condition. Even after the enlarged gland has been removed there is often a degree of incontinence for some time, but it will subside. Unfortunately there are many men still suffering from extensive war injuries in the region of the bladder which cause incontinence in some degree or other.

Incontinence due to nervous disease. The involuntary passage of urine may occur in some diseases of the spinal cord. In the early stages of the disease known as locomotor ataxia there is often a false incontinence, that is, a chronic distension of the bladder with overflowing. It may be first noticed by bed-wetting at night. In the disease called disseminated sclerosis the bladder is small and contracted and the urine is ejected in spurts without the power to control it.

Incontinence due to nerve injuries. Injuries to the back in which the spinal cord is damaged, such as fractures, dislocations and crushing accidents or gun-shot injuries are usually followed by a period during which the urine is retained in the bladder and only escapes by overflowing. This may last for as long as two months, and may be followed by ordinary incontinence in which the bladder works as it does in a child before the age of voluntary control and it will have to be re-educated until full control returns.

Incontinence in childhood. For treatment of BED-WETTING see the article under that heading.

Retention of Urine. By retention of urine is meant that a person is unable for some cause to pass urine in the ordinary way. There are many causes for this inability to void water. It may be due to obstruction, such as the increase in size of the prostate gland, or swelling in the region of the bladder due to inflammation, or to some sort of tumour or growth. Any of these will cause obstruction to the flow of urine by pressing on the passage by which the urine escapes from the bladder. Again, there may be an obstruction in the passage or urethra itself, such as a foreign body or a stone. The passage may be ruptured or narrowed by previous disease (stricture) or swollen by acute inflammation. Retention of the urine may be due to lack of tone in the muscle walls, a condition which is generally due to some nervous disease, but in this case there will be other symptoms to show what the disease is. There is retention in many forms of poisoning such as toxic poisoning in such diseases as typhoid fever, appendicitis, syphilis, etc., or due to poisons such as arsenic, mercury, lead, belladonna, etc.

There may also be an inability to pass urine due to spasm of the muscle guarding the exit from the bladder. Here the muscle which is in spasm is holding itself tightly contracted instead of opening and closing as it normally does. This may happen after an operation round the entrance to the bowel or in the region of the bladder itself.

Diverticula. These are pouches in the wall of the bladder which are lined by mucous membrane. They are usually only discovered when the bladder has been examined by the instrument called the cystoscope.

Rupture of the Bladder. This is usually met with in adult males. A *full* bladder is easily ruptured by any form of violence applied to the lower part of the belly, such as a blow, kick, a crush by the wheel of a vehicle, or a fall on a projecting object. In fractures of the pelvis the bladder is often torn or penetrated.

Foreign Bodies. Objects of all kinds have been found in the bladder. Such articles as hair-pins, pencils, etc., are quite commonly introduced by the patient into the urethral passage. As a result of diseases of the pelvic bones and in parts of the body near the bladder, such objects as pieces of bone may find their way into the bladder.

Tumours of the Bladder. These usually occur between the ages of 40 and 60. Like all tumours, they are divided into two main classes : simple or innocent tumours and malignant or life-destroying growths. Of the simple tumours the most common is the *papilloma*, which is a growth of the lining membrane of the bladder. It may vary in size from a split pea to that of an orange.

Cancer. It is rare to find a cancer beginning in the bladder ; it has usually spread from a malignant growth in other organs.

Stone or Calculus. Most of the stones found in the bladder started in the kidney and increased in size after entering the bladder. Stones of the bladder are usually freely movable, but may be fixed in the opening of the passages leading from the kidneys to the bladder, or from the bladder to the external world, or in " diverticula " in the bladder wall.

Fistula. Is a communication passage between the interior of the bladder and some other organ. It is usually the result of an injury or disease. Fistulas in the bladder are of three sorts. First, there is the fistula which sometimes forms after an operation for removal of the prostate, or which may be made intentionally when the passage through the urethra is permanently obstructed and cannot be opened up again. This fistula allows the urine to escape through the skin of the abdominal wall to the outside. Secondly, there may be a fistula between the bladder and some part of the intestines. This is usually due to injury or to inflammation which has led to the rupture of the wall of the bladder. There may be a fistula communicating between the bladder and the vagina in women. This may follow an operation of tearing of the vagina due to some such cause as a pessary, or be due to some large growth. (*See* URINARY SYSTEM ; URETHRA.)

BLAIN. Blain is a term sometimes applied to a blister or a pimple. The most common type of inflamed blister is chilblain. (*See also* CHILBLAIN.)

BLAND. This term is generally applied to foods of a mild and soothing nature, such as milk and arrowroot, etc. Invalids are usually given bland substances while they are ill or recovering from a severe illness.

BLASTOMYCOSIS. This is a rare, very chronic disease caused by the yeast fungus, and occurs generally in men who have been concerned with the handling of straw or grain. The skin is usually affected, especially that of the face ; the backs of the hands and forearms are the next commonest sites. Sometimes the disease spreads to the blood and thence to the lungs and other internal organs. There are one or more raised-up sores, which may look like warts, and which rapidly become studded with tiny abscesses, which break, ulcerate, and finally heal up and leave a scar.

The outlook of this disease is not altogether favourable. Even if the disease is only in the skin, it is most intractable to treatment ; improvement may occur, but a cure is rare. Even after improvement, recurrences are frequent. When the disease spreads through the system, it is fatal.

BLAUD'S PILLS. These pills are a very useful and popular way of taking iron in anæmic conditions. They leave no bitter taste in the mouth, can be bought anywhere and are easy to swallow. They are an old formula, particularly useful for anæmic persons whose digestion is weak.

BLEACHING POWDER. *See* CHLORIDE OF LIME.

BLEB. For a description of blebs and blisters *see* BLISTER.

BLEEDERS. There are certain unfortunate families where the male members have a peculiar state of the blood which causes them to bleed excessively from the smallest scratch or wound. In popular language these people are called " bleeders," and in medical terms, *hæmophilics*. It has been generally considered that only the men in hæmophilic families were "bleeders," but it seems likely that the women may in some cases bleed more easily than is usual, without their bleeding being definitely uncontrollable as it is in the case of the men. The tendency is, however, carried down in the female line and the sons of a woman from one of these families may be "bleeders." It used to be said that the tendency was only transmitted by the female line, and that only the daughters of bleeders must not marry, but of course this is absurd. There would be no families of bleeders if there had not been a married male "bleeder" somewhere within a few generations, so it may be taken for granted that no member of a hæmophilic family should marry and beget children. This is, perhaps, a little too severe, because the trouble does show a tendency to die out of families.

Treatment. It goes without saying that "bleeders" should be protected in every way possible from anything that might cause bleeding, since once bleeding starts it may be found impossible to stop it. They should not enter dangerous occupations, but should be trained to some such occupation as that of a clerk or shop-keeper. No teeth should ever be extracted, and of course no surgical operation should be allowed. It sometimes happens that the condition is not very well understood, and the relations will allow a boy to have a tooth pulled out, or some little operation like circumcision or the removal of tonsils be performed, without telling the operator that the child comes from a bleeding family, and the truth is only discovered when it is too late to save the child.

Once the bleeding has started, the usual methods for stopping bleeding must be tried. They are pressure by a tourniquet or tight bandages. The application of bandages wrung out in very hot or very cold water, or the application of adrenalin solution ($\frac{1}{1000}$) on cotton-wool. The patient should be taken to a doctor or hospital at once, as a transfusion of blood from a healthy person may have to be carried out and injections of calcium into the veins.

If a "bleeder" is not lost in childhood and reaches the early twenties, the condition will usually improve, and it is likely that before long science will be able to discover something to cure, or at least assist, this unfortunate class of people along the lines of other diseases, in which there is something missing from the blood. (*See also* HÆMORRHAGE.)

BLEEDING. All forms of bleeding are described under the title HÆMORRHAGE.

BLEEDING or BLOOD-LETTING. Bleeding a patient is a procedure which is not often resorted to nowadays, except in certain cases of heart and lung disease, when there is more blood in the veins than can conveniently be circulated. (*See also* Cupping.)

BLENORRHŒA. This is the term applied to any excessive discharge of mucus or phlegm from a mucous membrane. (*See also* Mucus ; Mucous Membrane.)

BLINDNESS. By blindness is meant a complete, or nearly complete, loss of the power of seeing, and to be blind is one of the worst afflictions from which a human being can suffer. The saddest part of blindness, however, is that the majority of cases could have been prevented if care had been taken at the proper time, since they are due to diseases of the eyes which have been neglected. The causes of blindness are numerous, beginning with the defect of being born blind, and going on to all the various diseases of the eye itself, either local or in the course of some general disease, and finally the cases that are due to accident or injury. (*See also* Eyes ; Vision.)

Born Blind. The first cause, that of being born blind, owing to complete absence of the eyes, or to some defect of the eyes, is fortunately very rare, as it is naturally incurable. But it is frequently said that many children are " born blind." This is quite a mistaken idea, and the sooner it is discredited the better for a great number of babies who are condemned to life-long blindness through the ignorance or carelessness of their mother or attendant. The cause is a disease known as Ophthalmia neonatorum, which is described under Ophthalmia ; Blindness of the Newly-born, which is due to the child's eyes becoming infected at birth by a discharge from the passages of the mother due to the disease called gonorrhœa. " It has been calculated that this disease accounted for one-third to one-half of all the persons in blind asylums, so destructive of sight it is : but now that it is more vigorously dealt with and is notifiable by doctors and midwives its incidence has been kept down." This was written in 1930. In a general report written recently it is said that " Ophthalmia neonatorum remains the most frequent and the most distressing cause of blindness, seeing that these cases must be regarded as *almost entirely preventable*."

Diseases of the Eye will be discussed under their various headings. In injuries to the eye, the treatment naturally depends on the extent of the injury. Briefly, the other chief causes of blindness are *trachoma, glaucoma,* and *conjunctivitis. Syphilis,* both inherited and acquired, is a very important cause, which accounts for nearly one-third of all cases of blindness.

Tobacco Blindness. Tobacco blindness is found chiefly among working-men, and is caused either by smoking or chewing tobacco in a quantity of not less than three ounces a week. The symptoms rarely occur before the age of forty, though the person may have smoked for years. The poison was accumulating in the system. Women are as likely to be affected as men when they smoke the same amount of tobacco. Other things that seem to have an influence on the ease with which the tobacco affects the sight are the age of the smoker, sleeplessness, prolonged anxiety, the overuse of alcohol, and general weakness from any cause. Some people also seem to be more easily upset by tobacco than others ; that is, they are more susceptible to the effects of tobacco. Smoking on an empty stomach is blamed for some cases. (*See* TOBACCO.)

BLISTERING. Blistering is sometimes carried out as a remedy in the treatment of cases such as lumbago, rheumatism, neuritis and other painful conditions due to inflamed nerves. Irritating substances are applied to the skin which raise a blister at the point where they are applied. After the blister has formed, the " nagging " pain from the nerve is usually much relieved. The blister will not be very painful. When it has formed sufficiently, the blistering substance should be removed, and once the blister has burst, some bland soothing ointment should be applied.

BLOOD. Blood is the fluid which circulates through the heart, the arteries and the veins, and supplies nourishing material to every part of the body. In the veins it is dark red, and in the arteries bright red ; but when exposed to air it becomes thickened and divides into a red clot and a yellowish watery fluid called *serum*. The amount of blood in the body is now considered to be roughly one-twentieth of the total weight of the body, and in a healthy person, the blood consists of 78% of water and 22% solids. In the body the blood-vessels form a completely closed channel through which the blood ceaselessly circulates, and never escapes except in case of an accidental escape which we call bleeding or hæmorrhage. It is, however, always collecting new substances and discarding other substances through the walls of the blood-vessels by a process which is technically known as *osmosis*.

The first duty of the blood is to feed the body, which requires a large number of different substances to keep it in health, each one of which must be present in the blood and must be carried to the part of the body where it is required. In addition, the materials for all the *secretions* or juices which the body forms through its various organs are obtained from the blood. Some of these secretions for which the materials are obtained from the blood are used for the special purposes of digestion, etc., but in some cases, notably that of the secretions of the *thyroid* and *suprarenal glands*, they are poured back into the blood where they carry out the purpose for which they were destined.

Again, the blood acts as a carrier of oxygen to the tissues from the lungs. The red colouring matter, or *hæmoglobin*, of the blood is the agent by which this carrying of oxygen, or *oxidization*, is performed. Heat is also distributed throughout the body by the blood, which receives heat at various points in its route and thus helps to keep the whole body at an even temperature. For instance, in passing through the muscles and glands, which are heat-producing bodies, the blood picks up heat, which is cooled off in the *capillaries* or little blood-vessels near the surface of the body.

Blood, as well as feeding the body and providing the materials with which the various organs of the body carry on their own specialized work, has also the very important duty of ridding the body of waste matter, and is therefore an important part of the drainage and scavenging system of the body. *Carbonic acid* formed in the tissues is not wanted by the body and is carried to the lungs and there is breathed out ; other waste materials are changed into urine, sweat, urea, etc.

In appearance, the blood is a red, sticky, non-transparent fluid. It is composed of a pale yellowish fluid called *plasma* in which float enormous numbers of minute bodies called *corpuscles* and *platelets*. The blood corpuscles are red and white in colour. A method of estimating the numbers of these corpuscles has been invented by means of which the number of red and white corpuscles in a cubic millimetre (roughly a pinhead) of blood is calculated. The average number of red cells is round about 5,000,000, and of white cells is 10,000. The red corpuscles are called *erythrocytes* and the white ones are *leucocytes*.

The red blood corpuscles are circular discs which contain hæmoglobin, a compound of iron which has the power of attracting and combining with oxygen, the part of the air which is absolutely necessary to keep us alive. By means of this power the red cells act as carriers of oxygen from the lungs to the tissues. These red cells are always being renewed, and the old dead ones are destroyed by the liver or spleen and are got rid of by means of the bile.

The white blood corpuscles are larger and very much fewer in number than the red ones. They possess the power of moving about in the blood-stream and are often described as the scavengers of the body, as they are able to eat up and destroy invading foreign bodies, such as germs. An invasion of germs into the blood causes a great increase in the numbers of these white blood corpuscles. They make their way to the point of invasion and wage war on the intruders ; this process is called *phagocytosis* and it is by means of it that the body is protected from infection by germs.

The *blood platelets* are disc-shaped bodies, which are colourless and smaller than the red corpuscles. Their origin and duty is not definitely known, but they are thought to play a part in the clotting of the blood.

The blood *plasma* is the watery fluid which contains the corpuscles and platelets. It is the nourishing substance which feeds the tissue cells of the body. (*See* TRANSFUSION OF BLOOD.)

Blood Heat. The normal temperature of the blood is about 100° F. When taking the temperature with a thermometer, however, the heat is judged to be about 98·4° F., as it is not easy to take the temperature of the actual blood itself. It is the constant circulation of the blood which keeps the body at the same temperature.

BLOOD - POISONING. A condition of poisoning of the blood, due to the presence of germs or the poisons or toxins they produce. Blood-poisoning may arise from an infected wound or any other source of infection causing fever and other symptoms. (*See also* SEPTICÆMIA.)

BLOOD - PRESSURE. By blood-pressure is meant the force with which the blood is pumped along the arteries by the heart's beating. The strength of the heart's muscle, the elasticity of the walls of the arteries, and the volume of blood in the arteries are all important factors in determining the blood-pressure. In diseases which are accompanied by great weakness, such as anæmia and heart failure, the blood-pressure is *lower* than normal, whilst in many other diseases it is *higher* than normal. In middle-age and old-age high blood-pressure may be a troublesome and even dangerous condition.

The blood-pressure is measured by an instrument called a *sphygmomanometer*. The normal pressure varies at different ages and it is usual to say that the normal pressure for any individual is 100° F. plus half the age in years. A pressure of 155 or over is high blood-pressure or *hyperpiesis*. This condition may be constitutional, caused by disease, or due to an increased volume of blood from overeating or over-drinking. There may be temporary high blood-pressure from strong emotion, anger, pain, or exercise.

The symptoms caused by high blood-pressure are breathlessness on exertion, palpitations and a feeling of discomfort in the region of the heart, dislike of lying on the left side, headaches, giddiness, noises in the ear, irritability and loss of the power of concentration. In worse cases there may be bleeding from the nose, numbness and tingling in the limbs or cramp and coldness in the legs. There may even be temporary blindness and a stroke.

Where high blood-pressure is present the patient should moderate his manner of living, so as to avoid mental and physical strain and he should obtain a sufficient amount of rest. The diet should be cut down. Meat and alcohol are best avoided and smoking should be cut down to a minimum. Fish, poultry, eggs, fruit and vegetables are the best foods.

Low blood-pressure or *hypopiesis* may be merely an individual peculiarity, for one person may have a blood-pressure lower than the average, just as another may have a higher one. But it may be due to disease of the suprarenal glands, such as Addison's disease. It may be the result of severe loss of blood, chronic weakness as in cancer, some forms of heart disease, and conditions like myxœdema and diabetes. It is also frequently present in states of anaphylaxis and intestinal obstruction. The condition often comes on suddenly as in shock or fainting and is then only temporary, or it may be long continued. The blood-pressure is said to be low, if the reading is below 110 in an adult.

The patient will complain of weakness, a perpetual tired feeling, sleeplessness, headache and giddiness. In an acute attack such as shock after an accident, a quick means of raising the pressure for a short time is to give an injection of adrenaline solution. Ephedrine sulphate tablets taken by mouth thrice daily are very useful and in Addison's disease the new treatment by a gland preparation called eucortone should be tried. Rest is a very necessary part of treatment. The diet should be mixed with a sufficiency of vitamins and at least three pints of liquid a day. Iron and arsenic tonics will be given for anæmia and if the low blood-pressure is due to weakness of the heart digitalis may be prescribed. Where the low blood-pressure is due to bleeding or shock the patient must be kept warm and may require injections of salt solution into the veins.

BLOOD-SPITTING. Blood-spitting should always be taken seriously and the cause ascertained by a doctor. Streaks of blood in the sputum may be only from soft gums (due to pyorrhœa) or from blood from a varicose vessel in the nose or the upper part of the throat running down into the mouth. When it is more than just a streak it should be carefully noted whether the blood is coughed up or vomited up ; even a slight cough may bring up a large quantity of bright and frothy blood, and this is practically always from the lungs and is a sign of tuberculosis of the lungs, though in a few cases it may be due to heart disease causing congestion in the lung. Vomited blood is usually dark in colour, owing to the action on it of the digestive juices ; this blood is usually due to bleeding from an ulcer in the stomach, and the affected person often feels faint before the blood comes up ; as a general rule dark blood will also be passed from the bowel in such cases.

BLOOD TRANSFUSION. Taking blood from one person

and injecting it into another. (*See also* BLOOD ; TRANSFUSION OF BLOOD.)

BLOOD - VESSELS. The blood-vessels are the arteries and veins which carry the blood to and from the heart. The *arteries* lead from the heart and branch off in every direction carrying a supply of good blood containing oxygen to every part of the body. The *veins* lead to the heart and carry the waste products of the

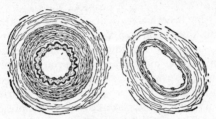

Blood-vessels
A. Artery; B. Vein

blood and the carbonic acid back to the heart. They are stronger and tougher than the arteries and the blood in them is dark-bluish red, whereas in the arteries it is bright red. The blood-vessels are liable to disease from the influence of the poisons that may be present in the blood. Their walls may become thickened, and it is possible for them to lose their elasticity. They become liable to break or become obstructed by clots. (*See also* ARTERIO-SCLEROSIS ; ARTERY ; BLOOD ; BLOOD-PRESSURE ; CIRCULATION OF THE BLOOD ; etc.)

BLOODLESSNESS. Bloodlessness, or *anæmia* as it is more generally termed, is a state in which there is not enough, or not strong enough blood in the body. There are several types of this condition and the causes may be under-nourishment, hæmorrhage, cancer, wasting discharges, poisons, etc. (*See also* ANÆMIA.)

BLUE DISEASE. Cyanosis or deep-purplish colouring of the skin is a symptom of malformation of the heart. Babies with this discoloration are said to suffer from blue disease.

BLUSHING. This is a sympton usually arising from general nervousness. The circulation of the blood is greatly influenced by the nervous system, and when an emotion, sometimes pleasurable, sometimes painful, is experienced, the blood-vessels and the small arteries suddenly become dilated, thus causing a hot flush to be felt on the skin.

BOILS. A boil is a festering sore which may appear on any part of the body. It is generally very painful to the touch, with a core in the centre. (*See also* ABSCESS ; CARBUNCLE ; FURUNCLE.)

BODY. The study of the make-up or structure of the body is called *Anatomy*, and of its working or functions is *Physiology*. The entire bony structure of the body is the skeleton, consisting of the *skull*, which includes all the bones of the head, the *spinal column* or backbone, to which are attached the *shoulder girdle* with the ribs below, and, at the lower end, the *pelvic girdle*. The legs are attached to the pelvic girdle and the arms to the shoulder. The backbone supports the body in the upright position, the ribs form a protective cage in which the breathing apparatus and the heart are found, together with the upper parts of the abdominal organs. The pelvic girdle similarly protects the lower abdominal and reproductive organs. The backbone also serves as a protective channel for the spinal cord. The skull contains and protects the exceedingly delicate substance of the brain and the organs of sight, hearing, smell, and taste. The bones of the body are covered with muscular tissue or flesh. The main part of the body between the head and the lower limbs is called the trunk. It has been seen that its walls are formed of bony and muscular tissue and it contains two large cavities, the chest or thorax, and the abdomen, which contain the organs or viscera as they are called. The limbs, or appendages, are attached to the trunk. The whole body is protected by an outer covering called the skin or epidermis, which in turn is protected at points of friction by a growth of hair or nail.

BONE, AND BONES. There are 206 bones in the human body, and these, together with cartilage, or gristle, form the general framework of the body, which is called the skeleton. In appearance, fresh bone is pinkish-white in colour, with a deep red centre. If a bone is broken across, it is seen to consist of two kinds of tissue. One sort is dense and compact in texture, and is called *substantia compacta*; the other sort is a network of spongy fibrous tissue, and is called *substantia spongiosa* or cancellous tissue, owing to its resemblance to lattice-work. The outer part of the bone is always formed of the hard, dense tissue, while the inner portion is of the spongy material. On examination under a microscope it will be seen that the two sorts of tissues are really the same porous material, except that, in the inner tissue, there is less solid matter and the pores, or spaces between the solid particles, are larger. In the living body, the bones have vessels running through them and are coated with a fibrous membrane called the *periosteum*. Through the spongy bone in the middle of the long bones of the body, runs a cavity which is filled with a material called the *medulla ossium* or marrow. In the long bones the marrow is yellow in colour, whereas in the other bones, and in the ends of the long bones, it is red. The periosteum is full of small blood-vessels which run into numerous tiny channels in the outer bone substance called *Haversian canals*, and thus carry nourishment to the bone. If a bone is broken it will be seen to bleed from these minute vessels. A large artery runs through the marrow and is called its nutrient artery. It is accompanied by one or more veins. There is also a nerve supply.

Bones Classified. The bones of the body are divided into four classes : long, short, flat and irregular. The *long* bones are the bones of the limbs and are employed in movement. They are levers consisting of a body, or shaft, and two ends, which fit into joints and are movable in these joints. At each end they are

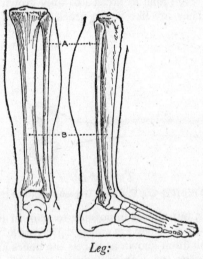

Leg:

A. Fibula; B. Tibia

covered with cartilage or gristle, while the joint is lubricated with a fluid called *synovial fluid* and is thus able to glide easily, without undue friction, over the cartilage-covered end of the other bone with which it connects in the joint. The long bones of the body are the humerus, the ulna and radius in the forearm, the femur (or thighbone), tibia and fibula in the leg. The bones of the finger and toe and the collar-bone or clavicle.

The *short* bones occur in the parts of the skeleton where strength is required, and they are compact and strong bones with a limited range of motion. The bones of the wrist, ankle and instep are short bones. The *flat* bones are bones which are meant to protect delicate structures or provide broad flat surfaces suitable for the attachment of muscles. They are the skull bones, the shoulder-blades or scapulas, the pelvic bones, the breast-bone or sternum, and the ribs. The *irregular* bones are so called from their shape, which makes it difficult to describe them with any of the other groups. The jawbone, the spine and some of the bones of the skull are irregular bones.

Bones, Composition of. Bones are composed of both animal and mineral matter in a proportion of about 33% animal or organic matter to 66% mineral or inorganic matter. The inorganic matter is chiefly calcium phosphate.

In young children the amount of mineral matter in the bones is nearly the same as the amount of animal matter, and their bones are, therefore, soft and flexible rather than brittle. These young bones are not very liable to break like fully grown bones, but they bend easily. They are like young green shoots of trees which are

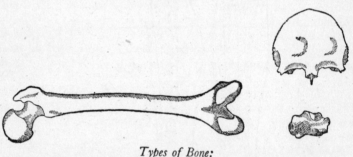

Types of Bone:
A. Long (Femur); B. Short (Trapezius); C. Flat (Front)

very easily bent but almost impossible to snap in two with a clean break like old wood. They are called " greenstick " fractures therefore. In the condition known as rickets the bones are very soft also.

Bone, Diseases of. It sometimes happens that a child is born without one or other of the usual bones, and such absence may be found in generation after generation, or only in isolated cases. The bones most often absent are leg or arm bones. The most common disease of bone is *rickets*, which is a chronic disease seen in young children and due to faulty feeding and bad hygienic conditions. Acute inflammation of bone, which is called *osteomyelitis*, is a serious condition in which the bone is very tender and the patient has a high temperature and becomes very ill. *Chronic inflammation* of a bone may be due to tuberculosis. Various tumours arise in bone and are usually of a dangerous type. *Periostitis*, or inflammation of the covering of the bone, may be acute or chronic. All cases of disease of bones require to be seen by a doctor.

BONE-MARROW. Marrow is the soft substance found in the middle of bones. It has something to do with the production of red blood corpuscles and is used in the treatment of some kinds of anæmia. It can be taken raw in sandwiches or on toast, or in a preparation made with glycerine. (*See also* SUPPLEMENT ON DIET AND INVALID COOKERY.)

BORACIC ACID. Boracic acid or boric acid may be obtained as white crystals or as a white powder. It is used largely to keep wounds, ulcers and sores from becoming infected. A solution of boracic acid may be employed as an antiseptic wash. Boracic lint is used a great deal for dressing wounds. Boracic powder when mixed with starch forms a useful dusting powder for infants. For unpleasantly smelling perspiration of the feet a solution of boracic acid should be used and a little of the powder dusted into the socks or stockings may do much to prevent this condition. An ointment may be made up of 1 drachm of boracic acid with vaseline to make an ounce.

BORAX. Borax, or sodium borate, consists of transparent colourless crystals, with a sweetish taste. It is an excellent antiseptic and is one of the chief ingredients of many of the popular mouth washes. As a lotion for the eyes, 10 grains are dissolved in a fluid ounce of warm water. It has been given in cases of epilepsy as a substitute for bromide in order to lessen excitability. The glycerine preparation of borax is a very good application as an emollient for sore nipples.

BORBORYGMUS. Borborygmus is the medical name for the rumbling noises often made by the bowels.

BOTULISM. This is a very severe variety of food poisoning due to the presence of the germ called the Bacillus botulinus. The toxin is present in the infected foods, particularly such foods as sausages, tinned foods, ham, fish, and canned vegetables, especially vegetables. The onset of symptoms usually occurs a few hours after the infected food has been eaten. The patient may complain of headache and usually the vision becomes blurred. There is considerable weakness in the arms and legs, but there is usually no pain and the mind is quite clear. The voice may become very weak. The tongue is furred and the temperature is usually lower than normal. The acute stage of the disease usually lasts for about 3 or 4 days. The patient should be kept in bed and the stomach immediately washed out with warm normal saline. An injection of morphine should be given as soon as possible as this delays the action of the toxin. A botulinus antitoxin should be prepared and given to the patient. Convalescence is generally very slow, and disturbances of vision may persist for weeks after the other symptoms have disappeared. Attacks of botulism very often prove fatal, and usually several people are affected who have partaken of the same food. Foods, when being prepared or canned, should be heated to an adequate temperature as the bacilli and spores are killed by heat.

BOUGIE. A bougie is a slender, rod-like surgical instrument which can be introduced into any of the external passages of the body such as the urethra, for the purposes of examining them. Medicated bougies are used in the treatment of vaginal discharges, etc.

BOUILLON. The French name for a clear extract of meat. Beef-tea is the usual bouillon for invalids. Bouillon is also used for the broth on which bacteria are fed in test tubes when they are being cultivated in a laboratory for any purpose.

BOVINE TUBERCULOSIS. Bovine tuberculosis is the form of consumption which cows have. It can be transferred to human beings, especially babies and delicate people, by drinking unpasteurized cows' milk from infected cows. The best milk dealers now have their cows tested periodically for tuberculosis, and are therefore able to assure their customers that they are obtaining milk from healthy cows. (*See also* TUBERCULOSIS.)

BOWEL. The bowel is now more often called the intestine, or intestines, and will be described under that heading.

BOW LEG. Bow legs or bandy legs are nearly always the result of forcing a weakly or rickety child to walk at too early an age. (*See also* RICKETS.)

B.P. The initials B.P. when they appear in connection with any drug preparation show that the drug is mentioned in a book called the British Pharmacopœia. This book gives a very detailed account of most drugs used in medicine, including the origin, standard of strength in active principles, dosages to be used in various conditions, as well as methods of preparation, etc. Drugs which are used in prescriptions must conform to the British Pharmacopœia standard unless there is any particular reason for not doing so. The initials B.P.C. stand for British Pharmacopœia Codex, which includes various drugs and preparations additional to those mentioned in the British Pharmacopœia.

BRACHIAL. The term brachial means anything to do with the arm. The brachial artery is a continuation of the axillary artery, which extends along the inner side of the arm. (*See also* ARM.)

BRACHYCEPHALY. This means shortheadedness. Certain races of people, such as the Germans, are born more short-headed than others. In various sorts of idiots the skull may be brachycephalic.

BRADYCARDIA. Slowness of the heart. In certain diseases the heart-beat is abnormally slow, and it is always very marked in the condition known as heart-block. A common cause of bradycardia is general weakness and lack of vigour. (*See also* HEART; PULSE.)

BRAIN. The brain includes all that part of the great nervous system of the body which is enclosed in the skull. The normal weight of the brain is from 40 to 50 ounces ; it is slightly heavier in men than in women, the average weight in men being from 49 to 50 ounces, and in women from 44 to 45 ounces.

Divisions of the Brain. The largest part of the brain consists of the " big brain " or " cerebrum," which occupies about

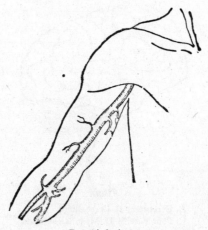

Brachial Artery

two-thirds of the total area of the skull and consists of a mass of nervous tissue thrown into many folds. The " little brain " or " cerebellum " lies at the back of the skull and is also thrown into folds, but these are very fine and delicate as compared with those of the big brain and resemble in appearance the fine leaves of a fern. Uniting the two halves of the little brain is a wide band of nervous tissue, called the " bridge " or " pons," and this " bridge " is continuous below with the enlarged upper end of the marrow of the spine, which is called the " bulb " or " medulla." These are the four chief structural divisions of the brain : the " big brain," the " little brain," the " bridge," and the " bulb."

Nerve Centres in the Brain. Attached to the under-surface of the brain, mainly to the " bridge " and to the " bulb," are twelve pairs of nerves, by means of which we are able to use our special senses of smell, sight, taste and hearing. These nerves also control the movements of the face muscles, the movements of the eyes, the movements of chewing and the movements of the head and neck. They are numbered in order from one to twelve. Although each nerve has its own independent sphere of action, yet the combined action of two or more nerves may be necessary to produce one particular effect.

The complicated paths by which each part of the brain is linked up with every other part, and the means by which all parts of the body are brought into communication with the brain, cannot be described here. But in a few words, the brain, taken as a whole,

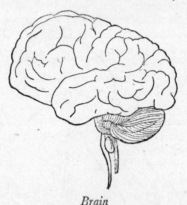

Brain

A. Cerebrum; B. Cerebellum;
C. Pons Varolii; D. Medulla oblongata

consists of a countless number of nervous elements, consisting of nerve cells and their two types of processes. One type of process carries messages or impulses towards the cells ; the other type carries impulses away from the cells. By means of these two sets of processes the different parts of the brain and spinal nervous system are brought into relation with each other and with every other part of the body. (*See* FACIAL PARALYSIS.)

The grey matter of the Brain. The nerve cells in the brain form what is called the grey matter. Through much painstaking experimental work done mainly by British scientists, it has been made possible to map out certain parts of the grey matter of the " big brain " into various areas and to predict what will happen if one or other of these areas is injured or diseased. One such area is called the " motor " area, because when we wish to move our limbs or any part of our bodies, it is this area of the brain which enables that movement to be carried out, i.e. the message is sent from this area down through the brain to the spinal cord, then is transmitted along a nerve and finally reaches the muscles, which obey the message they have received by contracting, thus causing the required movement to take place. If this area is damaged, the side of the body on the opposite side to that damaged is paralysed, because the path taken by messages from the motor area crosses to the opposite side of the brain at the level of the " bulb." Other well-defined areas of the grey matter are those concerned with the appreciation of sensation. The area for sight, for example, is situated at the back of the brain, and if this part of the brain is injured or destroyed by disease, no matter how perfect our eyes may be, we become blind. There is a special and very important area of the brain which enables us to recognize the position of our limbs in space, without the aid of sight ; and the same area tells us the position, size and shape of objects with which our limbs may come into contact. The ease with which we are able to distinguish the various objects in a pocket, for example, without using our eyes, is entirely dependent on this area of the brain. If it becomes damaged in any way, we lose this power. But the greater part of the " big brain " is composed of what are known as " silent areas," because nothing is known about them. They are presumed to be concerned with the intelligence and mental well-being of the individual, since large parts of these areas can be destroyed without in any other way apparently causing ill-effects, but the intelligence suffers. These " silent areas " are situated in the foremost part of the " big brain," and it has been noticed by many that in disease of this part of the brain the intelligence suffers first.

The *little brain* controls our balance and so enables us to alter our position in space as the need arises. If there is disease of one side of the " little brain," this state of tone is lost on the whole of the side of the body corresponding to the side of the " little brain " affected, and the limbs on that side feel " floppy," and are clumsy and awkward in their movements. Balance is badly maintained and in walking the person tends to fall to the side of the damaged " little brain." In advanced disease of the " little brain " these signs are so obvious that the untrained eye can see them, but in the early, and the only curable stage, it requires the services of a specialist to detect slight signs of disease.

Diseases of the Brain. The brain is liable to suffer from the same types of disease, broadly speaking, as any other organ of the body, but owing to the special nature of the tissue of which it is composed, the results of such disease processes are of a peculiar character. In order to understand this, it is necessary to appreciate that the brain is enclosed in a box—the skull—which cannot expand. Therefore, anything which increases the size or weight of the brain or its coverings will cause a certain amount of extra pressure inside the skull and this pressure not only produces pain, but many other symptoms, as well as destroying the delicate nervous tissue. Another important point is that the essential elements of the nervous system, the nerve cells and their processes, once destroyed, never re-form ; their place is taken by scar tissue, which is incapable of receiving, conducting, or transmitting messages or impulses. So if a nerve cell dies, or is killed by some disease process, that unit of the nervous system can never be replaced. It has not yet been discovered whether each unit is at work all the time, but a loss of only a few nerve cells can often be shown under the microscope when there have been many symptoms of diminished nervous activity during life.

To say where a disease is present in the brain may be almost impossible, or on the other hand, may be very simple. If there is some disorder of the " little brain," for example, the signs are so definite and unmistakable, that it is only a question of determining the nature of the malady. Similarly, if one of the areas of the brain whose special action is known, such as the " motor " area, becomes diseased or injured, certain signs (in this case, signs of paralysis of the opposite side of the body) occur, which enable the nerve specialist to say with certainty that something is amiss with this particular region of the brain. In the " bridge " of the brain or the " bulb," where many of the nerves coming out of, or entering the brain are attached, and where many conducting paths are crowded together, destruction of these will cause interference with the normal action of the movements controlled by these nerves and conducted along these paths, so that it is a comparatively simple matter for one who knows the structure of the brain to say when this region is damaged. But in the " big brain," where so many " silent " areas exist, of whose action and conducting paths we know nothing, it may be almost or quite impossible to decide where the disease is, until it reaches an area whose action gives us some information.

Treatment of Brain Diseases. From the point of view of treatment it is of the greatest importance to establish not only the position of the disorder, but its nature. There may be some failure in development ; our disorders may be the result of injury, or of infection by a microbe which causes a reaction known as inflammation ; animal parasites may make our bodies their temporary refuge ; our tissues may wear out before the normal span of life is over, a process which we call degeneration ; finally, tumour growth may take place and destroy or replace normal tissues. The brain is not exempt from any one of these misfortunes, but from the practical standpoint some are vastly more important than others. For failures in development, which may be of any degree from such slight ones as cause only weakness of one side of the body and limbs up to those in which the child has so little brain developed that it is a complete idiot, we can do nothing except to ensure that the most is made of such intelligence as is present, and of such movements as are possible. For the sake of the fathers and other children it is best that such children as are mentally unfit should be looked after in special homes.

Injuries to the Brain are always serious and should never be treated lightly. If the brain has been only slightly damaged, the injured person recovers from unconsciousness and is then said to have had *concussion*. If there has been extensive damage to the brain tissues, on the other hand, unconsciousness deepens into what is called coma, a state in which the breathing becomes noisy and hurried and from which it is impossible to rouse the person. In cases of only slight damage to the surface of the brain, what is called concussion, the danger is that if the patient does not take care to lie up in bed until such time as his doctor permits him to get up, he will develop a severe headache, which may persist for months. A long period of rest in bed, after even a few minutes' complete loss of consciousness from head injuries, is essential if this headache is to be avoided.

The infections of the brain which give rise to inflammations are so many and varied that it is impossible to consider them here, except to say that as the majority of these infections do not attack the essential elements of the brain, the nerve cells, but rather the tissues supporting them, and their fatty coverings, the diseases produced by these infections, though they may be disabling, are in many cases consistent with long life. Treatment may stay the progress of these diseases, but cannot cure. (*See also* CEREBRO-SPINAL MENINGITIS ; MENINGITIS.)

The wearing out or premature dying off of nerve cells before the rest of the body cells is one of the characteristic features of old age. The failure of memory for recent events is a well recognized picture of the elderly. But sometimes this wearing out of the nerve cells occurs at an earlier age and then the picture is a sad one. In association with the failure of memory, weakness of the will develops and all the patient's mental activities become lessened. These patients become as children and are as easily led, and it is in these cases that unscrupulous relatives or attendants find their opportunity to influence the unfortunate victim to alter a will so that they may benefit. (*See also* MENTAL DISEASE.)

Tumours of the Brain. The brain is one of the commonest positions in the body in which tumours may develop. During the last twenty years surgery has made such wonderful strides that if the signs of tumour formation are detected early enough, there is every chance that an operation on the brain can be undertaken and the tumour—if not situated too deeply in the substance of the brain—removed, at least in part. In any case, the operation of opening the skull will relieve the patient's symptoms and prevent his going blind, which is the inevitable result of leaving the skull intact. In many cases it is possible for the specialist in brain diseases to say exactly where the tumour is lying, from the signs he is able to observe. It may be that certain nerves on one side of the brain are not acting as they should owing to pressure from the tumour, or an area of the brain which can be recognized from the results of damage to it may be pressed upon. The important thing is that the early recognition of the presence of a tumour is absolutely essential if any hope of a complete cure can be promised or even attempted. (*See also* MENINGITIS; CONCUSSION.)

Brain Fag. Any excess of mental strain or worry may cause the brain to feel fatigued. Over-indulgence in alcohol, sexual excesses, or the abuse of drugs may be the exciting cause. The symptoms are generally restlessness, insomnia, and the inability to concentrate on work or reading. Treatment consists of rest, nourishing foods, and plenty of open-air exercise with a sufficiency of sleep.

Brain Fever. This is an old-fashioned term for meningitis. (*See also* MENINGITIS.)

BRAN. Bran is the outer covering or husks of any cereal. It contains little or no food value, but is taken in the form of biscuits to provide " roughage."

BRANDY. Brandy contains 40 to 50% of alcohol, and good cognac may contain as much as 60%. This spirit is largely used in medicine as a stimulant, and is prepared by the distillation of the juice of grapes. Brandy is considered to be very rich in energy-giving and restorative properties. (*See also* ALCOHOL.)

BREAST. The term breast is commonly used for the front part of the chest, including the two *mammæ* (breasts) and the breast-bone, but in medical language the term breast means one or other of the mammæ or glands which furnish milk. In the female the breasts are two large hemispherical prominences which lie to the right and left of the breast-bone on the front of the chest. In child-hood there is little difference to be seen between the breasts of girls and boys, but at the age of puberty they enlarge very considerably in the female but not in the male. When the body has attained its full growth the breasts remain stationary, too, until pregnancy takes place, when they immediately begin to swell. During the period of lactation or nursing, the breasts are swollen and reach their largest size. After weaning they return to a smaller size, but will usually remain larger than they were before childbearing. Other changes take place at this time which will be more fully described under the headings of PREGNANCY and CHILDBIRTH. The female breasts shrink after the menopause or change of life, and in old age become completely atrophied.

The breasts are composed of glands and vessels imbedded in fatty tissue. In the centre of each breast is a small eminence called the nipple. It is a deep rose colour, and is surrounded by a circle of pink called the areola. This areola remains a delicate pink colour until pregnancy has become established when it changes to brown and remains brownish for the rest of life. The nipple is perforated in fifteen to twenty places by the openings of the milk-bearing ducts. On the areola are various small prominences which are really sebaceous glands, and contain a fatty substance that acts as a protection to the skin of the nipple during suckling.

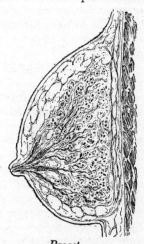

Breast
Section of Female Breast showing Milk Glands and Ducts.

The mammary gland for giving off the milk is a very complicated arrangement. In the depths of the breast the milk is gathered in very tiny vessels. Several of these unite together to form little bundles no larger than a pinhead. These bundles unite again into bigger vessels called *lobules*, and the lobules converge together in groups to form *ampullæ*, or the reservoirs, which contain the milk and which lie under the areola and have direct connection with the nipple by way of tubules or ducts. The arrangement has been compared to a bunch of grapes of which the stalks are hollow. The ducts from the various ampullæ do not unite, but discharge their milk from the nipple by means of small ducts. As well as the complicated milk-secreting apparatus the breasts are well supplied with nerves, arteries and veins, and have numerous lymphatic glands which connect with the axillary glands in the armpit.

BREAST, ABSCESS OF. Breast, or mammary, abscess nearly always arises from mastitis or inflammation of the breast. If pus-forming organisms find their way into the inflamed area suppuration begins and an abscess forms. These abscesses occur in one of three situations. They may be just under the skin or nipple and the pus may not burrow far inwards, in which case the abscess will quickly come to the surface and may be opened, causing little pain or discomfort. If, however, the pus forms deep in the substance of the breast, it may track in every direction and involve the whole breast. The typical signs of suppuration are present and the patient is in great pain and becomes very ill. A third sort of abscess may have nothing to do with lactation, but may start in the region behind or below the breast, when it is called a *submammary or retromammary* abscess, and may be due to injury to the breast, or to disease spreading from the lungs to the breast. It may be very chronic. *Cold abscesses* due to tuberculosis may occur here. These *submammary* or *retromammary* abscesses may in time point and come to a head below the breast or in the armpit. The treatment of breast abscess is the same as for other abscesses. (*See also* ABSCESS ; MASTITIS ; TUBERCULOSIS.)

BREAST, DISEASES OF. The female breast is subject to various diseases, most of which are painful and some of which are severe. Most of these diseases are related to one of the periods during which there is extra activity in the breast, namely at puberty when the breast begins to develop, during suckling or about the time of the change of life. Acute inflammation or *mastitis* occurs most often in the early days of the nursing period, although it is not rare to find it in the breasts of babies in their first few days of life. This condition in the infant readily yields to treatment and all that is necessary in most cases is to cover the part with a pad of sterile dressing such as gamgee tissue. In mastitis occurring after childbirth, a more serious condition is present and care must be taken that it does not develop into a breast abscess. Mastitis and abscess may become chronic and very troublesome. Cysts and glandular tumours may arise in the breast. Cysts may be due to chronic mastitis or may be caused by the retention of milk in women who are or have recently been nursing. Adenomata or glandular tumours may occur in the breasts of younger women whether they have borne children or not. They may be perfectly painless, small, not very hard lumps, or they may be exceedingly painful. In every case of trouble in the breast, especially if there is a lump of any description, a doctor should be consulted at once. Only if the patient comes early to the doctor can she be sure that the condition is not cancer, and if it is cancer, early removal will give a very good chance of permanent cure. (*See also* BREAST, ABSCESS OF ; CANCER ; MASTITIS ; PAGET'S DISEASE.)

BREAST FEEDING. Breast feeding is the natural method of nourishing the infant, and the normal mother's milk contains in proper quantity and proportions all the food materials necessary to keep the infant healthy. It also has the advantage of being in most cases germ free. Suckling her child also aids the mother's system to return in a natural way to the normal. It is therefore the duty of the mother both to her child and to herself to feed the child as Nature intended. Only in cases of grave necessity should the infant be put off breast feeding.

BREATH, OFFENSIVE, HALITOSIS. The breath of a perfectly healthy and cleanly person is, practically speaking, odourless. In certain cases of disease, however, and in all cases of neglect of the cleanliness of the mouth, the breath acquires a more or less offensive odour. This is often, unfortunately, more noticeable to other people than to the offender himself.

The causes of bad breath are very varied, though in practice they are limited to a few common reasons. The most frequent, probably, are local conditions, such as lack of cleanliness, decayed teeth, pyorrhœa of the gums, chronic tonsillitis and sinusitis, and other mouth and nose conditions. Most of these causes of unpleasant breath can be avoided by strict attention to cleanliness.

Chronic constipation is almost equally an offender in producing bad breath. Gases produced from decay of the food which is retained in the intestine are absorbed into the blood and may be given off by the lungs. Indigestion, with furred tongue, will also produce bad breath. In these cases temporary relief may be obtained by replacing one odour by another, i.e. by putting a small drop of oil, such as oil of cloves, on the tongue, or by eating cachous, but for permanent benefit the cause must be treated.

Many general diseases give a characteristic, not necessarily disagreeable, odour to the breath ; this is often very useful in diagnosis. For instance, in blood-poisoning the breath is sweet, in diabetes and acidosis fruity ; in others, such as certain nose troubles, gangrene of the lung, cancer of the larynx, and acute fevers, the breath is terribly offensive.

BREATHLESSNESS. Breathlessness, or shortness of breath (dyspnœa), can only be considered a disease, or rather a symptom of a disease, when it is present while the patient is at rest. It indicates that the body is not being supplied with sufficient oxygen for its needs, and this may be due to disease of the lungs, or air passages, or of the heart. Adenoids, which is a common affection of children, causes them to go about with the mouth open, thus producing breathlessness ; croup, which is also seen chiefly in children, often causes alarming breathlessness. Asthma is a condition in which this complaint is one of the chief symptoms.

In almost every disease of the lungs such as pneumonia, consumption, bronchitis, etc., shortness of breath is present, and in pleurisy the patient makes the breathing quick and short in order to avoid the pain of deep inspirations. Practically all affections of the heart, including the fatty heart of corpulent persons, cause breathlessness ; and anæmia is also a common cause, especially in young women.

The treatment naturally depends largely on the immediate cause of the complaint, but in order to relieve the patient of the distressing symptom of breathlessness, complete rest in bed is advisable, and propping up with pillows may be beneficial.

BRIGHT'S DISEASE. *See* NEPHRITIS.

BRINE BATHS, or baths in very salty water, are found to be very invigorating for patients suffering from rheumatism or debility. (*See also* BATHS ; SEA BATHING.)

BRITISH PHARMACOPŒIA. *See* B.P.

BROMIDES. The bromides of potassium, sodium, ammonium, calcium and iron are used a great deal in medicine. Externally, they have no action whatever; but internally, they act by powerfully depressing the nervous system.

BROMIDROSIS. Bromidrosis is a condition in which the sweat of the body has a very disagreeable odour. (*See also* SWEAT, DISAGREEABLE.)

BRONCHI. The plural of bronchus. The bronchi are the air passages in the lungs. After the air has been breathed in through the nose it travels to the lungs by way of the *trachea* or windpipe. The windpipe divides into two smaller tubes, one of which leads to each lung. These are the right and left *bronchi* or bronchial tubes. When the bronchial tubes reach the lung they in turn divide into numerous smaller tubes which again divide, branching like a tree until the substance of the lung is permeated with these little air vessels. The very smallest bronchi are called *bronchioles*. Inflammation of the lining of the bronchial tubes is the well-known disease called *bronchitis*. Bronchitis becomes serious when the walls of the smaller bronchioles are affected, since the air is hindered in its passage through them to the air cells, or *alveoli*, of the lung and breathing becomes difficult. Spasm of the muscular tissue of the bronchioles with swelling of the mucous membrane of the bronchial tubes is the cause of the breathlessness, which is the characteristic symptom of asthma.

BRONCHIECTASIS. Bronchiectasis is a condition in which one or more of the bronchi become enlarged and dilated, and a cavity is formed inside the chest. The condition is usually due to a previous attack of pneumonia or broncho-pneumonia, or to the inhaling at some previous time of a foreign body such as a piece of sponge, or tooth, or bit of bone. The widened area of the bronchus once formed is liable to collect matter which quickly decomposes, with the result that the breath and expectoration have a very disagreeable odour. The patient is overtaken by severe bursts of coughing in the effort to expel the matter which has collected in the bronchiectasis. If the condition is not very bad the same treatment as for bronchitis is carried out, but it may be necessary to have operative treatment, such as artificial pneumo-thorax, or else lobectomy or removal of the affected lobe of the lung. Recently improvement, though not cure, has been brought about by washing out the cavity with antiseptics introduced by means of the instrument called the bronchoscope.

BRONCHITIS. Bronchitis is well known to everyone, because it is almost a national disease in the British Isles. Our climate makes us very liable to it, and it will be the fate of a great many of us to have the chronic type, or " winter cough " in our old age.

Acute Bronchitis. Bronchitis in its acute form is a feverish cold with cough and sore chest. It is contagious and can be caught by others who come in contact with the sufferer. It is an acute catarrhal inflammation of the windpipe and larger bronchial tubes and is, as has been said above, very common in wet climates like ours. In healthy adult people it is rarely serious, but in very young children and aged people acute bronchitis is always a serious disease and is often fatal chiefly because of the lung complications which so often accompany it.

Acute bronchitis usually starts as a common cold and then extends down the air passages. Very often it follows an attack of influenza or infectious diseases like measles and typhoid fever. Many people are very prone to it and the slightest exposure to cold and damp or the germs of other people's colds will bring on an attack.

Symptoms. An attack of acute bronchitis starts as an ordinary cold, and then gradually extends, first to the larynx, where the vocal cords are affected, causing huskiness on speaking. There may be pain on swallowing and on talking and the throat will feel " raw." This feeling of " rawness " extends with the inflammation to the windpipe and larger bronchial tubes and produces a dry cough which is very painful. General symptoms are fairly well marked : there is a feeling of illness, heaviness and tiredness with pains in the back and an aching feeling in all the joints. Bronchial signs begin with a feeling of tightness and rawness in the upper part of the front of the chest. At first the cough is very dry and the expectoration is scanty, but after a few days the material coughed up becomes yellowish and abundant. With the loosening of the cough the pain grows less.

Course. After about a week the light fever present usually disappears and the cough becomes loose.

In children the risk of the disease spreading is much greater, and it then spreads downwards to the smaller portions of the bronchial tubes.

Treatment. To lessen the risk of other people catching the cold, the patient should sleep alone and, when possible, there should be an abundance of sunlight and fresh air. A " bronchitis kettle," e.g. a kettle containing a solution of eucalyptus or pinol, should be kept near the fire so that the vapour containing one of these oils is being continually given off. The room should be kept at a constant temperature of about 65° F., but must be well ventilated. The old-fashioned coal fire is still a good way of ventilating a room. Drinks of hot lemonade and a mustard plaster on the chest are very useful. The patient must remain in bed, and drink as much bland fluid as possible. The dry cough is usually very trying, and for this the kettle will be found very useful. Dover's powder, in 5 grain doses three times a day after meals, together with syrup of codeine, or heroin linctus in doses of one teaspoonful every four hours, are the medicines usually prescribed to quieten the cough. An expectorant cough mixture is also given.

Inhalations, such as a teaspoonful of Friar's Balsam in a jug of hot water, are very useful for the dry cough. The water should not be too hot, and in practice the best way to be sure of a suitable temperature is to pour boiling water in the jug and to wait for five minutes by the clock before adding the Friar's Balsam and inhaling. Care must be taken not to inhale before the end of the five minutes as, if the vapour is too hot, the larynx may be scalded and the inflammation rendered worse than before. It is also important that one should not go from a moist atmosphere to a dry one or to a different one after the inhalation, but should remain in the same temperature. The best way to avoid this is by inhaling just before settling down for the night, though the inhalations can be repeated more often when the patient is confined to bed in a room with a constant temperature.

After one or two days the expectoration becomes more free, and then the various expectorant mixtures such as ipecacuanha wine, etc., are very useful.

In children the amount of the discharge is sometimes so great that it is difficult to bring it up. If there should be any difficulty in breathing, or should the colour become dusky, an emetic such as salt and water, or a tablespoonful of tincture of ipecacuanha, should be given and repeated if necessary. This procedure will bring up quantities of phlegm, and greatly relieve the condition.

BRONCHO-PNEUMONIA. Pneumonia which affects the bronchial tubes as well as the lungs is called broncho-pneumonia.

Pneumonia proper usually starts in the lungs, whereas broncho-pneumonia affects more particularly the smaller *bronchioles*. It is more often found in children than in adults, whereas pneumonia is more frequent in older people. (*See* PNEUMONIA.)

BRONCHOSCOPE. A bronchoscope is an instrument for examining the interior of the larger bronchial tubes, by means of a tube passed down the back of the throat through the larynx and the windpipe.

BRONZING. In certain diseases, especially in Addison's disease, the skin becomes pigmented and has a decidedly bronzed appearance. It is also a symptom in exophthalmic goitre, diabetes, and chronic arsenic poisoning.

BRUISES. A bruise is caused by a damaging of the soft tissues under the unbroken skin. It may be of any severity, from a very slight injury to an extensive, deep-seated, and intensely painful one. In extreme cases dangerous or even fatal bleeding may occur from damage to an important organ of the body. People who suffer from scurvy, hæmophilia ("bleeders"), and fat and anæmic females, are liable to be bruised from very trivial causes. (*See also* BLACK EYE.)

BRUIT. Bruit is a French word meaning noise, which is used to denote any abnormal noise heard when listening to the heart with a stethoscope. The more usual name in English is a murmur.

BUBO. Inflammation or swelling in a lymphatic gland. The term is usually employed in connection with swellings in the groin due to venereal diseases or plague. It may, however, be applied to swellings in other lymphatic glands.

BUBONIC PLAGUE. This is an acute infectious fever caused by the germ called Bacillus pestis, which is communicated to man by means of the brown and the black rat. It is more pre-valent in the East than in any part of the world, but occasionally cases appear in England, the germs no doubt being carried by rats from ships.

Death may occur at any stage of the disease ; but in cases which improve, convalescence may be very prolonged. Plague is a disease with a very wide range of symptoms and which may be divided into various types. (*See also* PLAGUE.)

BULIMIA. Bulimia is the medical name for hunger which is more extensive than it should be under normal conditions. It occurs in some forms of insanity and is also a symptom of diabetes.

BUNION. Inflammation of a *bursa* of the foot, usually in the neighbourhood of the big toe, is a very common complaint and can be very painful and crippling. It may be due simply to the pressure of badly-fitting footwear, such as boots or shoes that are too narrow or too short, but very often the big toe is already deformed by gouty heredity or arthritis and the bursa which forms to protect the joint becomes inflamed by some extra pressure.

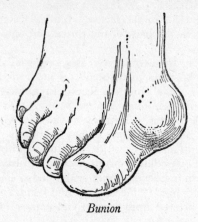

Bunion

Bunions must be treated like other forms of *bursitis*. (*See also* BUR-SITIS.)

BURNS AND SCALDS. A *burn* may be caused by dry heat, such as fire or touching a hot metal ; by lightning or an electric current ; by corrosive acids, such as nitric acid or vitriol ; or by corrosive alkalis such as caustic potash, caustic soda or quicklime. A *scald* is caused by moist heat, such as boiling liquids, steam, hot oil or tar. The extent of the damage varies from a mere reddening of the surface of the skin to a charring of the deep tissues. The chief dangers from burning or scalding are shock and blood-poisoning. Even the smallest burn is very painful. The best treatment is to spray on a 2 per cent solution of tannic acid in warm water ; the tannic acid coagulates the surface and prevents the absorption of poisons. Medicated paraffin (ambrine) and 1 per cent picric acid solution in hot water are also useful.

BURSA. A small enclosed sac containing clear sticky fluid. These little bags of fluid are found in various parts of the body where two parts would rub on each other.

BURSITIS. Inflammation of a bursa is known as bursitis. In acute inflammation the bursa becomes distended with fluid, and the tissues in the neighbourhood become swollen, hot and red. The treatment is similar to that of an acute abscess, hot fomentations and rest being necessary. If pus forms in the bursa it must be let out. In certain occupations the bursa in a particular region may be subject to repeated irritation and a condition of bursitis may become chronic. The commonest forms of chronic bursitis are " housemaid's knee," " miner's elbow " and " weaver's bottom." One form of " tennis elbow " is a bursitis. In these chronic forms of bursitis the movement which causes the irritation to the bursa must be avoided and the part rested. Iodine painted on over the region of the bursa will help to reduce the swelling, and an elastic bandage for support may be very useful.

Persons who habitually carry weights in the same way, like

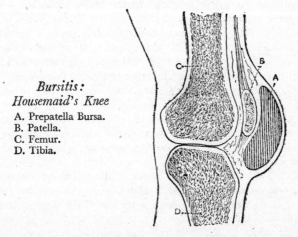

Bursitis:
Housemaid's Knee

A. Prepatella Bursa.
B. Patella.
C. Femur.
D. Tibia.

porters, are subject to bursitis in various parts of the back and shoulders. The form which is common amongst the porters at Covent Garden is called a " hummy."

BUTYRIC ACID. An acid with a sharp, bitter taste which is contained in butter. This acid may form in the stomach owing to indigestion, and its presence generally imparts a very unpleasant odour to the patient's breath.

CACHEXIA. In medicine the term is applied to conditions in which there is much wasting and general loss of flesh, due to some serious disease such as tuberculosis, cancer or syphilis.

CADAVER. Cadaver means a dead body, but it is applied especially to the dead body of a human being.

CÆCUM. The cæcum is the first part of the large intestine or bowel. It forms a large pouch with its closed end pointing downwards and its open end communicating directly with the colon. Its average size is about 2½ inches long and 3 inches broad. The appendix is attached to the cæcum. (*See also* INTESTINE.)

CÆSAREAN SECTION or OPERATION. This is an operation by which the child is removed from the mother's body through an opening which is made in the abdominal wall. It is frequently necessary to carry out this operation in cases where the child cannot be born in the natural way without endangering the life of the mother. The death-rate from Cæsarean section is very small, and if it is properly carried out no serious complications are likely to arise. It gained its name from the fact that Julius Cæsar was born in this manner.

CAFFEINE. This powerful substance is found in the leaves and beans of the coffee tree and in the leaves of common tea. In character it is slightly bitter to the taste, and is composed of colourless, silky crystals which melt easily in cold water. Excessive tea drinking may cause indigestion, but this may be due to the tannin in the tea and not to the caffeine. It is a well-known fact that tea and coffee are stimulants and increase the mental activities, but very excessive indulgence may cause trembling of the muscles and " nervousness."

In bronchial asthma, caffeine citrate may be given before bedtime and during the night. It is useful in dropsy due to kidney disease, heart failure in pneumonia, nervous headache, and also in cases of diarrhœa.

CAISSON DISEASE. This is a condition which occurs in divers, and in others who work under high atmospheric pressures. Symptoms do not develop until after the diver returns to normal atmospheric pressure.

Symptoms. In the mildest forms there is headache, also giddiness and fainting which may pass off without any ill effects. In the more severe cases there are agonizing pains in the limbs, joints and trunk, known by the workmen as " the bends," from the position in which the limbs are held. As a rule, the milder forms, including the " bends," generally recover without any permanent ill effects. Even cases of complete paralysis may recover in a few days, though usually improvement is more gradual.

In order to prevent the occurrence of this disease the workers should pass from the atmosphere of very high pressure to the normal one by means of a series of air-locked chambers, where the pressures are gradually lowered, staying a definite time in each chamber.

Treatment. When symptoms of caisson disease do occur, the patient should be placed in a chamber and the atmospheric pressure raised to that at which he was working. He should then be very gradually brought back to the normal atmosphere.

CAJUPUT OIL. Oil distilled from leaves of certain plants grown in Batavia and Singapore. Used externally, it is a stimulant and irritant and is often rubbed into the skin in the treatment of chilblains, rheumatism, and chronic inflammation of the joints. In small percentages it is soothing and is, for example, the chief ingredient in the soothing oil called gomenol.

CALABAR BEAN. A powerful drug known as physostigmine or eserine salicylate is obtained from the calabar bean. Physostigmine applied locally to the eye causes the pupil to contract and is used extensively by oculists in the treatment of certain eye disorders, especially glaucoma.

CALAMINE. The natural zinc carbonate when washed and pulverized forms a smooth powder which is known as calamine. It is an excellent drug for skin diseases and may be made up as a lotion, or prepared with vaseline and used as an ointment.

CALCIFEROL. The pure substance that has been isolated as vitamin D and is the product of the action of the ultra-violet rays of light on a substance, ergosterol, contained in most living cells and food-stuffs. (*See* VITAMINS.)

CALCIUM. Calcium is best known as quicklime, limestone or chalk. Calcium chloride is used to increase the clotting power of the blood. It may be given by injection into the muscles to gain a quick effect. To arrest intestinal bleeding, 30 to 60 grains daily have been given internally, accompanied by rectal injections containing 60 grains to two pints of water. It is employed in itching skin affections such as urticaria, pruritis and prurigo. It is useful in chilblains, small doses being taken frequently. Calcium carbonate and calcium phosphate in equal parts, a teaspoonful thrice daily, is an excellent remedy for diarrhœa of gastric origin. Lime water is used in the preparation of milk for infant feeding, as it reduces the size of the curds ; 1 to $\frac{1}{2}$ teaspoonful should be used.

Used externally the prepared chalk of calcium may be used as a dusting-powder. Calcium mixed with equal parts of linseed or olive-oil is well known as Carron oil, after the famous Scottish ironworks where it was first used. This is applied to burns, but tannic acid is now thought to be a better remedy.

CALCULUS. Calculus is the term applied to a stone-like material found in the body, particularly in cavities of the body. These stones or *calculi* usually form in the bladder, kidneys, ureters and sometimes in the pancreas. So long as the calculus stays in the cavity in which it has formed it may give rise to no symptoms whatever, but immediately it begins to pass out from the cavity intense pain is generally set up. (*See also* GALL-STONES.)

CALLUS. A callus or callosity, like a corn, is a thickening. of the horny layer of the skin, sometimes to many times its normal size.

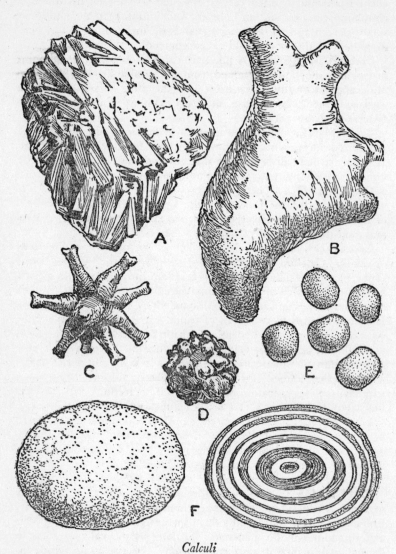

Calculi

A. Oxalate (Crystalline type); B. Phosphatic from Pelvis of Kidney;
C and D. Calcium Oxalate (Mulberry); E. Small Calculi from Bladder;
F. Mixed Uric Acid and Calcium Oxalate (External View of Section).

Treatment. On the feet they occur when badly-fitting shoes are worn ; not only shoes that are too tight, but those that are too loose can produce callosities, following blisters due to the constant friction. The remedy here is obvious. They also occur in some deformities of the feet where one part of the foot has to take all the pressure. It will generally be found that with properly fitting shoes, calluses gradually disappear, but if any further measures need to be taken, the treatment described under CORNS will be found suitable.

CALOMEL. Mercurous chloride, more commonly known as calomel, is a heavy white powder used as a purgative. It is a useful remedy for an overloaded liver and for dyspepsia generally, though some people find it rather upsetting or depressing. It should be given at bedtime, and be followed by a morning glass of salts. (*See also* CHOLAGOGUE.)

CALORY. Calory is the name given to a heat-unit ; the amount of heat required to raise the temperature of one kilogram of water from 0° to 1° C. In special diets the amount of food eaten is carefully measured out in calories.

CALUMBA is an excellent example of a simple bitter and may be prescribed with salts of iron. It is useful in dyspepsia and may be given as a mild, appetizing tonic in convalescence. (*See also* BITTERS.)

CAMOMILE. The flower-heads of Anthemis nobilis, the properties of which are due to an oil, camphor, and a bitter substance it contains. It is useful in coughs and for in-

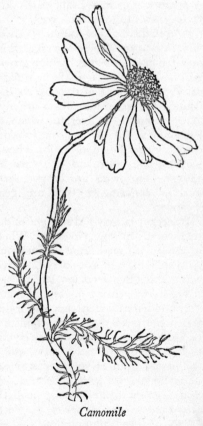

Camomile

fantile colic. A large cup of boiling water is poured over about a dozen of the flower-heads and left by the side of the fire to infuse for 10 or 15 minutes. The infusion is then strained, sweetened and served hot. Camomile is also extensively used as a hair-wash.

CAMP FEVER. An old popular name for typhus fever.

CAMPHOR. Camphor is a white crystalline substance obtained from the camphor laurel which grows in Formosa and Japan. Its stimulating effects make camphor a favourite ingredient in many liniments. It is constantly being used in the treatment of chronic rheumatism, lumbago, neuralgia and in the chest complaints of children. The liquid preparations with various substances added, such as thymol and carbolic acid, are excellent local remedies for neuralgia, and may be dropped into a tooth for the relief of toothache. Camphor ice rubbed into the skin is very useful for chapped hands. A mixture of camphor salicylate and sodium sulphate may be taken before meals to ward off a cold.

CANCER. The human body is subject to tumour growths of various sorts. These are divided into two classes, benign growths and malignant growths. Benign growths are all the cysts and tumours which do not shorten life. Malignant growths are those which cause a great deal of damage to the body and eventually lead to death. The general health is greatly impaired and the organ, such as the stomach or liver, in which the cancer is growing becomes less and less able to carry on its work until the day comes when it can no longer function at all. They are also apt to spread to other parts of the body and to return after they have been cut out. Malignant growths are of two sorts, sarcomas and carcinomas ; but for convenience they are generally referred to simply as " cancer."

Cancer is largely a disease of middle and old age but does sometimes occur in young people. When younger people are attacked by cancer it usually runs a much quicker course than in older persons, and may be considered an acute disease. In older persons, when it is discovered too late to operate upon successfully, it can still often be held at bay and alleviated for a number of years.

It is often said that cancer is a disease of civilization. It is true that there is a larger proportion of cases in the so-called civilized countries than amongst the less civilized races, but it is by no means unknown amongst native races, and as it is so much more a disease of old age than of youth it is possible that in civilized countries more people are kept alive until the cancerous age. The same thing applies to the increase in the number of deaths from cancer. It is obvious that as fewer people are allowed to die from other causes, such as consumption, in these days, and more people are kept alive to the age of fifty, there must be an increase in the number of deaths from cancer until some means is discovered of curing cancer at a later stage in its course.

It may be pointed out here, however, that cure of cancer after it has taken a good hold can only amount to getting rid of the tumour by some such means as surgically cutting it out or shrivelling it up by radium or X-rays, and great damage may be done to the surrounding parts before the cancer is discovered. By far the more important thing is to prevent cancer from occurring at all, or to discover its presence at a very early stage.

Different kinds of Cancer. The difference between carcinoma and sarcoma is one of the character of the cells of which they are composed. The whole human body is composed of millions of cells. These cells are described in a separate article and it is sufficient here to state that the life of a cell in the body is like the life of the body itself. The cell begins, grows and develops and finally dies and is succeeded by other cells. Like bodies there are normal cells and abnormal cells, that is, well and sick cells. There are also cells of different types, like people of different races. The two most important groups of cells are first the group containing the cells forming the skin, the linings of the mouth and various organs and passages of the body and the glands. The other group consists of the cells forming the connective tissue or generally the flesh ; and the tissue composing such parts of the general framework of the body as the bones, muscles and gristle. A malignant growth of the first group of cells is called a *carcinoma* and of the second group a *sarcoma*. Both sorts of growth are popularly grouped together and called *cancer*.

Of carcinomas and sarcomas, the carcinomas are by far the more numerous and are the more dangerous. Sarcomas develop in the tissue surrounding bones, muscles, etc., whilst carcinomas attack glands, organs such as the stomach, and soft parts like the lip, and the skin itself. Skin cancers are called epitheliomas, and are described separately under the headings CANCER OF THE SKIN and EPITHELIOMA.

As well as the breast and womb, stomach and rectum, which are the most frequent sites, cancer is found frequently in the intestines, gall-bladder, liver, larynx, tongue, œsophagus (the passage from the mouth to the stomach) and in bones. Cancer of the skin, and epitheliomas (including smoker's cancer) are described separately under their own headings.

Occupational Cancers. Certain occupations have a greater risk of cancer than others, and in these cases the cancer is almost certainly due to constant irritation of a part either directly, or as the result of a frequently used chemical substance. For example, in the Lancashire cotton-mills male workers get a form of cancer called mule-spinner's cancer. This cancer arises in the scrotum and is due to constant irritation of the part by the constant saturation of the clothes with the lubricating oil used. Precautions are now taken to prevent this form of cancer. Chimney-sweeps, and gardeners to a very small extent only, are also liable to cancer of the scrotum and cancer of the skin, due to the soot they work amongst. Workers with rubber may get cancerous growths on the skin, and all workers with tar products, such as creosote, benzine and paraffin are liable to cancer. (*See also* CANCER OF THE SKIN.)

Causes of Cancer. The causes of cancer are as yet unknown except that constant irritation of a part seems to be directly responsible for a certain number of cancers, such as the trade cancers. Why this should be so is not known. In the case of cancer of one of the internal organs, such as the stomach or intestines, cancers seem to arise on the site of old, standing inflammations such as chronic ulcers, and in cases where chronic poisoning of the body by toxins and abnormal germs has been going on for a long period of years, thus causing the part to be thoroughly unhealthy. Some authorities think that under-nourishment of the body in respect to vital substances like vitamins opens the door to cancer. A blow on a soft part such as the breast may be quickly followed by cancer. It is thought by some workers on the subject of cancer that there may be a definite cancer germ, which like other germs gains admittance to the body and settles in a weak spot, and in 1925, Dr. W. E. Gye and Mr. J. E. Barnard were able to photograph living organisms which they found present in cases of both carcinoma and sarcoma. Other workers, however, were unable to confirm their observations. They are continuing their researches into the causes of cancer in company with a great band of skilled medical research workers all over the world, who are working under such bodies as the Medical Research Council, the Cancer Research Fund and the British Empire Cancer Campaign. Much work also is being done in the great hospitals and in private laboratories. It would seem that it is only a question of time until the cause of cancer is known and then its prevention and cure by medical means may become comparatively simple.

Treatment of Cancer. As has been said previously, the only successful treatment for cancer at present known is complete removal at an early stage by operation, and as so much depends upon the earliness of the operation, not an unnecessary day should be wasted after the diagnosis has been made. Some authorities prefer treatment by " deep " X-rays or radium as a means not only of slowing the growth and rendering the patient more comfortable, but actually of cure, though operation has the most advocates. Radium treatment does better than operation, however, in some cases such as cancer of the tongue. The truth is that both radium and X-ray

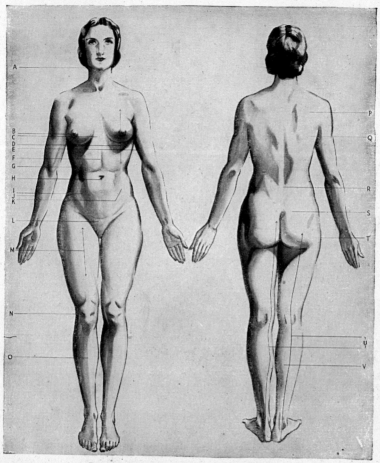

Letters indicate the centres of the areas where warning pains may occur

A, Mumps, toothache, neuralgia, tonsillitis, pharyngitis, laryngitis, diphtheria, scarlatina, adenitis.

B, Mastitis, cysts, malignant disease of breast; pregnancy.

C, Dyspepsia and other stomach diseases, bronchitis, aneurism, angina pectoris, influenza.

D, Pleurisy, pneumonia, shingles, neuralgia, muscular rheumatism.

E, Rheumatism, neuritis, angina pectoris—usually left arm.

F, Dyspepsia and other stomach diseases, duodenal ulcer, pancreas disease, pneumonia, diaphragmatic pleurisy.

G, Liver diseases, gall-stones, gall-bladder diseases (especially at x), pneumonia or pleurisy, floating kidney.

H, Gastric ulcer, hernia in children.

I, Appendicitis, colitis, disease of right ovary.

J, Writer's cramp, etc.

K, Colitis, constipation, diseases of left ovary, obstruction of bowel.

L, Bladder diseases, diseases of ovaries or womb, inflammation of pelvis.

M, Diseases of ovary or womb, neuralgia, renal colic (one side), psoas abscess, inflamed glands in groin.

N, Loose cartilage, disease of knee-joint, disease of hip-joint.

O, Rheumatism, bone disease, phlebitis, neuralgia, neuritis.

P, Gall-stones, liver diseases.

Q, Liver pains, pleurisy, pneumonia, herpes zoster (usually right side).

R, Diseases of womb or ovaries, lumbago.

S, Sacro-iliac diseases.

T, Hip-joint disorders.

U, Sciatica.

V, Muscular cramp, locomotor ataxia, neuritis, varicose veins, phlebitis, intermittent claudication.

See also frontispiece.

II.—THE EAR AND THE EYE

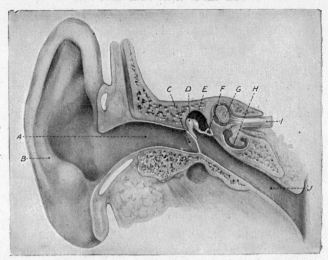

THE EAR

A, External Meatus (passage of ear).
B, Outer Ear or Auricle.
C, Ear Drum.
D, Malleus.
E, Incus.
F, Stapes.
G, Cochlea.
H, Semi-circular Canal (organ of balance).
I, Acoustic Nerve (nerve of hearing).
J, Eustachian Tube.

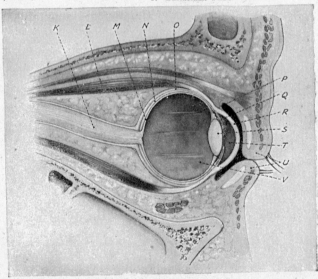

THE EYE

K, Optic Nerve (nerve of sight).
L, Muscle of Eye.
M N O, Inner, middle and outer layers of the Retina.
P, Conjunctiva.
Q, Iris.
R, Cornea.
S, Lens.
T, Aqueous Humour.
U, Eyelids.
V, Vitreous Humour.

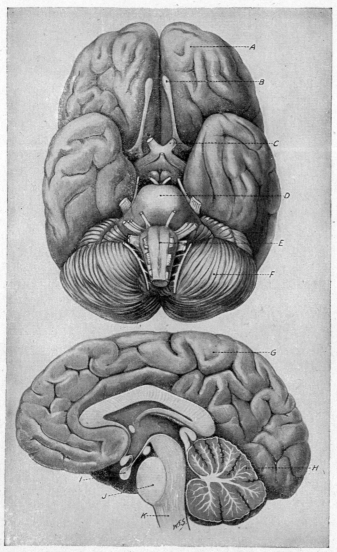

Under Surface of the Brain

A, Frontal Lobe.
B, Olfactory Bulb (from which emerge the nerves of smell).
C, Optic Nerve (nerve of sight).
D, Pons Varolii.
E, Medulla Oblongata.
F, Cerebellum.

Section through the Brain

G, Cerebrum.
H, Cerebellum.
I, Pituitary Body.
J, Pons Varolii.
K, Medulla Oblongata.

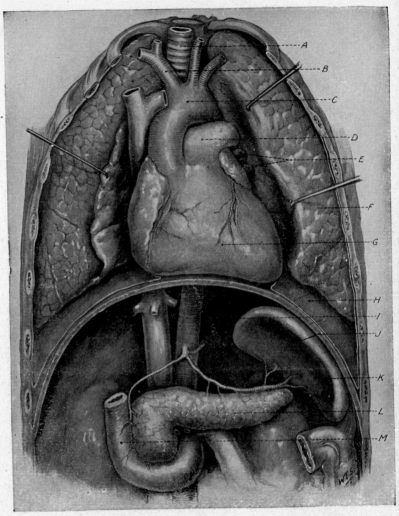

A, Trachea or Windpipe.	F, Lung.	J, Diaphragm.
B, Innominate Artery.	G, Heart.	K, Spleen.
C, Aorta.	H, Pleura.	L, Pancreas.
D, Pulmonary Artery.	I, Abdominal Aorta.	M, Duodenum.
E, Pulmonary Veins.		

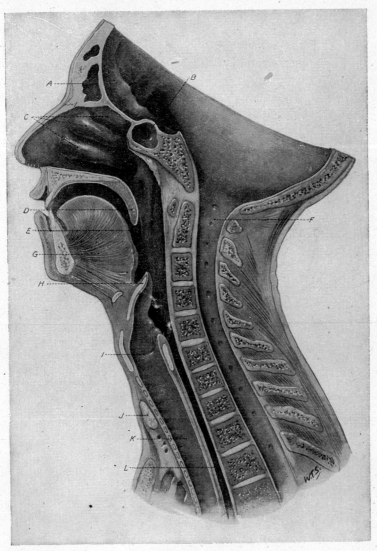

A, Frontal Sinus.
B, Sphenoidal Sinus.
C, Superior middle and inferior turbinals.
D, Soft Palate.
E, Tonsil.

F, Spinal Cord (leading from the Brain and containing the Spinal Cord. The brain and spinal cord have been removed in this illustration).

G, Tongue.
H, Epiglottis.
I, Vocal Cord.
J, Thyroid Gland.
K, Trachea or Windpipe.
L, Œsophagus or Gullet.

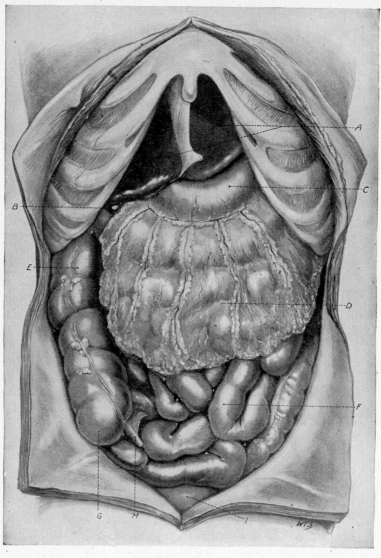

A, Liver.
B, Gall Bladder.
C, Stomach.
D, Omentum covering the Intestines.
E, Colon (Large Intestine).
F, Small Intestine.
G, Cæcum.
H, Appendix.
I, Urinary Bladder.

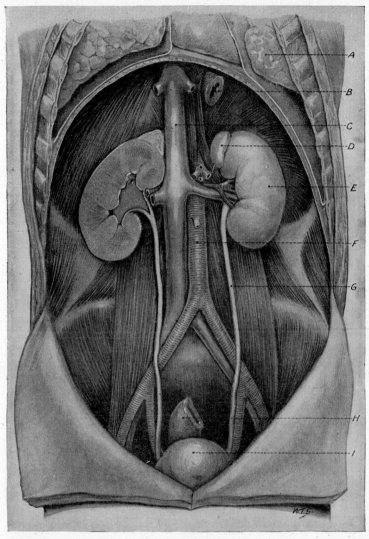

The Kidneys are shown in their positions on the posterior wall of the Abdomen, the right Kidney being cut open to show its Pelvis and the Ureter coming from it

A, Lung.
B, End of Œsophagus.
C, Vena Cava (the great vein of the Abdomen.)
D, Suprarenal Gland.
E, Left Kidney.
F, Abdominal Aorta.
G, Ureter.
H, End of Large Intestine.
I, Urinary Bladder.

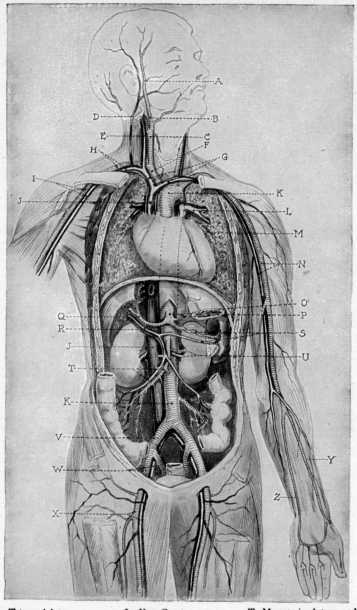

A, Temporal Artery.	**J,** Vena Cava.	**T,** Mesenteric Artery and Vein.
B, External Carotid Artery.	**K,** Aorta.	
C, Common Carotid Artery.	**L,** Pulmonary Artery.	**U,** Renal Artery and Veins.
D, External Jugular Vein.	**M,** Pulmonary Veins.	**V,** Common Iliac Artery and Vein.
E, Internal Jugular Vein.	**N,** Brachial Artery and Vein.	
F, Innominate Artery.	**O,** Cœliac Axis.	**W,** External Iliac Artery and Vein.
G, R. and L. Innominate Veins.	**P,** Gastric Artery.	
H, Subclavian Artery and Vein.	**Q,** Hepatic Artery.	**X,** Femoral Artery and Vein.
I, Axillary Artery and Vein.	**R,** Portal Vein.	**Y,** Radial Artery.
	S, Splenic Artery and Vein.	**Z,** Ulnar Artery.

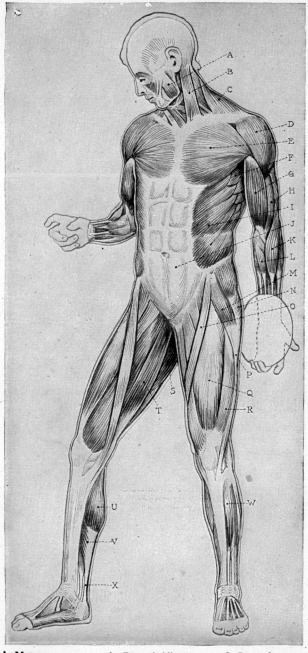

A, Masseter.
B, Sterno-mastoid.
C, Trapezius.
D, Deltoid.
E, Pectoralis major.
F, Serratus magnus.
G, Biceps.
H, Triceps.

I, External oblique.
J, Rectus abdominalis.
K, Supinator longus.
L, Flexor carpi radialis.
M, Tensor fasciæ femoris.
N, Gluteus medius.
O, Sartorius.
P, Ilio-tibial band.

Q, Rectus femoris.
R, Vastus externus.
S, Gracilis.
T, Abductor longus.
U, Gastrocnemius.
V, Soleus.
W, Peroneus longus.
X, Tendo Achillis.

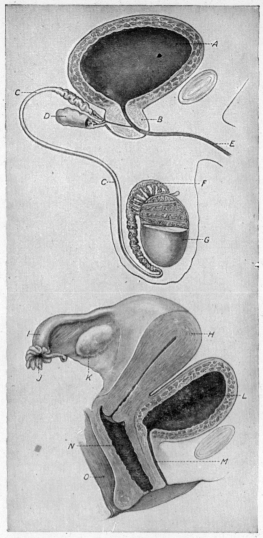

Male

A, Urinary Bladder.
B, Prostate Gland.
C, Vas Deferens.
D, Seminal Vesicle.
E, Urethra (leading to Penis).
F, Epididymis.
G, Testicle.

Female

H, Uterus or Womb.
I, Fallopian Tube.
J, Fimbria or opening of Fallopian Tube.
K, Ovary.
L, Urinary Bladder.
M, Urethra.
N, Vagina
O, Rectum.

XI.—THE HEART AND THE LUNGS

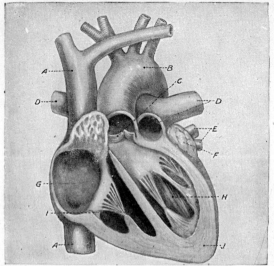

THE HEART

A, Vena cava (superior and inferior).
B, Aorta.
C, Semi-lunar valves of the aorta.
D, Pulmonary artery.
E, Pulmonary veins.

F, Left auricle (only partly visible).
G, Right auricle.
H, Left ventricle.
I, Right ventricle.
J, Muscular wall of the heart.

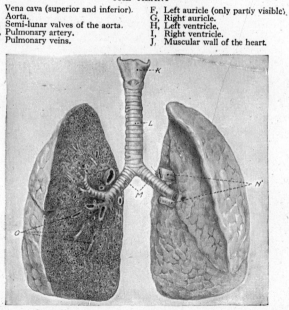

THE LUNGS

K, Cartilage of Larynx.
L, Trachea or Windpipe.
M, Right and left main Bronchi.

N, Blood-vessels of the Lung.
O, Smaller Bronchi of the Lung.

XII.—THE DIGESTIVE SYSTEM

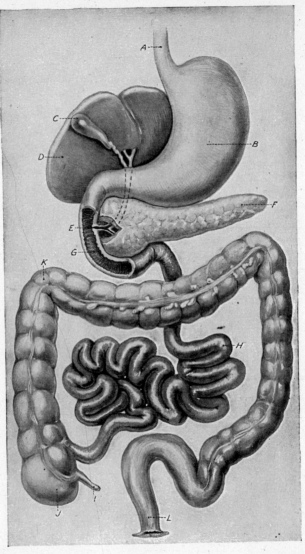

A, Œsophagus or Gullet.
B, Stomach.
C, Gall Bladder.
D, Liver.
E, Ampulla of Vater (where

the ducts of the Liver
and Pancreas enter the
Intestine).
F, Pancreas.
G, Duodenum.

H, Small Intestine
I, Appendix.
J, Cæcum.
K, Large Intestine.
L, Rectum.

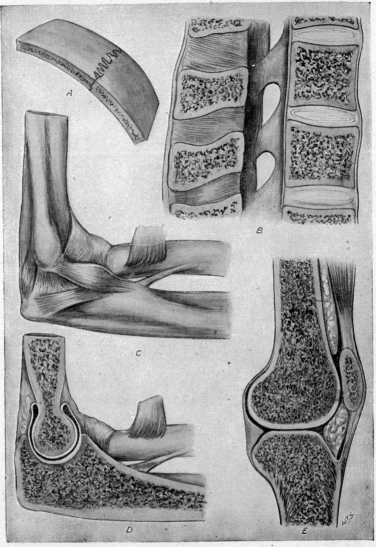

A, Immovable Joint (between bones of Skull).
B, Intervertebral Joints (between the Vertebræ of the Spine) showing, on the right, the **Inter-**vertebral discs of cartilage between the bodies of the Vertebræ.
C, Elbow-joint (hinge joint), showing ligaments holding bones in place.
D, Section of Elbow-joint, showing joint cavity and synovial membrane lining.
E, Section of Knee-joint, showing patella, or knee-cap, on the right.

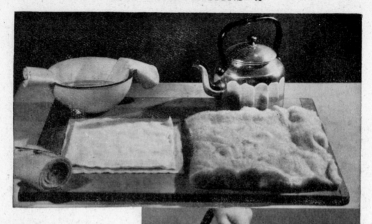

Above: Requisites for a Hot Fomentation. Towel in basin, boiling water, bandage, lint and mackintosh, cotton wool.

Right: Boiling water poured on lint placed on towel in basin.

Below: Towel twisted round lint, twisting out the hot water.

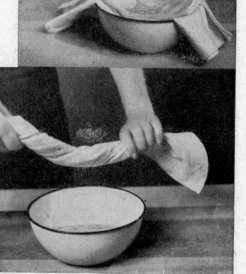

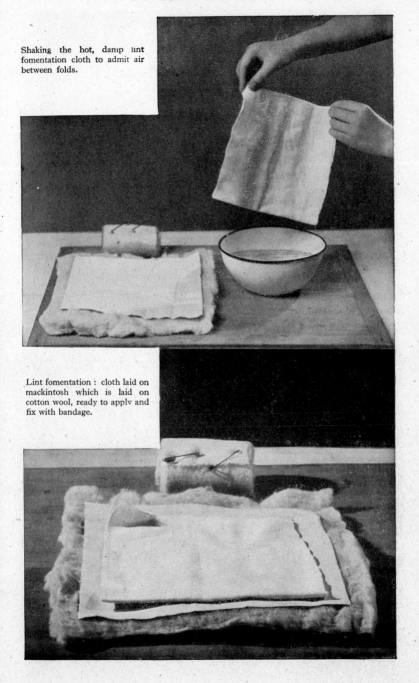

Shaking the hot, damp lint fomentation cloth to admit air between folds.

Lint fomentation : cloth laid on mackintosh which is laid on cotton wool, ready to apply and fix with bandage.

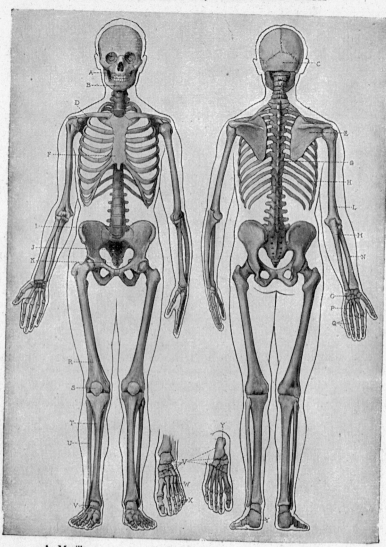

A, Maxilla.
B, Mandible.
C, Occipital Bone.
D, Clavicle.
E, Scapula.
F, Sternum.
G, Vertebræ.
H, Ribs.

I, Pelvis.
J, Sacrum.
K, Coccyx.
L, Humerus.
M, Ulna.
N, Radius.
O, Carpus (8).
P, Metacarpus.
Q, Phalanges.

R, Femur.
S, Patella.
T, Tibia.
U, Fibula.
V, Tarsus.
W, Metatarsus.
X, Phalanges.
Y, Os Calcis.

treatment do very well in early cases of cancer, but one does not know yet how long such cures last and operation is more certain, at any rate, up to the present, so the patient should choose the safer course. In late cases of cancer where little can be done but perform " palliative " operations to make the patient more comfortable, a great deal can be done by X-rays and radium to relieve the patient of some of his miseries ; even in those cases where a cure is impossible the skilful administration of pain-deadening drugs will render the latter stages more bearable both for the patient and for his family and friends. (*See also* BREAST, CANCER OF ; CANCER OF THE SKIN ; EPITHELIOMA.)

CANCER OF THE SKIN. The skin, like every other part of the body, is afflicted with cancer. Cancer of the skin arises from an overgrowth of a group of the cells making up the skin tissue. For some reason, these begin to grow rapidly, using the neighbouring healthy cells for food, and often spread to other parts : in short, they behave like an invading army of lawless marauders—an army that is too often, alas! victorious over the law-abiding body cells.

CANCRUM ORIS or CANKER OF THE MOUTH. This is a disease of the mouth which generally appears in childhood between the ages of one and five. The patient is usually in a very debilitated state owing to some such disease as measles, diphtheria, scarlet fever or whooping-cough. Deep, foul ulcers appear on the inner side of the cheek and may spread rapidly and pierce through the cheek. The gums and lips may be similarly affected. The temperature is usually very high, and in cases where there is general blood-poisoning or broncho-pneumonia the patient may even die. The disease is due to germs and to poor hygienic surroundings. An intramuscular injection of sulpharsenol is usually given by the doctor.

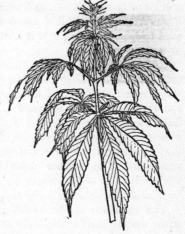

Cannabis Indica

CANITIES. A term applied to blanching or whitening of the hair. (*See also* HAIR.)

CANNABIS INDICA. Cannabis Indica is an Indian hemp from which a powerful drug is obtained, which is also known as *hashish* or *bhang*. The drug is obtained from the dried flowering tops of the plant Cannabis sativa from which the resin has not been removed. It acts as an antispasmodic, and a narcotic or sleep producing drug. The patient may have a sensation of mild intoxication, feeling very gay and pleased with everything. This drug is used extensively in the East, and when it is taken in moderation it causes no harm. When taken to excess it leads to loss of appetite, trembling of the limbs, and insanity; but very large doses have been recovered from, and no death from cannabis indica is on record.

It is used in medicine in the form of a tincture or of an extract, and may be administered in cases of neuralgia and migraine. It is also useful in the treatment of colics, whooping-cough, and painful menstruation.

CANNULA. A tube used for withdrawing fluids from the body. A double cannula is used to wash out a cavity of the body :

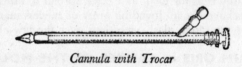

Cannula with Trocar

one tube being used for the inflow of a fluid and the other tube for the outflow.

CANTHARIDES. Cantharides is obtained from various species of beetles known as Spanish Fly or of Mylabris. It contains a powerful poison called cantharidin. Cantharidin is very largely used to raise a blister, and it is of all drugs the most commonly used as a counter-irritant.

CAPILLARIES. The tiny blood-vessels of the body are called *capillaries*. They continue the circulation of the blood between the smallest arteries and the smallest veins, called the *arterioles* and the *venules,* and are so small that they cannot be seen with the naked eye. The capillaries form dense networks throughout the tissues of the body. They are thickest in size just under the skin, and smallest in the linings of the organs deep in the body, and in the brain. The number of capillaries in any given organ depends upon the need of that organ for blood. The denser the network of capillaries the greater is the supply of blood.

The structure of the capillaries is interesting. They consist of walls made up of a single layer of cells whose margins are joined together with a cementing substance. The capillaries branch out from the walls of the arteries and veins, and from the arteries they obtain their supply of blood which has taken up oxygen and nutritive blood. The walls of the capillaries have the characteristic of being able to pass oxygen, carbonic acid and nourishing materials from the blood through their walls into the tissues for the purpose of feeding the tissues, whilst similarly the capillaries can collect waste materials out of the blood which they return to the veins for destruction and excretion from the body. The white blood-corpuscles or leucocytes, which protect the body by attacking disease germs which have found their way into the blood-stream, are able to pass through the capillaries, backwards and forwards between the blood and the tissues. (*See also* ARTERY ; BLOOD ; LEU- COCYTES ; VEINS.)

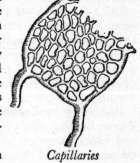

Capillaries

CAPSICUM. Capsicum is also known as Guinea pepper or Pod pepper. The dried ripe fruit of the plant when powdered is called red or cayenne pepper. It is used in medicine in the form of an ointment or tincture. The ointment is used as a counter-irritant and may be useful in the treatment of chest affections, rheumatism and sciatica. (*See also* CHILLI PASTE.)

CARAWAY. This is the name of the dried ripe fruit of the Carum carvi. The fruit yields an oil with an aromatic odour and a spicy, pleasant taste. The oil is used in medicine and as a flavouring agent. A few drops may be taken as a means of soothing an irritated stomach.

CARBOHYDRATE. One of the largest and most important groups of substances from which the body obtains its food is the group of carbohydrates, which are so called from the fact that they contain carbon, hydrogen and oxygen, all of which are necessary to the maintenance of health. Of these three elements, carbon is the means by which the energy and heat of the body are provided for. In the body it is burnt up, producing heat and energy. It follows, therefore, that at different times the body will require different amounts of carbohydrates. In winter more will be required than in summer, and the individual who has to perform much physical exertion will need more than the person who leads a sedentary life. The labourer will need more than the clerk. This is well seen by the craving that athletes often have for sweets or sugar after an outburst of strenuous exercise. (*See also* DIGESTION.)

CARBOLIC ACID. Carbolic acid or *phenol* is obtained by distilling and purifying coal-tar. Carbolic is a powerful caustic and irritant, and when applied to the skin in concentrated form will cause burning and pain. A white spot may appear on the part, which becomes red when the acid is removed. Externally, carbolic is largely used as a deodorant and disinfectant. The raw acid may be used for disinfecting drains, bed-pans, etc. A weak solution is used to wash wounds to keep them antiseptic, and mosquito bites may be relieved by the application of weak carbolic. It is also useful in keeping the mosquitoes away. Carbolic cleanses, heals, disinfects and allays pain. Because of its deadening effect a strong solution will relieve itching from any cause. Carbolized gauze and carbolized lint are also prepared and used frequently for dressings for wounds.

Poisoning by Carbolic Acid. Immediately on swallowing, an intense burning pain may be felt in the mouth, gullet and stomach, and white ulcerated areas may appear in the mouth. The skin becomes cold and clammy, and breathing gradually becomes more and more feeble and finally stops. Treatment consists of washing out the stomach several times with 10 per cent. alcohol and water. Apomorphine is a suitable emetic. White of egg, and large doses of any harmless oil may be given. Chalk and lime water and caffeine are also antidotes. The patient must be kept as warm as possible by the use of hot-water bottles or electric pads. Medical aid should be called in as early as possible.

CARBON MONOXIDE. Carbon monoxide is a very poisonous, odourless gas. It is the dangerous gas given off from the exhaust of a motor-car or from a geyser in a bathroom. In extreme cases death may occur very quickly and artificial respiration may prove of no avail. The presence of this gas is very treacherous in coal mines, as miners may go on working in a poisoned atmosphere without being aware of it. Many people who have gone to sleep in a room heated by charcoal braziers, or having otherwise breathed air overcharged with carbon monoxide, have gradually become unconscious and died from the poisoning.

When entering a room filled with gas in order to rescue a person, the mouth and nose should be covered with a damp cloth and the windows should be thrown open immediately. On no account should a naked light be used. The person should be dragged or carried out into the fresh air and the clothing loosened as much as possible and artificial respiration started. The doctor should be called as soon as possible and inhalation of oxygen gas should be given when necessary.

CARBONIC ACID. Carbon dioxide is a gassy product commonly known as carbonic-acid gas or carbonic acid. This gas must be given off by the body if health and life are to be continued. Any atmosphere which is overcharged with carbonic acid may produce symptoms of headache, loss of appetite and lack of energy. When it is inhaled in a pure form, death results from asphyxia. It is of great value if breathing is difficult in the new-born child, and it has been given to stimulate the breathing in cases of opium poisoning and pulmonary collapse.

Carbonic acid snow may be made from the gas which has been allowed to escape from a cylinder into some suitable receptacle or tube. The snow can be moulded so as to form a pencil, which may be applied to birthmarks, port-wine stains, lupus or rodent ulcers. The application is usually for about half a minute or a little longer. (*See also* ANÆSTHETICS, LOCAL.)

CARBUNCLE. A carbuncle is an inflammatory condition of the skin and tissues under the skin, and is usually due to infection by a germ known as the staphylococcus. The carbuncle usually starts as a simple boil or group of boils, often at the root of a hair on the skin, but it rapidly spreads to the tissues around and under the original boil and may become very large. Pus forms at several points, and if the carbuncle is left without proper attention the skin may become riddled with sinuses and the whole region

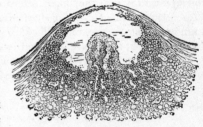

Carbuncle

may become a soft, boggy mass of pus and dead tissue, which will leave a very unsightly hole when the carbuncle finally heals up. In cases that are at all severe the patient becomes very ill with a high temperature, rapid pulse rate, constipation and furred tongue. The condition may rapidly become dangerous to life. Cases where there are two or more carbuncles at the same time, or where the carbuncle is on the lip or face or behind the ear, are especially dangerous to life.

Treatment. The treatment is, in the less severe cases, the same as for a boil. Hot applications, such as antiphlogistine or poultices, should be continued until the matter comes to the surface, when it may be allowed to escape through small incisions, while the wound is sprayed twice daily with hydrogen peroxide to remove the dead tissues, and is dressed with boracic fomentations. As soon as the condition is recognized, injections of manganese or a vaccine should be given and the general condition should be toned up in every possible way. The diet should be generous, and a tonic should be given. Alcohol in such forms as sherry or port is often beneficial. A sleeping-draught may be given if there is insomnia.

If the carbuncle is a bad one, the doctor may decide that surgical treatment is necessary. (*See also* BOIL.)

CARCINOMA. Carcinoma is the most frequent form of cancer. It has been described under the heading CANCER.

CARDIAC. An adjective meaning anything to do with the heart. The heart and its diseases will be described under headings beginning with HEART.

CARIES. The term caries means decay, and is usually used in connection with decay of teeth, or bones. (*See also* BONE NECROSIS.)

CARMINATIVE. Any drug which produces a feeling of warmth and which relieves the feeling of over-fullness in the stomach, is known as a carminative. Those which act chiefly on the skin are oil of turpentine, cade, camphor, menthol, oil of mustard, oil of cajuput, oil of eucalyptus, arnica flowers, and myrrh. Oil of peppermint may be taken internally for the relief of flatulence. Other examples of carminatives are aniseed, allspice, cloves, cinnamon, bitter orange, and dill. Dill water is a common carminative for children and it is greatly used to cover the taste of sodium salts.

CAROTID ARTERY. The two great arteries down each side of the neck are called the carotids, or common carotids, and

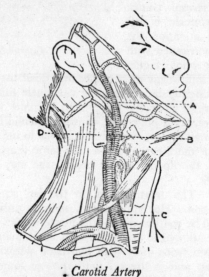

Carotid Artery
A. External Carotid; B. Internal Carotid;
C. Common Carotid; D. Jugular Vein.

by them blood is carried to the head and neck. The right common carotid artery rises from the *innominate artery* where it forks off from the *aorta* just behind the junction of the breast-bone and collar-bone. It travels upwards until a point at the level of the larynx or Adam's apple is reached, when it divides into two branches, the *external carotid* and the *internal carotid*. The left common carotid artery rises from the uppermost part of the *arch of the aorta* and travels upwards to the same distance as the right common carotid where it also splits into the left external and internal carotid. The external carotids supply the scalp, the face and the greater part of the neck, while the internal carotids feed parts within the skull and the cavities which contain the eyes. (*See also* ARTERY ; AORTA.)

CARRIER. It sometimes happens that a person may have in his body harmful germs to which his blood has grown so accustomed and has developed so many *antibodies*, that they do him no harm, but may be transferred to people whose resistance to them is not so strong and who therefore become victims of the infection. These harbourers of germs are known as " carriers."

CARRON OIL. Carron oil is a mixture of equal parts of linseed oil and lime water and is greatly used in the treatment of burns. This oil takes its name from the Carron Iron Works in Scotland, where it was introduced. Carron oil should only be applied if the skin is unbroken, but tannic acid or picric acid solutions are better treatment. (*See* BURNS.)

CARTILAGE. Cartilage, which is commonly known as gristle, is found in various parts of the body, chiefly in joints. The walls of the chest, the windpipe, the bronchial tubes, and the structure of the nose and ears are of cartilage. Most of the bones of the body develop from cartilage, which is replaced by bone as the infant grows older.

Certain joints of the hinge variety have small separate pads of cartilage, each of which is called a *meniscus*. These menisci are easily dislocated and cause pain and loss of power in the joint until they are replaced. The commonest of these dislocations are those of the semi-lunar cartilage of the knee and the cartilage of the jaw.

CASCARA SAGRADA. Cascara sagrada is a very serviceable drug for the treatment of chronic constipation, as one of its great advantages is that gradually increasing doses are not required. The liquid extract is very bitter, but this can be circumvented by taking the drug in capsule form, or the taste may be concealed by various aromatic substances, a well-known palatable preparation being cascara evacuant. The drug should be taken on retiring at night and continued for about ten days, gradually lessening the dose until finally the medicine may be stopped altogether. Constipation in a child will often be relieved by one to three drops in syrup, one to three times a day.

CASEATION. This term is applied to a form of degeneration, in which the structures of the body are converted into a soft, cheese-like substance, usually due to tuberculosis.

CASEIN. The chief protein constituent of milk, the curd, is known as casein. It is obtained from the milk by the action of acids and rennet, and is much the same thing as white of egg, but contains more nitrogen and a large amount of phosphorus. It constitutes the curd of milk, and in human milk the curd is much less firm than in cow's milk.

In order to obtain a light, easily-digested curd, milk may be diluted with soda water, and for a baby's bottle, the cow's milk may be diluted by adding some lime water.

CASTOR OIL. One of the most useful and indispensable drugs we possess is castor oil. It is exceedingly disagreeable to take in an undisguised form, but since it is so very valuable as a medicine the patient would be well advised to make up his mind both to swallow it and to keep it down when it is swallowed.

Castor oil is so useful because it is almost the only purge which will clear the bowel thoroughly with one dose of medicine, and it does not cause unpleasant griping pains. For this reason it is used when some doubtful article of food has been eaten and it is desired to get it thoroughly cleared out of the bowel before it can do further damage, or in cases where something is irritating the intestine which has not been removed by other aperients. It is given as a routine dose the night before an operation, so that no inconvenience will be caused by a loaded bowel at the time of the operation.

Castor oil can now be obtained in capsules and there are also many preparations of castor oil on the market in which the taste and smell are reduced to a minimum.

CATALEPSY. Is a condition in which there is a blind obedience to any suggestion made. People so affected will imitate any action seen ; they will repeat like parrots any short sentences spoken to them ; and they will allow their limbs to remain placed in any awkward position. In many cases there is also an obedience to orders, however absurd, or however dangerous their nature. This is something like the condition which is seen in people who have been deeply hypnotized, but goes beyond it. Catalepsy is more often seen in people suffering from a grave mental disorder, dementia præcox, but it may also occur occasionally in the course of some forms of hysteria.

CATAPHORESIS. *See* IONIZATION.

CATARACT. Cataract is a disease in which vision is more or less obscured because the lens of the eye becomes progressively more opaque, or, rather, intransparent. The patient " sees through a glass darkly."

Cataract is a very common disease ; it has been estimated that it is present in 96 per cent. of people over sixty, but it is usually so slight that it gives rise to no trouble. Sometimes, however, the density of the lens increases, and the patient has what is known as a *hard* or *senile cataract*. It begins usually about fifty-five or sixty.

Roughly speaking, there is only one symptom, that of increasing difficulty of sight. This is worse in a bright light. In the great majority of cases, both eyes are affected, though the cataract is not necessarily equally advanced ; this point is of considerable importance when treatment is to be decided upon. When the cataract is advanced, and practically the whole lens is affected, the appearance is as if the pupil were filled with ground glass.

The various treatments that have been tried to prevent or retard cataract are legion, and none of them is of the slightest use. Two palliative or " relieving " measures only need be noticed. One is a preliminary operation (iridectomy), which is favoured by some surgeons ; the other is the use of atropine drops in very weak strength, which assist in dilating the pupil, and so give better sight for the time being by illuminating the outer and less affected portions of the lens. Atropine must be used with very great care, and only under medical supervision, or a disease known as *glaucoma* might be caused.

Treatment. If vision is fairly good, it is often better policy to correct it as far as may be with glasses, and leave well alone. On the other hand, if vision is seriously interfered with, the proper course is to operate.

CATARRH. Inflammation of mucous membrane in any part of the body is known as catarrh, though frequently the word is used to describe a catarrhal cold in the head. When the mucous membrane of an organ is inflamed owing to the action of harmful bacteria or the presence of irritating material it usually gives off a wet discharge, as in the case of acute nasal catarrh or bronchitis, which is inflammation of the bronchial tubes. Catarrhal conditions of the bowel and stomach are very frequent both in temporary and chronic form. They are known as gastritis and colitis. Catarrh of the gall-bladder is cholecystitis. The term summer catarrh is sometimes used to describe hay fever, and catarrhal fever is usually influenza. Dry catarrh is the term used for a kind of bronchitis with cough and pain but no expectoration.

CATARRH, NASAL. Nasal catarrh or persistent discharge from the nose is often looked upon as a disease, and is popularly

5 *

supposed to be incurable. It is not, however, a disease, but only a symptom that something is wrong with the nose. A great many conditions can give rise to nasal catarrh and most of them are curable. The most frequent cause of nasal catarrh is repeated attacks of cold in the head, which is an infectious disease and is caused by quite a large number of different microbes, some of which are more virulent than others. When the microbes are of a mild type the cold usually clears up quite soon ; but when a more virulent type of microbe is responsible, such as the germs of influenza or pneumonia, it may not clear up and a chronic catarrh results.

Treatment. One of the best methods of treating chronic nasal catarrh is by a simple nasal douche. This should not be sniffed up the nose, but allowed to run through from a glass douche, or else syringed up by a rubber ball syringe. If the douche is sniffed up it may convey infection to the other parts of the nose and even to the ears. A favourite douche is to take equal parts of bicarbonate of soda, borax and common salt, and make them into a powder. A ½-teaspoonful of this powder to a ½-pint of warm water is douched up the nose once or twice a day. Some people prefer nasal drops of menthol in liquid paraffin, 10 grains of methol to 1 oz. of liquid paraffin. If these simple methods do not clear up the nasal catarrh after carrying them out regularly for three or four weeks, the nose should be examined by a doctor as there may be an infection of one of the air sinuses of the nose, or nasal polypi may be present, or the bone of the nose may be bent, preventing proper drainage.

CATGUT. Catgut is the material used for tying blood-vessels or stitching together skin and tissues in surgery. It is necessary for this purpose to use a material that can be thoroughly sterilized and which will also be absorbed in time. A material that is absorbed too quickly would not serve the purpose, nor would one that did not absorb at all. The guts or intestine of various animals has been found to answer the purpose almost perfectly, and the prepared material, from whatever animal it comes, is collectively called *catgut*.

CATHARTIC. *See* APERIENT.

CATHETER. Tubes of rubber or metal which are used for passing into a cavity through a narrow canal are called catheters. The most usual one is the urethral catheter, designed to pass through the urethra or canal through which the urine is discharged from the bladder.

CAUL. On the head of a new-born child there may be a sort of cap formed by the membranes with which it was covered in the womb. As a general rule the baby's head ruptures these membranes in passing and they are left behind, but occasionally a portion remains adhering to the baby's head. This is known as the caul. This membrane used to be considered to have magic powers and a dried caul carried by a sailor at sea was supposed to protect him from drowning.

CAUSTIC. Caustics are substances which are able to destroy tissues. They may be applied to the skin as a liquid or a solid. The most commonly known caustic is silver nitrate or caustic lunar which is greatly used to destroy warts.

CAUTERY. It is sometimes very necessary to destroy portions of tissue and this can be done by cautery much more efficiently than by the action of caustics. There are many kinds of cautery, but as a rule this operation is carried out by an instrument heated by an electric current, or in a flame. *Actual* cautery is carried out with a white-hot iron, while *button* cautery is carried out with an iron heated in hot water. In *galvanic* cautery a platinum wire is heated by electricity and applied to the part to be destroyed. The use of the cautery knife is not yet very widespread, but its possibilities in surgery are unlimited. One great advantage of the cautery operation is that it absolutely prevents bleeding from the tissues and a patient may have small portions done at a time in order to prevent the shock of one big operation. (*See also* DIATHERMY.)

CELL. Cells are the tiny particles of living matter of various sorts from which the whole human body is built up, just as a huge building is built of small stones. In the case of any building its stones can be seen, but in the body the cells are so minute that high-powered microscopes are required to see them. Under the microscope a single cell looks like a tiny drop of jelly with a speck in it. In the beginning our bodies start as a single cell containing this speck which is called the *nucleus*. The firmer substance of the cell is called the *protoplasm*. The nucleus contains still smaller particles called the *nucleoles*. The protoplasm of which the cell chiefly consists is able to move and to take substances into itself for food purposes. Its chief characteristic is that it *grows* and *multiplies*, and changes its form so that the one cell from which we start in our mother's womb increases itself with great rapidity through all the stages of larger and larger embryos until a complicated human body has been built up, composed of millions of cells of different sorts and uses and the baby is born. It continues growing by cell multiplication and differentiation and finally becomes a man or woman.

Cell reproduction and growth. Cells reproduce themselves by dividing. A change begins to take place in the nucleus which divides into two halves which are known as the daughter nuclei. Each of these daughter nuclei forms the nucleus of two new cells. These again divide, which makes four cells from the original one.

Division continues thus until masses of cells are formed. At an early stage the cells which are to form the organs, the bones and so forth of the body are differentiated from the others, and when they reproduce themselves they form other cells in their own likeness. As well as building the body and its various organs, the cells produce amongst themselves the various substances which are used in the mechanism of the body, the lubricating oils, the food digesters, etc. The life of cells is naturally not as long as the life of the body ; they die and are replaced unto many generations. They can also become ill or damaged and be repaired. It will be seen therefore that the cells are the agents by which the body is built up, and is kept in repair. Certain diseases of the body, noticeably tumours and especially cancers, are caused by irregular growth of certain cells. For some reason, or reasons, which have not been fathomed, they change the character of their growth.

CELLULITIS. When the cellular tissue under the skin becomes infected by harmful germs it becomes inflamed. The inflammation may be localized to a particular small spot, in which case a boil or abscess forms, or it may be general over a larger area but may not show any tendency to gather to a head in any particular spot. This condition is called cellulitis and shows that the tissues are successfully resisting the invasion of the germs. There will be an area of reddened skin with no very definite edges. The skin may be shiny and the region is swollen and tender.

Treatment. To treat the condition heat should be applied locally, either in the form of hot baths or fomentations, or in a dry form such as hot-air baths or hot pads. The part should be kept raised if possible and must be kept at rest. Counter irritation in the form of iodine, cantharides or mustard plaster may be applied. Cupping or treatment by suction bells is sometimes employed. The cellulitis may disappear without coming to active suppuration. But if suppuration arises it must be treated, as in the case of an abscess, by incision. (*See also* ABSCESS ; BOIL.)

CEREALS. The cereals have always provided an important source of food to the human race. The varieties which we make most use of include wheat, rye, maize, oats, barley, millet and rice. Owing to their deficiency of protein and fat, cereals and their food products should be supplemented with other substances such as milk, cream, nuts, butter or eggs, as for example, bread and butter, milk puddings, etc.

CEREBELLUM. The cerebellum is the part of the brain which lies below and behind the cerebrum. (*See also* BRAIN.)

CEREBRO-SPINAL FEVER is an infectious disease caused by a tiny germ which enters the patient's body through the nose and throat and from there reaches the nervous system, where it causes inflammation of the coverings of the brain and spinal cord. The disease often occurs in epidemics, especially in the winter and spring, and during an epidemic very large numbers of people may be attacked by the disease owing to the fact that certain people, known as " carriers," do not themselves fall victims to the disease, though they harbour in their noses and throats the microbes which can infect those with whom they come into contact. The disease can occur at any age, though in most epidemics young children are most frequently affected. Children are very liable to the disease, and it is particularly dangerous in infants between the ages of six months and three years. There are many and varied forms of the disease, but the acute type is by far the most common.

Symptoms. The patient has an intense headache, usually felt at the back of the head ; he feels generally out of sorts, and the temperature goes up. The earliest sign which may make one suspect the presence of cerebro-spinal fever is stiffness of the muscles of the back of the neck. This soon becomes very marked, and the patient finds that any attempt to bring the head forward gives him pain. He therefore lies in bed with the head drawn backwards and resents any attempt to make him bring the chin down towards the chest. There is very often a shivering attack at this stage, or in children, a convulsion.

Vomiting, not associated with the taking of food, may occur, but is more common in children than in grown-ups. The mental condition soon becomes typical of irritation of the brain ; the patient lies huddled up in bed, unwilling to move, disliking any interference, whether this be to feed him, to examine him, or even to talk to him. He may become delirious, talking utter nonsense, or he may lie in a condition of complete apathy, taking no notice of anything, the eyes being open and staring, with a peculiar vacant look. Young children are especially liable to lie motionless, this condition being interrupted at intervals by a distinctive cry, which can never be forgotten by anyone who has once heard it, so high-pitched and anxious is it. The cry is independent of any headache the child may have, and is quite purposeless, though no less distressing to those who have to listen to it.

In a considerable number of cases a rash appears over the body and arms during the first week of the illness. The rash may take the form of large rose-red spots, or it may look rather like a measles rash. The patient loses flesh rapidly, and at the end of a week appears quite wasted. Loss of sleep, which is the usual accompaniment of the severe headache, adds to the patient's misery. If the illness has not been diagnosed by the end of the first week and the

essential treatment has not been given, the outlook for recovery
is poor, but in few other illnesses, if any, is it possible for a patient
to be so ill and yet to recover completely, as in cerebro-spinal fever,
provided that the adequate treatment is forthcoming early enough.
The certain diagnosis is made by examination of the fluid which
surrounds the spinal cord. Some of this is taken by puncturing the
space between the spinal cord and its coverings in the lower part
of the back and withdrawing the fluid with a syringe. In cerebro-
spinal fever the fluid looks cloudy when it is withdrawn, owing to
the presence of many pus cells in it.

Treatment. As soon as the diagnosis is settled, treatment by
serum is carried out, and this is absolutely essential. The earlier
the serum treatment is given the better the hope of complete recovery.
Hence the extreme importance of early puncture of the spinal
canal. The serum is given into the canal, and the results of its
administration are often dramatic. The patient who has lain
apparently unconscious for several days may after one dose of
serum become quite normal mentally, and though weak and exhausted, presents quite a different picture to that seen before the
serum was given. Vigorous serum treatment is, however, essential
as relapses are common, and it is not safe to depend on one dose
of serum to establish a lasting improvement, even in mild cases.

A case of cerebro-spinal fever is best in hospital, as the illness
is not only an exhausting, but a distressing one to watch. If the
patient is nursed at home, the main trouble is to ensure that enough
food is taken to maintain his strength as far as possible. In the
early stages, when the patient is irritable and resentful of attention,
it may be very hard to persuade him to take even a liquid diet.
Raw eggs, beaten up in milk, freshly prepared meat essences, and
as much water as the patient can be induced to take should be
given in small quantities at frequent intervals. Later in the course
of the illness, when the patient is only semi-conscious, the act of
swallowing cannot be relied on, as some of the food may " go the
wrong way " and enter the lungs. Feeding by means of a nasal
tube, inserted by the doctor, three or four times a day, must then
be resorted to. According to the age of the patient, from a quarter
to half a pint of peptonized milk, or of beef essence, is given at
each feed. A raw egg may be given with the milk. The bowels
must be kept well opened. Tepid sponging often helps to soothe
the restless patient when the fever is at its height. Those in attendance
on the patient should pay great attention to personal cleanliness,
and should come into contact with as few people as possible whilst
they are in charge of the case, for fear of spreading the disease.
They should gargle the throat twice a day with either a weak

solution of permanganate of potash (a solution which is faintly pink is the right strength), or with a half-strength solution of peroxide of hydrogen. The latter solution can also be used to sniff up the nose, or the nose may be sprayed with a weak solution of iodine and menthol. Those in attendance on a case of cerebrospinal fever rarely themselves take the disease ; the danger is that they may give it to other people.

CERVICAL. This word is derived from the Latin, and literally means " the neck." It is applied to various glands and nerves which lie in the region of the neck, and there are also the *cervical vertebræ*. It is also used to denote the *cervix* or neck of the womb.

CERVIX. The cervix is the neck of the womb. It is a frequent focus of ill-health in women because it is so often torn during childbirth. If the tear is neglected and becomes infected with harmful germs, it may cause serious trouble, and very often a small tear will be responsible for the state of poor health which many women fall a victim to, in which there is a chronic slight discharge from the front passage and chronic feelings of discomfort and tiredness. An old and neglected cervical tear may become the seat of cancer at a later stage. A doctor should be consulted, as the condition is very amenable to skilled treatment.

CHAFING. When two surfaces of skin rub together it produces a condition of irritation known as chafing or intertrigo. (*See also* INTERTRIGO.)

CHALK. Chalk or calcium carbonate is used in medicine in many different ways. In the prepared form, which is calcium carbonate freed from most of its impurities by washing and drying, it is used as a dusting-powder, and it also forms one of the ingredients of many of the tooth powders. It may be used internally with great benefit in cases of diarrhœa and colitis, and also in chronic dyspepsia.

CHALK STONES. Chalk stones are often referred to as goutstones or *tophi*, and are found under the skin of gouty people. Although these deposits are called chalk stones they are made up of sodium urate. The most common site for these stone-like deposits is about the knuckles and the lobes of the ear. (*See also* GOUT.)

CHANCRE. A chancre is an ulcer which develops about four weeks after infection by one of the venereal diseases, usually syphilis. (*See also* SYPHILIS.)

CHANCROID. This term is applied to a soft sore, caused by venereal disease. (*See also* CHANGRE.)

CHANGE OF LIFE. Women have many ways of referring to the period when their child-bearing life ceases, but the most common popular name for it is the change of life. Doctors talk of it as the climacteric or menopause, or sometimes even the critical age. This last name is a very suitable one, because the change of life is always a critical age for women. Many women pass through the change with little discomfort ; some have a bad time for a couple of years, and then take a new lease of life and begin to enjoy themselves again ; while others, unfortunately, settle down to a life of invalidism and misery. Many of the sufferings of these women could be avoided with proper care and consideration during the critical age.

The chief physical change that takes place at this time is that the ovaries and other organs of reproduction cease to perform their function and become atrophied and shrivelled. This change occurs at different ages in different types of women, but it is somewhere between the ages of thirty-five and fifty-five—between forty-five and fifty being the most usual age. As a general rule, it may be taken that the earlier the menstrual periods start, the longer they will go on, and that the women in the same family are likely to have the change of life at about the same age. Certain factors make slight differences to the age at which the change may be expected. For instance, very early marriage may shorten the sexual life, and spinsters and childless women are likely to reach the change some years before married women who have had children and have led a normal sexual life. States of health in which the vitality is lowered may also bring on the change at an earlier age.

Physical Changes. It has been said above that some women pass through the climacteric without any particular discomfort, but these are in the minority. Most women feel discomfort in various degrees, and some women become upset mentally.

It is not always easy for a woman to know when she is approaching the change of life, and the first time a period is missed for a few days she may imagine that she has become pregnant. In most cases the periods cease gradually, either by becoming scantier until they finally cease or by missing three or four months at a time, then appearing again in a regular fashion for some more months until they again disappear for some more months. The time taken from the first irregularities until the final ceasing of the periods is usually between one and two years. In a few cases the periods stop suddenly and completely, and there is generally a large amount of disturbance to the general health with this type of climacteric. In the earlier stages of the change there may be an increased flow at the periods instead of the usual diminished flow. This excessive flow, or *menorrhagia*, as it is called, should cease after a few months. If it does not do so a visit should be paid to the doctor, as it may be the sign of some trouble, such as a fibroid tumour or even the beginning of cancer, and such conditions can be cured if taken in time.

The unpleasant symptoms which are very general amongst women at the climacteric are mostly due to the upset of the nervous system. These are flushes, nervousness and irritability, disturbances of the circulation causing " pins and needles," etc., and dyspepsia and neuralgia of various sorts. It is also noticeable that many women become unduly fat at this time.

Flushing. Of the symptoms of the climacteric the condition known as flushing is the most distinctive. It is a rush of blood to some part of the body, such as the face, or it may be a sudden hot feeling all over the body. These hot flushes may be followed by feelings of chilliness. Palpitations are also frequently present. The heart may suddenly be felt thumping rapidly, and the woman may feel breathless and alarmed for a short time. The attacks of palpitation may come on after exertion or at any odd time without rhyme or reason. In some women they come on at night and waken them up out of their sleep. These flushings are very unpleasant, but are in nowise dangerous, and always vanish after the change of life has become established. Ringing in the ears and dizziness are also frequently present.

Neuralgia. One of the most troublesome accompaniments of the change of life is neuralgia. It occurs in many forms. Sometimes it is merely fleeting pains in different parts of the body, or it may attack some particular part such as the breast. If pain occurs in the breast at this time it is as well to have an examination by a doctor, as cancer of the breast is liable to start at this age. Another painful form of this malady which is not uncommon at this time is neuralgia of the stomach, in which pains are felt in the middle region of the abdomen. Headache, especially one-sided headache, is common, and backache often occurs.

Obesity. The tendency to put on flesh about the time of the climacteric is distressing to many women. There are a few cases where the increase in weight is accompanied by dryness of the skin, falling out of the hair, dulling of the intelligence and slowing of the heart's action. In these cases there is some glandular deficiency in the thyroid gland or the pancreas which should be corrected by the administration of thyroid extract, or in certain cases, insulin. These remedies should, of course, only be taken under a doctor's care. (*See also* OBESITY.)

Nervous symptoms. As well as the physical changes that take place at the change of life there are mental changes. The sexual desires are diminished in most cases, though in happily married couples complete loss of desire rarely if ever takes place as a result of the menopause. On the other hand, some women, especially those of neurotic temperament, feel greatly increased desire, and in some cases become unable to control their emotions. These women may be such a nuisance that they have to be shut up in institutions where they can be cared for by specially trained nurses. Their behaviour, too, may cause the break-up of a home that has hitherto been happy. Forbearance on the part of the husband may tide over the dangerous period until the wife returns to a more normal frame of mind. At this time also, the unattached woman of this neurotic, over-sexed type often falls a prey to designing persons of either sex. She may rush into a hasty and disastrous marriage often with someone young enough to be her son, or she may land herself in other undesirable situations.

In many other ways the general health of a woman may suffer at the climacteric. She may have indigestion in various forms ; constipation may be troublesome, etc. All these conditions should be corrected in the ordinary way, but it is a very great mistake for a woman to consider herself an invalid at this period. Her life should be modified if possible so that she may go slowly, avoid as much worry as possible, and have extra rest when the need is felt. A placid and easy-going existence is the best at this period, but the slowing down should be regarded as temporary, just a well-earned rest before embarking on a new phase of life. Many women really begin thoroughly to enjoy life after the menopause, and their health improves almost as if the cessation of the reproductive functions had released more energy for the upkeep of the body.

CHAPS. Chaps are the sore cracks that come on the hands, face or other exposed parts of the body in frosty weather.

CHAULMOOGRA. Chaulmoogra oil is obtained from an evergreen shrub which grows in Burma and other parts. This oil is used a great deal in the treatment of leprosy, and it is also given for tuberculosis and rheumatism.

CHEIROPOMPHOLYX. This disease with the long name is quite common and can be very irritating. It chiefly affects the hands between the fingers, and may extend on to the backs or palms of the hands and up the arms. The feet are also frequently affected. Both hands may be involved. The disease consists in the development of small blisters filled with clear fluid, and almost embedded in the skin.

Treatment. Two different views are held as to the cause of cheiropompholyx—one that it is nervous in origin, and the other that it is due to infection by germs. Those who hold the first view leave the skin condition alone, and treat the complaint by tonics and other measures to improve the general health. Those who hold the second view treat the condition by frequent bathing with antiseptic solutions, such as weak mercury sublimate and the application of salicylic acid as an ointment or dusting powder. The possibility of *ringworm* or " itch " is always considered, and a proper examination made to exclude this. When the attack is over, the excessive sweating should be treated, and the hands " hardened " by resorcin or formalin soap. If the disease has spread to the backs of the arms and hands, it often appears to be more acute, and a soothing treatment is required. Calamine lotion or a simple dusting powder (talc, not starch) is preferable to the antiseptic treatment mentioned above.

CHEST. Chest is the popular name for the *thorax* or upper part of the trunk of the body. It is a framework of bone and cartilage in which are found the principal organs of breathing and circulation. The lungs and heart are vital to the maintenance of life, and are of soft, easily damaged material and require room for expansion. The chest therefore takes the form of a strong bony cage in which these vital organs are protected from injury and in which they have room to contract and expand freely.

The chest extends from the shoulders to the diaphragm. Its principal bony structure is the spine. From the spine the twenty-four ribs extend, curving round to meet the breast-bone or *sternum* in front. The first five ribs on each side extend directly from the spine to the breast-bone, the second five join into one bone before being attached to the breast-bone, and the last two on each side float loose in front, and are attached only to the spine, and not to the breast-bone. The ends of the ribs, where they join the breast-bone, are formed not of bone but of cartilage, which give them a certain amount of flexibility, and enables them to be moved by the chest muscles as they expand and contract in the process of breathing in and out.

The measurement round the chest in men is usually between 32 and 42 inches, but the girth is not so important as the difference between the measurements taken during breathing in and breathing out, which gives the range of movement of the chest. A good range of movement is conducive to good health. Many people are born with narrow chests which are not necessarily weak chests, but they should try to develop them by breathing exercises, correct posture and as much open air as possible, as the narrow or small chest is more liable to lung troubles than the broad chest. It is useful to accustom weak-chested children at an early age to sleeping with the window open at night.

The chest in old age or as a result of chronic bronchitis may become rounded, or, as it is called, barrel-shaped, through chronic enlargement. In this type of chest the range of movement will be very small, probably not more than one inch difference between breathing in and breathing out. Rickets in infancy is responsible for two common sorts of deformity of the chest. The condition called *pigeon-breast* is very common in rickety children, and there may also be bony swellings on the ribs where they join on to the breast-bone causing a condition popularly known as "rickety rosary." (*See also* HEART ; INTERCOSTAL ; LUNG ; RIBS, ETC.)

CHICKEN-POX. Chicken-pox or varicella is an acute infectious disease characterized by a typical rash and accompanied by fever. Infection is spread by direct contact, by a third person, or the germ may be inhaled. The organism which causes this disease has not yet been identified. Children are chiefly affected, but adults are also liable to infection. The incubation period lasts from 11 to 21 days, but symptoms generally make their appearance about 14 days after infection. The rash may be the first symptom, but in adults especially, the eruption of the rash may be preceded by headache, backache, discomfort and shivering.

At the beginning of the disease there may be a slight rash or flush, appearing one or two days before the true rash appears. The typical rash may appear on the second day. It attacks the front and back of the trunk of the body and the inner sides of the thighs, and later may spread to the face, scalp, and limb endings. The legs, forearms, feet and hands are generally involved to a lesser degree, and in very rare cases spots may appear on the mucous membranes of the mouth or throat. These spots very quickly become pustular and may burst in about 2 days' time. The rash comes out in crops for the first 2 to 7 days, so that spots in the various stages may be seen simultaneously on the body. The vesicles or spots finally dry up into a scab and a crust, which may take from 4 days to 4 weeks to drop off. Scarring does not occur unless the tissues of the skin have been destroyed, but on separation of the scab a slight redness may be present which usually fades and leaves a white spot which may last for years.

The temperature is usually only slightly raised, but in severe cases may be considerably high for a few days. Gangrenous chicken-pox, resembling smallpox, in which the tissues of the skin die, is to be met with in very debilitated children, and is sometimes fatal. In hæmorrhagic chicken-pox bleeding may appear under the skin, or there may be bleeding from the mucous membranes.

Chicken-pox is one of the milder diseases, and its course should be uneventful, except for the severe types. Complications do not, as a rule, arise, but cases of earache, inflammation of the kidneys, laryngitis, and various nervous complications such as neuritis, meningitis and encephalitis, sometimes occur.

Treatment. The patient should be put to bed until the temperature has returned to normal and all spots have reached the crusting stage. Usually the only treatment required, beyond that necessary for any mild fever, is a local application to ease the irritation of the skin. The patient must never be allowed to scratch. the spots. A dusting powder of equal parts of starch, zinc oxide and borax may be applied. During the period when the crusts are beginning to form the body may be sponged with warm water containing enough potassium permanganate to colour it pink. In the final stage, after the crusts have come away, zinc ointment may be applied to the tender skin which is left.

The period of quarantine generally lasts for about 20 days for those persons who have been in contact with the disease, and the patient must be isolated until the scab has come off, which usually takes from 3 to 4 weeks.

CHILBLAINS. This disease is only too well known. It occurs during the winter months only, and is found especially in children who are below par (though it may occur at any age). The patients are subject to colds and chills, and, though the heart itself may be healthy, the circulation is somewhat defective. Cold damp weather seems to favour the appearance of chilblains, rather than dry and frosty air ; and thin clothes and underfeeding are undoubted factors in their production. Tight boots and gloves, and the too-rapid warming of the hands after exposure to cold, are also blamed.

Treatment is conducted on three lines : general, local, and preventive, the last of which nowadays should be considered as of quite as much importance as the others. They all work towards the same end, that of improving the circulation, both local and general. Internally, cod-liver oil and tonics, such as Easton's syrup and Fowler's solution, are given to benefit the general health. Calcium preparations have become very popular of late years. Various ways of giving this have been tried, but the most convenient method is to use calcium lactate tablets, 5 grains, 2 or 3 to be taken 3 times daily. It was thought that calcium, which has an effect on the clotting power of the blood, might be an infallible remedy in cases of chilblains, and sometimes it does produce excellent results. In other cases, the effects are disappointing ; it is, however, well worth a trial.

The local applications recommended are too many even to name ; only those which have been proved worthy will be mentioned. When itching is the most prominent symptom, calamine lotion, menthol, or cold water applications seem to give most relief.

Iodine, in ointment, tincture or collodion, appears to be the most generally successful routine treatment, but must not be over-done, or an " iodine itching " may occur, which may be almost as troublesome as the chilblains themselves. A convenient method is to use the weak tincture of iodine (5 per cent.) as a paint for two nights, and on the third a mild ointment. This may be continued as long as the iodine causes no irritation. If the chilblains have broken, a mild ointment should be used, the object of treatment now being not to stimulate the circulation but to heal the ulcers. Cold cream, boric ointment, and ammoniated mercury in zinc paste are all good. Arctic explorers use an " ointment " of whisky and soap, which is said to be equally effective.

In very bad cases, hot-air baths and X-rays have been found useful, also electric treatment by the high-frequency current, but these methods are not within the reach of all.

The preventive method has been neatly summed up in a few words : prepare in summer for the winter. In other words, preventive treatment must not be given up as soon as the winter's crop of chilblains disappear. *All* cold must be avoided.

CHILD-BED FEVER. Child-bed fever is a popular name for the serious infectious disease that arises in women during the lying-in period after the birth of a child. It is described under its medical name of PUERPERAL FEVER.

CHILDBIRTH, PREPARATIONS FOR. In a normal case with a first baby, pregnancy can often be calculated to a definite date by counting nine months and one week from the first day of the last period before the pregnancy began. This should give the earliest date at which the baby may be expected. There are, however, often variations, usually in the way of arriving too soon, but with first babies it is surprising with what punctuality most of them make their appearance in the world. The date of " quickening " is also a guide, as it occurs half-way through the pregnancy.

Before the date of the expected arrival of the child, the mother, if she is wise, should have had several examinations either by her own doctor or at an ante-natal clinic to see that all is in order and going on well. The most dreaded complication of the later stages of pregnancy and the confinement and lying-in period is the condition called eclampsia, in which convulsive fits occur. This condition can usually be avoided if examinations of the pregnant woman's urine are made from time to time during the pregnancy, since the chief symptom that there is a danger of eclampsia is the appearance of albumen in the urine. The medical examinations may reveal other important matters as well. For instance, if the child is lying in the wrong position for birth, it may be necessary to turn it round in the womb. It will also be ascertained whether twins are present, and whether the bony ring surrounding the exit from the womb is larger than the head of the child. If it is not, and the condition is not discovered until the birth has begun, there will be serious trouble ; whereas, if the condition is known in time several things can be done.

When all these preliminary examinations show that pregnancy is progressing normally, it is the duty of the expectant mother to keep her health as good as possible, and to prepare for the approaching event with a quiet mind. The nurse or midwife should be engaged well beforehand, as the best ones quickly get booked up. She will advise as to the choice of a room for the confinement, and as to what to prepare in the way of waterproof sheets and other necessary equipment.

Equipment that will be needed.   For a well-equipped confinement which is to take place at home and not in a hospital, the following articles are desirable. A waterproof sheet about a yard and a half square, and an old sheet to use as a draw sheet. A couple of large rolls of cotton-wool and three binders. A special size of sanitary towel is provided by all the makers for use in confinements. Three dozen will be needed. Special surgical safety-pins are safer than the ordinary domestic ones if they can be procured ; several, both large and small, will be required for the baby's binder and the mother's. Green or castile soap and a clean nail-brush. A bed-pan, douche-can and three feet of rubber tubing to fit in. Strong scissors, two enamel bowls about a foot across, and two hot-water bottles. A roller towel is often useful, and linen thread will be required. A bottle of disinfectant—usually lysol, unless something else has been asked for by the midwife. Vaseline, methylated spirits, boracic powder for the baby's eyes, and a bath thermometer are other requirements. It will usually be found that some of these things, such as the waterproof sheeting, bed-pan and douche, can be borrowed from friends or hired from a chemist. A special tin of dressings for confinements can be obtained from the chemist, which will save a lot of trouble, if the expense is not too great.

The layette, or outfit for the baby, should be ready a couple of weeks before the birth is expected. A week or so before the date when the confinement is expected to begin, the room in which it is to take place should be thoroughly " spring-cleaned " and all unnecessary furniture and ornaments put away. The bed chosen for the confinement should be a single one and should not be too low, or it will mean a lot of stooping for the doctor and nurse.

The actual progress of the confinement is described in a separate article called LABOUR, and the after-events are described under the heading PUERPERIUM, which is the name for the period after the confinement before the mother is restored to her normal state of health—the lying-in period. (*See also* PREGNANCY.)

CHILL. A person usually complains of feeling chilly when they have been exposed to a draught, or when they have been out in the wet on a cold day. Shivering may be followed by symptoms of a common cold, with catarrh of the nose, and in more severe cases, influenza, pneumonia, or inflammation of the throat may result. Chill may be experienced in many diseases, especially in cases of malaria. The patient should be put to bed and kept warm with hot-water bottles and blankets, and hot drinks should be given. A very excellent drink is made up with whisky, lemon, sugar, and hot water. This should be given after the patient has been put to bed.

CHILLI PASTE. This is a paste made up of capsicum, hard and soft paraffin, and prepared lard. It is an excellent counter-irritant, and may be applied to the skin in cases of chronic rheumatism and neuralgia.

CHIMNEY-SWEEP'S CANCER. The form of cancer to which sweeps are especially subject is supposed to be caused by the fact that they work amongst soot, which causes irritation of the skin. (*See also* CANCER ; CANCER OF THE SKIN.)

CHIN-WELK. This is a popular name for the disfiguring blisters and pimples that are found on the chin in cases of BARBER'S ITCH, which is described under that heading.

CHIROPODY. By chiropody we mean the surgical care of the feet, which of course includes the treatment of corns and calluses. A person who specializes in the care of the feet is called a chiropodist.

CHIROPRACTIC. A system of medicine that lays down that all disease is due to maladjustments of the spinal vertebræ pressing upon the spinal nerves and that disease can be cured by correcting such maladjustments by manipulation. It resembles osteopathy, but has a rather more limited outlook. (*See* OSTEOPATHY.)

CHLOASMA. The development of patches of discoloration on the face, especially on the forehead, cheeks and on the skin around the mouth, is known as chloasma. These patches may be brown, yellow or black in colour, and may vary from the size of a sixpence to the size of the palm of the hand. They are often to be seen on the skin of pregnant women, or they may appear during the menstruation period. Chronic diseases of the womb may be responsible for the discoloration, or disorders of the liver may be the cause. People suffering from tuberculosis of the lungs often have these patches of discoloration on the forehead and upper parts of the cheeks.

CHLOROFORM. Chloroform is a colourless liquid, with a sweetish taste and a peculiar odour. It is largely used as a general anæsthetic. When breathed in it abolishes all sense of pain, and it is a particularly safe anæsthetic to give to young children or old people ; but it must be given mixed with plenty of air and by a doctor who understands its administration. A mixture which is known as A.C.E., containing alcohol, chloroform and ether, is used a good deal instead of pure chloroform, especially for operations which require that the patient shall be unconscious for a long time. Chloroform put up in small capsules may now be had all ready for use in cases of childbirth ; in this way the risk of an overdose is avoided. (*See also* ANÆSTHESIA.)

CHLOROSIS. Chlorosis, or " green sickness," as it is sometimes called, is a form of anæmia which occurs chiefly in young girls, though it has become rare in recent years, owing to the healthier lives they lead. A fuller description is given under the heading ANÆMIA.

CHOKING. For simple choking caused by a piece of food sticking in the throat or some such accident, an adult may be struck on the back between the shoulders, smartly but not too violently. A very young child may be lifted by the toes and held upside down for a few seconds. If these methods are not successful send for the doctor at once (*See* ASPHYXIA.)

CHOLAGOGUE. Cholagogue is the term applied to any substance which increases the flow of bile from the liver. (*See also* BILE.)

CHOLECYSTITIS. This is the medical name for inflammation of the gall-bladder, and is described under the heading of GALL-BLADDER, INFLAMMATION OF.

CHOLERA, ASIATIC. Cholera is an acute disease due to a specific organism known as the *cholera spirillum* or *Koch's bacillus.* The condition is characterized by very frequent watery stools, muscular cramps, suppression of urine and collapse. The germ is conveyed to man by means of infected water. Food and flies also act as carriers.

CHOLESTEROL. Cholesterol or cholesterin is the name of a substance which is present in the bile. It is found in the yolk of egg and in the blood. Gall-stones are frequently composed of cholesterol. (*See also* BILE ; GALL-STONES.)

CHOREA. Chorea is more popularly known as St. Vitus's dance. It is chiefly a disease of childhood, in which there are irregular and involuntary actions of the muscles of the face and limbs. (*See also* ST. VITUS'S DANCE.)

CHOROID, THE. The choroid is the middle of the three

coats of the eyeball, and lies between the white and the retina. In the front half of the eye it forms the ciliary processes, and beyond these, the iris. It is black in colour, and its use is to prevent " dazzling " and to ensure that objects are seen clearly. (*See* Eye.)

CHYLE. Chyle is the term applied to those ingredients of the food which, after passing through the stomach and being mixed with the gastric juices, are absorbed from the intestine, not by the blood, as is the case with the greater part of the absorbable ingredients of food, but by the *lymphatic glands*. The special lymphatics which deal with the absorption of chyle are called the *lacteals*, because of the milk-like appearance of their contents during the process of digestion. The parts of the food which are absorbed by the lacteals are the fats. The chyle is carried by way of the *thoracic duct* to the *left subclavian vein*, where it is emptied into the blood-stream. (*See also* Blood ; Digestion.)

CHYME. When food is well soaked with the gastric fluid and has been thoroughly mixed by the action of the stomach, the valve at the lower end of the stomach opens and the stomach contents are passed on into the *duodenum* in a form called chyme.

CICATRIX. The technical name for a scar. New scars are usually purplish or red, but after a time they become white and glistening. (*See also* Scar.)

CINCHONA BARK. This name is given to the dried bark of the stem and branches of cinchona trees, of which there are several varieties. *Quinine*, as well as other powerful drugs, is extracted from the bark. (*See also* Quinine.)

CIRCULATION OF THE BLOOD. The blood is circulated throughout the body by the heart and the blood-vessels. The different parts of the blood circulatory system are described in separate articles under the headings Artery, Blood, Capillaries, Heart, Vein. Only a brief description of them will be given here.

The *heart*, which is the central organ of the blood system, lies within the chest or thorax. It is a bag-shaped organ with a wall of muscle, and while the body is living it contracts at a definite rate, thus acting as a pump for pumping blood throughout the body. When this pump ceases its work the body ceases to live, and unless the heart's action is restored, death has taken place. The blood, pumped by the heart's contractions or beats, as they are called, flows into a system of long tubular vessels called *arteries*, and is carried by them to every part of the body. These arteries are branched in every direction to supply the limbs and outlying parts of the body with blood. Their branches are again branched, and so on until the smallest arteries are reached. These end in tiny vessels called *arterioles*, and the arterioles open into a net-work of infinitesimally small vessels called *capillaries*, which are only visible under a microscope. By the time the capillaries are reached the blood-stream has absorbed the oxygen from the air breathed in and

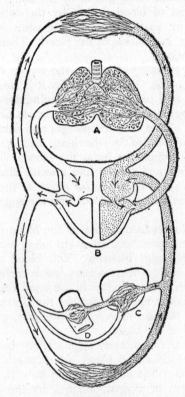

Circulation

Diagram showing circulation, Arterial blood to the left, Venous blood to the right. A. Lungs; B. Heart; C. Liver; D. Intestine; Capillaries at top and bottom.

nutriment from the various organs of the body where it is manufactured, and by means of the capillaries this nutriment is passed into the tissues of the body, and thus they are fed and enabled to carry on their work. The capillaries, as well as passing out nutriment into the tissues, collect from the tissues the waste materials which must be removed from the body in order to keep it in health.

These waste materials pass from the capillaries to tiny vessels called *venules*, which are in the same relation to the *veins* as the arterioles are to the arteries. The venules flow into the smaller veins, and the smaller veins join on to the main veins in a similar system to that of the arteries. By the veins, therefore, the bad blood containing the waste materials not required by the body is carried to the heart. This system of blood supply by the arteries and blood collection for return to the heart by the veins is known as the systemic or greater circulation of the blood. There are, however, two minor circulations.

In the lesser or *pulmonary circulation*, the venous blood enters the heart at the *right atrium*. From this cavity it is carried to the *right ventricle*, and from it is passed along the pulmonary arteries to the lungs, where it circulates throughout the whole tissue of the lung in the capillaries, giving off carbonic gas and other noxious substances which are exhaled by the lung, and receiving oxygen. After circulation through the lungs the blood, which is now reoxygenated, purified and turned into arterial blood, passes back through the *pulmonary veins* to the *left atrium* of the heart, whence it passes into the *left ventricle* and out into the systemic circulation again.

The other lesser circulation is that of the blood which circulates through the spleen, pancreas, stomach, small intestine and the greater part of the large intestine. This blood is not returned directly to the heart from these organs, but is carried by the *portal vein* to the liver, where it percolates in the small vessels of the liver, discarding toxic substances and leaving the organ by the *hepatic veins*, whence it is passed to the *inferior vena cava*, which conveys it to the *right atrium* of the heart.

The function of the circulatory system of the body is to convey to the tissues the fluid called blood, which contains the nourishment required to keep the body alive and in working order. This nourishment consists of oxygen obtained by the lungs from the air and nutritive substances obtained from the food. The way in which the nutritive substances are absorbed into the blood is described elsewhere. The second function of the circulatory system is to remove from the blood the impurities which it has absorbed from the system during its journey through the body. Two distinct sets of blood-vessels are used for these purposes. The arterial system conveys the pure and nutritive blood throughout the body and the venous system returns the impure blood to the heart. The heart serves the double purpose of dispatching arterial blood on its journey round the body and receiving back the impure blood, and also of dispatching the impure blood on its way to the lungs for purification and receiving it back for restoration to the main circulation.

CIRCUMCISION. Circumcision consists in the operation of the cutting off of the foreskin of the penis. This is quite a simple affair in baby boys, without any danger attaching to it, and is practised as a religious rite by Jews and Mohammedans. Among other people circumcision is usually done only when the foreskin is abnormally tight, but it would not be a bad thing if every male child were circumcised as a hygienic measure.

CIRRHOSIS. When the tissues of an organ have been chronically inflamed for a long time they may become fibrous and hard. This condition is known as *cirrhosis*. The organ which becomes *cirrhotic* is hindered in the carrying on of its work. The liver, kidney, heart and spleen are the organs chiefly affected, of which the liver is the most usually attacked.

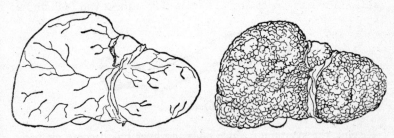

Cirrhosis of the Liver

A. Normal Liver; **B.** "Hob-nailed Liver."

CIRRHOSIS OF THE LIVER. This often goes by the names of " gin-drinker's liver " and " hob-nailed liver "—in the former case because of the belief that it is caused by the consumption of too much alcohol, and in the latter because the liver shrinks and develops a hard, knobby surface. It is thought that cirrhosis is frequently caused by the action of the common germs such as those which normally inhabit the bowels. They settle in the liver and cause a long chronic low infection of the organ. Or chemical irritants from a diet which is habitually rich in highly spiced foods such as curries may be absorbed by the liver and cause cirrhosis. It is believed that certain metallic poisons, particularly lead, will bring about this condition. The liver becomes congested with blood, first becomes very much enlarged, and then begins to shrink and harden. In some cases, however, it does not shrink, and has much the same appearance as a liver that has undergone fatty degeneration.

Symptoms. The majority of the sufferers from cirrhosis of the liver are males over forty, and it is more common amongst those working in the liquor trade and amongst commercial travellers than in other occupations. The patient usually has a feeling of discomfort in the pit of the stomach, with nausea, indigestion, sickness and vomiting. There may be bleeding from the stomach, the blood being either vomited or passed through the bowel. The patient sleeps badly, and very often looks thin and slightly yellow-faced. The urine becomes scanty and turbid, and dropsy with distended abdomen and enlargement of the legs are very often present.

Treatment. The diet should be of the lightest description, and meat should not be eaten. Fish, milk puddings and milk soup should form the greater part of the meals. The bowels must be kept open, and bicarbonate of soda should be taken daily in warm water to relieve the feeling of nausea. Treatment can only aim at

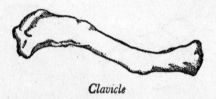

Clavicle

relieving the symptoms, since once the liver has become cirrhotic, nothing can be done to bring it back to its original state. No alcohol must be taken, and the patient should take as much exercise as possible. (*See also* DROPSY.)

CITRIC ACID. This acid is to be found in lemons and oranges, and they owe their sharp flavour to it. It is greatly used to provide cooling drinks, especially in cases of fever. This drink is particularly soothing for those suffering from an irritated stomach. Citric acid is also used to correct acidity of the stomach, as on absorption into the blood it is changed into an alkaline substance. It has been given internally in the treatment of rheumatism and jaundice.

CLAUDICATION, INTERMITTENT. This is a form of intermittent lameness associated particularly with arterio-sclerosis, though it may occur temporarily in other diseases which have a weakening effect on the walls of the arteries. The patient will feel intense pain in the legs after walking for a short time and will have to stop. Immediately he sits or lies down the pain ceases, only to return again when walking is resumed.

CLAUSTROPHOBIA. Dread of being shut up in an enclosed space such as a room with the door shut, or in a crowd.

This nervous dread is sometimes felt by persons who are the victims of neurasthenia. Such people may find it almost impossible to bring themselves to go into the carriage of a railway train or into a theatre or cinema. The opposite state, of being afraid of wide open spaces, is called agoraphobia.

CLAVICLE. The collar-bone, or clavicle, is a long bone lying in a horizontal position between the breast-bone and the arm. With the *scapula* it forms the shoulder. The collar-bone gives width to the shoulders and supports the arm, which joins on to its end at the tip of the shoulder and is thus held free of the body.

CLAVUS HYSTERICUS. A pain in the head felt by hysterical or neurasthenic people, who say that they feel as if a nail were being driven into their heads. (*See also* HEADACHE.)

CLAW FOOT (*Pes cavus*). A deformity of the foot in which the arch of the foot is very much exaggerated, so that the balls of the toes are brought near to the heel. The condition is seldom present at birth, but is usually due to some form of spinal disease. The very high instep makes it difficult to obtain suitable boots, and corns and callosities form easily. There may be severe pain in the instep. In early cases the condition may be corrected by putting the foot in plaster of Paris in a position to correct the deformity, followed by massage and exercises and the wearing of special boots.

CLEFT PALATE. The palate or roof of the mouth is formed by two plates, of bone in front and muscle behind, which normally join together in the middle line of the roof of the mouth. Occasionally, however, a child is born in whom the two sides of the roof of the mouth do not completely join up, with the result that a gap is left. This condition is called cleft palate, and if left untreated will cause great difficulty in feeding and speaking. The

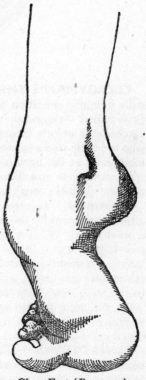

Claw Foot (*Pes cavus*)

only way to close the gap is by operation which should be done in early childhood, preferably during the first three months of life. If the gap cannot be closed by operation a specially prepared dental plate should be worn.

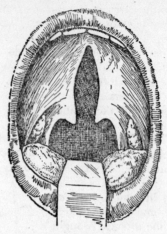

Cleft Palate

CLERGYMAN'S THROAT. Clergyman's throat is a chronically inflamed condition of the structures at the back of the throat. It is called " clergyman's " throat, but might as well be called teacher's or actor's throat, as it is in most cases found in people who use their voices in the pursuit of their daily work. The mucous membrane at the back of the throat is dotted with little dark red spots varying in size from a pinhead to a small pea. There may be a dry irritable cough and the voice becomes husky and weak.

Treatment. The treatment consists in rest of the voice, and a tonic treatment for the general health. As a temporary alleviation a good variety of throat pastille may be sucked at intervals. The well-known throat paint called Mandl's paint, which contains iodine, is a useful application to the throat. All unhealthy conditions of the nose and throat, such as enlarged tonsils, or deflected septum in the nose, must be attended to, and as the condition will recur when the voice is used again if the condition was originally due to faulty production of the voice, lessons in voice production and breathing should be taken.

CLIMACTERIC. Climacteric or menopause are medical names for what is commonly called by women the change of life. It may occur at any age between thirty-five and fifty-five, according to the type to which the individual woman's family belongs, and the process usually takes a couple of years. A full account will be found under the heading CHANGE OF LIFE.

CLINICAL. This term, which comes from the Greek, means literally a bed, and the word is used in connection with the bedside treatment of a disease. A *clinician* is a doctor whose opinions and teachings are based upon experience gained at the bedside of his patients. The term *clinic* is used to denote a place where medical instruction is given in the presence of the patient whose symptoms are studied and whose treatment is considered. A *clinical* thermometer is one which is used when taking the temperature of a patient.

CLOT. A solidification of the blood. In normal persons the blood clots on exposure to air at a perfectly definite rate of time, and this clotting time is useful as a test of the state of the blood. An abnormal clotting of the blood while in a blood-vessel is called *thrombosis*, and " clots " at the menstruation periods and after childbirth are common.

CLOVE. Cloves are obtained from the dried flower-buds of a species of myrtle grown in the Indian Archipelago. The oil or the infusion of cloves may be used internally in order to relieve the colicky pains in indigestion. Cotton-wool dipped in oil of cloves and applied to the hollow of a decayed tooth, or a clove chewed, is generally found to relieve toothache. Cloves are frequently used in cookery because of their aromatic flavour ; they also impart a pleasant odour to the breath.

CLUB-FOOT. Club-foot or talipes is a deformity in which the foot is twisted so that it is no longer able to be placed upon the ground. The condition may be congenital (present at birth) or it may occur later in life as a result of paralysis or injury.

There are four varieties of club-foot : (1) *talipes equinus*, in which the heel is raised from the ground, causing the patient to walk on the ball of the foot ; (2) *talipes calcaneus* is the opposite condition, where the heel rests on the ground and the front of the foot is raised ; (3) *talipes varus* is the condition in which the sole of the foot is turned inwards, so that the patient walks on the outer edge of the foot ; and (4) in *talipes valgus* the foot is turned outwards, causing the patient to walk on the inside of his foot. These forms are usually combined, as in the condition of *talipes equina-varus*, where the heel is drawn up and the sole is turned inwards, or *talipes calcaneo-valgus*, where the heel rests on the ground and the sole is turned outwards.

Treatment. For the cases acquired at birth, treatment must begin in the early weeks of life while the bones are still very soft and pliable. The position of the foot must be corrected several times daily, the mother or nurse gently but firmly turning the foot to the normal position and holding it there for a few minutes. In addition to this, the muscles of the leg should be massaged daily.

A splint should be used to hold the foot more firmly in position, so that, as the child grows older, the bones will gradually assume

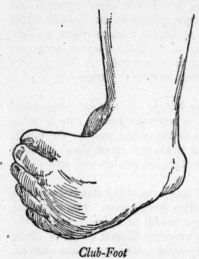

Club-Foot

a normal shape. If massage and manipulations are not carried out immediately after birth it may be necessary later on to resort to surgical operation. Tendons may have to be divided or parts of the deformed bones may have to be removed, especially in bad cases.

When the deformity is due to paralysis, treatment by massage and electricity may be found beneficial. For cases which are due to contraction of the muscles following an injury, operation may be necessary. In most cases it will be found necessary to wear a special apparatus in order to support the ankle and keep it in the correct position. Treatment is generally a very prolonged affair, and in order to get the best results, must be carried out regularly and patiently.

COAL-MINER'S LUNG. This is a condition which is common amongst coal-miners, in which the linings of the lungs become impregnated with particles of coal-dust. It is described under ANTHRACOSIS.

COCAINE. Cocaine is obtained from the leaves of two South American plants. The dried coca leaves have been used from time immemorial by the natives, who roll them up with a little lime and chew them. Cocaine is largely used in medicine to relieve pain, and a few drops of it may be injected under the skin as a local anæsthetic when a very small operation has to be performed. Operations on the nose and mouth may be carried out after painting a solution of cocaine over the part. Cocaine ointment is useful when applied to the skin in cases of itching, eczema and shingles, but it must never be used in cases where the skin is broken. Small doses of cocaine have been given to allay excessive vomiting, and it has been said to cure seasickness. A solution is used to soothe pain in the eye due to the presence of a foreign body, or slight operations may be carried out while the eye is anæsthetized with cocaine.

Poisoning by Cocaine. A single large dose may cause extreme mental excitement, delirium and convulsions. Taken habitually in small doses, the patient eventually loses all moral sense, and becomes a victim of sleeplessness. Death may result from sudden paralysis of the central nervous system.

Treatment. In cases of acute poisoning, the stomach should be washed out by means of a stomach tube. The poisonous effects are best counteracted by giving ammonia, digitalis, strychnine, amyl nitrite, or nitroglycerine, with strong coffee by mouth, or if the patient is unconscious, by injection into the rectum. Anæsthesia by chloroform and ether may be necessary to stop the convulsions. (*See also* ANÆSTHESIA.)

COCCUS. A coccus is the name given to spherical-shaped germs. The name is derived from the Greek for a berry. The commonest cocci are streptococci, staphylococci and pneumococci, of which accounts are given in the article on GERMS.

COCCYDYNIA. This is a condition where there is pain more or less severe in the region of the coccyx or end of the spine. Sitting, walking, and moving of the bowels may cause pain which is sometimes described as being excruciating. There may be a history of an injury to the coccyx caused by a blow or at childbirth, but sometimes the condition is a nervous one.

COCCYX. The coccyx is the name given to the last bone of the spine which is composed of four rudimentary vertebræ, and corresponds to the tail in animals. In early life the joint between

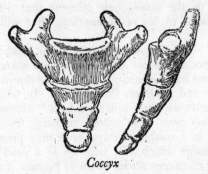

Coccyx

the coccyx and the *sacrum* is movable but it becomes fixed in later life. It sometimes happens that the coccyx is slightly bent inwards and this may be the cause of backache. A coccyx that is too long may cause discomfort after sitting for a lengthy period. The coccyx may be damaged or displaced by sitting down suddenly on something hard. A displaced coccyx can be returned to position, but is apt to slip out again. In a few cases rigidity of the coccyx may cause difficulty in childbirth. (*See also* COCCYDYNIA ; VERTEBRA.)

COD-LIVER OIL. This is a very valuable and easily digested form of fat. Not only is it very easily absorbed into the blood by itself, but it seems also to aid the absorption of other foods. It is made by purifying the oil obtained from the livers of cod-fish. Scottish oils are said to contain the most vitamins, the oil obtained from Newfoundland ranking second, then the Norwegian. Owing to its richness in vitamins A and D, cod-liver oil is invaluable in the treatment of rickets, or in wasting diseases such as consumption, or general debility.

COELIAC DISEASE. This is a disease of childhood shown by the passage of large, pale, offensive stools, and by gradual wasting ; the cause appears to be some failure in the power of the body to absorb fats and starches. There are usually some mental changes in the child, precocity, irritability, and sometimes hysteria. Deficiency symptoms appear, due to the lack of fat absorption. The treatment is dietetic, a diet being prescribed high in protein and low in fat, and with no carbohydrates. Underdone meat, dried milk, white of egg, broth, and later small amounts of bacon and butter, with crisp toast and rusks. Over-ripe bananas seem to be helpful, and orange juice, yeast extract, essogen, advita, for their vitamin value.

COLD, THE COMMON. The common cold, which is sometimes called by the technical names of *coryza* or acute nasal catarrh, is the commonest ailment that afflicts mankind, and no one seems to hit upon anything that will rid us of the plague.

Symptoms. The symptoms of cold in the head are well-known to everyone. Sometimes an attack starts with shivering and chilly feelings down the back, sometimes with a sore throat and sometimes with headache and stuffiness in the nose. In whatever way the attack starts, however, there will soon be a " streaming " nose and perhaps watering eyes. The watery discharge from the nose may be cleared up in a couple of days, or it may progress to a thick yellowish discharge which will take up to a week to get rid of. Sometimes the discharge settles down to become a chronic catarrh of the nose which may be quite difficult to deal with.

Causes of " colds." Cold in the head is an infectious disease caused by a variety of germs. The severity of the cold depends largely upon the degree of harmfulness of the germ and to the degree of susceptibility of the individual. Some people are much more liable to catch colds than others, and this is the reason that people with colds should treat themselves as infectious, as indeed they are, and keep out of crowded places, refrain from visiting sick or delicate persons and, if they must go about amongst their fellows whilst in the " streaming " stages, be careful to cover the mouth and nose with a handkerchief when sneezing or coughing. The cold that is slight in their case may be serious in their neighbours. A couple of days off from the office may not matter to them whereas to another it may spell disaster.

Treatment. Many people have their pet ways of trying to prevent the catching of colds by taking precautions when they have been with a person who has a cold or when colds are epidemic. These certainly do good and may mean a slight cold instead of a severe one. Such methods are : spraying the rooms with disinfectant, burning disinfectant vapours, putting eucalyptus, Friar's balsam or some such preparation on the handkerchief ; or on the other hand, spraying the nose and gargling. This routine of spraying and gargling does ward off many colds, but the day will inevitably come when the most careful person will fall a victim. A healthy mode of life and fresh air in the house without draughts are really the best preventives. The teeth, nose and throat should be examined if the tendency to catch cold is very marked.

When the cold has actually been caught, and is in full swing, simple treatment will relieve the discomfort and the cold should run its course very quickly. If the person recognizes in time that a cold is coming on, he may cut short the attack by taking a hot bath and retiring to bed with hot drinks and something to cause perspiration—a couple of aspirin or similar tablets or a Dover's powder. If the symptoms have subsided by the morning begin taking a tonic, and be careful to avoid catching new infection or a chill for the next few days. If, however, the cold is well developed, follow the same treatment or use any of the favourite cold remedies such as ammoniated tincture of quinine, a few drops of camphor on a lump of sugar, or two aspirins every four hours (if in bed or confined to the house only). If the throat is sore, gargle at intervals with salt and warm water or some simple gargle such as glycerine of thymol. For the sore nose and nasal discharge, inhalations are of the greatest assistance. Menthol crystals, Friar's balsam, or oil of eucalyptus may be used by the method of pouring boiling water over the crystals or liquid in a bowl and holding the head over the bowl, while breathing in the scented steam. A large towel placed over the head and bowl forms a tent to keep the steam from escaping. Soothing substances such as chloretone inhalant may be sprayed in vapour form into the back of the nose with pleasant effects, by a special spray called an atomizer. Or an ordinary liquid spray may be used with glycerine of thymol or some such substance. Black-currant jujubes are a favourite thing to suck during a cold if the throat is at all irritable.

When the cold is over, tone up the general health with a tonic and remember that colds *are* infectious. (*See also* INFLUENZA.)

COLIC. Colic is the term used to denote pain due to irregular or violent contractions of muscular tissues in the body. The most usual form is that due to spasmodic contractions of the bowel and is called *intestinal colic*. There may be *gastric colic* in the stomach, *biliary colic* due to irregular contractions of the bile ducts, *renal colic* in the kidneys, etc. The cause of colic is usually some kind of irritation such as indigestible food in the stomach or a stone obstructing a duct. The muscular walls of the ducts try to pass on the stone by their contractions and pain results. When muscular tissue is fulfilling its ordinary function without opposition from irritating substances there is no pain.

Treatment. Colic may be so severe that morphia will have to be administered, as in the case of biliary colic. Atropine is the most useful drug for counteracting the tendency of muscles to go into spasms. The most common form of colic is intestinal colic due to constipation, undigested food or to a chill. Sips of hot water with peppermint or ginger in it or a dose of chlorodyne may relieve the pain, but castor-oil should be taken afterwards to remove the cause of the irritation. Frequently a hot-water bottle held to the part will be all the treatment necessary to relieve the pain temporarily.

If colic does not yield to simple remedies quickly, it is always best to call in a doctor, as it is impossible for the ordinary person to be sure of the cause of the pain.

The commonest cause of colic in babies is cold, and this should be remedied by giving sips of warm water and applying heat to the abdomen, taking great care, however, that the fomentation or hot-water bottle is not too hot for the delicate skin of the infant. Children whose extremities are exposed in cold weather are apt to suffer from colic. The blood circulating in the head and feet is more exposed to extremes of temperature than that in the big vessels of the trunk and therefore should be protected in cold weather by caps and socks.

COLITIS. By colitis is meant inflammation of the large bowel or intestine. The condition is described according to its nature as mucous colitis, catarrhal colitis and ulcerative colitis.

Mucous Colitis. The distinguishing feature of this condition is the passage from the bowel of quantities of membraneous-looking material which consists entirely of mucus. Mucus is the slimy material which exudes from the mucous membranes or linings of the various organs or passages of the body. In the case of mucous colitis the mucus is from the lining of the large intestine, and it may be due to a catarrhal condition of the bowel or to a nervous condition in which too large a quantity of mucus is being given off.

Symptoms. The mucus passed in mucous colitis is very varied in character. It is sometimes passed in long bands of a ribbon-like appearance, which may be mistaken for segments of a tape-worm. It may be of considerable thickness and bear on its surface the marks of the folds of the intestine, or it may be in the shape of a tube surrounding portions of the stool, so that people are led to believe that they have passed pieces of the bowel itself. It occurs most commonly in females. Before, the disease becomes fully established there is generally a history of poor health dating from an attack of some illness such as influenza. Patients who subsequently develop mucous colitis have often been subject to occasional attacks of cramp in the bowels, usually lasting a day or two, dyspepsia, flatulence, etc. The main symptom is that of constipation of a very severe nature requiring the constant employment of purgatives to overcome it. The motions are generally hard masses often covered with glairy mucus. At other times the motions are ribbon-shaped or have a pipe-stem character, indicating spasm of the intestine.

Treatment must aim at three things : overcoming the tendency to constipation ; improving the patient's nutrition ; stimulating and strengthening the nervous system.

The patient should be confined to bed at first in severe cases for at least six weeks, if possible among strange surroundings. Visits from friends and relations should be forbidden, but the surroundings must be cheerful. The diet must be ample and nutritious, well cooked and daintily served, consisting chiefly of eggs, raw or lightly boiled ; soups, meat jellies, custards, finely-minced beef and mutton, calves'-feet jelly, fish souffles, pounded chicken, crisp toast or biscuits with plenty of butter. The patient must avoid green vegetables, starchy foods, fruits, pastry and cheese.

The bowels must be made to open regularly every morning, and this can be done by suitable doses of castor-oil continued without intermission for several months. It must be given in doses sufficient to produce a soft motion, and the quantity will naturally vary in different individuals. Where castor-oil is too unpalatable, sulphur and cream of tartar, half a dram of each mixed with a little syrup of lemon, can be substituted. Liquid paraffin is sometimes very useful. Irrigation of the bowel is often useful as it washes away the tenacious mucus which clings to the walls of the intestines. Plombières treatment is also useful if it can be obtained. (*See also* IRRIGATION OF THE BOWEL ; PLOMBIÈRES TREATMENT.)

Acute Catarrhal Colitis. Acute attacks of inflammation of the bowel are usually due to the eating of some doubtful article of food or something else which " disagrees " and are part of a general stomach and intestinal upset.

It is as well, therefore, to treat the matter with care at the beginning in order to avoid such a complication.

Ulcerative Colitis. Colitis in which the bowel ulcerates is a not uncommon disease of middle life ; it is very difficult to cure and is of serious import. It is not known what causes it, but as it closely resembles tropical dysentery it may be due to some similar germ. It begins gradually with increasing diarrhœa in which mucus, pus and blood are passed. The number of stools increases to as many as twenty a day. The patient soon becomes desperately ill and wastes away, often dying of exhaustion if the disease cannot be stopped in time.

Treatment. The treatment is the same as for mucous colitis, but when the patient recovers he must always be careful what food he eats, and must confine himself to food which leaves little residue in the bowel, such as milky foods, fish and chicken. Meat, vegetables and fruit are better entirely avoided. Constipation must also be guarded against by taking some intestinal lubricant such as liquid paraffin. (*See also* DIARRHŒA ; DYSENTERY ; ENTERITIS.)

COLLAPSE. This term is applied to a condition of extreme exhaustion. It may follow some prostrating disease such as pneumonia, cholera, infantile diarrhœa, etc. Any condition in which there is a great loss of fluids from the blood-vessels may bring about a state of collapse. The state of collapse is very similar to the condition of surgical shock. The main difference between the two lies in the onset, which is more gradual when the state is due to some disease.

Symptoms. The face is pale and haggard and the eyes are sunken and glassy. The body may be covered with cold sweat, while the temperature is generally reduced to 95°–97° F. The voice is very weak, and the pulse feeble. The patient may be quite conscious but unable to pay attention to what is going on around him, while in other cases unconsciousness may occur.

Treatment consists of keeping the patient as warm as possible. He should be allowed to lie on his back with his head low, and medical advice should be sought. Hot-water bottles should be placed at the feet and sides and warm blankets should be used to cover him. Stimulants should only be administered under medical supervision in cases suffering from collapse resulting from bleeding, or when bleeding is likely to occur.

COLLAR-BONE. The medical name for the collar-bone is the clavicle, and it is described under that title.

COLLES' FRACTURE. Colles' fracture is a break in the radius at the lower end just above the wrist. This type of fracture is usually caused by a fall on the hand when the arm is outstretched to save oneself, and the end of the bone may be impacted, or driven on to the upper part. Colles' fractures usually unite without leaving much deformity of the arm, and the arm is fit for use in three or four weeks.

COLLODION. This is a thick liquid made by dissolving gun-cotton in ether and alcohol, or with acetone. When painted on the skin the ether rapidly dries, leaving a thin protective film. This forms an excellent covering for small wounds after they have been thoroughly cleansed and dried, but it must not be used on discharging wounds. Collodium callosum, which is collodion used in conjunction with salicylic acid, is a rapid and painless solvent for corns and warts.

COLLOID. This is a name applied to a type of cancer in which the tumour is filled with a glue-like substance. It affects chiefly the internal organs.

COLLYRIUM. A lotion for the eyes is called a collyrium, and the one most commonly used is a solution of boracic acid.

COLOMBA. Fissures or cracks in any part of the eye are called *Colomba*.

COLON. The large bowel or large intestine is called the colon. It is described under the heading INTESTINE.

COLOUR-BLINDNESS. Some people are unable to distinguish between colours, and are called *colour-blind*. The degree of colour-blindness varies, the commonest form being the inability to distinguish between red and green ; blue-yellow colour-blindness is much more uncommon, and total colour-blindness very rare. The condition is very much more common in men than in women, and occurs equally in all races. It is apt to run in families, several brothers, perhaps, being affected ; or it is sometimes transmitted from grandfather to grandson, the son escaping the defect. Colour-blindness may exist in one eye only, the other having normal colour-vision.

COMA. Coma is a state of deep unconsciousness. It is usually a matter of serious importance. Poisoning by various poisons which take effect on the nervous system, such as alcohol, prussic acid, opium and any of the sleep-inducing drugs such as those derived from barbituric acid (like veronal), cause coma. Certain injuries to the brain which cause pressure on the brain, such as fracture of the skull or brain tumour, may bring on coma. There may be coma in very severe attacks of influenza, malaria, sleeping-sickness and even measles. Coma is also a symptom of severe

6*

diabetes. Coma vigil is the name given to a state which occurs with severe fevers in which the patient lies muttering to himself often with his eyes open but is really in a state of unconsciousness.

Treatment. When a person is found lying unconscious without any obvious cause and cannot be wakened, a doctor should always be sent for, even if it is suspected that the cause is really heavy drinking, because it may be a state of coma due to some disease or poison which is threatening the patient's life. The coma of diabetes can now be dispersed almost immediately by an injection of insulin. (*See also* DIABETES.)

COMPRESS. A compress is a folded cloth, wet or dry, applied firmly to a part of the body for relief of inflammation, or to prevent hæmorrhage. A compress wrung out in ice-cold water is a very good way of treating a sprain or for the prevention of " black " eye.

COMPRESSION. Compression of the brain is due to a piece of bone or a clot of blood pressing on the brain. In some cases a tumour, or inflammation of the outer coverings of the brain, may be causing the compression. It is a much more serious condition than that of concussion, and the treatment of the case will depend on the exciting cause. (*See also* BRAIN.)

CONCEPTION. Conception means to become pregnant. (*See also* PREGNANCY.)

CONCUSSION. Concussion of the brain is almost always caused by a fall or a blow. If the concussion is slight, the patient may be able to understand what is being said to him, but in more severe cases the patient may relapse into a state of unconsciousness.

Treatment. The patient should be laid on his back and all clothing should be loosened, and plenty of fresh air is necessary. The patient must be kept perfectly quiet until the arrival of the doctor, and no attempts should be made to arouse him. (*See also* BRAIN.)

CONDYLE. By condyle is meant any rounded eminence such as occurs in the joints of many of the bones, especially the jutting-out pieces at the outer and inner sides of the elbow or the knee.

CONDYLOMA. A wart-like growth or tumour often found near the opening of the anus. Growths of this type can be removed by the use of caustics or by surgery.

CONDY'S FLUID. A useful disinfectant named after an English physician, Henry Bollmann Condy, who lived in the 19th century. One part of sodium or potassium permanganate dissolved in 500 parts of water will make an efficient disinfectant.

CONFINEMENT. This term is used in connection with childbirth, usually to denote the lying-in period. (*See also* CHILDBIRTH ; LABOUR ; PUERPERIUM.)

CONGENITAL. This term is used in connection with any disease or condition which is present at birth. Many congenital deformities of the body are due to accidents before or during birth. Conditions, such as congenital dislocation of the hip, may not be noticed until the child starts to walk. Some congenital deformities of the hands and feet include club hand ; polydactylism, that is, the presence of extra fingers or toes ; overgrowth of one or more fingers or toes ; and club-foot. Syphilis is one of the most common congenital diseases.

CONGESTION. When any abnormal amount of blood collects in any organ or part of the body, causing swelling of the part, it is said to be congested. The condition may be due to some weakness of the circulation, but often it is an early symptom of inflammation. It becomes a serious condition when the lungs are affected.

CONJUNCTIVA. The conjunctiva is the thin membrane lining the eyelids and covering the white of the eye. It continually " sweeps " the eye by the involuntary closure of the lids, and keeps it moist and free from friction by mucus poured out by its glands on to the surface. It is well supplied with blood-vessels, and this character, together with its constant exposure to the air, render it very liable to attacks of inflammation, which is called conjunctivitis.

CONJUNCTIVITIS is caused by anything that irritates the conjunctiva ; there are many forms. The three chief symptoms of conjunctivitis are pain, running of the eyes, and congestion of the blood-vessels. The pain is generally described as smarting, scalding, or itching. *No eye trouble, however slight it may seem to be, should in any circumstances be treated as of no account.*

Treatment. In treatment, the *cause* as far as possible must be corrected. The eyes should be rested and protected from any irritants such as smoke, bright lights or cold winds. Warm antiseptic washes are used several times daily ; these serve both to wash away the secretion and germs, if present, and are also very soothing to the inflamed eyes. Special symptoms, such as pain or twitching of the eyelids, are relieved by cocaine locally, or a chloral and bromide mixture. A soothing ointment is applied to the edges of the lids.

Every case should be treated as if infectious ; it is impossible to be too careful. Any dressings should at once be burnt. The patient should never be allowed, as sometimes happens, to use the same towel over and over again to wipe away the discharge ; and, of course, no other person, especially a child, should be allowed access to towels, etc., used by the patient. These details may seem unnecessarily troublesome ; but, if carefully attended to, a great deal of eye trouble would be avoided.

The general health is often at fault and should be carefully regulated. Treatment with laxatives and tonics often helps greatly. The food should be good, nourishing and plain, and plenty of time allowed for sleep. A daily warm bath is helpful in increasing the action of the skin. The patient should be in the fresh air as much as possible, provided that the eyes are protected from sun, wind and dust.

Simple Conjunctivitis is caused by any persistent irritation, such as a dusty or fume-laden air, eye-strain, working in a too brilliant light, the misuse of alcohol, etc.

Treatment. The treatment is according to the cause, which should be removed, and the eyes should be frequently bathed with a mild alkaline lotion, such as weak bicarbonate of soda in warm water.

Angular Conjunctivitis is a very chronic form of conjunctivitis in which the reddening of the eyes is especially noticeable in the corner. It is treated by zinc drops or ointment.

Catarrhal Conjunctivitis or Pink Eye is very contagious, and the disease may attack several members of a family, or run through a school. In addition to the usual symptoms, a dislike of light is present, and adults generally suffer a good deal of pain.

Treatment. The disease is easy to treat, as it usually recovers of its own accord in a week or two. Frequent washing with an antiseptic lotion and the use of an antiseptic ointment are all that is necessary.

CONSTIPATION or COSTIVENESS is the very common condition in which the bowels do not move often enough or are not completely emptied when they do move. The number of motions required for health varies for different people. The majority of people have the bowels opened once a day ; but two motions a day are quite usual, and some other people have only a motion every other day without apparently feeling any bad effects.

Symptoms. The symptoms that can be caused by constipation are numerous. The complexion becomes sallow and " muddy," the tongue is furred and the breath may be offensive. The appetite will not be good. There may be sick-headache, giddiness, mental depression and sleeplessness. In fact, almost any symptom of ill-health may be present in a mild form. As a general rule pain is not present with constipation unless aperients have been taken, when the pain is due to the contractions of the bowel which they cause. If there is great distension of the abdomen with gas, it means that there are harmful germs at work, and the condition will need treatment. Any sudden or violent pain, especially with sickness and collapse or a rise in temperature, should be attended to at once by a doctor, as it may mean ulceration or obstruction in the bowel. Pain at the actual moment of passing the motion may be due to piles.

Treatment. The treatment of chronic constipation where there is no definite disease causing it, is the treatment of the general state of health and the regulation of the diet and daily habits. The most important thing will probably be the daily exercise. A certain amount of exercise is absolutely necessary for everyone who does not obtain sufficient muscular exertion in the course of his day's work, and in this respect it may be remarked that housework in a small house, except on days when washing or strenuous cleaning is done, does not amount to sufficient exercise for many women. They need a brisk walk as well. The object of the exercise is to stimulate the working of the liver so that it will produce and send into the intestine enough bile to secure proper digestion of the food. It goes without saying that the call to the stool should be answered as soon as it occurs. In most persons' lives it is convenient to so train the bowel that the call comes at the same time every day, and it should be at a time that is likely to be a convenient one. This training can be begun in the very earliest days of babyhood.

The question of diet is, of course, of the greatest importance in the treatment of constipation. As a general rule it will be found that the diet of the constipated person is too solid, too concentrated and too easily digested. A certain amount of irritating matter or roughage is required to force the bowel to make the effort to get rid of it. This roughage is best obtained from porridge, brown bread, green vegetables, and certain fruits like brambles, figs, or prunes which are not entirely digested. After roughage, fluid is necessary. This may be taken with the meals or in larger quantities between meals. Very few people living in towns drink a large enough quantity of fluid in the day. Some people may need more fat in the diet, and this is obtained by taking butter, cream, salad oil.

If attention to the diet, exercise and daily hygiene do not cure the constipation, it will then be necessary to use some simple aperient. These are fully discussed in a special article on aperients.

CONSUMPTION. Consumption is the old name for the disease which is now called tuberculosis. Consumption of the lungs is called phthisis; consumption of the skin is called lupus. All forms of consumption except LUPUS are discussed under the heading TUBER-CULOSIS.

CONTRACEPTION. This term is derived from two words :

contra, against, and conception, to conceive. It is applied to the prevention of conception, or birth control. (*See also* SEX HYGIENE.)

CONTRACTED FINGERS. The condition in which the fingers become contracted is known as Dupuytren's contracture, after a famous French surgeon who died nearly a hundred years ago. It is often hereditary and is found in succeeding generations of the same family, usually amongst the males. The skin and tissues beneath it in the ring and little fingers of one or both hands, become thickened and drawn together, so that the fingers become folded over into the palm of the hand. It is not known why the condition arises, but cases are found in gouty and rheumatic people and in people who use their hands a great deal as well as in cases where there does not appear to be any reason for the condition. It is thought by some authorities that a glandular deficiency may cause it and some cases have done very well on treatment by extract of thyroid gland.

Treatment. In early cases massage may give relief and even stop the condition from getting worse, but when the fingers become really deformed the tissues beneath the skin may have to be operated on, and in the case of a manual worker it may be advantageous to remove the little finger entirely. (*See also* FINGER.)

CONTRACTURE. Contracture means the permanent shortening, distortion or deformity of a muscle, or of various muscles, such as Dupuytren's contracture. Contraction is the term used for certain forms of temporary shortening.

CONTUSION. A bruise is medically termed a contusion. This term generally means that the skin is unbroken but that swelling and discoloration are present. When the skin is broken it is referred to as a contused wound.

CONVULSION. A convulsion, commonly called a fit, is a violent irregular motion of the whole body or of part of the body, due to involuntary contractions and relaxations of the voluntary muscles, and may be compared to an earthquake in the system. The most common convulsions are those which occur in infancy and are called infantile convulsions ; those occurring during attacks of St. Vitus's dance called choreic from its other name of chorea ; those due to epilepsy ; to lockjaw (tetanus) ; or advanced kidney disease (uræmic convulsions). Women also suffer from convulsive fits during the latter stages of pregnancy (eclampsia) and during the menopause (climacteric). All these will be found under the diseases which cause them.

COPAIBA. The oil of copaiba is largely used in cases of gonorrhœa as a disinfectant and stimulant.

COPPER. Copper sulphate, more commonly known as blue

vitriol or blue stone, is of considerable value in medicine. Used externally, the sulphate is applied as a caustic to reduce growths on the skin and an ointment of copper citrate is useful in the treatment of ulceration of the eyelids.

Poisoning by Copper. Large doses of salts of copper violently irritate the stomach and intestines. Treatment consists of washing out the stomach by giving large quantities of warm water followed by white of egg or milk. If the pain is very severe, opium may be prescribed to allay the irritation.

CORN. A corn or clavis is a circumscribed overgrowth of the horny layer of the skin, occurring as the result of prolonged pressure due, of course, to the use of improperly fitting footwear. The corn has a deep core or " eye," while the surrounding parts are overgrown, and there may be a varying degree of inflammation.

Treatment. The true remedy for corns is correctly fitting shoes. Without them all other measures are temporary and palliative only. When a corn has formed, relief from pressure and consequently from pain is given by the well-known corn-plaster, which consists of an adhesive ring of cotton-wool which surrounds the corn. Strict attention to cleanliness of the feet, by daily bathing, also to some extent relieves the pain.

To remove the corn, it should first be softened by a thorough soaking in hot soapy water, to which sodium carbonate (washing-soda) is added in the proportion of 2 tablespoonfuls to a basin of water. Soakings on several successive days may be necessary before the corn will soften. It should then be rubbed down as briskly as possible with pumice-stone or a friction cloth.

The central core and the surrounding callosity can also be softened by various medicaments. A rapid method, which is best used only by a medical man, is to place a drop of liquor potassæ, 15 per cent., or strong acetic acid on the corn, and rub in as vigorously as can be borne.

Slow, but painless, methods consist in the use of milder horn-dissolving agents, the chief of which is salycilic acid, used either as a " medicated plaster " or as a paint in combination with collodion. The plaster consists of a small centre of salicylic plaster, surrounded by an ordinary corn-plaster. The medicated part should be placed over the corn, and the whole kept in place by a narrow strip of surgical plaster. It should remain in place for three days ; it will then be found that the superficial part of the core and the surrounding horny part will have softened, and may easily be removed.

" Soft " corns occur in any position between the toes, and even after what seems to be a complete removal are exceedingly apt to recur. Cleanliness of the feet is here even more important than in the case of hard corns, especially if there is much sweating of the feet. The most suitable application is spirits of camphor, which should be painted on at night ; during the day zinc oxide or talc powder should be used, and wool placed between the affected toes. A powder containing starch (as do many toilet powders) should not be used, as it is apt to irritate a damp skin. These are, naturally, only palliatives ; the most satisfactory method is surgical removal which, however, may need to be repeated if the corn recurs.

CORNEA, THE. The cornea is the window of the eye. It is a transparent membrane covering the iris and the pupil. At the side of the eye it joins the white. It is well supplied with nerves, and so is extremely sensitive.

Ulceration of the Cornea. An ulcer may occur at any point on the cornea, and, when it heals, an opaque scar is left. Sometimes the ulcer eats through the cornea and damages other structures in the eye. Any degree of damage to the sight, from a mere cloudiness to complete blindness may be caused.

Keratitis. The term keratitis is used to denote inflammation of the cornea without ulceration. The most important form of keratitis affects children at about the age of puberty, sometimes several members of the same family, and girls rather than boys. The cause in the great majority of cases is congenital syphilis, other signs of which may be present. Injury is quite frequently the exciting cause which lights up the disease.

Symptoms. Two common forms of the disease are seen. In the *mild* form the eyes easily tire, and vision is blurred. Greyish spots are seen on the cornea. The patient recovers in a few weeks. In the *severe* form the symptoms are much more acute ; pain, especially, may be very distressing. The cornea becomes obscured by closely-packed blood-vessels which from their appearance are called " salmon patches." In the course of a few weeks the patient is practically blind, but recovery takes place in 6–12 months. The outlook is generally good, unless complications occur.

Treatment. The eye is treated by atropin drops. Anti-syphilitic treatment is given, and the general hygiene is carefully regulated. A difficulty in many cases is that the patient loses interest in everything but his own " hopeless " condition. Both he and his family should be made to realize that this despairing frame of mind is quite unnecessary, as his blindness is only temporary.

CORPUSCLE. The blood-cells are called corpuscles. (*See also* BLOOD.)

CORROSIVE. A corrosive substance is one which destroys tissues or any part with which it comes in contact. There are a large number of substances of a corrosive nature and many fatal accidents have occurred through drinking them. These poisons include the strong acids, strong alkalines and caustics. The more important acids include oil of vitriol or sulphuric acid, hydrochloric acid, nitric acid, oxalic acid, acetic acid and carbolic acid.

The more common alkalies which act as corrosive poisons include : caustic soda, caustic potash, washing soda in strong solution and ammonia. Among the caustic salts are zinc chloride, silver nitrate and chromic acid.

Symptoms of corrosive poisoning come on very quickly after the acid has been taken. There is intense pain in the mouth, throat and stomach, followed by vomiting, which is usually blood-stained. There is generally great difficulty in breathing and the patient may die of collapse in a short time.

Treatment. The doctor must be sent for at once and, if possible, the nature of the poison should be stated ; this may be ascertained from the label on the bottle from which the poison was taken. *On no account should an emetic be given, as this will cause further injury to the already damaged tissues and may cause perforation of the stomach.* Soothing liquids such as milk and white of egg, or a wineglassful of olive oil in the same amount of warm water, or gruel may be given. The antidotes for the common types of poisoning are set out under POISONS.

Shock must be guarded against by keeping the patient as warm as possible. Strong tea or coffee, warm but not hot, may be given later as a stimulant.

CORROSIVE SUBLIMATE. This is a salt of mercury known also as perchloride of mercury, mercuris chloride or bichloride of mercury. The chief use of this substance is as a disinfectant or antiseptic. It is one of the most powerful of all the antiseptics and even in very dilute solutions will kill virulent germs, but it must not be used on metal instruments because it corrodes them.

Cases of poisoning by this substance should be treated promptly by giving white of egg. An emetic should be given in this case as, in spite of the name of the poison, it does not act as a corrosive but as an irritant. (*See also* MERCURY POISONING.)

CORTEX. The outer layer of an organ is called the cortex. The *cerebral cortex* is the thin layer of grey matter on the surface of the *cerebrum.* (*See also* BRAIN.)

CORYZA. The medical name for nasal catarrh—running at the nose. (*See also* COLD, THE COMMON.)

COSTIVENESS. Costiveness is another name for constipation. This term is often applied to small children. (*See also* CONSTIPATION.)

COTTON-WOOL. Cotton-wool is made of the hairs of the seed of the cotton plant. It becomes absorbent after the fatty and oily substances have been removed ; this is termed " absorbent cotton-wool " and it is used extensively in medicine.

COUGH. Cough is an important symptom in many diseases, and may be the chief thing the patient complains of. In other diseases, however, the cough may be so slight as to be hardly noticed by the patient and yet be important enough to lead the doctor to the correct diagnosis of the disease.

Varieties of Cough. In diseases of the throat, the cough is usually hoarse, barking and "croupy." In ulceration or thickening of the mucous membrane of the throat, the cough may be husky and imperfect.

Cough in diseases of the Lungs. In *bronchitis* the cough is at first short and dry and may be painful. As the secretion is increased it becomes moist, and may also be paroxysmal.

In *tuberculosis* cough is an early symptom. At first it is dry and hacking, later it becomes loose and is accompanied by expectoration mixed with slime and matter. It is often most severe in the morning.

In *pneumonia* the cough is infrequent, short, dry, restrained and associated with severe pain in the side. In acute *pleurisy* the cough, although it is usually present, is seldom so noticeable as in acute pneumonia.

The paroxysmal cough of *whooping cough* is very characteristic.

Enlarged glands at the root of the lung may give rise to very severe and persistent coughing.

Diseases of the Heart. Inflammation of the membrane lining the heart (pericarditis) is sometimes accompanied by a painful cough. Aneurysm is usually associated with a dry and brassy cough. Any condition in which the heart's action is feeble, may give rise to a troublesome cough.

Cough in diseases of the Abdominal Organs. The so-called " stomach " cough is associated with indigestion. It appears to be due to irritation of the back part of the throat and upper part of the food-pipe (œsophagus) caused by dyspepsia. It is common in children and is often associated with the presence of enlarged tonsils and adenoids.

Nervous Cough. This term is applied to all forms of cough in which no definite cause of irritation can be discovered. It is often a mere habit, and it may be associated with emotion, especially that caused by speaking in public.

Hysterical Cough. Cough is fairly common in cases of hysteria. It may be very severe and persistent and give rise to anxiety as to the condition of the lungs.

COUNTER-IRRITANT. Irritation of the skin in order to relieve pain or congestion of some part of the body is known as counter-irritation. This may be carried out by means of rubbing the skin with the hand, or by artificially producing a blister or redness by means of a drug. Counter-irritation is often applied to the chest in cases of bronchial catarrh by rubbing camphorated oil well into the skin. The number of diseases that benefit by counter-irritation are numerous, but this method appears to be especially beneficial in chronic inflammatory conditions such as rheumatism and bronchitis.

COURSES. This is a popular term for the menstrual periods which occur in women. (*See also* MENSTRUATION.)

COW-POX. This is believed to be a form of smallpox among cattle, but which may be communicated to human beings who come in contact with it. It is a relatively mild disease showing none of the severe symptoms of smallpox. There is usually a slight rise in temperature, and a sore generally appears on whichever part of the body has come in contact with the diseased cow ; generally on the hand through the process of milking. It was noticed that persons who had suffered from cow-pox did not develop smallpox, and it was this observation which led Jenner in 1796 to carry out, for the first time, vaccination of man with cow-pox lymph obtained from the hand of a dairy-maid. The lymph which is used nowadays is taken from the sores on a tuberculin-tested calf and, after being mixed with glycerine and water, is stored in a cool dark room before being used. (*See also* VACCINATION.)

CRACKS. Cracks may occur in several parts of the body and where they are present should always be healed up as soon as possible, not only because they are usually painful, but also because they make an open doorway for the entrance of germs into the blood. The most common cracks are those on the hands and lips. Cracks on the skin of the hands are called chaps, and are described in a separate article.

CRAMP. Cramp is a painful spasm of any muscle. The muscles which are most often subject to cramp are the muscles of the legs and feet. The attack may be due to lying or sitting too long in a strained position. As a rule the cramp passes off quickly. Exposure to cold, general debility, fatigue or gout are some of the conditions which may produce cramp. Cramp is also used loosely to mean any colicky attack in the abdomen. Cases of drowning from cramp are usually due to heart failure. In cramp in a limb, the best way to relieve the pain during an attack, is to stretch the affected limb. This may be very difficult and extremely painful, but it is well worth the effort. If the victim is unable to do this, the affected part should be rubbed energetically until the spasm gives way.

CRANIAL NERVES. These consist of twelve pairs of nerves, which come from the brain itself. They control the senses of sight, smell, hearing, speech, etc., also all movement and sensation about the head and neck.

CRANIUM. The cranium is that part of the skull which contains the brain, though the whole skull is often wrongly referred to as the cranium. The bones that form the skull are divided into two classes, the cranial and the facial. (*See also* SKULL.)

CREEPING PALSY. This is a popular term which is used by many people when they are describing symptoms of diseases such as disseminated sclerosis, spinal meningitis or general paralysis of the insane. It is a vague term and has no real medical significance.

CREOSOTE. Creosote has the same action on the body as carbolic acid, and has been used externally as an antiseptic. Creosote is largely used as an inhalation in bronchitis and lung complaints.

Creosote is taken internally for vomiting and flatulence and it has been much employed in the treatment of tuberculosis and asthma.

The ointment of creosote is made up with creosote, hard paraffin and white soft paraffin. It is used in various skin diseases such as dermatitis and inflammations of the skin.

Is a powerful antiseptic, and the well-known disinfectant lysol is made from it. Jeyes' disinfectant also contains cresol. It is used in surgery and in domestic life as an antiseptic. A tablespoonful to $1\frac{1}{2}$ pints of water is a convenient strength for disinfecting instruments, linen, drains, etc. For the hands, one tablespoonful to $2\frac{1}{2}$ pints will be found strong enough.

CRETINISM. A cretin is a child who suffers from a peculiar form of idiocy, owing to the absence or deficiency of the juices of the thyroid gland. (*See also* DUCTLESS GLANDS.)

Cretinism seems to be more prevalent in certain parts of the world than in others, and it may be possible that atmospheric and geographical conditions play some obscure part in the non-development of the gland. Cases are very common in Switzerland, Northern Italy, and France, but cases have been known to appear in England and America.

Symptoms. If a child is born with the thyroid gland undeveloped, nothing unusual is noticed until the child reaches the age of about nine months. It will be noticed then that the child is backward, and physical as well as mental signs begin to develop. The head appears to be large and flat, and the tongue is unusually large and tends to protrude. The hair becomes thin, and the skin appears to be very dry. The abdomen is seen to be very prominent and the back is curved in. Speech, if it develops at all, is very late.

and defective. Quite a number of these children die young, but there are many who grow up. They are never anything else but idiots ; and they remain dwarfed, rarely attaining the height of four feet.

Treatment. Treatment should commence immediately the condition is discovered. Continuous administration of thyroid gland extract is necessary to make up for the deficiency in the patient. The child will, under this treatment, begin to react very quickly, and so long as the treatment is kept up will reach almost normal standard.

CRISIS. The word crisis as used in regard to illness means a turning-point, and is used to mark the moment in severe illness when the patient suddenly takes a turn for the better and the high temperature drops quickly.

It has been explained that crisis means the rapid drop of temperature in severe illness, but it happens in some diseases that the drop of temperature is slow but sure, and the patient recovers very gradually. This sort of ending to an illness is described as an ending by lysis, not crisis.

CROTON OIL. Croton oil is an exceedingly powerful purgative, and is far too drastic in its action for ordinary purposes.

CROUP. This is a condition of difficulty in breathing accompanied by a harsh cough. It is due to a spasm of the muscles which guard and control the entrace to the lungs.

Causes. In young children the portion of the voice-box containing the vocal cords, which is known as the glottis, is so small that the slightest swelling which narrows the opening, or the presence even of a little mucus causing a blocking of the passage, will give rise during the night to attacks of suffocation which may be very terrifying.

Symptoms. The child is usually between the age of 2 and 5 years, and seems perfectly well during the day, though he may possibly have a slight cold. He wakes up suddenly about 11 p.m. with intense difficulty in breathing. His breathing is jerky, air is drawn into the lungs noisily and it makes a whistling sound. There is also a hoarse cough. After a period of time varying from a few minutes to an hour or more, the attack ends and the child falls asleep again as though nothing had happened. These attacks may be repeated night after night.

Although it is very alarming, croup is rarely fatal, and simple treatment is all that is necessary to stop the attack.

Treatment. The attack of difficulty in breathing which naturally inspires so much alarm is treated by applying to the front of the neck a sponge or handkerchief soaked in water as hot as possible, taking care not to burn the skin. The handkerchief should be wrung nearly dry. The water should be changed and the sponge or handkerchief kept hot until the suffocation has disappeared. Between the attacks the child should be kept in a warm room, and a steam kettle should be used. The bowels should be kept open regularly. The child must be kept as quiet as possible and all excitement and irritation should be avoided. If the condition of rickets is present this must of course be treated.

Other Conditions which resemble Croup are :

Congenital Laryngeal Stridor. This is a condition which is present at birth or just after. The difficulty in breathing is continuous and ceases after a few months. It does not cause any distress and is never fatal.

Catarrhal Spasm of the Larynx. In these cases there is some degree of cough or hoarseness present. The onset of the attack is fairly rapid, but not sudden as in false croup. The breathing is not jerky. It is never fatal.

Catarrhal Laryngitis (Acute laryngitis). In this case there is a history of a previous cold, difficulty in breathing and some degree of fever. The difficulty in breathing becomes steadily worse and lasts longer each time. The condition may be a simple sore throat or it may be due to diphtheria.

Whooping Cough. In this case there will be the characteristic " whoop."

Enlarged Tonsils and Adenoids. These may cause some obstruction to breathing and produce a noise very similar to that of croup. The treatment is to remove the tonsils and adenoids.

CROWING. This is also called laryngismus stridulus, laryngospasm or croup, and is a form of convulsion affecting the muscles of the throat, causing the patient to make a crowing noise rather like the whoop in whooping cough. It is a condition which affects children between the ages of 6 months and 2 years. It is found to occur in children who have rickets, and adenoids are frequently found to be present. (*See also* Croup.)

CUBEBS. This drug is obtained from the dried unripe full-grown fruit of a plant known as the piper cubeba which is grown in Java. It is largely used as a remedy for bronchitis or chronic sore throat. Asthma is sometimes relieved by smoking cubebs cigarettes.

CURD. When milk enters the stomach, the part of the milk called caseinogen is fermented into solid casein thus forming a curd. (*See also* Casein.)

CURETTAGE. This term is applied to an operation in which the interior of the womb is scraped with a *curette*. A curette is an instrument shaped rather like a spoon with a long handle, which varies in size according to the circumstances of the case.

One of the commonest causes for this operation is the removal of fragments of the products of conception, which if left in the womb would result in inflammation and infection. It frequently has to be performed after a miscarriage.

CURVATURE OF THE SPINE. The normal movements of the spine are forward, backward and sideways, but if any exaggeration of these movements appear, curvature of the spine may result. For full particulars *see also* SPINAL CURVATURE.

CUSPARIA. This drug is an aromatic bitter more familiarly known as angostura. (*See also* BITTERS.)

CUTICLE. The cuticle is popularly used to refer to the layer of skin which grows round the base of the nails, but it is really the outer covering protecting the whole skin of the body. (*See also* SKIN.)

CUTIS. The true skin. (*See also* SKIN.)

CUTS. A cut, however small, should be thoroughly cleansed before one tries to stop the bleeding, in order to avoid a septic (poisoned) wound. The simplest way is to hold the injured part under a running cold water tap for a few minutes. The surrounding parts should be washed away from, never towards, the wound. Broken glass, etc., should be removed if seen ; the cut should not be probed.

After washing, mild tincture of iodine should be dabbed (not rubbed) freely over the cut and the surrounding skin, and a clean dry bandage put on. A perfectly clean handkerchief is suitable. Sticking-plaster or ointment should not be applied.

Even fairly profuse bleeding may often be stopped by a firmly applied bandage ; boracic powder is sometimes useful. For more serious cuts, where the bleeding cannot be stopped, a tourniquet should be put on above the wound, and medical aid summoned at once.

CYANOSIS. This term is applied to a bluish discoloration of the skin which is due to the blood not being properly mixed with oxygen in the lungs. It may be a symptom of heart disease, or lung disease such as pneumonia, but by far the most frequent cause is a disturbance of the nervous system, owing to the presence of poison in the body. When people begin to look blue (or cyanosed) it is generally a sign that some illness is beginning, though in some cases it may be very slight indeed. There is a type of person who is always cold, and rather blue looking, but these people are generally the unhealthy type, and there may be no definite symptom of heart disease causing the blueness. Certainly a weak heart is known to produce blueness round the lips, etc., but every case of blueness is not due to heart disease. Very often the unfitness which produces cyanosis is caused by poisons due to habitual constipation, and the blueness will disappear as soon as the body has been cleared of the poisons. Rheumatic people very often show signs of blueness just before they are going to have an attack of their condition ; so also do people who have recurrent attacks of malaria. Many women have a blue and cold appearance just before the commencement of the menstrual period.

In certain conditions cyanosis may prove a very grave sign ; but, again, there are degrees of this condition which may go on for years without causing any disturbance to the patient.

CYSTITIS. This means inflammation of the bladder. It is usually due to infection by a germ, together with a lowered state of health. Some types of germs are so powerful that they alone will cause inflammation of the bladder, but these are not common.

The causes which tend to lower the body resistance are, injury or congestion of the bladder wall and stagnation of the urine.

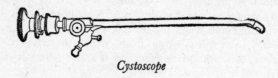

Cystoscope

Stagnation of the urine may be due to a variety of causes in the passage from the bladder to the exterior (the urethra), such as stricture (narrowing of the passage), enlargement of the prostate gland which surrounds the neck of the bladder, the presence of stone or other foreign body ; and also to various conditions affecting the nerve supply to the bladder.

Congestion of the bladder may be due to inflammation of the neighbouring structures such as the womb, to tumours of the bladder, etc. Damage during pregnancy or after childbirth is also quite a common cause.

The actual cause, the presence of virulent germs, may arise in the urethra ; or the germs may descend from the kidneys down the ureters. Germs are more liable to enter the female bladder from below—than the male—because the female urethra is much shorter than the male. The passage of a catheter may be followed by inflammation of the bladder.

Symptoms of Acute Cystitis. Pains in the lower part of the belly, also agonizing pain in the bladder and at the end of the penis in the male, after passing water. Water has to be passed frequently and urgently. The water contains an abundant deposit of slime and pus with perhaps blood in varying quantities.

Treatment. Rest in bed and food consisting of a milk diet are necessary. The pain is much relieved by hot hip-baths, of which two or three a day may be taken lasting for 20 minutes. Hot fomentations should be applied to the skin over the bladder. The bowels must be kept open with suitable aperients. Alcohol in any form is not allowed. The catheter should not be passed while the condition is acute, nor should any attempt be made to wash out the bladder. Sedative medicines should be given.

Chronic Cystitis. Here there is some pain, but usually much less than in the acute stage. There is more a feeling of weight in the lower part of the belly. There may still be a desire to pass water frequently and to evacuate the bowels. Damp and cold, sexual and alcoholic excesses will make the discomfort worse.

The water is cloudy, smells offensive and may be difficult to pass. It often contains pus and blood and is frequently alkaline. Of the complications of cystitis the most serious is infection of the kidneys.

Treatment. This depends on whether the germ causing the cystitis makes the water acid or alkaline. When the water is acid the germ is either that of gonorrhœa or one known as the Bacillus coli, a germ which normally lives in the large intestine. Drugs are given which tend to make the water alkaline. Citrate of potassium and bicarbonate of soda in large doses are given three times a day. The patient should not get up from bed till the condition has cleared up, as relapses are common. After a few days the water must be made acid. Making the water alkaline has prevented a great deal of activity on part of the germs, and has relieved the symptoms, but the only effective disinfectant of the bladder known is hexamine or urotropine, and it will only work when the water is acid. The water, then, is made acid by giving sodium acid phosphate, and the hexamine is given in fairly large doses. There may be a temporary aggravation of symptoms such as some discomfort and frequency in passing the water, so the patient should be warned of this in order to prevent disappointment. The hexamine is usually effective in clearing up the infection. In the case of gonorrhœa, of course, the local infection must be treated at the same time.

Local treatment may be carried out by washing out the bladder. An antispetic fluid is introduced by way of the urethra into the bladder two or three times a day. The bladder is washed out again and again until the returning fluid is quite clear. The fluid is usually silver nitrate. (*See also* BACILLURIA ; BLADDER.)

CYSTS. Cysts of one sort or another are tumours or swellings filled with fluid or semi-solid substance. They grow in almost any part of the body and vary in size from little pea-sized lumps to great unsightly growths, which are very disfiguring. Some sorts of cysts are dangerous to life, but many are harmless, though ugly and uncomfortable. A few varieties will be mentioned below. The commonest variety of cyst is the *sebaceous cyst* or *wen*, which is formed by the blocking of the sebaceous or fat glands of the skin. These wens may grow in any part of the body, but are most common on the face, neck and head. A curious variety of cyst is the *dermoid cyst*, which is present at birth, but usually does not develop until later in life. It is usually found on the face and contains such substances as skin, hair and even teeth. *Hydatid cysts* are important

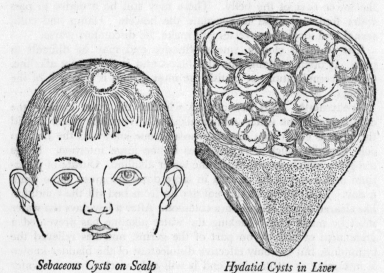

Sebaceous Cysts on Scalp   *Hydatid Cysts in Liver*

cysts which are caused by a worm resembling the tapeworm. This worm inhabits the intestines of sheep and dogs and is conveyed to human beings by these animals. They usually occur in the liver or lungs. *Ovarian cysts* of various sizes are fairly common in women, and in some cases grow to astonishing sizes. For further information about any of these varieties of cysts look under their own headings.

DACTYLITIS. This word literally means inflammation of the finger (from the Greek word dactyl, a finger). It is a condition which starts in one of the small bones of the finger and is nearly always tuberculous in origin. It may be a sign that tuberculosis is present in some other part of the body, so it is necessary that the general health should receive attention. Dactylitis may also occur in children owing to inherited syphilis.

DALTONISM. This term is applied to colour-blindness. The condition was named after John Dalton, an English chemist, who died in 1844. (*See also* COLOUR-BLINDNESS.)

DANDRUFF. Dandruff, or scurf, is due to a mild chronic inflammation of the skin of the scalp. The inflammation may be present for many years, the only disturbance being a slight itching. The head is " scurfy," i.e. the horny cells of the scalp are shed in large numbers and form scales ; and there is a tendency for the hair to come out. Each fallen hair is replaced by one thinner and weaker, until the hair is seriously thinned. Finally, the hair roots become atrophied, and baldness results.

This is one of the commonest of skin diseases ; it has been estimated that one in every three people is affected. It is chiefly due to local causes, the commonest being neglect of washing, brushing, and combing, with the consequent accumulation of cells and dried perspiration upon the scalp. Too vigorous brushing and combing, the use of harsh drying shampoos and lotions, the excessive use of oils, and anything which hinders the natural perspiration of the scalp (tight hats or head-dresses, " transformations," etc.), also cause the condition. Many sorts of germs are found upon the scalp, and these, though they do not cause the inflammation, help to keep it up when it has once started. Hence borrowed or dirty brushes and combs should never be used. Some people, such as those with tender skins, which turn red and are irritable on very slight provocation, are specially liable to dandruff. Acne or rosacea, oily skins, a tendency to kidney or rheumatic troubles, defective digestion ; other scalp troubles, such as boils, seborrhœa, and wounds are frequently accompanied by dandruff.

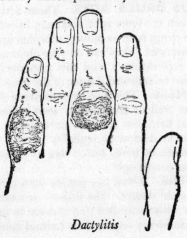

Dactylitis

Treatment. This long list of causes shows that the treatment must be general and preventive, as well as local. The *preventive* treatment consists in avoiding anything harmful to the scalp, and due attention to the hair. The *general* treatment consists in regulating the diet and attending to the ordinary rules of hygiene.

The milder cases of dandruff should be cured by regular care of the hair. If possible, it should be washed daily, and the juice of half a lemon mixed with the final rinsing water.

The cure of a well-established case requires endless patience and care, as the condition is very obstinate. Ladies with long hair would be well advised to have it cut, as the applications of medicaments to a scalp covered by long hair is not only very tedious and difficult, but the resulting appearance is far from attractive.

Many substances have been used, such as sulphur, salicylic acid, resorcin, iodine, pyrogallol, etc. (Fair-haired people should avoid the use of any but the first two, as the others darken the hair.) The most valuable of these is sulphur, which may be applied as an ointment or emulsion, the latter being the cleaner method. The preparation is applied at night and well rubbed in, and a linen cap worn. A bathing-cap, so often advised, should *not* be worn ; it is most unhealthy for the scalp. The sulphur is allowed to remain on for ten days and then washed off ; after which the treatment is repeated until the cure is complete.

Since light treatment and X-rays produce such wonderful results in other cases of chronic inflammation, it was hoped that they would be equally successful in cases of dandruff, but the results have been disappointing. Improvement may occur at first, but the condition soon relapses, and may even be aggravated.

DANGEROUS DRUGS ACTS. These acts were passed by Parliament between the years 1920 and 1923 in order to prevent the sale of dangerous drugs such as opium, morphia and cocaine except in special circumstances. They can only be obtained from a chemist with a medical prescription ; and this prescription may only be used once and must be renewed if more of the drug is to be obtained.

DAY-BLINDNESS. This is an irregularity of the sight, in which objects cannot be well or comfortably seen either by daylight or by strong artificial light, but are seen more clearly and comfortably by a half-light, as in shadow or twilight.

It is not a disease in itself, but a sign of disease, and may be caused by various conditions.

DEAD FINGERS. There are people who suffer from what is popularly called dead fingers. The fingers, and sometimes the toes, may suddenly go white and cold and remain so for a short period and then just as suddenly regain their normal colour. The disease is considered to be due to a disturbance of the nervous system. Particulars are given under its medical term RAYNAUD's DISEASE.

DEADLY NIGHT-SHADE. *See* ATROPINE and BELLADONNA.

DEAF-MUTISM. This means that a person can neither hear nor speak. It may date from birth or be acquired at an early age, and in nearly every case the deaf-mutism exists because the child cannot hear and so has never learned to speak, as speech comes from the imitation of sounds heard. The most usual cause of deaf-mutism dating from birth (*congenital deaf-mutism*) is a defect in the development of the internal ear ; this may be hereditary and is said to be comparatively common in children who are the result of marriages between near blood relations, such as first cousins. Deaf-mutism acquired at an early age may be due to a variety of diseases, such as meningitis, scarlet fever, mumps, and inflammation of the internal ear.

Treatment. The first thing to do in the treatment of deaf-mutism is to make sure that the condition is not due to some disease of the ear, which ought to be treated. If the deaf-mutism is due to a defect of development of the ear no treatment will be of any avail, and the child should be sent to a special school for deaf-mutes, of which there are a number in different parts of the country, such as Manchester, Edinburgh, and several schools under the London County Council. Teaching speech by signs is now out of date, as it restricts conversation to those who are acquainted with the deaf and dumb alphabet. Nowadays deaf-mutes are taught by lip-reading and by the sense of touch : the pupil watches the movements of the teacher's lips and at the same time places his hand over the teacher's throat to feel the movements of the larynx. Although the education of deaf-mutes is a long and tedious business, the results usually obtained make it well worth while. (*See also* DEAFNESS.)

DEAFNESS. This may be due to blocking of the outer passage (external meatus) of the ear by wax, to blocking of the middle ear (the little space behind the drum) by catarrh or inflammation, or to disease of the internal ear (nerve-deafness). Many persons, when they become deaf, say that there is deafness in their family, and make little effort to get cured ; but an extremely small percentage of cases of deafness is due to any family influence. Deafness is common, much more common than most people imagine, and it is much more easily treated in its early stages than in its late stages, when it is almost always incurable. Wax can be removed easily by syringing the ear with a solution of bicarbonate of soda in warm water ; this dissolves the wax, which the stream of water washes out. Catarrh of the middle ear is usually an extension of a cold in the nose up the little tube that leads to the ear to the middle ear itself.

It is often brought on by violent blowing of the nose when one has a cold or by using a nasal douche and sniffing it up the nose too hard.

Catarrh of the middle ear is best treated by inhalation of menthol or Friar's balsam (1 teaspoonful to a pint of boiling water); a specialist can clear the ear by blowing the catarrh away with a little silver eustachian catheter; but this is a difficult procedure that needs much practice. Inflammation of the ear and chronic discharge from the ear cause deafness, but require treatment by a doctor to get them well. Internal ear-deafness (nerve-deafness) is usually due either to old age, or to a poisoning of the nerve of hearing by tobacco or quinine, or by the poisons of such diseases as mumps or syphilis. It takes a lot of strong tobacco to cause internal ear-deafness, but this cause is not uncommon.

Artificial Aids to Hearing. Many people rush to use an artificial aid to hearing without due consideration. No artificial aid can bring back the hearing to normal, for the reason that the aid itself is bound to have a restricted range of hearing. People prefer electrical types, because they are inconspicuous. These are often useful in middle-ear deafness (especially the kind called otosclerosis), when the deaf person cannot hear another person speaking unless he raises his voice. An ordinary hearing-trumpet (a useful one is the " banjo " type) does not need new batteries or renewals, but has the disadvantage of being more conspicuous; except for this disadvantage, the hearing-trumpet is often the best type of hearing aid.

The new valve-amplifier type of electrical aid is often useful in nerve-deafness. But the ears should always be examined by an ear specialist before getting an artificial aid, so as to get a correct diagnosis of the type of deafness. One has known a person to buy an expensive electrical artificial aid to hearing when all that was the matter was merely a plug of wax in the ear.

DEATH. When death takes place two things occur : (1) the circulation of the blood through the body, and (2) the act of breathing, stop. Changes take place in the cell tissue and, consequently, in the appearance of the dead person.

That the circulation has really stopped may be ascertained by listening carefully for the heart-beats. For the breathing, a looking-glass may be held before the face and note taken whether it becomes misty, or a feather may be placed on the upper lip and we may watch carefully for the faintest fluttering.

Those in attendance should close the eyes and mouth, bandage the jaw and straighten the limbs.

A few hours after death the body is cold. Bruise-like marks on the back show that congestion of blood is taking place ; during the next few hours the muscles stiffen, to relax again in about four days. A greenness on the abdomen two or three days after death shows that decay has begun.

Duties of Relatives. It is the duty of the relatives personally to report the death to the local registrar of births, marriages and deaths ; if a doctor was in attendance during the last illness, written notice must be accompanied by the doctor's certificate of the cause of death. They must sign the register in the presence of the registrar. Failing any relative who was with the dead person when death took place, or attending on him, the duty of informing the registrar falls on some other relative. Failing any relatives, it falls on someone present at the death, then on the occupier of the house, then on someone living in it, or the person arranging for the funeral. The body must not be buried until the registrar has given a certificate ; this is handed to the clergyman at the funeral.

Sudden or violent deaths and deaths in prison are matters for the coroner. It would be the duty of anyone witnessing a sudden or violent death or finding a dead body to inform the police. In Scotland the Procurator Fiscal holds a private inquiry and the Lord Advocate may order a public inquiry.

Cremation. Anyone wishing his body to be cremated after death should leave written instructions to this effect. If he forbids this form of burial, it cannot take place. Regulations for cremations and disposal of the ashes are made, under Act of Parliament, by the Home Secretary, and certificates by two doctors are required before cremation can be carried out.

DEBILITY. Debility is a term used to describe a state of health which is very much below normal. The term is a very wide one and many people use it when there is any form of weakness present in the system. Debility may be used to describe a state of the part of the body which is most affected ; for example, there is a state of *general* debility which may be caused by insufficient or improper food, lack of exercise, unhealthy surroundings, or many other causes such as exhausting illnesses or poisoning. *Nervous* debility usually owes its origin to some nervous worry which the patient has had for a long time. Financial or business worries or love affairs which have not turned out satisfactorily will often cause nervous debility. *Cardiac* debility is a term applied to persons who are suffering from some weakness of the heart. It does not mean that the heart is diseased, but it may be in a temporarily weakened state as a result of a severe illness. Any form of debility should be treated with adequate rest, plenty of fresh air, good and nourishing food and a proper amount of exercise and tonics.

DECLINE. When this term is used it generally means that the patient is gradually losing strength and that the body is wasting away. The word is popularly used in connection with consumption, but "decline" may occur in many other wasting diseases such as nephritis, nervous debility or in certain infections of the lungs.

DECOCTION. This word is derived from the Latin, which means to boil down. In dealing with medicine, a decoction is made by boiling a drug or drugs for a certain length of time and afterwards adding water if necessary. There is a difference between a decoction and an infusion. A decoction is actually boiled ; but an infusion is made by pouring boiling water over a substance just as in making tea.

DEFECTIVE VISION. There are two sorts of blindness and defective sight : in the first there is an easily recognizable defect in the eye ; in the second, however, there is no obvious cause in any part of the eye. It has been happily described as a " disease in which the patient sees nothing and the physician sees nothing!" The term *amblyopia* is used to mean this latter form of defective sight. (*See also* AMBLYOPIA ; BLINDNESS ; VISION.)

DEFICIENCY DISEASES are a group of diseases due to the lack of an essential element in the food called a vitamin ; vitamins A, B, C, D and E are different varieties of vitamin, the lack of which causes different diseases. The first disease that was recognized to be due to vitamin deficiency was scurvy, which is caused by lack of vitamin C, which is present in fresh vegetables or meat. Scurvy formerly used to break out in ships on long voyages, and it was found that it could be prevented by taking daily a small amount of lime juice as it was called. (In reality it was lemon juice from Mediterranean lemons, which were called limes by mistake ; lemon juice, it has been found, contains much more vitamin C than does lime juice.) Vitamin B, when lacking, causes a disease known in the East as beri-beri, in which the affected person has severe neuritis and eventually various forms of paralysis. At the siege of Kut, during the Great War, it was observed that the soldiers who had hand-milled (unpolished) rice escaped beri-beri, but those who fed on white (polished) rice contracted it ; the reason for this was that the " germ " of the rice, and also of wheat contains something that prevents beri-beri. Vitamin B_2, when lacking, causes pellagra which, however, is rare in this country ; but deficiency in vitamins B_1 and B_2 causes various disorders such as constipation and anæmia, and pregnant women and nursing mothers appear to require it particularly. It is also contained in yeast, oranges and tomatoes. Rickets, the third deficiency disease to be recognized, was at first thought to be due to an absence of vitamin A, the existence of which was made known only after vitamins B and C were discovered. Vitamin A was, however, confused with vitamin D, because they are present in almost the same substances. Rickets is now known to be due to deficiency in vitamin D, and the relation of this vitamin to sunlight is explained when it is realized that almost all living cells contain a substance (ergosterol) which when irradiated by ultra-violet rays becomes an anti-ricket substance. It was shown by the Commission to Vienna after the Great War that rickets could be prevented by the administration of cod-liver oil, by exposure to sunlight, and by exposure to ultra-violet light. The chief source of vitamin D is cod-liver and halibut-liver oil. Vitamin A (the fat-soluble vitamin) is derived from the green chlorophyll of plants, and so appears in milk, butter, animal fats and fish-livers—the fish get the chlorophyll from the animalculæ floating on the surface of the sea. The deficiency diseases directly due to lack of vitamin A (xerophthalmia, hemeralopia) are rare, but deficiency of this vitamin is responsible for a lowering of resistance to infection. Vitamin E is related to reproductive capacity, but is still a matter for research. Any ordinary diet of eggs, meat, green vegetables and seed germs appears to contain sufficient vitamin E. In this country an ordinary good mixed dietary is the best preventive of vitamin deficiency, as such a dietary will normally contain enough of the various vitamins to prevent any of the deficiency diseases developing.

DEFORMITY. Any abnormal condition of the body whether congenital (present at birth) or acquired later in life may be termed a deformity. Deformity may arise from many causes. When present at birth, it may be due to faulty development of the child in the womb ; it may be the result of some injury to the body at birth ; or it may be caused by disease.

Certain deformities such as extra toes or fingers seem to run in families, but such deformities are very easily got rid of if attended to at birth and no discomfort or unhappiness is caused when the child grows up. Those which are most common are club-foot, dislocation of the hip, cleft palate, hare-lip and wry-neck. Other congenital deformities may not be so easily treated and may even be so bad as to prevent a normal life being led.

Deformities due to injuries are very extensive indeed and may include scarring of the skin and shortening of the muscles, and damage to the bones. Many people are so badly scarred by burns that the tissues are destroyed, leaving very disfiguring marks. Skin-grafting has done much to prevent ugly deformities, especially on the face ; this is carried out by taking skin from a healthy part of the body and causing it to grow over the disfigured parts.

When muscles have been damaged they usually shorten during the process of healing. This condition may be treated by massage ; but, as a rule, a surgical operation is required to put matters right. Broken bones always cause a certain amount of deformity and unless they are properly reset, a considerable amount of deformity will result. It is advisable to have X-ray photographs taken after a fracture has been reset in order to make sure that the bones are in the correct position.

Various diseases are responsible for causing deformities of the bones and by far the most common is tuberculosis. It attacks the growing bones of young children and may even destroy part of the bone ; the ligaments also become diseased, thus causing the bones to assume abnormal positions. Most of the cases of humpback are due to tuberculosis of the spine and many displaced hips are due to the same cause.

Rheumatoid arthritis is a disease which affects many of the joints in the body. Very serious deformities are caused by this inflammatory condition and many people become altogether bed-ridden by it. However, the chief general disease which leads to deformity is rickets. This condition causes the bones to become soft and, as soon as any pressure is put on them—for instance, when the child begins to walk—the bones become distorted and many serious deformities are thus produced. Humpback, curvature of the spine, bow-legs, knock-knee and deformity of the pelvis are a few of the conditions which may arise through rickets. Many women are prevented from having children or, at least, have a difficult and dangerous time at childbirth because of the damage done to the pelvis by rickets in early childhood.

Paralysis due to some nervous condition may cause serious shortening of the muscles. Infantile paralysis, especially, is the cause of many permanent deformities. The limbs gradually waste away through not being moved or used, and a withered arm or leg is often one of the results of this condition. Surgeons who deal with cases of deformity are known as *orthopædic* surgeons, and surgeons who build up parts of the face or body are known as *plastic* surgeons.

DELHI BOIL. This is one of the many names applied to an Oriental sore. The condition is described under the heading ALEPPO BUTTON.

DELIRIUM. This is a mental disturbance which is marked by excitement, bodily restlessness and flights of the imagination and accompanied by senseless chattering. Delirium occurs in many disorders, but is a particularly distressing accompaniment of any high fever.

DELIRIUM TREMENS. This is not the result of a very large single dose of alcohol ; it occurs in those people who are steady drinkers, never drunk, but never completely sober. It comes on very often if, owing to such unforeseen circumstances as an injury, or attack of pneumonia, all alcohol is suddenly stopped. Delirium tremens is really a variety of acute insanity which is marked by delirium with trembling and excitement, and in which there is great anxiety, mental distress, sweating and pain. It lasts only a few days, and with proper treatment recovery is the rule ; but any further indulgence in alcohol renders the patient liable to another, and probably a fatal attack.

DELIVERY. By delivery is meant the stage of childbirth during which the child actually passes from the womb of the mother. In a normal delivery the head of the child comes first, and the rest of the body usually comes away within the space of a few seconds. After delivery has taken place, the mother should rest in bed for at least a fortnight ; but if this is not possible, daily rests should be taken and all heavy work should be avoided. Falling of the womb and its complications very often occur because the mother has neglected to take sufficient rest after her child has been delivered. (*See also* CHILDBIRTH ; LABOUR.)

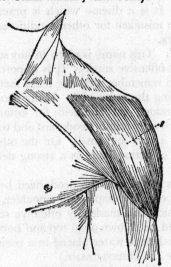

A. *Deltoid Muscle*

DELTOID. This is the name given to a thick muscle of the shoulder. It derives its name from its likeness to the Greek letter delta Δ.

DEMENTIA. This is a permanent loss of mind which results from destruction of certain nerve cells in the brain. It must be distinguished from *amentia*, a condition in which the mental powers have never developed. Dementia may be the last stage in some other mental disorder, or it may occur as the result of the wearing out and breaking down of the nervous system in old age, or the specialized cells of the nervous system may be starved of blood through disease of the arteries of the brain and so perish. The chief causes of disease of the brain arteries are excessive consumption of alcohol, chronic disease of the kidneys and syphilis.

Dementia Præcox is a mental disorder which causes, in its late stages, the most profound dementia. This mental disorder begins as a rule in adolescence or early adult life, and mostly in persons who have a family history of established mental disease. Before the onset of dementia præcox, the patient nearly always shows some signs of mental peculiarity.

DEMULCENT. A demulcent is the name given to any substance which has a soothing effect on the skin, particularly on raw surfaces such as a sore throat.

DENGUE FEVER. This is a type of fever which is very common in most tropical countries, and which usually commences with great suddenness. It is a disease which is practically never fatal and it must not be mistaken for other conditions, such as measles, malaria or influenza.

DEODORANT. This name is given to any substance that deodorizes or destroys offensive smells. It is important when dealing with this matter to remember that the mere fact of covering up a smell is not removing the cause of it. Many deodorant substances also act as disinfectants ; carbolic acid, for instance, is a powerful disinfectant, but it is only mildly deodorant and will not be of much use in covering up a very foul smell. On the other hand, chloride of lime is capable of acting both as a strong deodorant and as a disinfectant.

In the sick-room the air can be deodorized by burning a piece of thick brown paper. The paper will smoulder, thus giving off a pungent smoke which will mask any offensive smell in the room. The windows should be thrown open top and bottom to allow fresh air to come in. Buckets of water placed in a room will remove the smell of paint. (*See also* DISINFECTANT.)

DEPILATORY. This is the name given to any drug or method by which hair is removed from the body. Many depilatories are composed of sulphide of barium, but the effect produced by the use of this substance is temporary and the hair will grow again in the course of a week or two.

DEPRESSANT. This is the name given to a group of drugs which cause a depressing effect on various organs of the human body ; in other words, these drugs act upon these organs either through the brain centre or through the nerve supply and cause them to stop working. For example, when chloroform is given, it depresses the brain and eventually causes the patient to become unconscious. Many drugs are given to depress the action of the heart, and the same rule applies to the drugs which act upon various other centres of the body.

DERBYSHIRE NECK. A swelling of the neck known as goitre has long been associated with Derbyshire ; hence the term Derbyshire neck. This condition seems to occur more often in mountainous districts than in others. (*See also* GOITRE.)

DERCUM'S DISEASE. *See* ADIPOSIS DOLOROSA.

DERMATITIS or INFLAMMATION OF THE SKIN. When the skin is irritated in any way, whether from outside or inside, it behaves like all the other parts of the body in like circumstances : it makes a protest. To this is given the name dermatitis, or inflammation of the skin, or just skin trouble. The greater the amount of the irritation, and the more sensitive the skin, the more severe is the resulting inflammation.

The first stage is that of *erythema* or redness, due to the walls of the blood-vessels dilating or relaxing. The next is that the relaxed vessel walls allow fluid to be poured out into the tissues of the skin ; this results in the cells of the horny or topmost layer of the skin, instead of being shed as invisible single cells when their work is done, sticking together and coming off as noticeable *scales*. If the amount of fluid is greater, it flows out between the cells on to the surface and dries there, forming what are called *crusts*.

If the fluid is poured out more rapidly than it can make its way to the surface, it makes little pools in the epidermis, or upper layer of the skin. These form tiny blisters, and are called *vesicles*. Larger blisters sometimes occur, which are called *blebs* or *bullæ*. In some cases the fluid produced is actually so great as to wash off the outer layer of the skin, leaving an inflamed red surface from which drops of fluid are continually seen oozing. This was formerly called weeping eczema, but is now better known as *moist* or *weeping dermatitis*.

In very chronic inflammation the whole skin layer and the tissues underneath become thicker and harder. This process is called *keratosis*.

In view of these different results which may be brought about by irritation of the skin, and remembering that one or another, or two or three together, may be seen at the same time, it is easy to understand the great variety of skin " pictures " that may be found, the difficulty of treating them, and the patience that must in many cases be exercised by both doctor and patient if a good result is to be obtained. There is, at present, no one-day cure for dermatitis.

Sometimes dermatitis occurs in which one form of reaction is the chief, and it is convenient to recognize and treat this. It must always be remembered, however, that it is the *cause* of the dermatitis that is of importance, not the *form* it takes.

Treatment. The treatment of dermatitis or inflammation of the skin has already been discussed from the local point of view ; that is, as far as regards applications to the skin itself. The aim in treatment is to take away what the skin has in excess, and to supply what it has not ; for instance, to remove discharge, scales, or thick-ened skin ; to supply fat to a dry skin ; to relieve itching and heat. It is hoped by these means that the skin will be sufficiently put at rest to cure itself.

Diet. As, however, the skin takes such an important part in getting rid of waste products of the body, it should not only be put at rest from without but also from within. A generation or so ago dermatitis was treated almost too much by dieting, and in most cases from the point of view of experiment rather than of exact knowledge. It was known that some articles of food produced a rash in some people, but " idiosyncrasy " was not heard of then, and the tendency was to forbid anything that had ever been known to cause·dermatitis ! The result was that many patients suffering from skin trouble were restricted most rigidly to a few articles of diet and, as is now known, quite unnecessarily. Each case must be decided on its own merits. Mutton may cause, or increase dermatitis in one patient, and beef be quite harmless ; while in another the exact opposite is the case. And so with all the other foods that have been forbidden from time to time—fish, cheese, porridge, fruit, etc. etc. Sometimes a patient knows quite well that a certain article of food increases his skin trouble ; but in doubtful cases a skin test may be used. The patient may then have a reason-ably plentiful and varied diet, and be quite certain that he is safe from adding to his skin trouble.

A special word must be said about alcohol. It is sometimes said that alcohol " goes to the head," or " goes to the legs," according as to how an individual is affected by its use ; but it certainly " goes to the skin " in all cases. It has a greater power than any other food of increasing the circulation in the skin, and so flushing and warming it. Any form of dermatitis is rendered worse by alcohol, especially the more acute forms, and those in which itching is found. It must therefore be avoided whenever possible in such cases.

Soap and Water. It was once commonly believed that soap and water were bad for skin diseases, and the old belief is still widespread. Doubtless, years ago, when the water-supply was not so pure as it is now—possibly drawn from wells, and containing a large quantity of salts as well as other irritating ingredients—this may have been true. It is still true in some places where the water is very hard. A moderate use of soft water, however, though it may cause a slight increase of irritation in an acute dermatitis, more than compensates for this by removing scales, discharge, and germs from the skin. An oily dressing may need to be used afterwards if the skin tends to crack and dry.

DERMOGRAPHIA (Skin-Writing). Dermographia is a peculiar condition in which one is able to write or draw a pattern on the skin, and the result is immediately shown in vivid red raised marks. The patterns usually remain quite visible for several minutes, then gradually fade.

This peculiar condition often accompanies urticaria or nettle-rash, but the patterns usually itch, while in true dermographia the patterns do not itch. Nothing can be done for this condition ; it is one of those medical curiosities which is due perhaps to some disorder of the nervous control.

DERMOID CYSTS. This is the name applied to growths found in the body which contain structures that really belong to the skin. For instance, skin itself may be found growing inside, or hair, etc. (*See also* CYSTS.)

DESCENDING COLON. Part of the large intestine. (*See also* INTESTINES.)

DESQUAMATION. Derived from a Latin word meaning to scale, the term desquamation is used to describe the peeling of the skin which follows certain diseases. In scarlet fever, peeling of the skin is one of the most common symptoms ; in severe cases considerable loss of hair may accompany peeling. Desquamation of a branny appearance follows the fading of the spots in measles.

DESUDATION. This term is applied when any unusually violent sweating takes place. The term is also applied to a slight skin rash which appears, due to sweating. Children very often suffer from this condition when they are too warmly clad. The skin should be dusted with a powder, consisting of zinc oxide and starch. (*See also* SWEATING, DISAGREEABLE.)

DETERGENT. This name is given to any drug or substance which is used for cleansing or purifying. Soap, for example, is a detergent. Many alcoholic preparations are used to cleanse greasy skins.

DHOBIE ITCH. This is a Hindu name for ringworm of the

body. It is a disease which is very common in the tropics, and it derives its name from the belief that clothes become infected while being washed. The washerman in India is known as the dhobie. Full description of the disease is given under RINGWORM.

DIABETES (DIABETES MELLITUS). Diabetes mellitus is the medical name for the disease which is commonly known simply as diabetes, or sugar diabetes. It is, unfortunately, a fairly common disease after middle-age and used to come sooner or later to a fatal ending ; but with the newly-discovered treatment by *insulin*, diabetic people can now lead useful lives and live to die of other causes at a normal age.

Symptoms. A typical case of diabetes is a wasting disease, with the well-recognized symptoms of passing large quantities of urine (polyuria), thirst and hunger, together with sugar in the urine (glycosuria). If the malady is left untreated it will continue to get worse, until the patient falls into a fatal coma or state of unconsciousness. There are, however, all shades of severity of the disease, from a condition in which there is merely a trace of sugar in the urine, to one in which the symptoms are so pronounced as to make the patient seriously ill.

It is usual to regard everyone who continually has sugar in the urine as diabetic ; but it must be emphasized that sugar in the urine, especially when it is only temporary, is not of such great importance. It is really quite a frequent occurrence. Some cases are due to leakage of sugar from a faulty kidney, and many untreated cases of persistent and fairly well-marked sugar in the urine never develop into true diabetes. The exact amount of sugar present can only be measured after a meal of carbohydrate has been eaten, and where diabetes is suspected this examination is well worth doing, because in many cases it will save the person, who is merely suffering from the simple condition, an unnecessary amount of bodily and mental anguish. The onset of the disease is gradual, and either the frequent passing of urine or a marked thirst may be the first things to direct attention to the condition. It may set in more rapidly after a sudden emotion, injury, or severe chill. The thirst is often very distressing. Large quantities of water are required to keep the sugar in a liquid state, so that the body may get rid of it in the urine. The amount of fluid taken is in proportion to the amount passed as urine. The digestion remains good and the appetite may be enormous. The tongue is usually dry, red and glazed, and the saliva is scanty. The gums become swollen. In spite of the enormous amounts of food consumed, the patient usually becomes very thin and wasted, the skin is irritable, and there is constipation.

Complications.—Coma: The most serious complication of severe diabetes is coma or unconsciousness, which is caused by poisoning of the blood, or *acidosis,* caused by the faulty chemistry of the body. In a typical case of coma there is difficulty of breathing, the pulse grows weak, and the patient gradually loses consciousness, sinks into a deep coma, and dies, sometimes within twenty-four hours. The coma may come on without any warning, or there may be headache, thick speech, and a staggering gait before the coma comes on. In other cases there may be weakness, giddiness, and livid hands and feet, especially after exertion, preceding the onset of the coma.

Skin Eruptions: In diabetes, boils and carbuncles are very common. Eczema and intolerable itching are very often present. Profuse sweats may occur, and in certain cases there may be " bronzing " of the skin. In extreme cases the extremities may become gangrenous.

Other Complications: Diabetic persons are very liable to lung and tuberculous troubles, and are often carried off with an attack of pneumonia. There may be some degree of kidney trouble causing swelling of the feet and ankles, but general water-logging of the tissues is rare owing to the amount of urine that is passed. Neuritis, neuralgia, numbness, and tingling in the limbs are common. A diabetic person is often morose, and some become restless and anxious to a degree. In diabetes the sexual function is impaired and impotence is common, and is usually an early symptom. It is rare for a diabetic woman to conceive, and if she does she generally has an abortion, but a diabetic mother may bear a healthy child. There is, in fact, no known instance of a diabetic mother having a diabetic child.

Treatment of Diabetes by Diet. Diabetes is due to a change in the organ called the pancreas, and from the nature of things this change must be progressive if left untreated, otherwise the condition would never have manifested itself. This progressive tendency may be checked by dieting, but may unfortunately be made worse where the diet is unsuitable. In some cases the tendency to become worse is very marked and even suitable dieting will fail to check it. These are the cases where the preparation called *insulin* is necessary. As a general rule dieting is sufficient for slight cases.

The fasting is not really starvation, since as much tea, black coffee and beef tea as are required may be taken. Smoking may be allowed. When there is no more sugar in the urine the patient can start on a very little protein and a little fat. It is essential to know how much energy the food contains, and it is also desirable to give plenty of bulk in the food to ease the pangs of hunger.

Insulin Treatment. As has been stated above, the first hope

7*

of the diabetic patient is in diet, but if this fails insulin must be resorted to. It must be remembered, however, that it may take some months to find a suitable diet on which the patient does not lose weight and on which his general condition does not get worse. The strength of insulin preparations is measured in " units " according to its effect on the sugar in the blood. Unfortunately, patients vary in their response to insulin, so that the present " unit " of measurement is not very accurate, but it is the most satisfactory way of measuring the strength of insulin that has yet been discovered. Most preparations of insulin are such that a cubic centimetre of the liquid contains 10 or 20 units of insulin.

· **Symptoms.** Insulin poisoning may appear when insulin is being given in too large doses. The face usually flushes with a sweating which may be very marked ; the patient feels giddy and has a distinct sense of physical coldness about the limbs and there may be blanching of the face. Sometimes the first symptom is a feeling of nervousness or distinct tremulousness, so that the patient finds it impossible to co-ordinate his movements, e.g. if he tries to write he sprawls on the paper. There may be some vague feelings of apprehension—a fear of some disaster about to take place. Later, confusion and delirium may occur, with finally collapse and unconsciousness. Convulsions are rare.

These symptoms usually come on from 1 to 3 hours after an injection of insulin, but not infrequently may be seen from 4 to 6 hours, or even 12 hours after injection.

Sugar given by mouth will quickly relieve all the symptoms, so that there is little or no danger associated with the use of insulin if the patient is carefully warned to take sugar whenever any symptoms, such as those described, follow on injection. Any kind of sugar will do, but glucose is the best. The patient should carry with him some barley sugar, and he soon begins to recognize the symptoms, and by taking the sugar can prevent their further development.

Should the patient be unconscious the sugar must be given by injection into the veins and the collapse treated on the usual lines by stimulation with suitable drugs (strychnine, camphor, hot coffee, etc.).

Effect of Insulin on the Diabetic Condition. The insulin acts by restoring the diabetic patient to a normal individual. The food must be regulated and the necessary insulin dosage discovered and taken with the utmost regularity. When this is done, the blood sugar can be kept at a normal value. Many patients with long-standing diabetes are able to resume work, and appear to be as fit as the average person.

Insulin is required in cases where the diet treatment does not effect an improvement, and in patients where the diabetic condition is associated with definite symptoms such as :

Eye changes, which often end in blindness ; neuritis of various degrees ; intense local and general irritation ; weakness of the limbs, and pains in the back and sides ; diabetic gangrene.

It is important, of course, to be certain that the case is one of sugar in the urine due to diabetes, and not a case of *renal glycosuria*, where the sugar leaks through into the urine from the kidney. In this case the insulin will only lower the blood sugar still further and may give rise to signs of insulin poisoning.

Contraindications to Insulin Treatment. Insulin does not cure diabetes : the disease is essentially progressive in nature. In the young, however, there is definite evidence that recovery of the cells of the pancreas may take place when the disease is controlled by insulin, though no cases of a cure have yet been recorded.

The aim is to arrange a diet and to give the patient the necessary amount of insulin to keep his urine sugar-free.

As a rule the best results are obtained by placing the patient on a fixed diet which is calculated to be sufficient in all respects, and then to give increasing doses of insulin until satisfactory results are obtained.

For years after the discovery of insulin patients were kept on a diet rich in fats and poor in carbohydrates, but it is now recognized that it is better to have a diet comparatively rich in carbohydrates and poor in fats. This plan, indeed, enables the insulin dosage to be reduced, as a diabetic is less sensitive to insulin on a diet containing much fat but little or no carbohydrate. Small doses of insulin have been found to be more effective with plenty of dextrose (sugar) than are large doses with a smaller intake of dextrose.

DIABETES INSIPIDUS. This is a chronic disease in which there is a great increase in the amount of urine passed, but it does not contain sugar as does the water in ordinary diabetes. It is rather a rare disease. It is sometimes popularly called " drinking diabetes," the word drinking not referring to alcoholic drinking but to the fact that one of the chief features of this form of diabetes is a terrible and unquenchable thirst, so that the victims drink quarts of water or other liquids which seem to pass straight through them without appeasing their thirst. The condition is most common in early manhood, and sometimes it seems to run in families, especially in families where there is a marked tendency to nervous or mental troubles.

Symptoms. The two most noticeable symptoms which are also present are the increase in the amount of pale-coloured urine passed and the noticeable and distressing thirst. The beginning of the disease may be very slow and practically unnoticed or it may come on very suddenly. The frequency with which the patient has to make water causes distress and discomfort during the day and loss of sleep during the night. There may be as much as 20 pints of urine passed in 24 hours. *At first the amount of urine is greater than the amount of fluid swallowed, the extra amount coming from the food and from the tissues of the body. Later on this ceases to be so. As has been said above, there is no sugar in the urine. The thirst is very great, and there is a case on record of a young man who drank 70 pints of fluid daily and passed about 80 pints.

The mouth, tongue and throat are dry and parched and the appetite is usually increased. The skin is dry and harsh. The temperature is generally below normal, and in the early stages the digestion may be good. The condition may be caused by damage to the brain or nervous system. There may be pains in the back and the legs or a tingling and itching in the skin.

Treatment. At times the condition is so slight that it may be regarded as an annoyance rather than as a disease, but in severe cases the patient gets gradually worse. The muscles waste and the digestion fails, while the patient becomes drowsy and finally falls into a state of coma which lasts until death. The blood should always be tested for syphilis. No attempt should be made to reduce the amount of fluid swallowed by the patient, but it is sometimes useful gradually to leave meat and salt out of the diet. Hypodermic injections of pituitary extract are very useful and sometimes have a really dramatic effect in relieving the condition. Cure sometimes takes place of its own accord. (*See also* DUCTLESS GLANDS.)

DIACETIC ACID. This is an acid present in the urine in certain stages of diabetes and other diseases. If diacetic acid be permitted to continue to accumulate in the body it may lead to a very serious condition. It is important, therefore, to have a test made of the urine if there are any signs of acidosis in the body.

DIAGNOSIS. Diagnosis is the art of being able to distinguish one disease from another.

DIAPHORETIC. This is the name given to any drug or treatment which causes the skin to sweat freely. Turkish baths or hot-air baths are very good examples of a diaphoretic, and certain drugs may be given which act on the nerve centres and produce an increase of sweat. (*See also* FEVER ; SWEATING.)

DIAPHRAGM. The diaphragm is the dome-shaped muscular partition which separates the space of the abdomen from that of the chest. It is more popularly called the midriff. It is the chief muscle used in breathing, and when air is drawn into the lungs the diaphragm is able to be expanded. Singers and athletes are trained to breathe through the diaphragm rather than the chest.

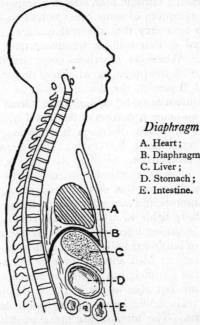

Diaphragm

A. Heart;
B. Diaphragm;
C. Liver;
D. Stomach;
E. Intestine.

DIARRHŒA. The condition where the bowels move too frequently and the motions are of too soft a consistency is known as diarrhœa. It is not a disease in itself, but rather a symptom of various diseases. It may be brought on simply by taking too strong medicines or by eating unsuitable food or too much fruit. Damp and cold will bring on diarrhœa in some people, and various nervous conditions may be responsible for an attack. Nervous excitement such as that experienced by students just before an examination is a well-known cause of diarrhœa.

By far the most common cause, however, is eating tainted or indigestible food. These foods set up irritation in the bowel and may be accompanied by severe colicky pains and much wind. In such a case, the first thing to do is to get rid of the irritating substance in the bowel, and this is done by taking some opening medicine. A large dose of castor oil should be taken, and when the bowels have been thoroughly purged, a chalk or bismuth mixture may be taken to clear up the diarrhœa. If there is much pain or exhaustion, a doctor may prescribe opium, which is very soothing to the irritated bowel. The diet for the next few days should be as simple as possible and should contain such things as arrowroot and corn-flour, etc.

When treating chronic diarrhœa it is important to bear in mind that it is a symptom of some other condition and not a disease in itself. It is necessary that the real cause of the diarrhœa should be discovered so that suitable treatment may be given as quickly as possible. Whenever diarrhœa continues in spite of the most simple forms of treatment, or whenever undue straining occurs, or when blood is passed, the doctor should be called in so that the proper treatment may be carried out. Great harm is often done by treating an acute condition of the bowel with opening medicines. For diseases of which diarrhœa is symptom, *see also* Cholera ; Colitis ; Dysentery ; Enteritis ; Influenza ; Typhoid Fever.

Summer Diarrhœa. Summer diarrhœa is also termed summer or infantile cholera, epidemic gastro-enteritis and infective diar-rhœa. Epidemics of this disease occur in almost every country during the summer and autumn months. Infants and young children are particularly liable to attacks of this condition, which is due to the bowels becoming infected with germs through eating bad food. In the case of bottle-fed babies, dirty milk or bottles are the greatest source of danger. Milk should never be left uncovered, especially during the hot weather, but should be stored away in a cool place where flies are not able to get at it. It should be sterilized, and bottles and teats should be thoroughly boiled before being used.

Symptoms. The motions are green in colour, slimy and foul, and of frequent occurrence ; in severe cases there may be blood-stained mucus as well. There is usually a high fever and the tem-perature may be extremely high, or it may be below normal. Con-vulsions are common and the child may pass into an unconscious state. An attack of this disease begins very suddenly and it is very severe while it lasts ; the child quickly becomes wasted and shrunken, and in severe cases, death may occur within 24 hours.

Treatment. As soon as the symptoms are recognized, all milk should be stopped and the child should be given cold boiled water or whey and water for 24 hours ; this will often cut short a serious attack. The rectum should be washed out very gently by means of a fine catheter with weak solutions of bicarbonate of soda at least once a day. If, in spite of these simple measures, the illness continues, the doctor should be called in immediately as it will be necessary to take further steps in the matter of treatment. In-jections of normal saline may have to be given in order to make up for the large amount of fluids which are being lost.

DIATHERMY. Diathermy is a form of electricity which is used both medically and surgically in the treatment of disease.

DIGESTION. The various articles of food which make up the average individual's daily diet can be divided into three main classes known as *proteins, fats,* and *carbohydrates.* Many of these substances are very complicated from a chemical point of view and are not, generally speaking, easily dissolved by the body juices, so that before they can be absorbed into the blood they must be split up into a simpler form. In the human body these splitting-up changes are brought about by chemical bodies known as *ferments* or *enzymes* of various kinds. There is a special ferment for each particular class of food, and it will not split up any other type of food. The object of these ferments is to break up the food into simpler forms which can be absorbed into the system. After they have been thus absorbed, some of these simpler bodies are picked out by the various organs of the body from the blood-stream and are *built up* into living matter, while others are *burnt up* to provide heat and energy.

Alimentary Canal. The digestive tube as a whole is known as the *alimentary canal.* It starts at the mouth and ends at the anus ; it is divided up into many different portions.

The mouth is the first portion of the alimentary canal to be considered. It is a cavity containing teeth and saliva. The teeth are primarily meant to bite into the food and to grind it into small particles so that the saliva can come into contact with as much of it as possible.

Digestive Juices. The digestive juices of the body (enzymes and ferments) are prepared by means of various glands : a gland is a structure which has the power of separating or forming certain materials from the blood which is flowing through it. Many of the membranes which line the hollow organs of the body also have the power of forming special materials, and therefore they are called " secreting membranes."

Salivary Digestion. As is the case in all the fluids of the body, most of the saliva consists of water—just over 99 per cent of it. The remaining very small fraction consists of mineral salts and organic matter.

The substance in saliva which takes an active part in digestion is one of the ferments known as *ptyalin.* Many of the foods we eat contain a large proportion of starch (such as bread, rice, potato, etc.), which will not dissolve in water. No food is of any use to the body until it has been turned into a state in which it can be dissolved. Starch therefore, as such, is useless as a food. This ferment or enzyme, known as ptyalin, has the power of doing this : it converts the insoluble starch into a soluble variety of sugar known as maltose. In the mouth this change begins as soon as the saliva mixes with starchy foods. The unchanged starchy substances are swallowed, together with some saliva, and the change of starch into sugar is continued in other parts of the digestive tube for a short while in the stomach, but completely in the intestines, where it is reinforced by a powerful ferment from the *pancreas*—a gland, incidentally, which is very similar to a salivary gland in structure. The saliva acts only on starchy foods.

The term *enzyme* or *ferment* is applied to various substances existing in small quantities in different parts of the digestive system. An enzyme has the effect of causing a chemical change in the digestion of the food with which it is associated to proceed more rapidly than it otherwise would.

Swallowing into the Stomach. Food, then, is masticated in the mouth and thoroughly mixed with the saliva. It is collected into a mass known as a bolus by the muscles of the tongue and of the cheeks, and then passed between the tongue and the roof of the mouth till it reaches the back of the mouth. So far all these arrangements are " voluntary," that is to say, they are under the control of the conscious will and can be stopped at any time. Once the food reaches the back of the mouth, the presence of the food will cause the swallowing machinery to come into play, and thereafter the passage of food and its further digestion is entirely beyond the control of the will.

The food has to pass into the food-pipe without touching the back part of the nose or entering the windpipe. The back of the nose is shut off by means of the soft palate. The contraction of the muscles at the back of the throat forces the food over a flap of cartilage at the entrance to the windpipe directly into the food-pipe or œsophagus. If one presses the " Adam's apple " during the act of swallowing, it is easy to understand how this is lifted up and the entrance to the windpipe, situated just behind the Adam's apple, is raised and comes forward so that food is shot across it.

As soon as the food enters the upper portion of the food-pipe the circular muscles in the walls of that tube contract just above it and force it downwards. In front of the mass of food the muscle becomes relaxed by means of a nervous reflex which is aroused by the presence of the food, so that a regular wave-like motion is set up, a narrow portion being behind the mass of food and pushing it down, and a wider part in front into which the food is forced. The force of gravity enters into the passage of food into the stomach but little, and it is owing to the muscular contraction that one can swallow solids, and even liquids such as water, when standing on one's head.

When the food-pipe is not engaged in swallowing, it is not a hollow tube, but is flattened, its front and back walls being together. In order that the act of swallowing may take place with regularity and ease, the mass of food must be sufficiently large to be within the grasp of the contracting muscles ; it is on this account that some people find difficulty in swallowing a pill, especially if it be a small one, unless food or drink be taken at the same time.

The Stomach. The stomach is a membranous and muscular bag, about ten inches in length from right to left, situated against the front wall of the abdomen and just beneath the partition which separates the abdominal cavity from the chest. This partition is a muscle known as the diaphragm. The shape of the stomach is very variable, the larger portion, just next to the heart except for the diaphragm, is the larger, and is known as the cardiac portion. When an individual is standing up the shape of the stomach is roughly that of the letter " J " The food-pipe enters the stomach at the top of the letter " J " which is known as the *cardiac orifice,* and the narrow end of the stomach joins up with the intestines by a narrow entrance known as the *pylorus.* Food enters the stomach by means of the upper opening, the cardiac orifice, and after being thoroughly mixed with the digestive fluid of the stomach, passes through the lower opening into the small intestine.

Gastric Juices. The only important ferment in the stomach itself is *pepsin,* which acts on the complex protein foods. Pepsin is only active in the presence of acid, and in the stomach this acid is that known as *hydrochloric acid.* The pepsin does not break down the protein entirely, and more changes have to take place in the small intestine before it is ready to be taken into the blood-stream.

The digestion which takes place in the stomach chiefly prepares the protein part of the food for the further action of the much more powerful ferments of the pancreas and intestine. The only other important ferment in the stomach is *rennin,* which has the property of clotting milk.

Commercially this ferment is sold as Rennet. It is prepared from the fourth stomach of a calf and is used to make junket.

The walls of the stomach are capable of being stretched a great deal. It can thus adapt itself to the quantity of food it contains and at the same time be always in contact with the food so as to act upon it.

Peristalsis. Regular wave-like or rhythmical muscular contractions pass down the walls of the stomach. These regular waves of contraction are known as " peristalsis," and by means of them the food is forced all the way down the intestinal canal. It is only in the large intestine, under normal conditions, that waves of contraction are seen to pass backwards, e.g. towards the small intestine, and these movements are referred to as " anti-peristalsis."

The Sphincters. At each end of the stomach the circular muscles are thickened and contracted so that there is no way through them. These areas of circular muscle are known as *sphincters* and they serve as doors to keep the cavity of the organ closed.

Gastric Glands. The mucous membrane or lining of the stomach is smooth and soft when the organ is moderately distended ; but it is drawn up into folds when the stomach is empty. It is covered with cells which make " mucus " to keep the surface moist, and its thickness is due to the fact that it is made up of glands which are like a long tube in shape. Their duty is to make gastric juices and they are accordingly known as *gastric glands*.

Gastric juice consists of water, to which are added the pepsin, rennin, hydrochloric acid and various salts such as phosphates of calcium, magnesium and iron, and the chlorides of sodium, potassium and calcium.

Pepsin is the active part of the gastric juice. In the presence of hydrochloric acid it has the power of acting on the protein foods. It can be obtained in a dissolved state by washing the lining membrane of the stomach with water, or it may be bought in the solid form from the chemist. " Peptonized milk " is milk which has been in contact with pepsin for some time at body temperature. The protein part of the milk is thus partially broken down or " digested," and so it becomes more suitable for invalids in whom the powers of digestion are weak owing to their illness.

Chyme. The fluid contents of the stomach are known as " chyme," from the Greek word meaning " I pour," because it is " poured " into the intestine and bowel. It consists of saliva and starchy foods in various stages of digestion. Protein food in various stages : undigested fat in the form of globules, mucus from the mucous glands, and a residue of undigestible substances.

Much information as to the processes which take place in the stomach has been obtained from human beings who have had an injury or a surgical operation on the stomach. Food vomited has been carefully analysed, and processes have been studied with the aid of X-rays. For these the patient is given what is known as a " bismuth meal." This is a food which contains a great deal of bismuth or a barium compound. This meal will not allow X-rays to pass through it, and so the outline of a hollow organ containing it is shown up on a screen when examined with the aid of the X-rays.

There is very little material absorbed into the body directly from the stomach. Even water passes through the stomach practically without any lessening in quantity. Alcohol, on the other hand, is readily absorbed, and this is the reason for the rapid effect of alcohol when it is swallowed on an empty stomach.

How Digestion Starts. The pouring out of gastric juice is usually started by the mental effect of seeing, tasting and smelling appetizing food. The next important thing in stimulating digestion is the actual presence of food in the stomach. Some foods are more active than others in this respect : meat extracts and meat juices are very active ; while others, such as milk, bread, white of egg, etc., are much less active.

Digestion in the Duodenum. The inner side of the small intestine is covered with a multitude of small projections which give the surface a velvety appearance. Their duty is to absorb food rather than to change food into a form which can be dissolved.

Digestion and the Large Intestine. After the chyle (the term applied to the contents of the small intestine) has passed along the whole length of the small intestine it enters the large intestine through an opening which is guarded by two folds of mucous membrane. These folds prevent, to some extent, the flow of the contents of the large intestine back into the small one. They form a kind of valve which is known as the *ileo-cæcal* valve.

The movements of the intestine are of two distinct types : one is *peristaltic* and consists of waves of contraction passing progressively and slowly down the intestine. The effect of these waves is to drive the contents slowly onwards. The other type of movement is known as *rhythmic segmentation.* A short length of intestine suddenly breaks up into a number of small segments or portions, and each segment undergoes a similar change. This happens many times and their combined effect is to produce a thorough mixing and absorption.

In the large intestine practically no digestion occurs, but there is a large absorption of fluid, both from the food and the watery and unused portions of the digestive juices. At the end of the small intestine the bowel contents are very watery, but the action of the large intestine makes the residue become more and more solid.

Putrefaction occurs only in the large intestine, which acts mostly as a storehouse. Some absorption, however, does take place as is shown by the absorption of water. There is also some evidence to show that people who are very ill can be kept alive by means of a glucose solution passed into the rectum.

The contents of the large intestine are bacteria, bile mucus, unabsorbed food and excess of digestive juices. The bacteria form nearly half of the solids excreted.

The fæces are the excretions of the large intestine. Their colour is mostly due to the bile in them, and the mass should be semi-fluid in consistence. The presence of food in the stomach has a marked reflex action in making the rectum contract. This tendency is most marked when food is placed into a stomach which is completely empty, hence the most suitable time to empty the bowels is directly after breakfast. The bowel is also a creature of habits and is far more likely to work efficiently if it is made to contract and expel its contents at the same time every day.

DIGITALIS. This is the name of a powerful medicine obtained from the purple foxglove plant which is to be found growing in our woods and hedgerows. Nowadays it is grown specially because of the digitalis obtained from it.

DILATATION. This is the term used when any hollow part of the body becomes stretched or dilated. Dilatation of the heart occurs when there is an increase in the size of one or more of the heart organs ; this usually happens through weakness of the muscles of the heart. In dilatation of the stomach there is usually a great deal of gas in the stomach which is causing it to be blown out.

DILL-WATER. This is an extract which is given to relieve flatulence and pains in the stomach. It may be given to the smallest child without any danger. A teaspoonful of dill-water, slightly warmed, will be found to give considerable relief in flatulence (wind) of young infants.

DIPHTHERIA. Diphtheria is a very infectious disease which attacks the throat, and sometimes the nose and larynx. Not only does the germ of this disease cause the membranes of the throat to become very inflamed and swollen, but it manufactures poisons which are carried by the blood-stream to the rest of the body. These poisons may set up dangerous consequences such as heart weakness and paralysis. The chief characteristic of the disease, however, is the formation of a " membrane " at the back of the throat which is caused by the lining of the throat becoming so inflamed that it dies and forms an extra covering as it were. This membrane is greyish or yellowish-white in colour and it is very firmly fastened to the throat. Other inflammations of the throat may look like diphtheria, but true diphtheria is diagnosed by the presence of a germ which has the special name of Klebs-Loeffler bacillus. This germ is named after two German doctors who were the first to discover, at the end of the nineteenth century, that diphtheria was actually caused by its presence.

The majority of cases of diphtheria seem to break out during the late summer months, especially if the weather has been dry. It will be found that by about the beginning of September the number of cases will begin to increase, and the highest peak is reached in

November. After that, a fall in the number of cases takes place. Immunization of children against diphtheria is to be recommended, as it definitely prevents outbreaks.

How Infection is Carried. The germs of this disease may be carried from one person to another, and the disease is so infectious that even doctors and nurses may become infected from their patients.

" Carriers." In a large percentage of the cases of diphtheria, the germs simply disappear after the patient recovers from the disease, but there are still a great number of patients who harbour the germs for a long period. These people are called carriers, and in this way it is possible for the germs of the disease to be passed on.

The Importance of the Membrane in Diphtheria. The membrane in diphtheria is formed by changes in the tissues as they are killed by the activity of the growing germs. At first it is firmly attached to the back of the throat ; and it is by the way the membrane is attached that the true diphtheria membrane can be distinguished from the membranes that are not due to diphtheria and can be pulled off the throat without causing any bleeding.

The Antitoxin Treatment. The diphtheria antitoxin is now administered by the doctor as soon as he sees a case that looks as if it might be diphtheria, while at the same time, he takes a specimen of the matter at the back of the throat and sends it to a bacteriologist to be examined, to see if the special germ of diphtheria is amongst them. If the germs are present the treatment is continued, and if they are not, no harm is done. The reason for this haste is that the membrane grows with great rapidity, and the day, or even few hours, required for the examination of the specimen will make a great difference to the patient's chances of recovery.

Symptoms. The period between the catching of the disease and the time when the symptoms first show themselves (the incubation period) varies from two to seven days : more usually two. At first the patient has the usual feverish symptoms of chilliness, fever, and aching pains in the back and limbs. The temperature does not usually rise above 99°–101° F. A young child may have convulsions at the beginning. The throat at first is only slightly sore and there is little difficulty in swallowing. The membrane usually appears first on the tonsils at the sides of the throat.

Treatment. Measures must be taken to prevent the spread of the malady. Diphtheria is best treated at hospitals ; but if the patient remains at home, the room in which the patient is kept should be clear of carpets, curtains and superfluous furniture. The room must be kept warm (67 degrees F.) and well ventilated. A steam kettle is useful. Only the nurse, the child's mother and the doctor should visit the patient. The strictest quarantine should be employed against the other members of the household.

The local treatment is not so important now that antitoxin is used, but the mouth should be frequently rinsed out with glycerine of thymol or a weak boracic acid solution. Nasal diphtheria requires prompt disinfection of the breathing passages, for which a very weak antiseptic solution is suitable.

When the voice-box is involved, a steam kettle is essential, and when there is obstruction the operation of *tracheotomy*, in which a tube is inserted into the windpipe, must be performed ; or intubation, in which a tube is inserted between the vocal cords, thus keeping them permanently apart. Hot applications to the neck are very comforting in the case of young children ; in older children ice poultices may be found to be preferable.

Diet and General Treatment. Food must be liquid, such as milk, beef juice, barley water, ice-cream, soups, etc. If swallowing is too difficult, the fluid must be given in a tube. As much water as possible must be drunk, and the bowels must be kept open by means of a dose of calomel at night and salts in the morning. If the circulation fails it must be stimulated by drugs such as coramine or camphor, and an injection of salt solution into the bowel, which is allowed to remain there instead of being passed out again, is very useful.

DIPLEGIA. By diplegia is meant paralysis on both sides of the body. This is a rare condition, as paralysis is usually one-sided. In children, however, it sometimes occurs as the result of injuries at birth. (*See also* PARALYSIS.)

DIPLOPIA. This is the medical name for the condition more commonly known as double vision. (*See also* DOUBLE VISION.)

DIPSOMANIA is a condition in which there is an intense craving for drink at intervals, leading to a drinking bout lasting a few days. During this time the patient is seldom sober. He is quite unable to resist the impulse to drink. After the bout is over, he returns to his normal life and remains without the slightest craving for alcohol until the craving suddenly returns after an interval and again he must drink wildly. Very often in between the bouts the patient not only takes no alcohol, but actually dislikes it. Before a bout is due the patient becomes miserable, very irritable and has sleepless nights. Then the craving for alcohol appears with rapidly increasing force. Nothing is known about the nature of dipsomania. It is quite different from the chronic drinking that results in delirium tremens, and perhaps has some relation to a mild type of true mental disorder.

DIRT EATING. This is a peculiarity which may occur among people who are insane. They not only eat dirt,·but all sorts of odd things such as lumps of coal, etc. Dirt eating is known technically as *pica*, from the Latin word meaning magpie.

DISCHARGE. The word discharge may be applied to many normal workings of the body. For instance, sweat is discharged from the sweat glands, and urine is discharged from the bladder ; but, as a rule, when we speak of discharges from the body we do not refer to these normal ones, but to others that appear from wounds or disease.

It should be remembered that most discharges are of an infective nature, so that dressings which are removed should be destroyed by burning. People suffering from a cold should be very careful with used handkerchiefs ; they should soak them in an antiseptic solution. It is a very good thing to use soft paper handkerchiefs when suffering from a cold ; in this way they can be burned immediately after use.

DISEASE. Disease is commonly used to mean that one, or some, of the organs or systems of the body are not working properly. This may be because the part was ill-formed or deficient in some way from birth, in which case the disease is called *congenital*. Congenital diseases are also often *hereditary*, that is, they descend from generation to generation in the same family. A *constitutional* disease is one in which the whole body or the whole of one of the systems of the body is involved, such as anæmia. An *idiopathic* disease is one for which the cause is unknown, and a *venereal* disease is one which is due to sexual intercourse, usually promiscuous.

It is important to distinguish between actual disease and the natural reactions of the body. Disease should be treated with a view to curing and getting rid of it ; but things that are sometimes symptoms of disease are also the body's natural reactions to unnatural states it finds itself in from time to time, and therefore must not be interrupted. For instance, a sneeze is a symptom of approaching influenza, which is a disease, and the sooner it is got rid of the better, but a sneeze is also the body's way of getting rid of a piece of dust which has lodged on the mucous membrane or lining of the nose where it is not wanted. If one sneeze does not do the trick and get rid of the unwanted dust particle, a whole series of sneezes will follow until it is got rid of. The same is true of conditions like diarrhœa and sickness. In diarrhœa the bowel is trying to get rid quickly of something that is hurting it, and vomiting is the stomach's way of returning quickly something that is irritating it, but repeated sickness and diarrhœa over days or longer means that the irritating substance remains there or that disease has set in. These matters must be left to people's common sense to a certain extent.

Organic and Functional Disease. The chief divisions of disease are mainly organic diseases and functional diseases. An organic disease is one in which some change has taken place in an organ whose working is upset, and the changes can be seen by the naked eye or by a microscope. A functional disease is one in which the working of the organ is upset but nothing can be seen to account for it.

Occupational Diseases. By occupational diseases we mean diseases which would not have been contracted by the individual if he had not been following that particular trade or occupation. In some occupations there is a definite danger from certain diseases as, for instance, lead-poisoning amongst painters, anthracosis or silicosis amongst coal miners, a certain sort of cancer amongst cotton-spinners, etc.

DISINFECTANT. Any substance which is able to kill the germs of disease is known as a disinfectant. Many people refer to antiseptics as disinfectants, but an antiseptic does not kill germs—it is used to prevent their growth. When treating a wound, an antiseptic is used to keep the wound clean and to prevent the growth of any germs, but when germs are actually present, such as in many infectious diseases, it is necessary to use a disinfectant in order to destroy them. The clothes used by the patient and all utensils used in the sick-room should be thoroughly disinfected. Among the more common disinfectants are carbolic acid, creolin, lysol, naphthol, formaldehyde, chlorine and potassium permanganate.

DISLOCATION. Dislocation usually refers to the displacement of a joint from its natural position. This may be caused by injury to the bones and ligaments which keep the joint in position, or it may be due to disease. Tuberculosis, for instance, is a disease in which the ligaments and bones may be gradually worn away, thus giving rise to dislocation. In some cases the bones may never have developed at birth, and so when any strain is put upon them, dislocation takes place.

Like fractures, there are two types of dislocation, simple and compound. In the first type there is nothing but a straightforward dislocation, while in the second the skin is broken and a part of the bone may protrude through. Surgeons usually divide dislocations into two classes: (1) congenital, which means present at birth, or (2) acquired later in life as the result of an accident.

The parts of the body which are most liable to become dislocated are the shoulder, the hip, the jaw, the knee-cap, the finger-joints and the elbow. The jaw may be dislocated as the result of a blow, or it may occur after a yawn. The collar-bone or shoulder-blade is very commonly put out as the result of a fall from a horse, and so on.

Once a joint has been dislocated, it is very apt to slip out again, and it is not ususual for a person to become quite expert at readjusting his own particular dislocation ; but this should not be tried on another person by any unskilled person.

Symptoms. The symptoms of a dislocation are loss of movement of the particular joint, but much depends on the type of dislocation which takes place. As a rule, it will be found that when the injured limb is compared with the normal one, there is some difference in length. Sometimes shortening takes place, while in other cases the limb may have lengthened. There may be some

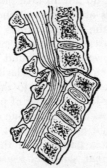

Dislocation of Spine, showing compression of Spinal Cord

pain and swelling around the joint, especially if the dislocated bone is pressing on some nerve.

Treatment. Immediate treatment consists of applying cold water cloths to the part in order to relieve the pain, and absolute rest is necessary until the proper medical advice can be obtained. It is unwise for an unskilled person to attempt to put the dislocated bone back into place, as great damage may be done by tearing nerves and vessels. After the limb has been adjusted to its normal position, care must be taken in using it.

DISPLACEMENT. Displacement of various organs of the body often occurs through injury or disease or, in some cases, the bones of the body may become displaced through the habit of standing and walking badly. The stomach may become displaced owing to weakness of the muscles, and the kidneys may be very movable, and descend lower than they should be normally.

Displacement of the womb is a very common complaint in women, especially in women who have had children. This condition can be corrected by operation, or relief can be had by wearing a special belt. (*See also* ABDOMINAL BELT.)

DISSEMINATED SCLEROSIS is a very common disease of the nervous system, and certainly the most common one in people between the ages of twenty and thirty-five. The exact cause is still unknown, but what occurs is a scattering of patches of changed nervous tissue throughout the brain and spinal cord. Although the fatty coverings of the essential parts of the nervous tissue in these patches are destroyed, and their place taken by a firm supporting tissue, the vital part of the nervous elements survives for a long time after the destruction of its fatty coverings, and so the course of the disease is, in general, a long one. The changes in these patches of nervous tissue do not all take place at one and the same time ; first one patch is attacked, and then another, so that the symptoms from which the patient suffers depend, practically by chance, on whichever part of the nervous system is first stricken.

In actual practice, however, it is found that certain parts tend to be involved with a remarkable regularity. The earliest effects of the disease which take the patient to the doctor are very often seen in the eyes. A very large number of patients with this disease complain first of rapid loss of vision in one eye. This may produce complete blindness in that eye for a short time, but it is good to be able to reassure such a patient that the vision will return, in nearly every case to normal, within a few weeks. The incident of the loss of vision in one eye often occurs years—even as many as twenty years—before any other signs or symptoms of disseminated sclerosis appear, and very often the patient, when seen with the fully developed picture of the disease, has completely forgotten that such an incident ever happened. Similarly, a patient may for a short time see two things instead of one, years before the apparent onset of the disease, and may forget the incident, but the double vision is part and parcel of the disorder.

Other early incidents (the word " incidents " best describes these symptoms, because they are fleeting, a feature which is almost peculiar to this disease) are sudden loss of power in a limb, which power returns within a week or a fortnight ; sudden attacks of numbness and tingling in an arm which lasts for a week or so and then disappears ; prolonged attacks of giddiness or vomiting, for which no ascertainable cause is present ; any of these may be one of the modes of onset of disseminated sclerosis. When the disease is advancing, stiffness of the legs and difficulty in walking become noticeable. This stiffness varies from time to time ; it may be so severe one month that the patient is forced to keep his bed, but within a month he may be walking again. This variation in severity is one of the chief characteristics of the disorder. The speech becomes altered, and the patient begins to speak in a jerking, " staccato " manner, but this type of speech is only heard in advanced cases. Most victims of this disease develop a trembling of the arms, which is most marked on movement towards an object, and is often noticed first in performing such fine movements as threading a needle. This trembling increases as the disease advances. The mental outlook of the patient is fortunately a happy one. The patient with disseminated sclerosis is surprisingly cheerful ; even when unable to walk, he does not seem to suffer mentally. A frequent and favourite expression of these patients is " Well, what's the use of being anything else but cheerful, doctor ? " Although periods of improvement lasting sometimes for many years occur, the disease must be said to be a hopeless one, inasmuch as it cannot be cured. The periods of improvement may be so long, however, that a patient may go for ten or fifteen years between his attacks. The only treatment which assists in improving the patient's condition is arsenic, and this is given as a matter of routine in every case. Where there is much stiffness of the limbs, massage is of great service. Patients with disseminated sclerosis should avoid over-exertion, but should not stay in bed as long as walking is possible. The vaccine treatment which was hailed as a cure for this disease is now discredited ; it has recently been suggested that the disease may be due to some lack of vitamins, but this has yet to be proved.

DISTENSION. It is not unusual for the stomach to become distended or blown out with food and with gases, or for the bladder to become distended with the presence of too much urine. As a rule, these states of distension do not last for very long, and they can be relieved quite quickly. Should distension of the stomach or any other organ become a chronic state, it would be advisable to consult the doctor, especially where there is any feeling of discomfort.

DISTILLED WATER. To make distilled water, ordinary tap water is heated and the vapour is collected drop by drop as it condenses. Distilled water is used if any chemically pure substance is required ; for example, a chemist always uses distilled water for doing accurate scientific work. It is rather unpleasant to drink, as it has a flat, mawkish taste ; but either boiled or distilled water is used a great deal in the East.

DISTRICT NURSES. District nurses are a highly trained body of nurses who are able to provide skilled attention by daily visits to patients who are unable to afford a permanent nurse or who are unable to go to hospital. The district nursing system was founded

220 DISTRICT NURSES

in commemoration of Queen Victoria's Diamond Jubilee. A district nurse, or Queen's Nurse, as they are called, usually visits each patient twice a day. She takes temperature and pulse and makes notes regarding the condition of the patient. She washes the patient, or gives a bed-bath if necessary, and makes the bed; but it is not within her province to do any cookery or housework. Anyone requiring the services of a district nurse should find out the address of the local nurse, or write to the General Superintendent, Queen's Institute of District Nursing, 57 Lower Belgrave Street, Westminster, London, S.W.1. But the doctor in attendance will usually tell the patient when a nurse is necessary and give the nurse her instructions.

DIURETIC. A diuretic is a drug which has the power of increasing the flow of urine from the kidneys. In certain diseases where the usual output of urine is very much below normal, it is necessary to give diuretics to encourage the flow of urine. When the urine has not been able to leave the kidneys it becomes concentrated and unhealthy, and as a result the body becomes poisoned by the waste materials which are normally got rid of in the urine.

Water is one of the best diuretics if only a mild stimulant to the kidneys is required. Many people do not drink sufficient water during the day to allow the kidneys to be well flushed out. Of course, if the kidneys are diseased, more complicated measures have to be taken and diuretics should be given with great caution and only under medical care.

Caffeine, which is contained in coffee and tea, is a good diuretic and it is especially valuable in heart diseases where there is an excess of water in the body (dropsy). Theobromine is a more powerful diuretic and it is not so likely to keep the patient awake as caffeine. It may be given in cachets in doses of 1 to 5 grains.

DIVERTICULITIS. A diverticulum is a blind pocket which sometimes forms in the walls of the soft organs of the body such as the large bowel (colon) or bladder. These pockets or pouches are quite common and in a great many cases give rise to no discomfort or symptoms of any sort. Occasionally, however, they may get inflamed through the collection in them of waste materials, and this inflammation may give rise to symptoms and is called diverticulitis. This may be serious enough to require an operation. (*See also* INTESTINE.)

DIZZINESS. Dizziness in itself is not a disease, but it may be a sign that the body requires overhauling. There are so many different ways in which dizziness might be caused that it would be difficult to give more than a few here.

When a person is feeling bilious it is not unusual for him to feel dizzy just before sickness begins, and the feeling generally goes when the biliousness disappears. Over-smoking may cause slight dizziness, and certainly indulgence in too much alcohol causes the head to go round. Some people cannot stand on heights without feeling dizzy, while others feel dizzy at the thought of going on board a ship. Certain forms of heart disease may cause dizziness, and sometimes inflammation of the ears may be the cause.

In the majority of cases it is advisable to keep the bowels open and to eat nothing but the most simple forms of food. Alcohol and tobacco should be cut down or, better still, avoided altogether. If the dizziness does not go, it is a sign that something is wrong and the doctor should be consulted.

DOG BITE. *See* BITES and HYDROPHOBIA.

DORSAL. Dorsal is the adjective applied to the back. The word is also used in connection with the back of any other part of the body. For example, the back of the hand is the dorsal part of the hand, and so on.

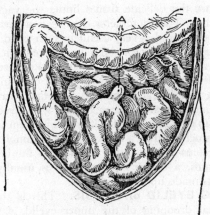

A. *Meckel's Diverticulum*

DOUBLE VISION. The ordinary act of seeing, which takes place whenever we look at anything, is the result of the two eyes working exactly together. It happens in certain diseases, and sometimes as a result of alcoholic excesses, that when one thing is looked at, two images of it are seen, that is, each eye has its own vision of the object and the two are not welded into one image as they are in healthy sight. This condition is called double vision or diplopia. (*See also* DISSEMINATED SCLEROSIS ; ENCEPHALITIS LETHARGICA.)

DOUCHE. A douche is an application of a stream of water to the whole or part of the body. It may be applied outwardly in the form of a jet or jets of water as in the Vichy douche and Aix douche, so called after the two famous spas, or inwardly into various cavities of the body such as the ears, nose and vagina. The external douches are mostly used together with massage for chronic diseases of the joints and muscles, and to stimulate the flow of sweat.

Internal douching is used for purposes of cleanliness and disinfection and to relieve congestion in the neighbourhood of the part which is douched. Of these douches the most generally employed is the vaginal douche for conditions in which there is a discharge or where the organs are congested and painful. These douches should be used at a fairly hot temperature, 100 degrees being about right. A tepid douche may give rise to a chill and so do more harm than good. The disinfectant used should be very weak as the purpose of the douche is rather to wash away germs and the mucus which is always present in inflamed conditions, than to kill the germs ; and with an antiseptic that may be strong enough to injure the delicate tissues lining the vagina or nose as the case may be. The Plombières douche is a means of washing out the large bowel, and is very useful in such conditions as colitis. The stomach and bladder can also be washed out, and also the womb, but these can only be done by trained experts.

DOVER'S POWDER. A powder which contains ten per cent. each of opium and ipecacuanha. It was first introduced by an English physician named Thomas Dover, who lived between the years of 1660–1742. This powder has always been a very popular one, and it is much used as a remedy for a common cold, or when there are symptoms of bronchitis. Because of the large amount of opium it contains, a doctor's prescription is usually necessary in order to have it made up at a chemist's.

DROOPING EYELID or PTOSIS. This is the name given to an abnormal drooping of the upper eyelid, caused by some deficiency in the muscle which raises the upper eyelid.

DROPSY. Dropsy is the name given to an unusually watery state of the tissues of the body. In every healthy person there is a certain amount of leakage of the watery part of the blood into the flesh, but when dropsy occurs, this normal state is very much exaggerated. The fluid part of the blood is controlled by a complicated system of tiny vessels known as the lymphatics, and if obstruction takes place in any of these vessels it is obvious that swelling is bound to appear, and the larger the vessel the larger the amount of swelling or dropsy will occur. Another cause of swelling is too great a flow of fluid out of the blood-vessels, in which case the lymphatics are not able to pass it along quickly enough, and dropsy takes place.

Dropsy a Symptom, not a Disease. There are very many

causes of the state of dropsy in the body, and it is not a disease in itself, as many people seem to think, but merely a sign that something is wrong in the body somewhere. There are also various forms of this condition, which may range from a small swelling caused by a bee sting, to the great swellings which cover the whole of the body ; but both states are true dropsies, the only difference being the quantity of swelling. In the case of a bee sting, the poison causes the blood-vessels to open more widely than usual, and a greater amount of fluid is poured out into the skin, thus causing a swelling (or dropsy) to appear over the place stung.

Again, many other conditions cause the blood-vessels to open, and it is natural to suppose that the more poisoned the vessels become, the greater will be the amount of swelling. Many people who suffer from rheumatism find that they swell up very easily, and it is thought to be due to poisons in the system. In very hot weather it is not unusual for the hands and feet to swell up; this is caused by an extra flow of fluid from the blood-vessels which the lymphatic glands are not able to carry away at once.

Dropsies of Heart and Kidney Disease. In certain diseases of the heart, dropsy occurs all over the body. Some of the worst forms of dropsy belong to this form of heart disease. There are several explanations for this excessive watery state of the body, but there is no doubt that blocking of the blood-vessels, and also of the lymphatic vessels, owing to the inability of the weakened heart to do its usual pumping of the blood, may cause this excessive swelling to take place. It is no unusual thing for a person to become intensely dropsical owing to heart disease, and when the heart condition is restored to normal, the swellings may disappear within a few days.

The dropsy caused by disease of the kidneys is not so severe as that caused by heart disease, and it seems to appear in certain parts of the body instead of all over. The legs very often become swollen, and the face, especially the eyelids, is largely affected.

Treatment. The same treatment will obviously not apply to all cases of dropsy. The cause of the condition will have to be taken into consideration, but the dropsy itself may be so distressing as to require special treatment apart from the disease which is causing it. For the slighter degrees of dropsy no special treatment need be given beyond treating the cause of the condition. Once the cause is removed, the dropsy will naturally disappear.

When the dropsy is due to heart disease, complete rest in bed is absolutely necessary, and such drugs as digitalis or salyrgan, which tend to increase the flow of urine, are usually given. The diet is generally kept as dry as possible and very little salt should be allowed.

The treatment of the dropsy caused by disease of the kidneys is usually the same as the disease. (*See also* NEPHRITIS.) Some of the excess fluid may be taken off by the operation of tapping, and this may require to be done repeatedly. It is not advisable to give drugs which increase the flow of urine when the kidneys are diseased, as this may set up irritation and aggravate the condition.

The general treatment of dropsy depends on the cause, and a doctor should be consulted without delay in order that the cause may be discovered, as far-reaching consequences may result if the condition is neglected.

DROWNING. At some time or other most of us will come in contact with drowning, or at any rate with accidents on the water. A person taken from the water, even though he may have been in some time, is not necessarily dead, and although there may be no sign of life, it is the duty of those around to endeavour for at least two hours to restore life. The means used will be found in the article on ARTIFICIAL RESPIRATION. After the emergency measures have been carried out and the person has begun to come round, he may be given hot tea or coffee or sal volatile to safeguard against sudden collapse. He should be put to bed with hot-water bottles and kept warm and quiet in a darkened room until he has a good sleep. (*See also* ARTIFICIAL RESPIRATION ; ASPHYXIA.)

DRYNESS OF THE MOUTH. The mouth is kept in a moist state by a constant flow of saliva, which is the fluid which is poured into the mouth from the salivary glands. It happens for various reasons that the flow of saliva is sometimes interrupted. The cause should be searched for and overcome. Dry mouth or " xerostomia " is a rare nervous disease found sometimes in people, usually women. Mouth-breathing or taking of drying-up medicines such as atropine for any length of time will cause a dry mouth. It is often present after operations or fevers, or any condition where the body is quickly losing its moisture. These temporary conditions can be helped by sucking glycerine and borax pastilles. (*See also* DIABETES INSIPIDUS.)

DUCT. The ducts of the body are the channels or tubes by which fluids are carried from one part of the body to another. As a rule the chemical substances, or secretions as they are called, of the various glands are poured into these ducts. For example, the fluid which goes to make up the saliva is carried to the mouth by the salivary ducts. Other ducts are the bile ducts leading from the gall-bladder and liver, the sweat glands all over the body, the lymphatic glands and so on. (*See also* DUCTLESS GLANDS.)

DUCTLESS GLANDS. Recent investigations have established the fact that all the bodily functions are under the control of powerful chemicals or drugs. Still more recently it has been shown that even the nerve impulses in certain nerves called the autonomic nerves actually cause the changes that occur at their nerve endings by setting free certain strong chemicals. The body and its work'ngs are therefore under the control of chemicals. Some of these chemicals are obtained from the food and are called *vitamins*, and others which are called *hormones* are manufactured in the body itself. All the tissues contain bodies which are able to set free chemicals which have a powerful effect. This can be seen especially in the way they behave when they are injured. There are, however, certain collections of cells in the body whose special work is to manufacture these chemicals and pour them into the fluids which circulate throughout the body, such as blood and lymph. Their action then becomes a general one involving the whole or part of the entire body. The substances which are manufactured by these glands are not collected together in a common tube or duct, but are taken away directly into the cells by the body fluids. In this way they are unlike the ordinary glands of the body, and so, in contrast to them, are called the *ductless glands* or *endocrine glands*.

At the present time a great deal of interest is being taken in these ductless glands or endocrines, and an enormous amount of work is being done on the subject of them, so that our ideas about them are being constantly changed and enlarged by new discoveries. Moreover, the relations between the various ductless glands are so complicated, that only parts of their fascinating story are yet clearly known. We must content ourselves, therefore, with a short description of the chief discoveries that have been made so far.

The Suprarenal Capsules or Adrenals are two small yellowish bodies which are found attached to the upper part of the kidneys. They consist of two parts, the *cortex* or bark, and the *medulla* or centre. From the medulla a very useful substance is produced which is called *adrenalin*. It can also now be manufactured artificially by the chemists. An injection of this substance has the same effect as would be produced by a stimulation of the part of the nervous system called the sympathetic nervous system. Recently a stronger substance of the same kind has been discovered in the medulla of the adrenals ; and also, from the cortex of the adrenals, another substance has been produced, which, although it is still only obtainable in an impure form, is able to keep alive people in whom the adrenals are diseased or have been removed. This substance has been given the name of *corticin*. Disease of the adrenals, which is called Addison's disease, is apt to be fatal and is associated with low blood-pressure, great weakness and a peculiar bronzing of the skin. Corticin is the only known thing which will relieve this condition. Another substance which is being obtained from the adrenals is an acid which is called *hexonuric acid* and is believed at present to be the same as Vitamin C.

The Carotid Gland. This is a collection of cells lying between the fork of the carotid artery where it splits into its two main branches at either side of the neck. It is now known to have a power of affecting the blood-pressure.

The Coccygeal Gland. A tiny collection of cells lying in front of the tip of the coccyx (tail) at the lower end of the backbone. Its use is still unknown.

The Gonads (testicle). The glands of the male reproductive system. Recently an extract has been prepared from the testicle which appears to have some power of restoring the sex characteristics which are under the influence of the chemical which is produced by the testicle. This, in its turn, is apparently under the control of the anterior pituitary gland. This gland also seems to be responsible for certain of the male characteristics, amongst which are the mental changes associated with puberty. Attempts are being made to use it to prolong the period of active sex life or delay old age. This work is still in the experimental stage. The extract which was used in earlier experiments was obtained from monkeys, hence it gained the popular name of *monkey gland* treatment.

Two extracts are now obtained from the ovaries of females, one from the ordinary ovarian substance and the other from the substance of the ovary during pregnancy.

The Pancreas. The pancreas, which in animals is called the sweetbread, contains special tissue which produces the substance called *insulin*. This substance controls the turning of sugar into energy by the tissues, and has also to do with the storing up of sugar in the form of starch which is called *glycogen*. People whose supply of insulin is deficient are subject to the disease called Diabetes Mellitus, or sugar diabetes, so called from the sweetness of the urine due to its containing large quantities of sugar. They are starved of energy because the greater part of the body's energy is obtained from the burning up of sugar and this can only take place in the presence of insulin. The result is that the sugar is poured out from the stores of glycogen, but, since it cannot be used, is given off in the urine. The patient accordingly becomes very thin and weak and may die. Insulin cannot yet be made artificially so efficiently as the natural insulin; though synthalin, an artificial imitation of insulin, may be useful if insulin cannot be given in certain cases.

Pineal Gland. This is a small gland situated in the brain. Tumours of this gland have been found where there is hypertrophy of the tissues of the sexual organs. Its uses are not, however, fully known.

The Pituitary Gland. This is a small gland lying in a hollow on the floor of the skull above the root of the nose, which, though small, is important enough to have been called " the leader of the endocrine orchestra." It consists of three parts : the anterior, or front, the intermediate, and the posterior or back part. The functions of the intermediate part are not clear. The anterior part is amazingly interesting, because it is known that its products control the growth of bones, especially the long bones. Over-production of its juices leads to the person being a giant. Too much pituitary extract in adults leads to growth of the lower face bones, hands and feet, a condition called " acromegaly." In addition, it is now certain that the extract of the anterior lobe causes the development and ripening of the sexual organs. Failure of this juice leads to the person remaining permanently in a condition of infantilism with regard to the development of the sexual organs. The pituitary extract is also associated in some way with the retaining of the fœtus, or unborn baby in the womb. During pregnancy a substance which resembles the pituitary extract is found in the urine, and at one time it was thought to be identical with it. It is used most successfully as a test of human pregnancy.

From the posterior part of the pituitary gland is obtained a secretion whose activities are well known, but whose place in the machinery of the body is not yet definitely known. Its chief activity consists of raising the blood-pressure by its action both on the heart and on the blood-vessels, and it is therefore very valuable in treating shock. It has also a very powerful action on the womb and causes it to contract, so it is used in midwifery. It also has an important action in regulating the water balance of the body, especially when the water balance is wildly disturbed as it is in Diabetes Insipidus, or water diabetes as it is sometimes called. It has, as well, some influence on the sugar chemistry of the body. These extracts cannot yet be obtained in a completely pure form. They are among the most powerful of known substances.

Spleen. While the main function of the spleen is to act as a reservoir for blood, there is some evidence to show that it produces a substance which has the power of causing a rapid improvement in the condition of the blood. This work is still in an early stage.

The Thymus Gland. The thymus is a large gland lying in the upper part of the thorax or chest. The gland increases in size until birth, when it slowly shrivels up. Its uses are quite unknown.

Thyroid Gland. The thyroid gland is a large gland situated in the neck just below the Adam's apple, but extending up both sides of it. This gland in early pre-historic man actually poured its material directly into the alimentary canal, so it is not surprising to find that an extract from it will work almost equally well whether taken by the mouth or as an injection. This is not true of the secretions of the other glands which only possess a feeble action, if any, when taken by mouth. An active extract has been abstracted from the thyroid and can be manufactured artificially. It is called *thyroxin*. The manufacture of it by artificial means is one of the great triumphs of chemistry. It is peculiar in that it contains iodine. Its main effect seems to be in connection with the chemical processes of the body, including those of growth. An absence of thyroid leads to failure to develop mentally and physically as in cretins and idiots. In older people failure of the thyroid has not quite such severe results, but it still leads to great stupidity and to various changes in the skin and hair, a condition which is known as myxœdema. Both conditions can be relieved by taking thyroid extract or

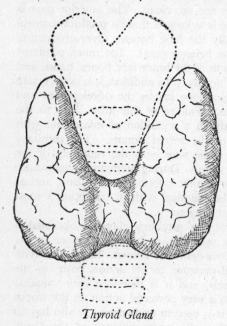

Thyroid Gland

thyroxin. Too much thyroid, on the other hand, will cause a speeding-up of the various processes of the body. The symptoms are loss of flesh, nervousness, flushing, and damage to the heart. This condition is called Graves' disease or exophthalmic goitre, because there is also great protrusion of the eyeballs and enlargement of the thyroid gland.

The Parathyroids. These are small collections of cells situated either actually in the substance of the thyroid gland, or just outside it. An active extract prepared from these tissues produces a large rise in the amount of the chemical called calcium in the blood. Moreover, injections of the extract are able to restore to the normal persons suffering from the peculiar train of symptoms known as tetany, a condition which, when it is very severe, may be fatal, and which is due to damage to or removal of the parathyroid glands. The details of this extract are not yet known.

Conclusion. All these ductless glands are closely related to each other in their workings, and disturbance of one leads to disturbance of the others, and to considerable confusion in the working of the body as a whole. As has been said, there is at the present time a great deal of research work being done on the subject of these glands, and all the time new discoveries are being made with

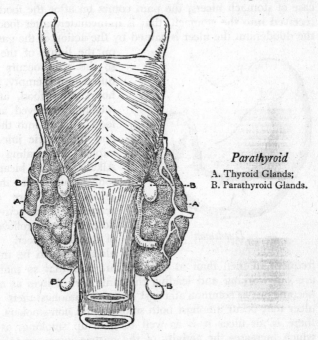

Parathyroid

A. Thyroid Glands;
B. Parathyroid Glands.

results in the treatment of disease which may be described as truly wonderful; yet there is still much that is equally wonderful to be unfolded in the future.

DUMBNESS. Dumbness means being unable to speak or to utter any of the sounds which make up words. There is a type of dumbness which is due to deafness, in which people are dumb because they have never been able to hear sounds. This type is explained more fully under the heading of DEAF-MUTISM.

When the hearing is good, dumbness is usually due to a disorder of the organs which produce the voice, or it may be due to some nervous disorder. Mentally-defective people are very often dumb, and certain hysterical conditions produce dumbness. Sometimes children suffer from a slight form of dumbness through such defects as tongue-tie or enlarged tonsils and adenoids. Sounds may be able to come, but words are prevented from being properly formed because of the obstruction in the throat. Stammering and lisping are really slight forms of dumbness, but these can generally be cured by careful training. (*See also* DEAF-MUTISM.)

DUODENAL ULCER. The duodenum or beginning part of the intestine is, like the stomach, subject to ulceration. In the case of stomach ulcers, the pain comes on after the food has been received into the stomach, that is immediately after food ; but in the duodenum the ulcer is caused by the action of the gastric juices

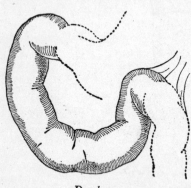

Duodenum

on the lining of the stomach, so the pain occurs when the duodenum is empty, about two hours after food, and is immediately relieved as soon as food is taken into the stomach and the gastric juices are occupied in dealing with it. Alkalis such as bicarbonate of soda counteract the gastric juices, which are acid, and render them less active, so large doses of alkalis relieve the pain of duodenal ulcer. Duodenal ulcers used to be much more frequent in men than in women, but now that so many women are out working and leading the same sort of lives as men it has become just as common amongst women as amongst men. Duodenal ulcer may occur amongst both smokers and non-smokers, but when there is an ulcer it is as well to give up smoking, as anything which increases the activity of the gastric juices, as tobacco does, will be bad for the ulcer.

Symptoms. Duodenal ulcer occurs at any age after childhood, but as it can be present for as long as twenty years without giving rise to more than a slight discomfort at intervals of months, or perhaps only for a few days in the spring and a few days in the autumn, it is not often diagnosed until middle-age, when the symptoms begin to get more troublesome. The pain, as has been said, comes on a couple of hours after food, or may only be thought of as a greater than usual hungriness as the next meal-time approaches. If a definite spot of pain is present it will be just to the right of the middle line of the abdomen and above the navel. There may also be an aching pain in the right side of the back, under the shoulder-blade. It is quite usual for people with duodenal ulcers to waken in the night with a pain which is immediately quietened by taking some food or alkaline powder or mixture. The appetite is usually good with this sort of ulcer, and the patient may remain fat and well-looking, in marked contrast to the person with a stomach ulcer who always becomes thin. The bowels are nearly always constipated, and when the ulcer is large and active there may be continuous bleeding from it with the result that the stools will be dark in colour. These dark stools, due to intestinal bleeding, are called *melæna*. The chief danger with duodenal ulcer is that the ulcer may be eating its way through the wall of the bowel and may break through or " perforate," as it is called, when a very serious situation arises with dramatic suddenness. Duodenal ulcers, unlike gastric ulcers, rarely turn into cancer.

Treatment. As has been said, duodenal ulcers may cause very little trouble for a great many years, and in fact the condition is more likely at this stage to be a *duodenitis*, or irritability of the duodenum, rather than a true ulcer, so that if all that is worrying the person is the slight discomfort before meals, it is a good thing to carry biscuits in the pocket and take doses of an alkaline mixture of magnesia, bicarbonate of soda and bismuth between meals. If, however, there are signs that the trouble is getting worse or is spreading to other parts, such as the gall-bladder, then a serious effort must be made to bring about a cure. This is a lengthy business if it is to be permanent and satisfactory, as the essence of the treatment is to rest the digestion, and this can only be done at the expense of the patient's strength for work. It is usual for the doctor to begin by putting the patient to bed for a month on a diet called the *Sippy diet*, after its inventor. This, in its earliest stages, is just as little food as will keep the patient going. The usual thing is a small glass of milk which has been citrated, every two hours, with perhaps Benger's food occasionally. Alkaline drinks are given in between times. This goes on for a fortnight, with the patient in bed. In the third week a little more food is added, such as a little thin bread and butter, raw egg in milk, junket, custard and jelly. Next week potato soup, cornflour, arrowroot, sago and tapioca may be added. In the fifth week a lightly boiled egg, white fish mashed up, thin toast or rusk with butter. For yet another week or fortnight the only addition to the menu must be finely-minced meat. After that there should be no more trouble from the ulcer, and in all but bad cases it should be cured sufficiently not to return if care is taken to avoid highly spiced and very hot food, too large meals, too long time between the meals, smoking, alcohol, and anything that is known to disagree with the individual. The alkalis should in some cases be continued permanently, a small amount of the powder or mixture being taken at intervals or one good dose each day. The surgical treatment of duodenal ulcers is not as satisfactory as that of gastric ulcers, though it may be necessary and result in an improvement in the patient's health and comfort. No operation, except in an emergency, should be undertaken until the medical treatment has had a thorough trial, and as will be seen from the account given above of the highly specialized treatment, a half-hearted attempt at the special diet while the patient tries to carry on his daily work will almost certainly be useless.

DUODENUM. The duodenum is the first part of the small intestine or bowel, and is connected with the stomach by a valve called the pylorus. It is eight to ten inches long. The gastric juices from the pancreas and the liver empty into it, and it therefore plays a great part in the digestive system of the body. At its lower end the duodenum joins on to the coils of the small intestine called the jejunum.

DUPUYTREN'S CONTRACTION. This is the name given to the condition commonly called contracted fingers, where the

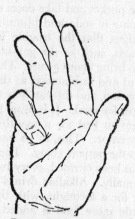

Dupuytren's Contraction

muscles of the little and ring finger contract and the fingers bend over into the palm of the hand. *See also* CONTRACTED FINGERS for a fuller description.

DURA MATER. This is the name applied to the outer covering of the brain and spinal cord. There are three coverings altogether, but the outer one, which is the strongest one of all, gets its name from the Latin words meaning hard mother. (*See also* BRAIN.)

DYSENTERY. Dysentery is an infectious disease of which the chief symptom is acute diarrhœa. There are several types of this disease, some being more severe than others, but in the main, the symptoms are all very much alike. Infection is carried by means of food and water ; flies and insects also play a large part in the spreading of this disease. Dysentery occurs in hot climates, and especially in Egypt, India, Irak and parts of America. During the Great War our troops out in the East suffered more from dysentery than any other disease, and no doubt it inconvenienced the men more than the enemy's shells.

Symptoms. The disease generally begins with a feeling of illness, loss of appetite, and a certain amount of diarrhœa, which gradually increases in severity and is accompanied by griping pains in the abdomen. At first the motions may be thin and watery, but very soon blood and mucus, or slime, is passed, and finally the motions consist of little else. The discharges from the bowels follow each other with great frequency, and the painful feeling of downward pressure which is always present, causes the patient to desire to go to stool all the time. Although the health may not be very greatly disturbed in a mild case of dysentery, it increases with the advance of the disease, and in severe cases the patient may die from sheer exhaustion and from loss of blood.

There is usually fever present, and the patient may suffer from thirst and scanty and painful flow of urine. At this stage the patient is usually very low and depressed and the discharges from the bowels become more offensive and are passed all the time.

If, on the other hand, the course of the disease is checked before it becomes too severe, the signs of improvement are shown by the number of motions which are passed. These become less in number

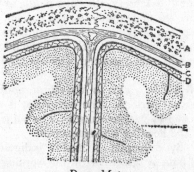

Dura Mater

A. Skull; B. Dura Mater; C. Arachnoid; D. Pia Mater; E. Brain.

8*

and more natural in appearance and the pains and straining become less severe. Convalescence is, however, a very slow business and attacks may come on again from time to time.

Preventive Treatment. In countries where epidemics of dysentery occur, it is of the utmost importance that steps should be taken in order to prevent the disease spreading. The water supply must be properly protected, and care must be taken to see that all the excreta of persons who are suffering from dysentery or who are convalescent from the disease is properly disinfected or burnt. All food should be protected from flies by placing netting over it, and only boiled water should be used for cooking and drinking and for washing food and food utensils. Constipation should be avoided, also the eating of unripe fruits.

Curative Treatment. The patient should at once be put on a diet consisting of albumin-water, rice-water, or light meat broth, and then arrowroot and cornflour. He should rest in bed and doses of castor-oil may be given along with opium to relieve the griping pains. In severer cases the drug which is most used is emetine, the extract of ipecacuanha. This is given night and morning for several days, the dose being lessened as the motions become more natural in appearance. Treatment depends on the type of dysentery present, and at the earliest opportunity the motions of the patient are examined in order to find out the exact type of germ which is causing the disease. A serum, appropriate to the germ found, is used ; other remedies which relieve the symptoms are carbonate of bismuth in large doses. Yatren is the name given to a mixture of various drugs, and this treatment is used if the diarrhœa still persists. The bowel is first washed out with an enema containing bicarbonate of soda, and then a warm, weak solution of yatren is injected into the rectum.

In the treatment of dysentery, the chief points to which attention should be given are the nourishment of the patient, and the proper care of his clothing and body, etc. During convalescence, red meat should not be given ; in fact, all rich food should be avoided. A change of climate will sometimes complete the cure when all other means fail.

DYSMENORRHŒA. This is the term applied to unusual pain at the menstrual periods. The complaint is a very common one and may be due to various causes. The subject is dealt with more fully under the heading MENSTRUATION.

DYSPEPSIA. By dyspepsia is meant indigestion, which includes any sort of pain or discomfort in the working of the digestive system. Dyspepsia is a symptom of the more serious stomach diseases such as ulceration, but it is also present in a great many people for some simple reason, usually a fault in their diet or mode of life, over-tiredness, etc. Some people are constitutionally dyspeptic, and though the condition may do them no harm, it may lead them to worry about their health more than is good for them. The subject of dyspepsia or indigestion is dealt with in the article on INDIGESTION.

DYSPHAGIA. The word dysphagia comes to us from two Greek words meaning difficulty in swallowing, and it is the term used whenever the act of swallowing cannot be carried out without difficulty. Dysphagia may be painful if it is caused by tonsillitis or any other throat complaint, but painless dysphagia is often experienced by people who are suffering from paralysis. Hysterical people may complain of difficulty in swallowing, but with them the condition does not usually last very long. (*See also* HYSTERIA.)

DYSPNŒA. Dyspnœa means shortness of breath and is an important symptom in certain diseases. (*See also* BREATHLESSNESS.)

EAR, THE. The ear is that one of the special sense organs of the body which enables us to hear ; it is also concerned with the sense of balance. It is usual to consider the ear under three divisions when describing it : the *external ear*, the *middle ear*, and the *internal ear*. The part of the external ear which stands out from the head and acts as a collector and receiver of air waves is called the *auricle*. It is so shaped that it can bring the sound waves to the passage, or *external meatus*, which leads from the outside to the middle ear. At the further end of this passage is the ear drum, which is set in motion when sound waves strike on to it. It vibrates, and by its vibrations the waves are conveyed across the tiny space behind the drum called the middle ear to the internal ear. It used to be thought that the sound vibrations were conveyed across the middle ear by the three little bones called *ossicles* of the ear, the *malleus*, *incus* and *stapes*. It is now considered more probable, however, that these ossicles have a damping effect upon violent sound vibrations and thus serve as a protection to the inner ear from too violent noise. The ear drum, also, has a much less important part in hearing than used to be imagined. A person can hear quite well with a perforation or hole in the ear drum so long as no suppuration is going on ; it does not do any damage to the hearing to have an opening made in the ear drum to let out inflammation.

The most important part of the organ of hearing is the internal ear. The third of the ossicles, which is called the *stapes* or stirrup, has its base attached to a membrane which closes the oval window of the middle ear, and movements of the stapes are communicated to a fluid called *perilymph*, which lies within the bony channels of the inner ear. The sound vibrations probably reach the peri-lymph through the membrane of another little window—the round window—into the inner ear. These movements are in turn communicated to another fluid, the *endolymph* which is found inside the small membraneous canal which lies within the long channels of the inner ear. Movements of this fluid stimulate the delicate nerve endings in the *cochlea* (so-called because it is shaped like a shell). The cochlea is the essential organ without which hearing cannot take place. It sends the vibrations on to the hearing centre in the brain where they are received and interpreted by the understanding. It will be seen from this description that the whole of the ear, or organ of hearing, is a very delicate and complicated piece of mechanism.

The Semi-circular Canals. The organ of balance consists of three little canals, called the semi-circular canals. They are situated deep in the temporal bone in communication with the internal ear. These canals lie in three different planes of the body, and movements of the endolymph in them stimulates delicate nerve endings, which help the brain to maintain the balance of the body. Diseases which affect the semi-circular canals, such as Menière's disease, upset the balance.

Diseases of the Ear. *Wax* (cerumen) in the outer passage of the ear (external meatus) usually causes deafness as well as discomfort; it is removed by syringing with bicarbonate of soda in warm water. A *boil* (furuncle) in the outer passage may be extremely painful, but is not serious; it is sometimes difficult, even for a doctor, to tell the inflammation caused by a boil from the inflammation caused by mastoid disease, but for one thing the person who has a boil is not very ill, though in pain, and is usually not deaf. A boil is treated by having a gauze wick, soaked in a solution of epsom salts in glycerine, pushed past it into the ear passage; this must be changed daily. *Acute inflammation of the middle ear* is always an extension up the little tube that communicates with the throat (the eustachian tube), of inflammation in the nose or throat, often helped by that dangerous procedure, sniffing a nasal douche up the nose. The best treatment of acute inflammation of the ear is to have the ear drum slit with a fine scalpel by a doctor; this lets out the inflammation before it bursts through the drum, making a big hole, and it soon clears up after this little operation. *Chronic suppuration of the ear* may go on for weeks, months, or years, and is a common cause of incurable deafness; it usually follows scarlet fever or measles in childhood. The most popular treatment is to drop in peroxide of hydrogen, but it is probably better to mop out the discharge thoroughly with cotton wool and then blow in boracic powder or 1% iodine in boracic powder, the latter being the latest treatment used successfully in America. Ionization is another useful method of treatment and is widely used in school clinics.

An ear should not be allowed to discharge for more than a month without having a serious talk with a doctor on the advisability of having an operation to stop the discharge ; sometimes it means only removal of adenoids, sometimes the simple mastoid drainage operation ; but either is better than long-continued ear discharge, which may in time even give rise to a brain abscess, and even when it does not, is a constant worry and a cause of persistent ill-health. Inflammation of the ear may go on to inflammation of the mastoid. This is a group of air cells in the bone behind the ear, which protects the delicate internal ear ; these air cells communicate with the middle ear and any inflammation can easily pass on to them. Unless this inflammation is relieved by an operation, meningitis or brain abscess and death may be the result. Many people are afraid of the word " mastoid " and dread this operation ; that is quite a mistaken idea and dates from the days when this operation was only undertaken as a last resort and at the last moment. The modern simple mastoid drainage operation, if performed early, before the inflammation of the mastoid has caused any complications, gives excellent results and is certainly not an operation to dread, while the patient has usually little or no pain afterwards. (*See also* DEAFNESS.)

EARACHE. Earache is a condition which should be treated with much greater care than it often is. How often does one hear that a child " has only earache "—as if earache were a thing of no importance. Far from being unimportant, earache is one of the aches for which there is almost always a definite reason.

Many things can cause earache. In a small child it may really be the pain from teething that is worrying him, or the child may have pushed some small body such as a bead into the ear. The most serious condition is that in which the pain is round and behind the ear in the part called the mastoid. This part may get infected after influenza or any of the infectious diseases such as measles, but especially after scarlet fever. Unhealthy noses and throats, enlarged tonsils and adenoids all may cause ear trouble of the sort that will later on lead to deafness.

In grown-up people there is sometimes a very slight dislocation of the little pads of gristle or cartilage, which lie between the ends of the jaws. This dislocation may cause excruciating pain in the ears until it is put right.

Treatment. The cause of the earache must be found and treated by a doctor ; but, before that can be done, the pain can be eased by lying down with a hot-water bottle, or hot bag of salt or sand pressed to the ear, or a few drops of warm glycerine dropped in, while some simple pain-deadening tablet such as aspirin may be taken. It may be necessary for the doctor to incise the ear drum and let out matter, a small operation which is soon recovered from and may prevent very serious mischief.

EASTON'S SYRUP. This is an old and well-tried tonic for general weakness, but more especially useful in cases where the nerves are fagged by over-work. The ingredients are quinine, strychnine and iron. When strychnine is contained in any mixture always be careful to shake the bottle well before taking the medicine, as strychnine is heavy and sinks to the bottom of the bottle. Easton's Syrup can also be obtained in tablet form.

ECCHYMOSIS. This term is used to describe bleeding which takes place just under the skin and is often the result of a bruise. The skin usually has a purplish appearance, gradually changing to green and yellow. (*See also* BLEEDING.)

ECLAMPSIA OR "FITS." Eclampsia is one of the most serious complications of pregnancy, and is characterized by severe fits. It does not come on in the early months of pregnancy and symptoms of it should be watched for after the fifth month, but it is not unusual for the first fit to occur actually during labour. The exact cause of eclampsia is not known, but it seems to have something to do with disordered chemistry of the body so that a poison is allowed to circulate in the mother's blood instead of being got rid of in the ordinary ways by which the body rids itself of waste products. What this poison is, is not known ; but it must be something that develops through pregnancy, as the condition of eclampsia only arises in connection with childbirth.

The earliest sign of eclampsia is the appearance of albumen in the urine, so it is necessary to keep watch on the way the kidneys are working during pregnancy. This is done by examining the urine periodically.

Warning Symptoms. There are several symptoms which give warning that eclampsia may occur, and if these are recognized in time the condition may be stopped from progressing to the stage of fits. The chief of these warnings is persistent headache, upsets of the eyesight, such as blurred vision, flashes of light before the eyes, and perhaps even blindness ; a greater degree than usual of stomach upset, and a lessening in the quantity of urine passed. If these warnings are neglected they may be followed at any moment by an eclamptic fit.

A typical Fit. In a typical fit the eyes enlarge so that the patient can hardly see, and the muscles of the face begin to twitch. In a short time the body goes stiff and remains fixed. The teeth are tightly clenched and the back is arched. The patient becomes blue from the inability to breathe owing to the spasm of the muscles used for breathing. This spasm of stiffness lasts any number of seconds up to a minute, when the muscles begin to contract and relax alternately and continue to do so for some minutes, after which the patient lapses into a coma, and may remain unconscious a few hours or even a few days. These fits recur again and again at intervals of a few hours, or may follow in quick succession.

Treatment. Eclampsia fits are always a serious matter, and are especially dangerous if they begin in the last three months before the child is born. If the condition is discovered before the fits begin it may be warded off, but once the fit is on the only thing that can be done is to protect the patient as much as possible from harm and treat the fit. Send at once for the doctor, and while he is coming try to keep the patient from hurting herself in her convulsions. Lay her on the floor, and place something, like a spoon or piece of wood, between her teeth if they can be unclenched enough. Turn her sideways so that the saliva will ooze away. When the unconscious stage arrives she may be put to bed.

The doctor in attendance will administer certain drugs, and aims his treatment at driving the poisons out of the system, but in most cases it is necessary to hurry on the birth of the child in order to save the mother.

ECTHYMA. This disease is a severe form of impetigo, in which the germ responsible for the disease makes its way into the skin and flourishes there. Ecthyma is most common upon the legs, between the knee and the ankle, and always indicates that the affected person is seriously run down in health. It usually attacks neglected, ill-fed children, but is also seen in adults whose living is poor, who are uncleanly, and below par generally. Lice and bed-bugs are frequent accompaniments of the disease, and probably help in its spread. The appearance on the legs is that of small ulcers, which have a characteristic "scooped out" appearance when the scab, which usually covers them, is removed. Each ulcer is surrounded by an inflamed reddish ring of skin, and leaves a scar when healing takes place.

Treatment. This is in itself very simple. Any milder antiseptic ointment serves as a dressing for the ulcer; and under cleanly conditions, where the patient has plenty of vegetables, fruit, and milk, and an iron tonic, he rapidly recovers. (*See also* IMPETIGO.)

ECTOPIC GESTATION. It sometimes happens that after pregnancy takes place, the fertilized ovum instead of developing normally in the womb, begins to develop in one of the organs outside the womb. This is known as ectopic gestation. The ovum may be arrested in the Fallopian tube and begin to grow in this small cavity ; when such a condition arises, it is very serious indeed.

The cause of the arrest of the passage of the fertilized ovum may be some obstruction in the Fallopian tube due to adhesions or possibly due to some former inflammation. As a rule abortion takes place between the sixth and twelfth week of pregnancy and there may be some serious internal hæmorrhage.

Generally there is a history of one menstrual period being missed, but very soon severe attacks of abdominal pains come on and there may be a continuous flow of blood from the vagina.

It is important that the doctor should be consulted at once, as an operation may be necessary in order to save the life of the mother. The condition is a very serious one and always requires surgical treatment.

ECTROPION.   Ectropion is a condition in which the eyelids turn outwards. It is a fairly common condition, and it is due to various causes.

ECZEMA. This very familiar word is derived from a Greek word meaning to boil over, burst out, or erupt. Naturally, using the word in its widest sense, *any* skin disease may be called an " eruption " or " eczema," but it really does not mean any one definite type of skin disease ; in fact, calling any skin rash " eczema " is much the same as calling any pain of unknown origin " rheumatism."

The more modern skin specialists have now discarded the term " eczema " for the term dermatitis, which means inflammation of the skin. (*See also* DERMATITIS.)

EFFERENT.   This is a term used to describe motion away from a centre, such as the course of a blood-vessel leading away from an organ or a nerve from the motor centre in the brain to the limb it moves.

EFFLEURAGE. This is the name given to the " stroking " movement used in massage. It is described under the heading MASSAGE.

EFFUSION. The word effusion (which means a pouring out) is used in medicine in connection with the pouring out of fluid from the normal stream into some other part of the body. One of the most common types of effusion is that which occurs in " housemaid's knee." There is usually a large swelling which is filled with fluid, and the same type of thing occurs in " miner's elbow." The popular phrase " water on the brain " simply means an effusion and a pleural effusion takes place when fluid collects in the chest, as in pleurisy. Treatment of effusions will naturally depend on which part of the body they appear in and according to their type. (*See also* ASCITES ; BURSITIS ; DROPSY ; PLEURISY.)

ELBOW. The elbow, or elbow joint as it really is, is the hinge joint formed by the bones of the upper and lower arms, that is to say the *humerus*, which is the single bone in the upper arm and the *ulna* and *radius*, the bones of the lower, or forearm. Of these the ulna is on the inner side of the arm and the radius on the outer side. The ends of the three bones are covered with smooth cartilage or gristle, and the upper ends of the radius and ulna together form a cup-shaped socket into which the rounded end of the humerus fits and is gripped snugly by them. The cartilage and lubricating fluid in the joint enable it to turn easily in the socket. The sharp point which is felt at the tip of the elbow when the arm is bent is the sharpened end of the ulna, and is known as the *olecranon process*.

Injuries and diseases of the Elbow. The elbow is a part of the body which is in almost constant use, and is therefore very liable to be accidentally hurt. A fall on the hand may dislocate the elbow. A common fracture of the arm is that of the humerus just above the elbow joint. In young children the ends of the bones, called the epiphyses, have not yet become joined in the same solid piece as the rest of the bone and are therefore very easily knocked off the main bone. The olecranon process which is the most exposed part of the elbow is easily broken across, but probably the most crippling accidents to the arm are the numerous forms of muscular injuries to which it is subject. These range in severity from simple strains to the tearing of the muscle from the bone to which it is attached, or breaking of its continuity, both conditions which lead to trouble and may be very difficult to cure. Almost every form of sport in which the arm is used has its own special form of injury, such as *tennis elbow* and *golf elbow*. These are terms loosely applied to several varieties of arm injuries which are apt to occur when playing these games. The little bursæ or bags of fluid which are found near joints to act as pads or shock absorbers, are a very frequent form of trouble in the arm and elbow. The most usual form of tennis elbow being due to chronic irritation of the bursa just above the elbow.

Treatment of elbow injuries. A stiff elbow is a frequent result of injuries of the arm and, as well as being very inconvenient to its possessor, is actually a danger to him when his work takes him amongst machinery, so above all things treatment should be directed towards restoring or preserving the movement of the arm from the straight position to that of bending the elbow to the shoulder. Massage, remedial exercises and electricity are all of use in these injuries. The elbow is concerned in movements of the arm involving the turning of the hand, lifting, and raising the wrist up and down, and these movements may be damaged by what may appear a trifling injury, and if the damage is allowed to become chronic a long spell of treatment and rest of the arm may be required to restore it to health, so that it is always best to attend to a slight injury when it appears, even if it means giving up tennis or whatever was the cause for the time being. People used to talk of "playing-in" their sore arms or "working-off" their muscle strains. This may make matters worse if real injury is present.

The elbow joint is subject to all the diseases that attack other joints, of which the commonest is arthritis. The arthritis may be simply inflammation of the joint due to infection or injury, or may be tubercular. It is important that it should be treated as soon as it appears, lest serious crippling results from letting the disease get a firm hold. (*See also* ARTHRITIS.)

ELECTRO-COAGULATION. Another name for surgical Diathermy. (*See* DIATHERMY.)

ELECTROLYSIS. Electricity applied to the skin can be made to have a destructive effect on the little glands at the roots of hairs, and is consequently used by beauty specialists and others to remove superfluous hairs. It is, of course, accompanied by a certain amount of pain, and in unskilled hands may be dangerous and lead to disfigurement. Where there is a heavy crop of "down" on the face electrolysis of the larger hairs may stimulate the growth of the down and so should be avoided, but for an isolated group of strongly growing hairs it is usually a successful though expensive way of having them removed. Each hair has to be operated on separately, and the treatment therefore is apt to be a lengthy one.

ELEPHANTIASIS. Elephantiasis is a very suitable name for this most uncomfortable and cruelly deforming disease. It may attack any portion of the body but it seems to favour the legs, causing them to become huge and ungainly like those of an elephant. This disease is caused by a tiny worm which gets into the blood and then passes on into the lymph vessels. These become blocked and the result is a gradual swelling up of whatever part of the body is affected. The disease is most frequently seen in tropical countries and it never seems to develop in cold climates.

Symptoms. The skin at first is smooth, but afterwards it becomes rough, coarse and thick, and is thrown up in folds just like the skin on the leg of an elephant. Attacks of fever occur at intervals, and although there is no pain there is a good deal of inflammation and swelling. The legs, arms, scrotum and breasts are the parts which seem to be affected more than other parts of the body. The scrotum (the bag containing the testicles) may be of great size, reaching almost to the ground.

Treatment. Surgical treatment is usually carried out and very often this means cutting off a limb or limbs. An elastic stocking should be worn and the leg should be raised up and rested as much as possible. This may help to delay the course of the disease, especially if injections of tartar emetic are given.

EMACIATION. Emaciation means a condition in which there is extreme loss of weight and wasting of the body. This may occur from excessive loss of fluid, in which case the wasting may take place very rapidly ; slow emaciation is usually due to the body not getting proper nourishment either through actual starvation from want of food, or because the body is using its nourishment in the wrong way.

EMBOLISM. An embolism is a plug of any sort which is floating in the blood-stream. Most often it is made of clotted blood which has broken off from a *thrombus,* or clotting of the blood in a vein, but sometimes it may be composed of other matters which are in the blood-stream, and which have probably broken off from some diseased part of the heart or of a blood-vessel. Air which has found its way into a vein may act in the same way as an embolus, or in countries where various sorts of worms find their way into the body, and especially into the blood, they may form a block in the circulation. Sometimes a very tiny particle of tissue from a diseased part may be infected with germs which increase in number to such an extent that they are able to dam the blood-stream. Whatever the cause of the clot or embolism the behaviour is the same. It floats in the blood-stream until it reaches some vital spot, when it causes sudden death, or it may remain in the blood-stream quite harmlessly, or again it may partially block some vein or attach itself to the wall of the blood-vessel, when it will probably cause an abscess.

The two cases in which fatal embolisms are most likely to occur are after childbirth and where there is a varicose condition of the veins, as in bad legs. After childbirth the blood in the veins of the womb is very liable to clot and form thrombosis, and there is no way that it can be foreseen that a small portion of clot will detach and cause serious trouble in one particular case while the great numbers of other mothers go unharmed.

In the case of thrombosis of the veins of the legs or elsewhere due to varicose veins, the treatment is always complete rest and keeping the leg still. In bad cases the leg is even enclosed in adhesive plaster to keep it absolutely motionless. This is partly because of the danger of embolism. Sometimes an embolism occurs where a limb has been kept still after a fracture, or a tiny embolism in the veins of the brain may cause sudden blindness or sudden paralysis of one side of the body. Surgical treatment—*embolectomy*—has recently been carried out successfully in a number of cases of embolism, the blood-vessel blocked being exposed and the obstructing embolus removed under local anæsthesia. *Fat embolism* may occur through fat getting out of the marrow of a long bone owing to a fracture, getting into the blood circulation and being carried to a vital part of the body, such as the brain, and causing a block there.

EMBROCATION. This is the name given to substances which are suitable for rubbing into the skin. They usually contain oil of some sort and some have alcohol as well. They are now more commonly known as liniments.

EMBRYO. By embryo we mean the fœtus in the womb up to about six weeks or two months after fertilization has taken place of the female element (ovum) by the male element (spermatozoa). After fertilization takes place the ovum grows rapidly in the womb, until at the end of the first month it is about a quarter of an inch long. At the end of the second month it is over an inch long and the beginnings of the human shape can be seen although it still has a trace of a tail. The eyes, ears and nose are forming and the limbs have begun to sprout. The head is particularly large for the size of the body and the brain is beginning to develop. Shortly after this the sex characteristics become recognizable and the embryo is henceforth called the fœtus.

EMETIC. An emetic is given in order to cause vomiting and this is one of the ways in which the stomach can be rapidly emptied. Nowadays emetics are chiefly used for cases of poisoning and the best ones are those which are in everyday use in the home, as quickness of action may mean the saving of a life. A tablespoonful of mustard stirred into half a glass of hot water will produce immediate and thorough results. Two tablespoonsful of common salt in warm water will act in the same way. If it is available, one of the best emetics is ipecacuanha wine. It is particularly safe for children, and it should be given in repeated teaspoonful doses until vomiting begins. Zinc sulphate (25 grains) mixed with a little ipecacuanha wine and dissolved in hot water is a very excellent emetic.

The ever-present and very popular method of producing vomiting by thrusting the fingers down the back of the throat must not be left out. In urgent cases this should be tried while an emetic is being prepared. Either the fingers of the sufferer or the fingers of another person should be gently pushed far down the throat, but no force or roughness should be used. This method does not always act, but it is worth while trying as it is so quick and requires no preparation.

Whenever an emetic has been given it is advisable to give a stimulant afterwards, such as coffee or brandy. This is especially

necessary if there are signs of collapse. Apomorphine is an emetic
which is given by injection and which produces excellent results ;
vomiting usually takes place within five minutes of injection but
its action generally causes nausea and prostration.

EMETINE. This is a drug which is derived from ipecacuanha
and is greatly used in the treatment of dysentery. It should not be
taken except under medical care, as prolonged use of the drug
leads to poisoning.

EMMENAGOGUE. An emmenagogue is a drug which is
used to regulate the menstrual periods. Ergot, potassium permanganate, aloes, etc., are used, and extracts of certain ductless glands
have been found to act as emmenagogues.

EMMETROPIA. A technical term used in connection with
refraction of the eye.

EMOLLIENT. Any substance which soothes, softens, or protects the skin is called an emollient. Ordinary cold cream, lanoline,
vaseline or olive-oil are a few of the more simple forms of an emollient. When there is any inflammation of the skin a more powerful
emollient will have to be used.

EMPHYSEMA. Emphysema is the name given to a condition
of the lungs in which the breath seems to be shut in and there is
much straining to breathe outwards. Such straining tends to

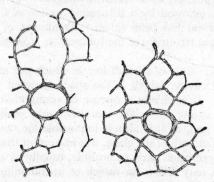

1. *Emphysematous and* 2. *Normal Lung Air Cells*

stretch the air-cells of the lungs and in some cases may even tear
them, and the chest becomes expanded and barrel-shaped.

The commonest causes of emphysema are asthma and bronchitis,
and it also occurs as the result of blowing wind instruments. It is
a condition which is found in elderly people who have suffered
from chest complaints all their lives, and each attack of bronchitis
aggravates the condition and makes it a little worse. Such people

should live in warm climates, or avoid attacks of bronchitis by taking great care of the chest. On no account should these people go out in cold or wet weather ; and fog, especially, is dangerous because it irritates the air tubes.

People who are subject to asthma should be very careful with their diet as certain foods tend to bring on an asthmatic attack which at once aggravates the emphysematous state. If the chest becomes irritated, a steam-kettle should be kept boiling in the room and Friars' balsam, added to the water, will be found very soothing.

People who suffer from emphysema should be very careful not to over-exercise or tire themselves in any way. Walking along dusty roads should be avoided as dust will tend to irritate the bronchial tubes. There is no cure for this condition, but by taking great care to avoid bronchitis and any strain on the lungs, the progress of the disease may be hindered. (*See also* ASTHMA ; BRON-CHITIS ; LUNG.)

EMPTINESS. The feeling of emptiness when one is hungry is a very natural one, but this feeling may occur as a symptom of indigestion, and many women experience it when they are pregnant.

When the feeling is due to indigestion it may be relieved by taking food in small quantities or some alkaline powder such as bicarbonate of soda ; but there are some forms of indigestion in which the relief is immediately followed by a distressing feeling of fullness, even if only a small meal has been taken. Treatment of the condition lies in the proper treatment of the indigestion. (*See also* DUODENUM ; INDIGESTION.)

EMPYEMA. This is a condition in which pus or matter forms in the pleural cavity, which is the space between the chest wall and the lung. It is chiefly a disease of young children, although it may occur at any age. The condition may really be regarded as an abscess, and, as it is almost impossible for the pus to escape through the thick wall of the chest, it is important that the condition should be cleared up as early as possible, usually by surgical means. The condition may follow an attack of pneumonia, or it may be due to tuberculosis of the lungs or cancer of the throat. Injuries to the chest, such as a gunshot or a knife wound, or any disease in the neighbouring organs, may spread infection and cause empyema.

Symptoms. If, after an attack of pneumonia, the temperature of the patient does not return to normal, it is usual for the doctor to suspect that empyema is present. There may be no special symptoms at first, but a rise of temperature is a sure indication that infection has spread. Symptoms generally associated with empyema are pain in the affected side, shortness of breath, sweating, and a temperature which varies night and morning. A cough may be present and very often the patient is irritable.

Treatment. The treatment of empyema is the same as the treatment of any abscess, namely, by opening and allowing the pus to drain away. To do this, it is necessary for the doctor to find out the exact spot in the chest where the pus is lying, and this is done by inserting a needle through the chest wall into the pleural cavity. A syringe is attached to the needle, and if pus is drawn off an operation is usually indicated. As soon as the pus is removed by operation or repeated aspiration with a syringe, the lung usually resumes its normal working order. In some cases the lung may

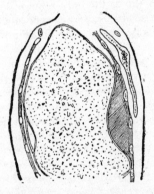

Empyema
Longitudinal section
through Lung.

fail to expand ; while in other cases, even in spite of operation, the infection may spread with fatal results. Empyema is a serious condition, and much depends on early and efficient treatment.

EMULSION. Emulsions are thick liquid preparations rather like milk in colour and usually consisting of oils, fats or resins. Milk and yolk of egg are examples of natural emulsions. As a rule, substances such as cod-liver oil are emulsified by the addition of glycerine, which not only hides the taste but makes it easier to digest.

ENAMEL OF TEETH. Enamel is the outer covering of the teeth and it is the hardest tissue in the body. It is white in colour, but when it is thin, the yellow dentine underneath may show through. Enamel is very readily eaten away by acids, hence the necessity of cleaning the teeth after taking vinegar and certain medicines, etc. (*See also* TEETH.)

ENCEPHALITIS means inflammation of the brain and this may occur in a very large number of ways. Many of the general fevers, such as scarlet fever, measles, mumps and influenza, may be complicated by encephalitis, but fortunately, only rarely does this happen. Much prominence has recently been given to that form of encephalitis which very rarely occurs after vaccination. Much more common is an encephalitis which results from extension of infection from the ear or the air cavities of the nose, through the bone into the brain. In these cases, the inflammation is confined to a relatively small area of the brain, pus is produced and an abscess is formed. The danger in this form of encephalitis is that the inflammation will not remain confined to one part of the brain, but will spread to the coverings of the brain—the meninges—and so cause meningitis, which is almost certain to prove fatal. Whilst the inflammation remains localized it is possible to operate and remove the pus, and this is the only hope of curing the condition. But prevention of these abscesses by proper and thorough treatment of all diseases of the nose and ear should be possible if the patients, with such troubles, are seen early enough.

Symptoms. The symptoms common to all the above forms of encephalitis are the general symptoms of any severe disturbance of the brain substance : severe headache, irritability, sleepiness, vomiting, convulsions. Later the drowsiness becomes more marked and the patient sinks into a coma from which he cannot be roused. Fever, sometimes accompanied by shivering attacks, is almost always present. Where the encephalitis is a complication of such infectious fevers as measles or scarlet fever, the signs of those diseases will be present and the inflammation of the brain being a general one, without any pus being formed, no operation will be of any benefit to the patient. Where the inflammation has extended into the brain through the skull from the nose or ear, the signs which the doctor can find from an examination of the patient will in all probability tell him in which part of the brain the abscess has formed ; generally an abscess forms near the place in the skull where the infection has penetrated. Thus, abscesses which are the result of disease of the nose are usually found in the foremost part of the brain ; whilst those which have followed disease of the ear are in one or other side of the brain or at the back of the brain, in the " little brain," or cerebellum. This information is essential if the surgeon is to find the abscess and remove the pus. It is sometimes difficult to obtain this information however carefully the patient is examined, because if he is so drowsy that he cannot understand what the doctor is trying to do, the patient may be unable to carry out the instructions given him which are an essential part of the examination. In that case, it may be necessary to operate on very slight evidence of where the abscess may possibly be found.

ENCEPHALITIS LETHARGICA is a curious and, although only recently discovered, a very common disease, known popularly, from one of its symptoms, as "sleepy sickness." Before 1917, no cases of this disease were known. Since then, there have been several epidemics of it in England and the disease has become scattered world-wide. There is at present no evidence to show that the disease is infectious in the sense that it can be conveyed from one human being to another, but we do know that whatever is the cause of the condition—and it is probably a microbe so small that it cannot be seen under the highest powers of the microscope—it gains entrance to the human body by the nose and throat. The symptoms have varied from time to time in the several epidemics, but for some years there have been no epidemics and the disease seems to have changed its character. In the epidemics, the symptoms were of sudden onset and after an acute illness, the patient, if he recovered at all, seemed for a time to get quite well and then developed certain signs and conditions which for some time did not appear to have any connection with the acute illness. In the cases which occur from time to time nowadays, no definite acute illness can be traced ; the symptoms of the conditions which were first thought to be sequels of encephalitis lethargica have turned out to be a chronic form of the disease itself.

In the acute attacks, feverish symptoms accompanied by a history of being unable to sleep for a night or two and a feeling of intense drowsiness during the daytime with "double vision" (i.e. seeing two things instead of one) was the common story. In more severe cases the patient would remain drowsy for days, or even weeks on end. From these attacks recovery occurred in about half the cases recorded. Since the epidemics, it is difficult to obtain a definite description of an acute attack from a patient who presents one of the chronic conditions associated with the disease. The most frequent, and unfortunately the most difficult to treat, of all these chronic stages of encephalitis lethargica is a weakness of movement, with slowness and difficulty in moving the arms and legs, which tends to persist. In typical cases, this condition resembles the "shaking palsy," though the shaking is not always so noticeable as it is in the true "shaking palsy." But there is the same mask-like expression of the face, the same slight bending forwards of the body, the same stiff movements of the limbs ; and in some, the same trembling of the limbs. Much can be done with drugs to assist these patients to overcome the stiffness of the limbs, but the trembling does not yield to treatment.

One of the most distressing features of this disease is its effect on the moral character of young people. Children who before they were attacked by it were normal, healthy, delightful creatures, afterwards may become young ruffians and pests to society. The

juvenile courts have recently been full of victims of this disease
who have come before the courts for thieving, destructive behaviour (e.g. smashing shop windows), attacks on younger children,
or sexual offences. In most cases the decision of the doctor that
the delinquent had suffered from encephalitis lethargica, has sufficed
to have him removed to a special institution for such cases, but
there must be many yet which go unrecognized. No child whose
behaviour suddenly alters for the worse should be condemned out
of hand as merely "naughty," until the possibility of an attack
of encephalitis lethargica has been excluded.

On adults, the mental effects are not so disastrous from the legal
point of view, but the complete mental outlook may be altered.
In cases which recover after severe symptoms, considerable reduction of mental capacity and obvious mental change may persist.

ENCEPHALOID. This is the term applied to a form of
cancer which resembles the tissue of the brain.

ENCHONDROMA. An enchondroma means a tumour
composed of cartilage or gristle. (*See also* TUMOURS.)

ENDARTERITIS. Endarteritis is a condition in which the
inner coat of an artery becomes inflamed or thickened. There are
many forms of endarteritis, and it may affect many parts of the
body or may be concentrated in one place.

Changes in the inner coat of the arteries are found in tuberculosis ;
also in diseases of the kidneys and in syphilis. Atheroma is a form
of endarteritis in which one of the main arteries, called the aorta,
is usually affected. Arterio-sclerosis is a disease in which the chief
changes are found in the middle coat of the arteries, but the inner
coat may be affected as well.

There is another form of endarteritis, known as intermittent
claudication, which usually affects young people and which produces
very distressing symptoms. Burning pain is felt in the legs after
walking a short distance and the sufferer is forced to rest. The
pain usually passes after a short time, but commences again as
soon as a few more steps are taken. The disease is due to the fact
that the space inside the artery is affected and this prevents the
proper supply of blood reaching the limbs. (*See also* ARTERIO-
SCLEROSIS.)

ENDEMIC. A disease is said to be endemic to a country or
place when it occurs in that particular place more often than in
other places, and never completely dies out. For instance, such
diseases as cholera and plague are said to be endemic in India and
the Far East, because there are always cases of it in those parts.

ENDOCARDITIS. The word endocarditis means inflammation of the endocardium or membrane lining the heart. The

disease is more common in a simple form after attacks of acute rheumatism in some form or other, and in these cases treatment and rest will bring about a good recovery, but the danger is that the condition may not be treated until it has got a hold, and it may turn into a more severe form in which the heart will be damaged. The disease is fully described under HEART, DISEASES OF.

ENDOCRINE GLANDS. These are certain glands in the body whose function is to form and give off into the blood-stream substances which are very important to our mental and physical well-being. The endocrine glands include the thyroid gland, adrenal bodies, pituitary gland, parathyroid glands, pancreas, ovaries and testicles. An important article on the recent discoveries that have been made with regard to the ductless glands is to be found under the heading DUCTLESS GLANDS.

ENDOMETRITIS. This term is applied to the inflammation of the endometrium, which is the membrane lining the inside of the womb. There are two types of this condition, the acute and the chronic.

The acute condition is generally caused by the retention in the womb of some part of the *after-birth*, following a confinement or an incomplete miscarriage, or it may be due to gonorrhœa. When due to gonorrhœa, the disease usually spreads upwards from the neck of the womb during the menstruation period, which may stop abruptly and be followed by a discharge. There is usually a great deal of pain in the abdomen, and immediate medical care is necessary.

In treatment of the acute condition due to the retention of portions of the after-birth in the womb, the interior of the womb must be thoroughly cleaned out and disinfected, a slight operation which is known as " curettage," and, as a rule, the condition clears up and the offensive discharges from the womb cease.

Chronic endometritis may follow the acute stage or the condition may be chronic from the first. The inflammation may spread to the muscles in the walls of the womb, and there is considerable discharge from the womb composed of a mixture of pus and mucus. The general health may be very low and the patient may show signs of nervousness.

Treatment. Treatment must be directed towards improving the health of the patient so that she may be able to fight against the state of inflammation present in the womb. The bowels must be attended to and the diet should be light and nourishing ; no alcohol should be taken. Tonics of a suitable nature should be given and douches will help to keep the vagina clean. Curettage, followed by thorough disinfection of the womb, is the usual treatment carried out, but the condition is one that may take a long time to clear up. (*See also* PUERPERUM ; WOMB.)

ENEMA. An enema is used as a method of clearing out the bowel. It takes the form of an injection of fluid into the rectum which causes the complete emptying of the bowel in a few minutes. It is a very good way of obtaining results, but it is not wise to give an enema in cases of disorder of the bowel without medical advice. An enema is much safer than the indiscriminate use of medicines and pills, and very often a slight obstruction will yield to a simple enema which would cause severe pain if pills were indulged in.

For a simple enema nothing more is required than soap and warm water, but the addition of a tablespoonful of olive oil or castor oil will ensure better results. About an ounce of common soap should be dissolved in a pint of boiling water, add whichever oil is to be used, and stir briskly until soap is thoroughly dissolved. The patient should be placed on the left side with the knees drawn up to the abdomen and the buttocks projecting a little over the edge of the bed. Add cold water until the enema is at a temperature of about 98° F. which is quite warm to the touch but not hot. A Higginson's syringe is a very popular type of enema syringe sold in most chemists' shops, but any type may be used so long as it gives satisfactory results. The bone nozzle at the end to be inserted into the rectum should be well lubricated with vaseline or soap, and the other end should be dropped into the jug holding the fluid. All air must be squeezed out of the syringe before it is inserted into the rectum and this can be done by pressing the bulb of the syringe several times until a few drops of the fluid come through. The bone nozzle must be inserted into the rectum very gently and without any pressure, and the bulb of the syringe must be squeezed slowly and firmly so that the fluid comes through in a steady stream. The patient must make every effort to retain the fluid for a few minutes, and once the nozzle is gently withdrawn a towel pressed tightly against the anus may help to retain the fluid. The amount of fluid used for an adult should be about 16 ounces or two breakfastcupsful, and for children about one ounce (two tablespoonsful) for every year of age. For example, a child of five should be given five ounces, and a child of eight, eight ounces, and so on. Enemas to young children may be given by means of a glass syringe, which is more suitable for small amounts than the ordinary Higginson type.

Constipation is generally the complaint for which an enema is given without medical advice, but there are times when sickness calls for a more specialized type of enema.

A medicinal enema may contain nothing more than a few ounces of soothing substance and may be given to check severe diarrhœa, hæmorrhage, or to save the patient from collapse. For dysentery or summer diarrhœa in children, an enema consisting of starch and opium is a common remedy. If ulceration is present, a few crystals of potassium permanganate, or a small amount of sulphate of zinc, may be added to a cupful of warm water and injected. For shock and collapse due to hæmorrhage or any other cause, the patient should be given an injection of saline solution either directly into the blood-stream or it may be given as an enema per rectum. As an injection into the bloodstream can only be done by a skilled person, the enema can be prepared by mixing a heaped teaspoonful of common salt in a pint of boiling water. About a teacupful of this, when it cools to a temperature of 100° F. which is warmish but not hot, should be injected slowly into the rectum and repeated at intervals of three to four hours.

Children who suffer from threadworms should be given an enema in order to dislodge them from the large bowel. The enema usually given for this purpose consists of a solution of quassia, but a salt solution may be used consisting of a small teaspoonful of common salt in a cupful of water. Vinegar may be given (a teaspoonful in a cupful of water) or a turpentine enema (25 drops in a cupful of water) is sometimes used for threadworms.

In certain illnesses, when it is impossible for the patient to take food by mouth, nourishment may be given by means of an enema. Great care must be taken, however, that no irritation is set up in the bowel, otherwise no benefit will result. The enema must be very slowly administered and the amount of nourishment given at one time must never exceed 3 ounces. It is advisable to give only predigested food such as peptonized milk, peptonized beef-tea, and so on. (*See also* CONSTIPATION ; DIARRHŒA ; DYSENTERY ; SHOCK ; THREADWORM.)

ENEMA RASH. This is a skin rash which sometimes follows the administration of an enema and which requires very careful diagnosis to distinguish it from scarlet fever. The medical name for this condition is erythema scarlatiniforme.

The patient is " upset " and feverish, and these symptoms are followed perhaps immediately, perhaps in a day or two, by a rash which may be almost indistinguishable from that of scarlet fever. Sometimes it is more like a measles rash, but in these cases the diagnosis is much easier, as the other symptoms of measles are absent. Peeling starts early and is very profuse, large flakes of skin being thrown off. In severe cases the hair may fall out, and the nails shed in layers.

The condition is due to some " poison in the blood " ; possibly a definite poisoning, as from shell-fish or other food ; or from some drugs, especially morphia ; or after using ointment of mercury ; or sometimes, as its name applies, after an enema has been given.

One attack appears to make the patient more sensitive to other irritating substances and repeated attacks are common. Probably many cases of " repeated scarlet fever," for which patients have even been admitted to hospitals, were in reality due to erythema scarlatiniforme.

Treatment. The treatment of an attack is simple. Locally, all that is needed is a simple dusting powder. The bowels should be thoroughly well attended to, and " imperial drink," which is made up of lemonade and tartaric acid, is recommended to be taken in large quantities. Quinine, anti-rheumatic remedies, and tonics are generally given to build up the system and to ward off further attacks ; but a thorough investigation to find the cause is the really important part of the treatment.

ENTERALGIA. This is the term given to pain in the bowels. Griping pain may be felt in the regions of the bowels, especially if some irritation has been set up by food poisoning. The pain may be felt over the navel, but as a rule, the pain is of a griping nature and it may be difficult for the patient to state definitely where it is. (*See also* COLIC.)

ENTERIC. This was the name used for typhoid fever, but nowadays enteric fever is known to be caused by various germs, so the name typhoid fever is given, and for cases very similar in character but generally of a milder type, the names paratyphoid A and paratyphoid B are used. The term enteric, however, includes all three diseases. (*See also* TYPHOID FEVER.)

ENTERITIS. This word means inflammation of the intestines and the condition may be caused by various diseases or affections. Diarrhœa is one of the most common causes. Inflammations of the large intestine are given separately under colitis. (*See also* COLITIS.)

ENTEROCELE. When a hernia protrudes from the bowel it is known as an enterocele. (*See also* HERNIA.)

ENTEROPTOSIS. This word means the falling of the intestines and it exactly describes the condition. Owing to a lax condition of the muscles which support the bowels, these may drop into the lower part of the abdomen and cause much interference with the normal workings of the body. The condition is brought on by faulty habits of standing or by chronic constipation. Women who have had many children are commonly afflicted with enteroptosis owing to the laxness of the muscles, which fail to give adequate support to the abdominal organs.

Treatment. Massage of the abdominal muscles and wearing of a well-shaped abdominal belt will be found to give most relief. (*See also* ABDOMINAL BELT.)

ENTEROSTOMY. This is the name given to an operation by which an artificial opening is made into the intestine.

ENTOZOA. Any parasites which live within, and derive nourishment from the human body are known as entozoa. Worms which live in the intestines form a very important group of the many types of entozoa. (*See also* GERMS ; WORM.)

ENTROPION. This is a condition in which one or more of the eyelids are turned inwards. It is very troublesome and may set up irritation which often causes serious damage to the eye. It occasionally occurs in infants as the result of an error in development, but it is much more often seen in elderly people. In the latter, the lower lid only is attacked. The laxity of the tissues which occurs in old age allows the lid to turn in, or spasm of the lids may occur which aggravates the condition. If the eye is bandaged for any length of time in elderly people, entropion is very apt to occur ; hence many surgeons dislike covering the eye closely after an operation for cataract, but prefer a shade or dark glasses.

Treatment. The treatment of entropion varies with its degree. In minor cases, such as occur after bandaging, the bandage and dressings should be removed, and the patient told to stroke the lids gently from the lashes down, or up, as the case may be, so as to pull the lids out. Collodion (often sold as "nu-skin") is sometimes useful ; it is painted on the lid every two or three days, after the skin has been cleansed with alcohol or ether. A strip of surgical plaster to draw down the lid is also useful.

In many cases, however, and in all cases which are due to scars, such methods would be useless, and an operation is required to put matters right.

ENUCLEATION. This is the name given to a surgical operation in which a diseased part of the body such as the tonsils or the eye, is shelled out from its surrounding tissue.

ENURESIS. This is the medical term for bed-wetting. The causes and treatment are fully described under the heading BED-WETTING.

ENZYME. Enzyme is the name applied to a chemical ferment which is produced by living cells in the body. Enzymes are present in the saliva and in the gastric juice and in various other secretions of the body. Enzymes play an important part in the process of the proper digestion of our food. (*See also* DIGESTION.)

EPHEDRINE. This is a drug which is very useful in cases of asthma and other allergic diseases such as hay-fever and urticaria ;

relief is generally experienced in about twenty minutes after administration. This drug is extracted from the Chinese drug Ma Huang, which was known and used over 5,000 years ago, and is still sold in Peking drug shops in small brownish green sticks.

EPHELIS. Ephelis is a technical name for sunburn.

EPHEMERAL FEVER. This is the name applied to a short attack of fever which usually lasts for a day or two. It may occur about the third or fourth day after childbirth, and is often called milk-fever.

EPICANTHUS. This is the name given to a fold of skin which in some people covers the inner corner of the eye ; it generally looks like a half-moon of skin round the inner corner, but may be practically straight. It exists normally in some Eastern nations, but in Europeans is considered, if at all exaggerated, to be a deformity. A small degree of epicanthus is often seen in children, one of whose parents has a high-bridged nose ; it is found that as the child grows, the nose grows also, and as the bridge rises, the fold of skin is gradually drawn away from the eyes until they look quite normal.

If this does not happen, and treatment is called for, an operation involving the removal of a small quantity of the superfluous skin is carried out. There are several varieties of this operation.

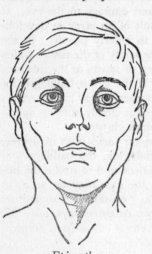

Epicanthus

EPIDERMIS. Epidermis is the name given to the outer layer of the skin. (*See also* SKIN.)

EPIDIDYMIS. The epididymis is a structure which is attached to the upper part of each testicle, and it is the beginning of the duct which conveys the secretion of the male organ of conception.

EPIDIDYMITIS. Epididymitis is the inflammation of the epididymis. It is generally the result of infection and it is a common complication of prostatic disease, but gonorrhœa is by far the most common cause. Tuberculosis is also a common cause of the disease.

Symptoms. At first there may be pain in the region of the groin and this has often been mistaken for appendicitis. There is usually some fever, and the epididymis rapidly swells and becomes intensely tender and the scrotum usually becomes red and swollen. The pain may be very severe and sickening in character.

Treatment. The most important line of treatment is rest. The scrotum should be raised and supported on a small pad placed between the thighs and either hot or cold applications should be made. The original cause of the inflammation should be treated.

EPIGASTRIUM. The large soft part of the body between the chest and the lower limbs which is called the abdomen or, in popular language, the belly, contains many of the most important organs of the body. It is important, therefore, to be able to describe roughly in what part of the abdomen a pain or swelling is situated ; so, for the purpose of making description easier, it is usual to divide the surface of the abdomen into different parts or regions. The epigastric region, or epigastrium, is the region which lies in the middle of the upper abdomen in front of the stomach. It is sometimes referred to as the pit of the stomach. (*See also* ABDOMEN.)

EPIGLOTTIS. The epiglottis is a leaf-like structure which stands at the back of the throat. It plays a very important part in

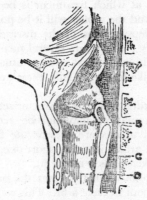

Epiglottis

A. Epiglottis; B. Vocal Cord; C. Œsophagus; D. Trachea.

the act of swallowing and it helps to prevent food from " going down the wrong way."

EPILATION. The removal of hairs is called epilation or depilation.

EPILEPSY was known to the ancients as the " falling sickness," doubtless on account of the rapidity with which a patient with epilepsy falls to the ground when he has a fit. This disorder has been well recognized for thousands of years, and it is one of the diseases which is viewed with horror and terror by lay people. For fear that their fits will be labelled " epilepsy," many sufferers refrain from seeking medical advice. This is wrong for two reasons : first, because epilepsy may be the symptom of some underlying disease of the brain, which if untreated will threaten life, or at all events be progressive ; secondly, because with suitable treatment " real " epilepsy can often be so controlled that no one except the patient is aware that he has in the past suffered from it. It is important to realize that true epilepsy, for which there is no underlying disease in the brain, begins at a very early age as a rule. About one-third of all cases begin before the age of ten, and three-quarters before the age of twenty. If a person above the age of twenty suddenly starts to have epilepsy, it is highly probable that there is some discoverable cause for it. Recently it has been found, for example, that a number of cases of epilepsy in soldiers were caused by the presence of tiny parasitic worms in the brain, which had been caught abroad.

Epilepsy often begins as infantile convulsions, and persistent infantile convulsions should lead parents to seek expert advice, for the younger the age at which treatment is begun the quicker the fits can be stopped, and the sooner will it be possible to discontinue the treatment. Epilepsy is one of the diseases to which there is a hereditary tendency ; sometimes several members of one generation are affected. Although great stress is usually laid by relatives on supposed causes like frights or falls, these are, as a rule, of little or no importance.

Epilepsy is a disorder which is characterized by attacks of unconsciousness, which may or may not be accompanied by convulsions. When convulsions are present the fit is described as a major fit ; when the attack is a very short one, unaccompanied by convulsions, it is spoken of as a minor fit.

Major Fits. In about half the cases the patient receives some warning that he is about to have a fit. This warning is a very brief one, and the patient does not have time to get to a place of safety before he falls as if shot. The warning may take the form of twitching of some part of the body, such as the thumb or forearm ; or curious sensations of " pins and needles " ; or a feeling of something queer in the stomach which seems to travel upwards towards the head ; or a giddy feeling. As the patient falls he sometimes utters a loud cry, which is so distinctive that it can never be forgotten by anyone who has heard it. By the time he has fallen he is unconscious and has become quite stiff, the head and eyes being turned to one side. The whole body appears rigid and the patient soon appears on the point of choking because he is not breathing. His face becomes blue, the veins in the neck become swollen and the pupils of his eyes are huge. Then the convulsions start and violent jerking movements of all the muscles of the body occur.

Air is drawn into the lungs, and is blown out with short puffs, the face soon resuming its natural colour. The jerking movements become slower, though not less violent, and then cease, the last jerks often being the most violent of all. The patient then lies with his limbs limp, his eyes open, though he is still unconscious, and he breathes deeply and noisily. At this stage he will often pass water without any knowledge of the act. After this state has lasted for about ten minutes, he recovers consciousness, recollecting nothing of what has taken place, and if allowed, will then probably fall into a natural sleep, from which he will waken after a few hours. This is a typical epileptic fit; but there are, of course, many slight differences in different cases.

Minor Fits take many forms, and their true nature is often unsuspected until a major fit occurs. There is, however, nearly always a brief loss of consciousness, often so slight that it is called a " faint," a " giddy turn " or a " sensation." The face turns pale in these, there is a fixed expression and anything that is being held in the hand is dropped. The patient may fall to the ground, or the whole thing may be over in a minute or so without a fall. Very occasionally water is passed in one of these minor attacks. The importance of the minor attacks is mainly because their true character goes unrecognized till a major attack occurs, but also because it is after these minor attacks that mental disturbances may take place which bring the victim within reach of the law. Whilst still in an epileptic state, that state known as " automatism," the patient may commit some crime during a maniacal outburst, of which, when he comes to himself, he has no recollection. Many times has this post-epileptic state been pleaded as a defence in a court of law, but it is a plea which a considerable amount of medical evidence is needed to support.

Epilepsy does not itself often cause death, but injury or death may be caused by the patient falling into the fire or amongst the traffic during a fit. Danger to life from the fit itself occasionally comes from choking, through vomiting before consciousness returns ; or if a fit occurs at night, by suffocation if the patient turns over with his face towards his pillow. The first danger can be guarded against by turning the patient on his side if he begins to vomit ; and the second, by making him sleep on a horse hair pillow, through which he can easily breathe. During the last stage of the convulsions, the tongue is often protruded and bitten, and measures must be taken to prevent this happening during an attack. The handle of a spoon, a piece of india-rubber, or a cork, should be forced between the teeth. Apart from this, there is nothing to do in the attack but to see that the patient does not hurt himself. The limbs must not be restrained, but all furniture with which the jerking limbs are likely to come into contact must be removed. After the attack the patient should not be roused. He should be left to sleep as long as he can, for patients who are roused immediately an attack is over tend to develop very bad headaches.

In many cases of epilepsy the attacks occur at certain times, either in the morning, or at night. When they occur only at night, they are usually easier to control than when they occur haphazard, or during the day.

Treatment. Although there are many people suffering from epilepsy who hold high public positions, as a rule there is some mental instability, if not deterioration, in those epileptics in whom the fits are not controlled. It cannot be too strongly emphasized that the drugs which are used to control the fits do not cause mental weakness or mental breakdown ; any mental change which takes place is due to the epilepsy and not to the remedies. This has been shown over and over again by the fact that patients who have taken huge doses of the appropriate remedies for years—for fear that the fits would return if they stopped taking the drugs—remain perfectly normal mentally ; whilst those patients who refuse to be treated, or who discontinue their treatment against medical advice, rapidly go downhill mentally. It is of the greatest importance to stop the fits ; if we can do this we can preserve whatever intelligence the individual possesses.

There is only one successful treatment for true epilepsy, and that is a strict observance of the drug regime laid down by the doctor for each individual case. It is important to anticipate the fits with the suitable drugs, so that if the fits occur mainly at night, the medicine is given in a single dose before going to bed ; if they occur only in the daytime, the dose should be given in the early morning. But the drug treatment applicable to an individual case needs to be carefully worked out. During the last few years the discovery of a new drug, luminal, has made the treatment of epilepsy more hopeful than it was in the past, since this drug seems to have a great value in controlling the fits. But the success of the treatment is very largely in the hands of the patient, for he must take the remedy with unfailing regularity for at least two years after the occurrence of the last fit. Then, very gradually, the dosage may be cut down. But many patients who have had epilepsy, and who have had their fits completely controlled, wisely prefer to go on taking a small dose of their particular remedy for years, rather than risk a return of the fits. It has recently been found that keto-genic diets (*i.e.* diets rich in fats and bringing about an increase of ketones in the urine) are useful in the treatment of epilepsy, about

6o per cent of cases so treated being improved and a large proportion of these cured. The best results are obtained in children. The extra fat is given chiefly as butter and cream, but also in other fat-containing foods.

Treatment of the general health is also of great importance. Patients with epilepsy should live in the open air as much as possible, and they should choose outdoor occupations in preference to sedentary ones. Farming or gardening is most suitable. Any occupation which involves situations of danger, such as work with machinery or on scaffolds, for example, must be avoided, and epileptics must not be allowed to bathe for fear of drowning.

EPIPHYSIS. It has been said elsewhere that the bones of young children are not made of the firm substance that we know as bone, but are made of gristle and cartilage, which is softer, and bendable. As the child grows older the bone begins to harden, or ossify, as it is called. The hardening process begins in spots, which enlarge until the whole bone is hard. Some bones, however, such as the bones of the leg and arm, are really made up of long shafts with two separate ends, which, when the bone is finally hardened, appear to be all in one piece. The hardening process, however, begins in the shaft and at each end of the bone and leaves bands of the softer material between the ends and shaft for some time after the rest of the bone is hardened. Each end of the bone is called an epiphysis, not an end, until the cartilage between it and the main bone has hardened. The cartilage which remains between the epiphysis and the shaft is called the epiphyseal line or epiphyseal cartilage. (*See* diagram on page 367.)

The importance of these epiphyses is that as long as the epiphyseal cartilage lasts it is a weak spot in the bone and is liable to be injured or be attacked by disease. This is why bone diseases are so very much more common in children than in grown-ups. If the epiphyseal cartilage is weakened through an injury or the debility of the child, germs which would otherwise have remained in the bloodstream may be able to settle in it, and cause suppuration or chronic inflammation, which is liable to spread to the bone itself, and may cause the very severe disease of childhood called osteomyelitis. Tuberculosis and syphilis often cause chronic inflammation of the cartilage. These bone troubles in young children are a serious matter and always require skilled treatment. With regard to the injuries to the epiphysis, the commonest one is for the head of the bone or epiphysis to be knocked off the main bone, and this requires much less force than would be thought necessary. It is what happens when a child is hurt by dragging on its arms, pulling it along the street, or lifting it up from the ground by its wrists. In spite of all that can be said to them, there are still people who will jerk a small child from the floor on to its feet by its wrists. (*See also* BONE ; CARTILAGE ; JOINTS.)

EPISCLERITIS. Inflammation of the white of the eye.

EPISPASTIC. This is the name given to a blistering agent of which the most widely used are preparations of cantharides or Spanish fly. (*See also* BLISTERING ; CANTHARIDES.)

EPISTAXIS. This is the medical term for nose bleeding. (*See also* HÆMORRHAGE.)

EPITHELIOMA AND " TRADE CANCER." This is the most usual form of cancer of the skin. It begins as a small hard lump or " plate " of growth ; or as a deeper hard nodule under the skin substance. This soon increases in size, and a yellowish-pink waxy-looking growth, with enlarged blood-vessels near by, appears on the surface. This unhealthy tissue soon breaks down and forms an ulcer, the borders of which are raised or rolled above the floor of the ulcer and remain hard and waxy. It very often commences at the junction of skin with mucous membrane (the membrane lining various channels of the body which communicate with the outside), as, for instance, at the lower part of the bowel, or on the lip ; if elsewhere, some definite chronic irritation seems always to be associated with its appearance.

It would be incorrect, however, to say that the irritation is the only cause of the cancer. For instance, *a few* workers in paraffin are afflicted with cancerous growths on the hands and forearms, but the great majority escape. *A few* sweeps are irritated by soot, and a " chimney-sweep's cancer " forms, usually on the scrotum ; but most sweeps are unaffected. The unknown factor, the " X," which determines that this paraffin worker or that sweep shall have cancer, is entirely unknown, though a tremendous amount of research work has been, and is still being, done on the subject.

To return : chronic irritation is in some cases a factor in causing cancer of the skin. Besides the paraffin and soot cancers already mentioned, cancer of the skin is found to occur among workers in X-rays, coal-tar, silver nitrate, arsenic, and many others, which go under the general name of " trade cancer." It may also occur in a number of chronic skin diseases, especially in people of later middle-age and old people ; it may occur in scars, moles, warts, burns, and chronic ulcers ; all these varieties of cancer, again, are probably the result of chronic irritation. An interesting form is that seen in Kashmir, where some of the natives carry a " fire-basket " slung from the waist. The skin of the thigh in one particular place is burnt day after day, a chronic ulcer forms, which may in time become cancerous, due to both the irritation of the burn and the constant rubbing of the soot on the affected part. If untreated, a skin cancer rapidly spreads to the tissues beneath the skin, infects the lymph glands, and finally leads to the death of the patient.

Treatment. If treated *early*, the cure can in most cases be guaranteed. It must be emphasized, however, that *early treatment is the only means by which it can be made certain that the growth will not return.* Too many ageing people disregard, for instance, a small sore on the lip, or treat it with some useless " cure-all " ointment for a few weeks, or a month or two, and are always " going to see the doctor next week." When, finally, the sore has grown to some size, they seek advice, often to be told that nothing can be done, or that only a palliative operation can be performed ; which last means, simply, that the surgeon will do what he can to make the sufferers comfortable till they die!

If seen in the early stages, treatment is often entirely successful. It consists in the thorough removal of the growth, and, very often, of the lymph glands in its neighbourhood. Nowadays it is followed by the use of X-rays and radium. An early cancerous growth of the skin, where it is judged that none of the lymph glands are yet affected, may be destroyed by X-rays or radium alone ; but even in these cases removal, followed by X-rays or radium, is considered to be the best treatment.

EPSOM SALT. Magnesium sulphate is commonly known as Epsom salt, because at one time it was obtained from the mineral waters of Epsom. Epsom salt acts on the bowels, and it is perhaps one of the most popular purgatives known.

EPULIS. This term is applied to a tumour growing from the jaws near the socket of a tooth. The usual treatment is removal of the growth by operation.

EQUILIBRIUM. By the equilibrium of the body we mean its power of balancing itself, so that it may remain upright or in any given position in which we wish it to be. This power of maintaining the balance depends upon the team-work of the muscles, which in turn depends upon the control and foremanship of the brain. A great many causes can upset the balance in a small degree, causing slight attacks of unsteadiness and giddiness, but when giddiness is present and continually and in a severe form, it must be suspected that there is trouble in the nerve centres in the brain or in the little semi-circular canals in the front part of the head which are actually responsible for keeping the body in an upright position. (*See also* EAR ; EPILEPSY ; MENIÈRE's DISEASE.)

ERECTILE TISSUE. In certain parts of the body there are

tissues which are very richly supplied with tiny blood-vessels, and when these vessels become engorged with blood, they cause the tissues to swell and become hard. This type of tissue is called erectile tissue. It occurs, for example, in the penis, which is largely composed of erectile tissue of this kind.

The interior of the nose is richly supplied with erectile tissue, and this plays an important part in the protection of our lungs. The fact that the membranes in the nose are able to swell up when they are stimulated by cold air, causes the passages of the nose to close up, and in this way any cold air is slightly heated in the narrow passages of the nose before it reaches the lungs. During a " cold in the head," however, the tiny blood-vessels in the nose may completely block up the air passages and make breathing a difficult performance.

ERGOT. Ergot is the spawn of a fungus found growing on rye, and it is a very valuable drug in medical practice. It acts on the muscle tissue of the blood-vessels, causing them to contract,

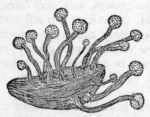

and this factor is made use of to check bleeding. But it is after childbirth that ergot is mostly used. By contracting the uterus the possibility of bleeding is much lessened, and the contracting movements are very helpful in causing the expulsion of blood clots from the womb.

Ergot (greatly enlarged)   **Poisoning by Ergot.** Poisoning by this fungus is known as ergotism. It is common in countries where bread is made from rye, or it may occur from an overdose of the drug. There are two types of poisoning : one in which the fingers and toes tingle and itch and finally become gangrenous or dead, and another which seems to affect the mentality. If an overdose of the drug has been given, the patient may show symptoms of sickness, dizziness and diarrhœa. An emetic should be given, followed by some castor oil and a stimulant such as strong tea or coffee, but, above all, the patient should be kept as warm as possible. (*See also* EMETIC.)

EROSION. The word erosion implies a gradual eating away, just as acid erodes and eats away anything it comes in contact with. In medicine, erosion may occur in the tissues and bones of the body from many causes. (*See also* BONE.)

ERRHINE. Errhines are drugs which cause running at the nose. Ammonia is an example of an errhine.

ERUCTATION. Eructation, or belching, means the sudden expulsion of gas from the stomach. Gas is formed in the stomach as the result of the fermentation of food which has not been properly digested. People who suffer from indigestion are very apt to belch after food has been eaten. (*See also* ACIDITY ; AEROPHAGY ; FLATULENCE ; INDIGESTION.)

ERUPTION. Eruptions of the skin are more commonly known as rashes. These may be caused by fevers, or they may be due to various diseases of the skin such as acne, impetigo, and so on. Eruptions on the skin sometimes follow the administration of certain drugs, or after an enema has been given. (*See also* ENEMA RASH ; ERYTHEMA.)

ERYSIPELAS. This disease is also popularly known as " the Rose," or " St. Anthony's Fire." It is an acute infectious disease due to a germ, the streptococcus, and is characterized by a spreading inflammation of a special area of skin, usually on the face, and by the general symptoms of a fever.

It is found all over the world, and at all seasons of the year, but is most common in temperate regions and in the spring. Occasionally epidemics occur. In the Middle Ages erysipelas was confused with poisoning by ergot. The germ clings to rooms, furniture, bedding, etc., and may be carried by a third person, but is readily killed by ordinary sanitary and disinfectant methods. Uncleanliness favours the development of the disease, as also do chronic alcoholism, chronic Bright's disease, wounds—whether large or mere scratches—and recent delivery, in which cases mother or child, or both, may be affected.

The disease appears from two days to a week after infection takes place, and lasts from two or three days to two or three weeks, the average being about a week or ten days. Relapses are fairly frequent.

Symptoms. In a typical case, which most frequently appears on the head and face, the commencement is abrupt. The patient feels cold and shivery ; possibly has a shivering fit or rigor, and an attack of vomiting. He often complains of intense headache. The temperature then rises sharply from the normal 98·4° F. to 104° F. or more. Very soon a sharply defined hot, tense, shining patch, which varies in colour from a bright scarlet to a dull brick-red, is seen on the skin. It may occur where there is a wound or scratch, or where the skin joins mucous membrane, as at the nostrils, or the corners of the eyes or mouth. A break in the skin is always present, though it may be so small as not to be noticed. The patch rapidly spreads, though it stops short at the chin, and never extends on to the front of the neck. The centre becomes paler. The edges are raised and hard, the patient complains of " burning " and pain, and the inflamed area is tender to the touch, and " pits " on pressure.

9*

The most tender area is the spreading zone just beyond the red margin. Nose-bleeding is common. Soon blisters appear on the inflamed area, which, in bad cases, take the form of blood-blisters.

The face is enormously swollen, so much so that the eyes cannot be opened. The glands in the neck are swollen and tender ; the mouth, throat, and nose may also be inflamed. After a few days, in ordinary cases, the inflammation ceases spreading, the redness disappears, the skin peels, and the temperature comes down to the normal. This may happen by a sudden fall (crisis) or by slow degrees (lysis). After the first feeling of illness, the patient is often very little disturbed, but even in mild cases there may be some delirium during the first few nights.

The outlook in most cases is favourable, but there are a few exceptions to this general rule. Chronic alcoholics and elderly persons, whose powers of resistance are poor, are prone gradually to go downhill and die from a slow general poisoning of the tissues, or toxæmia. In infants, the infection attacks the healing stump of the cord at the navel ; in this region it is very apt to spread inwards, and is almost always fatal. Erysipelas, associated with extensive wounds of the scalp, or after severe injuries, or of the passage leading from the womb after childbirth, or when the patient has kidney disease, is apt to take a serious course. Before antiseptic methods were used, erysipelas was one of the bugbears of surgery, and—especially after operations of any severity—not infrequently brought about the death of the patient.

In some cases the inflammation heals on the face, and spreads to the body and limbs ; it is called " wandering erysipelas." Sometimes the red colour is not present ; this condition is known as " white erysipelas." At first it may suggest a severe nettle-rash, but may be readily distinguished from this by the general symptoms. In the same way the ordinary form of erysipelas may closely resemble a dermatitis caused by exposure to some irritating substance, such as a poisonous plant, but the general symptoms of erysipelas serve to distinguish the two conditions. After many repeated attacks, a persistent swelling of the affected part may remain ; this is most often seen on the face or the leg.

Treatment. The treatment of erysipelas is simple, and very little beyond good nursing is required. The patient should be isolated ; the rest of the family and, still more, visitors must be kept out of the sick-room.

Locally, applications are used to prevent the spread of the disease, to guard against infection by other organisms, and to allay the symptoms. Numerous methods have been advocated to prevent the spread, which it would take too long to describe here.

One of the simplest and best is to paint a " barrier," one inch wide, all round the affected area, and one inch away from its margin, with the strong tincture of iodine, or liniment of iodine. The ordinary tincture of iodine is not sufficiently powerful. Care must be taken that the barrier is *complete* ; not the smallest area of skin must be left unprotected. To ensure this it is usual to paint the ring over two or three times, allowing each to dry before the next " coat " is applied. A second ring may be applied one inch beyond the first, to make doubly sure. This procedure is repeated for two or three days, even if the disease does not pass the barrier.

Ichthyol is also considered to be a very good application, either as ointment or lotion. This is spread over the whole of the affected area, and the blisters being pricked by a sterilized needle. Collodion and dusting powder, weak carbolic, or lead and opium fomentations are also advocated. In cases where the scalp is involved, the hair should be cut as close as possible. Ichthyol ointment is considered to be the best application when peeling is going on and itching is often troublesome.

As regards the general treatment, the patient should, at the first appearance of the disease, have a dose of calomel, followed in six hours (or the next morning) by a full dose of salts ; this thorough clearing of the bowels in the first instance often cuts short the disease. Laxatives (not strong purgatives) should be used as required, and plenty of water drunk during the whole course of the disease, so that both bowels and kidneys are flushed out, and not only do their own work efficiently, but to some extent put the skin at rest. The diet at first should be as for other fevers, that is, concentrated liquid nourishment ; when the fever has abated, the patient should have at first nutritious, though easily digested, food before he is allowed ordinary food ; and tonics should be given in convalescence.

If the fever is high, cold sponging or a cold pack are considered to be better than fever-reducing drugs (antipyretics). If the patient is sleepless or delirious, he may have narcotics ; morphia and hyoscine are very useful in cases where the delirium is severe.

There is no special remedy for erysipelas. Vaccines prepared from the patient's own germs are often useful, but the anti-erysipelas serum has proved disappointing.

The patient is considered to be infectious until peeling is quite completed. After recovery, he should take a hot bath followed by sponging with an antiseptic ; he should then have clean clothing and be moved into another bedroom. His clothing, bedding, etc., should be sterilized, and his former bedroom disinfected in the usual manner. (*See also* DISINFECTANT.)

ERYTHEMA or REDNESS OF THE SKIN. Erythema, which means redness, is a descriptive term applied to a group of skin conditions in which redness is the chief sign. It is the first sign of dermatitis, or inflammation of the skin, and shows that some irritation is present and acting on the skin, whether from within or without. The term erythema was formerly applied to very widely separated conditions, from bites of insects to the red and swollen skin over an abscess. Nowadays it is becoming much more restricted in its use.

The person is often feverish before the rash comes out, and frequently has a sore throat, or running nose, and red and running eyes, or pains in the joints. In these cases, where there is much disturbance of the general health, it is sometimes very difficult at first to distinguish erythema from scarlet fever, for instance, and until the diagnosis is certain, it is always wiser to treat the case as if it were infectious. No harm will be done if it is not.

Erythema is most common in young people, and is particularly apt to be found in those who have a rheumatic history. It is said to occur most commonly in spring and autumn, and occasionally groups of cases occur, which suggests that some forms may be infectious. The two main characters of erythema are redness and a fluid swelling of the skin, but it has many varieties. It may attack both legs, or both arms, and appear on exactly the same areas in each case. Some forms, indeed, occur so regularly that they have become recognized subdivisions of the main type.

ERYTHROMELALGIA. This is a condition in which the hands and feet become red and swollen, and very painful. The cause of the condition is not known, but it is thought that the nervous system may be at fault. The pain may be relieved by raising the limbs or by the application of cold.

ESCHAROTIC. An escharotic is a substance which is capable of destroying tissue. The commonest escharotics are sulphuric and nitric acids, caustic potash, and red-hot metals. (*See also* CAUSTIC.)

ESERINE. Eserine is also known as physostigmine, and it is greatly used in the treatment of eye conditions.

ESMARCH BANDAGE. This is an elastic rubber bandage which is used to control bleeding in amputations of the limbs. (*See also* BANDAGES.)

ESSENTIAL OIL. Essential oils or volatile oils form a very large and valuable group of drugs used in medicine. These oils may be divided into several classes ; for example, the oil of turpentine group, including camphors, are used chiefly for their action on the skin ; the group which are used to stimulate the kidneys include copaiba, oil of juniper, cubebs, oil of sandal-wood, etc. Oils which are used to aid digestion include oil of peppermint, anise, ginger, capsicum, nutmeg and cinnamon. Another group of essential oils are used in the treatment of hysteria on account of their peculiar odour. Valerian and asafetida are included in this group.

ETHER. Ether is a colourless, highly inflammable liquid which is used as a general anæsthetic. (*See also* ANÆSTHESIA.)

ETHYL ALCOHOL. Ethyl alcohol is what is known as absolute alcohol. (*See also* ALCOHOL.)

ETHYL CHLORIDE. When absolute alcohol is treated with hydrochloric acid, a very inflammable liquid known as ethyl chloride is produced. Ethyl chloride produces an intense feeling of coldness when it is applied externally to the skin, and because of this it is sometimes used for small operations such as the removal of warts, etc.

Ethyl chloride is also used to produce general anæsthesia for brief operations, and as it is very rapid in its effect it is especially useful for children. (*See also* ANÆSTHESIA.)

EUCALYPTOL. Eucalyptol is obtained from the oil of eucalyptus, and it is used as an inhalant in cases of bronchitis. It is less crude than oil of eucalyptus and is, therefore, less irritating to the mucous membranes.

EUCALYPTUS. Oil of eucalyptus is distilled from the fresh leaves of several species of gum tree grown in Australia. The oil is almost colourless, but some varieties are pale straw-coloured. It has a pungent smell which is very clean and refreshing. The oil is extensively used in the treatment of colds and influenza and it is one of the most popular remedies for bronchial catarrh. It is generally used by placing a few drops on a handkerchief, but this is only helpful in cases of a slight cold in the head. When there is much nasal catarrh, the oil should be inhaled or sprayed into the nostrils. The oil, when mixed with an equal quantity of olive oil, may be rubbed into the skin as a remedy for rheumatism. Eucalyptus oil has been given during cholera epidemics, and it has also been used in the treatment of measles, typhoid fever, and worms. Owing to its powerful smell it is often used to hide other offensive odours and it is sometimes given by mouth to correct bad breath.

EUGENOL. Eugenol is a colourless oily liquid used a great deal by dentists. It is the chief constituent found in oil of cloves.

EUONYMUS. Euonymus is the root bark of the wahoo or spindle-tree. It is used as a purgative and is also given where it is required to increase the flow of bile.

EUSOL. Eusol is a solution of chlorinated lime and boracic acid and it should contain no less than 0·5 per cent. of hypochlorous acid. Its name stands for **E**dinburgh **U**niversity **SOL**ution, having been evolved in the laboratories at Edinburgh during the war.

Eusol is used as a general antiseptic lotion for cuts and wounds and was of great value during the Great War, when it was invented for that purpose. It could be easily applied as a first dressing on the field to prevent sepsis, and could also be applied dry as a powder when water was not available. Similar solutions are Dakin's solution, chloramine-T, and so on.

EUSTACHIAN TUBES.   From the back of the nose there are two small passages leading on each side to the middle ear. These are called the eustachian tubes. Their chief use is to regulate the amount of air which passes to the middle ear, which is a very important matter in connection with the hearing, since the amount of

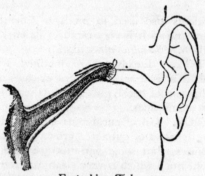

Eustachian Tube

air in the middle ear affects the position of the drum, which should be held just taut, and neither pushed outwards by too much air or allowed to sag by too little air being present. If catarrh is present in the eustachian tubes, as in the case of a common cold, it may cause the lining of the tubes to swell so much that not enough air gets past and there is a slight degree of deafness as a result. A catheter can be passed into the tubes by an ear specialist in order to make a passage for air. This is called inflation by the eustachian catheter. If the catarrhal condition is allowed to become permanent and to spread to the inner ear itself, permanent and incurable deafness will result. This catarrhal deafness is the most common form of deafness which is not hereditary.

In order to prevent catarrh spreading from other conditions such as adenoids or septic tonsils it is necessary to blow the nose properly. This should be done, not in the old-fashioned way of blowing vigorously down both nostrils at once, but by holding one nostril closed with a finger pressed on it while the other is blown gently; then closing that nostril in the same way while the other is cleared. (*See also* EAR.)

EUTHANASIA. This is the name given to the methods used to secure an easy and gentle death for persons suffering from some incurable disease. For example, it is usual for a doctor to try and give relief to a patient who is dying from cancer or some such painful disease by administering drugs, which have the power of producing sleep and mental ease.

EVIPAN. A drug which is a general anæsthetic, given by injection into a vein.

EXCISION. The operation of cutting out or excising any organ or part of the tissues of the body is often called an excision. An abscess is excised, or a breast which has to be removed is said to be excised. Any sort of a growth is excised and a joint may be excised; but no one talks of excising the appendix—it is " removed," nor the tonsils—which are " enucleated."

EXCITING CAUSE. This is a medical term used for the immediate cause of a disease.

EXCORIATION. This term is used to describe the loss of skin by rubbing or chafing.

EXCRETA or EXCRETIONS. The excreta or excretions of the body are the waste products of the body which are naturally discharged by it into the outside world. They are the fæces, the urine and the sweat. They must be got rid of by the body if it is to remain in health, and the process by which they are got rid of is called *excretion*. They are said to be excreted by the excretory organs.

EXOPHTHALMIC GOITRE or GRAVES' DISEASE. This is a disease of the thyroid gland in which the most noticeable feature is that the eyes become prominent and bulging. It was first described by an Irish physician called Graves about a hundred years ago. It is generally found amongst young women between the ages of fifteen and thirty years. When men get it they are usually older, between the ages of thirty and forty-five years being the most frequent age. A sudden fright, grief or shock, or the effects of a depressing disease or prolonged overstrain is a common starting-point for the disease, or, to be more correct, these disturbances may call it into activity. For a considerable time the patient may have had a feeling of weariness or exhaustion with no apparent cause, and have been nervous, irritable and restless.

Symptoms. As its name implies, there is a goitre or enlargement of the thyroid gland, which lies on the front of the neck rather below the middle. The eyes become prominent in nearly all cases, but sometimes only in a very small degree. They may, however, protrude so much that the eyelids cannot be closed over them and the patient has a staring look. The white of the eye is visible all round the iris or coloured part. Sometimes only one eye is affected and in this case it is usually the right one.

The action of the heart is disturbed and the pulse becomes rapid with palpitation. The patient is anæmic and becomes nervous and irritable with tremblings of the muscles and sleeplessness. Usually there is a history of other forms of nervous diseases amongst other members of the family, such as hysteria, epilepsy or St. Vitus's dance. There may be other symptoms in individual cases such as disturbances of the digestion, variable and capricious appetite, attacks of vomiting ; diarrhœa is fairly frequent, and loss of weight practically always occurs. Albumen and sugar may be present in the urine and more urine is passed than is customary, and more frequently than usual. The face is inclined to flush easily and there is much sweating and sometimes feverish attacks. In most cases the skin becomes browner than usual. It may be " tanned " all over or there may be brown patches on the cheeks. The hair becomes thin and poor and the nails brittle. The teeth tend to decay early in the course of the disease. There is always a good deal of nervousness which may go on to serious melancholia and depression.

Treatment. The treatment of exophthalmic goitre is primarily mental and physical rest. In severe cases the patient must be confined to bed, but a warm " stuffy " atmosphere is very injurious. The room should be light, sunny, and very well ventilated. A patient who is up should rest out of doors as much as possible. The diet should be chosen from among easily digested foods and should be liberal and nutritious. Red meat and alcohol in all forms should be avoided ; also coffee and strong tea, which act as stimulants, and in these cases increase the tendency to insomnia and nervous symptoms. Freshly-made weak tea is allowed, but pickles, spiced foods, chocolate, oatmeal and tobacco are generally forbidden.

Any sources of poisoning such as decayed teeth, diseased tonsils or nasal sinuses must be attended to. Iodine in milk is useful in some cases but others do not take it very well, and it should only be taken under a doctor's supervision. In urgent cases, where the heart or eye symptoms are very bad and the patient must continue at work for a living, the question of operation may have to be considered.

The thyroid gland itself is treated in various ways. There are two chief methods of operation : one consists in tying the arteries which supply the gland, and by thus starving it, diminishing the secretion. The other consists in removing part of the gland. Exophthalmic goitre has its ups and downs, and the operation is generally performed when the disease is fairly quiescent. Crile, the American surgeon, performs an operation which he calls "stealing the goitre." The patient is prepared for operation for a few days, until the routine is familiar and no longer causes apprehension. Then one morning she is given a sedative, followed by an anæsthetic, and recovers to find the operation over. This method is said to prevent the nervous symptoms which sometimes increase at this time. X-ray and electrical treatment are also frequently used.

EXOPHTHALMOS. Protruding eye balls. (*See also* Ex-ophthalmic Goitre.)

EXPECTORANT. Any drug which aids the removal of catarrhal matter and phlegm from the bronchial tubes is called an expectorant. These drugs are not all alike in their way of acting upon the body ; in fact, some have a very complicated mode of action. The only direct expectorants are those which can be inhaled as a vapour, thus causing the drug to come into close contact with the inflamed bronchial tubes. In this group are included the balsams such as Friar's balsam and balsam of tolu, eucalyptus, menthol, turpentine and benzoic acid.

An indirect expectorant is taken internally and its action is carried out by the blood circulation. Some drugs, such as senega and squills, are termed stimulating expectorants because they increase the flow of blood which in turn increases the amount of expectoration in the bronchial tubes and so aids its removal. Ipe-cacuanha is a valuable expectorant, especially in a dry cough, as it causes an outpouring of soothing sputum in the throat and gives great relief. (*See also* Bronchitis ; Cough.)

EXTRAVASATION. This term means the escape and flowing over into the surrounding tissues of any of the fluids of the body that are contained in an artery, or any vessel such as the bladder, etc. Extravasation is usually the result of a rupture, which may be brought about by injury or disease, or the break in the walls of a vessel or organ may be caused by internal pressure.

A good example of this is an ordinary bruise which shows the discoloration of the surrounding tissues owing to the blood escaping from the ruptured blood-vessels. Extravasation of urine takes place when the bladder or the urethra is ruptured, and bile may be extravasated from the intestinal tract owing to perforation. (*See also* Bladder ; Bruises ; Hæmorrhage.)

EXTREMITY. The word extremity is generally used in connection with the arms and legs. The arms are termed the upper extremities and the legs the lower extremities, but the word may be applied to the hands or feet.

EXUDATE. Exudate is the name given to pus or matter which exudes or comes from an inflamed area or from a septic wound. Exudates are found in large quantities in cases of pleurisy, which is an inflammation of the pleural cavity, or in the pericardium in pericarditis. (*See also* EMPHYSEMA ; PERICARDITIS ; PLEURISY ; SEPSIS.)

EYE, THE. Description. The apparatus by which we are enabled to see consists of the *eye* itself, the *optic nerve*, which is the special nerve supplying the eye, and the *occipital lobes* of the brain, which lie in the lower part of the back of the skull. The eye forms pictures of objects looked at, the nerve passes them on to the brain, and these receive the picture-messages and interpret them.

The *eyeballs* (*see* Photographic Supplement) each lie in a bony cavity in the front of the skull called the *orbit*. The eyeball is, roughly speaking, a round ball with a slight bulge in the front, which is the *cornea*. This is the membrane through which we see ; the window of the eye. It covers the *pupil* and *iris*. The pupil is the round black part of the eye, and is simply a hole in the centre of the iris, which is the coloured part of the eye. The *sclerotic*, or white of the eye, surrounds the pupil and iris. The cornea is, in health, a perfectly transparent membrane, through which the light passes. The sclerotic and the cornea together form the first coat of the eye. The sclerotic is composed of thick white fibrous tissue. Each eyeball is divided into two parts. First, a large division at the back, called the posterior chamber, which is filled with a perfectly clear jelly (*vitreous humour*), and secondly, a smaller division at the front, called the anterior chamber, which is filled with a clear watery fluid (*aqueous humour*). The division between the two chambers consists of the *lens* and the structures which hold it in place.

The *iris* or coloured part of the eye lies behind the cornea. It consists of a circular curtain of delicate muscle fibres, with the *pupil* in the middle. The muscle fibres are arranged in two layers : a circular layer, arranged in rings, which when it contracts makes the pupil smaller ; and a radially arranged layer (i.e. the fibres stretching from the pupil to the outer edge of the iris) which on contracting makes the pupil larger. The use of these muscles is to permit the required amount of light to reach the eye—more in a dim light, less in a bright light—so that the delicate retina shall not be damaged. The colour of the eye depends on the amount of colouring matter in the iris.

Eyelids. The eye is protected in front by the eyelids, which consist of a fold of skin strengthened by a very thin piece of cartilage, and lined by a thin transparent membrane, called the *conjunctiva*. When this reaches the inner margins of the lids it is folded on itself to cover the white of the eye as far as the cornea. It contains many glands which produce mucus ; this acts as an oiling fluid, and thus enables the eyeball to move easily and without rubbing in its socket.

Tear Gland. The eyeball is also oiled by the *lachrymal* or *tear gland*, which lies in the outer and upper part of the orbit. The tears bathe the front of the eye, and then flow away through two little tubes, called *canaliculi*. The entrances to these are situated just opposite to each other on the corner of the eyelids near the nose. They enter the side of a little bag, called the *lachrymal* or *tear sac*, which drains into the nose. If the tears are produced too rapidly, they flood the tubes and overflow on to the cheeks.

Diseases of the Eye are described separately under the headings BLACK EYE ; BLINDNESS ; CATARACT ; CONJUNCTIVITIS ; ECTROPION ; ENTROPION ; GLAUCOMA, etc.

EYEBROWS, THE. The eyebrows consist of ridges of slightly thickened skin, covered with strong hairs ; these are so arranged that the sweat from the forehead shall not trickle into the eyes and obscure or irritate them. Another useful purpose they have is shown by the way they are immediately drawn down as a protection when the eyes are exposed to strong light.

The eyebrows are one of man's prerogatives. Some birds have specially arranged feathers above the eyes, and the seal has a few stiff hairs ; but no animal, not even the higher apes, can lay claim to true eyebrows.

EYELIDS, THE. The eyelids are made up of four sorts of tissues : the skin ; the tarsus or " cartilage," which gives strength to the eyelids ; muscles, which control their movements ; and the conjunctiva, the thin moist membrane lining the eyelids. They act as a protective covering for the eyes.

The skin of the eyelids is finer than the ordinary skin of the body ; it has no hairs (except the eyelashes), and no sweat-glands. It is not firmly attached to the tissues underneath, as is the body skin, but moves easily over the tarsus. One result of this is that the blood-vessels below can be easily damaged, and that the blood flows out rapidly—hence the speed with which a " black eye " appears after a blow ; or fluid swelling of the lid arises in various acute conditions of the face, or in general diseases such as Bright's disease.

At the edges of the lids are the eyelashes, which are most important in that they keep the eyes free from foreign bodies, both solid and liquid, and also from the germs of disease. Behind the lashes are glands which produce an oily or waxy fluid ; this does not mix with the tears, but helps to prevent them from running over the margins of the lids and down the cheeks.

The eyelids are moved by two muscles, one of which passes round both lids, on the outside of the tarsus, and opens and closes the lids as required. The nerve to this muscle is the facial nerve, and when this is paralysed the lower lid hangs down, and tears run over the cheek. (*See also* ECTROPION.) The other muscle, or " lifter of the upper eyelid," is the muscle which carries out the involuntary blinking of the eye. This allows the moist inner surface of the upper eyelid to sweep the eye and keep it from becoming dried by exposure to the air, or injured by other organisms. It is supplied by the " eye-mover " nerve, so that *blinking* and *closing* the eye are carried out by two different mechanisms.

When the eyelids are closed in sleep the upper and lower lids exactly meet, so that the eye is protected and kept moist. At the same time the eyeball turns upwards, still further to protect the eye from possible injury.

The conjunctiva and the tear apparatus are described, together with their diseases, under their own headings.

EYESIGHT REQUIREMENTS NECESSARY FOR PUBLIC SERVICES. It is well known that candidates for the various public services must undergo a medical examination. What is not so well known is that in most cases eyesight tests are included, and disappointment has been caused to many candidates who are not aware of this, and whose eyesight falls short of the set requirements. It is therefore hoped that the subjoined list may be of use. (The precise *degree* of faulty vision allowed in certain cases is not given ; that is a matter for the oculist.)

Royal Navy. A naval cadet must possess perfect vision, both for distant and near objects, without glasses. Colour vision must be perfect. Squint, chronic inflammation of the eyelids, or other such faults of the eyes, *whether past or present*, disqualify.

Army. Candidates for Commissions are classified under three standards : (1) requires perfect vision in both eyes ; (2) requires perfect vision in one eye, and the second must be capable of considerable correction by glasses ; (3) requires that one eye shall be capable of perfect correction, and the other of considerable correction, by glasses.

Glasses are allowed, but only a small degree of *short-sight* is permitted. The colour sense is tested, but colour-blindness does not necessarily involve rejection.

Air Force. It is preferred that vision be perfect ; but in rare cases the very smallest degree only of faulty vision may be accepted. Colour vision must be perfect, and the field of vision not decreased.

British Mercantile Marine. The regulations here have not been laid down exactly, but a very high standard is required.

One eye must possess perfect vision ; a slight degree of imperfection may be allowed in the other. Glasses are not permitted. Colour vision must be perfect.

Police. Distant vision must be perfect, and glasses are not permitted. Near vision (as for reading) is not tested ; nor is there a colour vision test. Squint, inflammation of the eyelids, or any other eye troubles disqualify.

Railway Service. There is an eyesight test for all candidates, but whereas some degree of imperfection is permitted to clerks, etc., and glasses allowed, other grades, e.g. engine-drivers, must possess perfect vision and colour vision must be perfect. These grades are periodically re-tested, so that the high standard may be maintained.

'Bus Drivers. At present, drivers of public vehicles are only required to conform to the low standard laid down by the driving licence, i.e. to be able to read a moving number-plate at 15 yards distance. There is no test, so that a one-eyed or colour-blind driver is not debarred.

Civil Service, including Post Office. There are no definite regulations, each case being tested " on its merits." Imperfect vision incapable of correction by glasses would, of course, disqualify.

Indian Civil Service. Glasses may be worn, if necessary, but the corrected vision must be perfect in one eye, and only the slightest degree imperfect in the other. Only a slight degree of short-sight is permissible. There must be no disease of the eyes, and a squint that is at all serious disqualifies.

Teaching under Education Committees. Glasses may be worn, but the correction obtained must be high. A moderate amount of short-sight, *capable of correction*, is allowed, but astigmatism (q.v.) of more than a slight degree disqualifies.

Public Libraries. No sight test required.

Medical Officers. No sight test required, except for the Indian Medical Service, when the requirements are as for Army officers.

As a final note, it may be interesting to add that candidates for the *Church*, the *Law*, *Parliament*, or the *Universities* not only have no sight test, but that the totally blind (if their circumstances permit) may be admitted without question.

EYE TOOTH. The eye tooth, or canine as it is often called, is the third from the middle line of the upper teeth. It has a particularly long root which is directed towards the eye, and it often happens that an abscess at the point of this root cause will the eye to appear swollen and bruised or discoloured not unlike a " black eye." (*See also* Teeth.)

FACIAL NERVE. The facial nerve is the 7th cranial nerve

and it controls the muscles of the face, scalp and the ear ; curiously enough, one small strand of the facial nerve is the nerve of taste for the front half of the tongue. The facial nerve goes through a canal in the *temporal bone* close to the cavity of the middle ear and then spreads through the parotid salivary gland into a network that is distributed to the muscles of the face. It may be damaged in inflammatory conditions of the ear or in operations (especially the radical mastoid operation on the ear). A severe chill affecting the side of the face may also cause paralysis of the facial nerve (Bell's palsy), which, however, is only temporary. (*See also* FACIAL PARALYSIS.)

FACIAL PARALYSIS. Facial paralysis or Bell's palsy occurs most frequently in adults, though cases in children are not unknown, especially after diphtheria. In adults the commonest cause is neuritis or some inflammatory state of the facial nerve where it enters the skull just behind the ear. Other cases are due to disease in the middle ear, or the radical mastoid operation. It may also be due to direct injury of the nerve or to brain diseases such as meningitis, concussion or fractures of the skull. Facial paralysis due to inflammation or neuritis usually comes on fairly quickly and can be readily recognized after a few days.

Symptoms. Perhaps the person has been sitting in a draught and begins to feel pain behind the ear. Next day, or the day after, he may find that one side of his face is stiff and won't move properly. There may also be a rash on the face. The condition is nearly always one sided. On eating, the food may gather in between the tongue and the cheek because the muscles are not able to clear it away as one normally does without thinking of it in eating. The inside of the cheek may also be bitten because it falls flabbily within range of the teeth. The condition is tested by making the person laugh, wrinkle the forehead, whistle and close the eyes. The laugh will move the muscles of one side of the face only, the patient cannot whistle, the wrinkling of the forehead will be one-sided only ; the eye on the affected side will not close properly, and the eyeball rolls upwards when an attempt is made to close the eye. The senses of taste and hearing may be affected.

Treatment. Temporary facial paralysis usually clears up in about a month to six months' time. If it goes on longer it may become incurable, in which case a nerve-grafting or a plastic operation may cure the deformity. In the early days of the condition the patient should be kept in a warm room, not necessarily in bed, and if there is pain, heat should be applied over the region behind and in front of the ear which is painful. Blistering, at one time, used to be applied behind the ear, but is not used nowadays.

Massage and electricity in the form of mild galvanism are useful after the inflammation has subsided.

FACIAL SPASM. Spasms and twitchings of the muscles of the face are of two sorts. The first sort are real muscular spasms due to some irritation or injury of the facial nerve, while the second sort are nervous in origin and are called *tics*, under which heading they are described. (*See also* FIDGETS ; ST. VITUS'S DANCE.)

FÆCES. Fæces is the term applied to the discharges from the bowel, which consist of the part of the food which is undigested and other substances such as colouring matter (pigment) from the bile, and large quantities of bacteria. (*See also* STOOLS.)

FAINTING. Fainting is a temporary loss of consciousness which is also called swooning or syncope. It is due to the supply of blood to the brain becoming insufficient, thus causing a feeble action of the heart.

Treatment. The patient should be carried out into the open air if possible and laid flat on the back. Any tight clothing round the neck should be removed and also any tight articles of clothing such as a belt round the waist, or corsets. The face should be bathed in cold water and smelling-salts may be applied to the nose. The blood supply to the brain may be increased by raising the patient's legs. A few teaspoonsful of brandy or other spirits may be given if the patient is able to swallow. It is not advisable to force liquid down the throat of a person in a faint unless they are able to swallow naturally, as choking may take place. If it is not possible to carry the patient out into the open air, every care must be taken to ensure fresh air coming into the room by opening all the windows and doors. If spirits are not to hand, a teaspoonful of eau-de-Cologne or sal-volatile will serve the same purpose. Should the faint last long, or should the person be subject to frequent fainting turns, it is advisable to consult a doctor to see whether the cause of them cannot be cured.

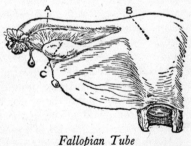

Fallopian Tube

A. Fallopian Tube; B. Uterus or Womb;
C. Ovary.

FALLING SICKNESS. Falling sickness is an old name for epilepsy, because people with this disease were noticed to fall to the ground frequently after giving a loud cry. (*See also* EPILEPSY.)

FALLOPIAN TUBES. These are two hollow tubes situated one on each side of the upper part of the womb, the purpose of which is to bring the tiny ovum (which is microscopic in size) from the ovary down into the womb. Inflammation of the Fallopian tubes is called Salpingitis, and is apt to be a serious condition which usually requires operation. (*See also* SALPINGITIS.)

FALSE PAINS. A few days before childbirth takes place, there may be colicky pains in the abdomen which are not true labour pains. These pains are due to contraction of the intestines and are very liable to occur if constipation is present. True labour pains are accompanied by other signs and are more regular in their occurrence. (*See also* LABOUR.)

FARADISM. The electricity produced from an induction coil is called faradism, or faradization when the current is applied to the body. This method of treatment is used to produce the contraction of muscles and stimulation of the nerves, and it is very beneficial in cases of paralysis.

FARCY. Farcy is another name for glanders, and the term is derived from the expression " farcy buds " or nodules which appear in the tissues underneath the skin. (*See also* GLANDERS.)

FASCIA. Fascia is the name applied to sheets or bands of tissue which surround and connect up the muscles of the body.

FAT. Fat is necessary to the body in order to produce heat and energy. Too much fat may be stored up in the tissues of the body instead of being utilized by the body as fuel, and this condition is known as Obesity. Obesity can be dangerous to life as well as a source of discomfort to the individual. Methods of treating this over-fatness will be found under the heading of Obesity. (*See also* DIGESTION.)

FAUCES. Fauces is the name given to the narrow opening between the mouth and the throat. On either side are the pillars of the fauces in which the *tonsils* are imbedded. Above the opening is what is known as the *soft palate*, and below lies the root of the tongue. During an attack of tonsillitis, the narrow opening, or fauces, is very often blocked up by the inflammation of the surrounding tissues and tonsils. (*See also* TONSIL ; TONSILLITIS.)

FAVUS. Favus, like ringworm, is a disease of the skin and hair caused by the growth of a fungus ; and again like ringworm, it is most common upon the scalp, though it may be found on the non-hairy skin, and affecting the nails. Its special feature is the production on the surface of rounded, sulphur-yellow, cup-shaped crusts, called *scutula*, which crumble readily. In some cases these are absent, and the disease then closely resembles ringworm, but can be distinguished from it by microscopical examination of the hairs.

Treatment. If favus attacks the non-hairy skin only, it is readily cured by the *constant* application of an antiseptic ointment, the time taken for a cure varying from one to eight weeks.

If only a small area of the scalp is affected, it can also readily be cured by pulling out the hairs with forceps, and thoroughly rubbing in an antiseptic ointment. In widespread cases there are only two methods which are of the slightest practical use, namely, X-rays and thallium. (*See* RINGWORM for details.) Conservative methods such as cutting the hair short and rubbing in an antiseptic ointment are so useless that even the risk of permanent baldness from X-ray or thallium is justified in the hope of a cure. It has been said that " children affected with favus get no education, and when they grow up no employment ; the boys drift into the criminal classes and the girls to the streets." Thanks, however, to the energetic co-operation of educational and medical authorities, the disease is gradually being stamped out in this country.

FEBRIFUGE. A febrifuge is a drug which is given to reduce fever. (*See* ANTIPYRETIC.)

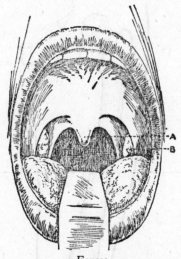

Fauces
A. Uvula; B. Tonsil

FEMORAL VESSELS. The main blood-vessels of the thigh are the femoral artery and the femoral vein.

The *femoral artery*, which is a continuation of the abdominal aorta, leaves the abdomen in the middle of the groin and travels down the upper leg to the back of the knee where it becomes the popliteal artery. After the femoral artery leaves the pelvis it can be felt as it passes into the groin and pressure can be applied at this point to stop bleeding. In the groin the artery is not situated very deeply, and so is liable to receive serious damage if anything pierces the groin.

The *femoral vein*. The corresponding vein to the femoral artery in the leg is called the femoral vein. The two blood-vessels run closely together for the whole of their course down the leg to the back of the knee. The femoral vein, or one of its tributary veins, are often the site of a *thrombosis* or clot of blood which may follow on from the condition called *phlebitis* in which there is an inflammation of the walls of the vein and the surrounding tissues. *Varicose veins*, which are veins in which the walls are abnormally dilated or stretched, are commonest in the leg too, and many of these veins go to join the femoral vein. The condition called *white leg* which sometimes arises after childbirth is also associated with the femoral vein. These conditions will be described under their own headings.

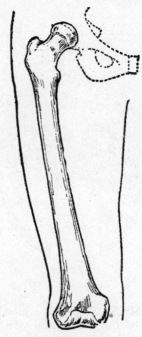

Femur

FEMUR. The femur or large bone of the leg is the longest and strongest bone in the body. It stretches from the hip-bone to the knee joint. The femur, like other long bones of the body has a body and two ends. The upper end of the femur has a large rounded head, which fits into the cup of the hip-bone, a narrower neck and two jutting-out pieces called *trochanters*.

The lower end of the femur forms part of the knee joint. It consists of two longish jutting-out pieces called *condyles*.

Fractures of the Femur. The femur, as has been said, is a long and strong bone. It therefore requires a considerable amount of violence to break it in any but the aged people. In old people, however, it is liable to snap near the upper end, owing to the brittleness of the bones in old age, and a fractured femur is always a very serious matter in an old person, and is frequently fatal owing to the complications such as pneumonia that may arise from the necessity of keeping the body flat in bed. This has a very bad effect on an already enfeebled circulation.

Treatment. In younger persons the same danger of pneumonia exists but more effective measures can be taken to prevent it. For instance, it is not necessary to keep them in bed for the same length of time, and some surgeons get them up and about on crutches with the leg in the special splint, called Thomas's splint, in a very short time. Great care must be taken with the setting of a fractured femur as it is very liable to shorten the leg and thus throw the whole body out of alignment. Unfortunately, the surgeon has often no choice between risking his patient's life by keeping him lying in an immovable position and letting him get up at the risk of shortening his leg.

FERMENTATION. Fermentation is produced by the presence of minute germs and yeast plants. Probably the best-known example of fermentation is the production of alcohol. A slight degree of fermentation is always present in the stomach, but this is only dangerous when it takes place in excess. The formation of gas in the stomach is a sign that too much fermentation is taking place owing to the presence of undigested foods, which should be removed by taking a suitable purge and regulating the diet. (*See also* ALCOHOL ; DIGESTION ; INDIGESTION.)

FERMENTS. Ferments are substances which when in contact with another substance are capable of bringing about chemical changes, and these changes play an important part in the digestion of our food. (*See also* DIGESTION.)

FERN ROOT. A preparation made from the root of the common male fern is used as a cure for tapeworms. (*See also* TAPEWORM.)

FERRIC SALTS. Ferric salts are preparations of iron which are chiefly used in medicine in cases of anæmia. Parrish's food,

Easton's syrup and Blaud's pills are iron preparations which are very popular ; they are very good for strengthening the blood and increasing the general tone of the body.

FESTER. Fester is a popular term used in connection with the formation of pus or matter. (*See also* ABSCESS : ULCER ; WHITLOW.)

FEVER. Fever is a condition in which the body-temperature is raised above normal. Fevers in general are discussed under the heading Infectious Diseases. In tropical countries to be "down with fever " usually means to have malarial fever. In this country, however, the disease which is spoken of as " fever " is scarlet fever.

FIBROIDS. Fibroid tumours of the womb or fibroids as they are often called, are much the commonest tumours in women. They are on the whole more common in young unmarried women and women who have not borne children than in mothers of families, and, indeed, they are one of the commonest causes of barrenness in a married woman. Often these tumours are small and cause no symptoms, so that their presence is not suspected, but on the other hand they may grow to enormous sizes. They have been found weighing anything up to 100 pounds.

Symptoms. As has been mentioned above, fibroids often cause no symptoms, or at least no symptoms that are sufficiently uncomfortable to attract notice. When there are symptoms the commonest ones are excessive loss at the menstrual periods, and swelling and increase in size of the abdomen. There may also be pain and discharge from the front passage. Sometimes the tumour is only discovered because the patient is being examined to discover the cause of obstruction to the working of the bowels or bladder, or to both, and in the course of the examination the large tumour in the womb is found.

Treatment. Small fibroids which are not causing discomfort or excessive bleeding require no treatment. If treatment is required the tumour can be removed by peeling it out of the womb, an operation which is simple and safe, and does not disturb the functions of the reproductive organs. If the growths are very large, very numerous, or show signs of turning malignant as they sometimes do at the change of life, the whole womb is often removed ; but this is a matter for the advice of a specialist.

FIBROSIS. By fibrosis is meant the development of a tough and leathery sort of tissue called fibrous tissue. Fibrous tissue most often develops where there has been some injury to the ordinary tissue of a structure to such an extent that it cannot hope to recover.

FIBROSITIS. Fibrositis or myalgia is a condition in which inflammation occurs in the muscular tissues of the body. Tiny swellings, or nodules as they are called, appear in the tendon coverings of the nerves, ligaments and similar structures which form part of the muscular tissue of the body. These swellings are very painful to the touch and they cause intense pain on movement of any of the muscles. There is often a certain amount of stiffness as well. The name "muscular rheumatism" is often used for fibrositis, and it is generally considered to be due to the same causes which produce other forms of rheumatism.

When fibrositis occurs in the back the condition is known as lumbago, and this form can be very crippling indeed. Another common type of this condition occurs in the neck (stiff neck), or the chest may be attacked (pleurodynia). There is also a very common condition of aching and stiffness of the muscles over most of the body. The pain may come on suddenly and, as a rule, there are intervals of pain until the condition is cured.

Fibrositis appears to occur more often in men than in women, and it is commoner after middle life. The condition is probably due to the presence of some infection in the body. Usually bad teeth or infected tonsils are the cause, or there may be some poisons present in the intestines owing to faulty diet. Attacks may also follow exposure to cold or wet, or prolonged fatigue or strain.

Treatment. If the pain is very severe the patient should rest in bed, but as a rule the milder attacks are not severe enough to compel complete rest. Heat applied to the body is the most soothing way of easing the pain, and this may be given in the form of a hot bath, hot fomentations, or hot-water bottles. Radiant heat baths or hot air baths are very good if they can be taken.

Massage should be carried out as it tends to increase the circulation of the blood over the affected part. The swellings or nodules should be looked for, and if these can be gently rubbed away, so much the better. Liniments may be rubbed into the skin to stimulate it, and a very useful one consists of methyl salicylate, menthol, oil of eucalyptus, and oil of camphor. An ointment made of methyl salicylate and lanolin is also very good. A combination of massage and heat can be given by going over the affected part with a warm iron. The skin should be protected by layers of brown paper, and only the very lightest pressure should be used.

Drugs such as sodium salicylate or aspirin may be given to help to relieve the pain. If the attack is severe, 15 to 20 grains of sodium salicylate may be given every three hours for the first twelve or twenty-four hours, then the dose should be gradually lessened.

The treatment so far has only dealt with relieving the pain, but this can in no way bring about a real cure. The cause of the fibrositis must be discovered, and this can only be done by a complete overhaul of the body, especially the teeth and tonsils. (*See also* RHEUMATISM.)

FIBULA. The fibula is the smaller bone in the lower leg. It lies on the outside of the leg and meets the larger bone of the lower leg, the tibia, at both ends. The tibia and fibula curve away from each other, however, in their course between their two ends. The upper end of the fibula is not part of the knee joint but begins just below it and can be easily felt as a lump sticking out from the bent knee on the outside of the front of the leg. At the ankle, however, it joins up with the ankle bone and the tibia to form the ankle joint. (*See also* ANKLE ; LEG.)

Fractures of the Fibula. The fibula is altogether a slighter bone than its fellow, the tibia, and is liable to be broken. But the strong tibia usually serves as a splint and saves the damaged fibula from serious displacement. By reason of the strength of the tibia the broken fibula need only be bandaged, not splinted during the day, and it reunites very quickly. The weight of the body may often be put on the foot as soon as three weeks after the break. Massage and passive remedial exercises may be carried out almost from the first.

FIDGETS. Fidgets is a word used to describe the jumpy and restless movements seen in children. It is always a sign that the child is in a highly nervous state, and the condition may be made much worse by allowing the child to become over-tired.

The more regular type of jerky movement may be due to " tic " or twitching of the muscles, which usually begins as a form of nervousness and later develops into a habit. In older people fidgets is generally a sign of over-tiredness. It should not be forgotten that chorea or St. Vitus's dance may be mistaken for ordinary fidgetiness. For a description of this disease of childhood *see* ST. VITUS'S DANCE.

FIG. Figs, as well as various preparations made from them, act as a mild type of laxative medicine. Syrup of figs is a well-known and very useful medicine for children, but the effective ingredient in it is really senna.

FILARIA. Filaria is the name given to a group of tiny worms which are responsible for producing disease in human beings. (*See also* ELEPHANTIASIS ; FILARIASIS.)

FILARIASIS. This is a disease which is common in tropical and sub-tropical countries, and it is caused by infection by tiny worms. The peculiar thing about these tiny worms is that they stay hidden away in the lungs and kidneys all day and only enter into the blood-stream at night when the mosquito is abroad to do its deadly work. But if a person who is on night-duty sleeps during

very high degree. The fingers of a Lancashire weaver will do things that would be impossible for instance to a farm worker.

Disease of the Fingers. The fingers are so greatly used and are in such an exposed position that they are very subject to injury and infection. The bones may also become tuberculous in childhood, a condition which is known as dactylitis. Rheumatoid arthritis frequently deforms the fingers of older people. Contracted fingers in which the little and ring fingers bend into the palm of the hand is often a hereditary condition, but may be the result of irritation

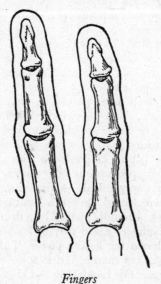

Fingers
Skeleton of Index and Second Finger of Left Hand

to, and over-use of, the fingers. "Writer's cramp" is a condition of nerve strain in which the fingers become useless for certain movements until they have had a prolonged rest. Whitlows are painful abscesses occurring in the hand. Raynaud's disease is a disease in which the fingers go "dead" owing to defective circulation. Various skin diseases affect the fingers such as itch, Baker's itch, cheiropomphlyx. All these different conditions affecting the fingers are described under their own headings. Gathered fingers are also described separately, as they are important because of the bad results they may have.

Fingers, Gathered. A gathered or poisoned finger is a very common occurrence with some people, whilst other people can get all sorts of cuts and scratches on their hands without any bad results.

Certain classes of people, too, have to be more careful than others when they get a slight injury on the hand. The most dangerous occupations as far as hand injuries are concerned are doctors, nurses and workers on the land. The first two groups because of the great danger they run of getting virulent germs into the cut, followed by rapid blood-poisoning which may mean the loss of the limb or even of life ; and the land workers because of the danger of infection with the germ of lockjaw (tetanus) which lives in the soil. Gathered or festering fingers are usually due to infection entering the skin by some very small and often unnoticed opening such as the minute opening made by a thorn or splinter. A larger cut which bleeds freely is not so liable to gather because the bleeding washes out the wound. The symptoms of a gathered finger are the same as for any other abscess : redness, soreness and heat concentrating in one spot and finally coming to a head with a collection of pus or matter.

Treatment. If there is a splinter or piece of dirt in the sore spot or under the nail where the gathering is, it should be removed if it can be seen. The finger should be soaked for long periods at short intervals in water as hot as can be borne with some mild antiseptic in it. Or it may be poulticed with antiphlogistin or hot fomentations and wrapped up until the abscess points, or comes to a head as it is commonly called. A tiny gathering will open and discharge of its own accord with this treatment, but any larger abscess will have to be carefully opened by a doctor. If the gathering is on the front of the finger a scar may be formed by unskilful treatment which may lessen the feeling power of the finger. In some occupations this may not matter, but to some workers it may be a distinct disadvantage. For bandaging the finger *see* BANDAGES.

FINGER-STALL. A loose covering for the finger, made of rubber or thin leather, is described as a finger-stall. It is worn to prevent irritation or infection to a cut or sore and it is especially useful to the housewife who has to go about her duties of washing-up, etc. The stall for this purpose could be made out of the finger of an old glove. The stall may be worn over a thin dressing.

FINSEN LIGHT. A form of light from which the heat rays have been excluded and only the blue and violet rays remain is known as Finsen light. It is used a great deal in the treatment of diseases of the skin. Dr. Finsen, a physician, was the first to discover the effect of such light and, while working in Copenhagen, he made much use of it in the treatment of lupus and other skin diseases. (*See also* LIGHT TREATMENT.)

FISH-HOOK WOUND. A fish-hook wound is a very troublesome thing to deal with, but the only way to extract the

hook from the finger is to push the hook *forward* until the point
and barb are seen quite plainly. The whole barb should then be cut
off and the rest of the fishing hook can be pulled out without further
trouble. A little iodine should be painted over the wound after it
has been thoroughly washed and a dressing applied in order to
prevent dirt from causing infection.

FISH-SKIN DISEASE. This is a disease in which the skin
has the appearance of the scales of a fish. It is technically known
as ichthyosis. (*See also* Ichthyosis.)

FISSURE. The term fissure has really two meanings in medical
language. In dealing with the anatomy of the body, fissure is
used to describe various clefts which occur in the region of the
brain, while in surgery the term fissure refers to cracks in the skin
or mucous membranes.

Anal Fissure. The commonest part of the body for a fissure
to appear is at the margin of the *anus*, which is the lower opening
of the bowel. The crack, which usually develops into a small ulcer,
is almost always caused by the passage of hard motions.

Symptoms. Although the ulcer may be very small in size,
it can create a life of misery until the place is healed. Every time
the bowels are opened, severe pain follows. The pain is not only
felt around the crack or fissure itself, but may extend up the back
and down the thighs and it may last for hours after movement of
the bowels has taken place. As a result, anyone who suffers from an
anal fissure refrains as much as possible from going to stool, thereby
setting up a vicious circle. Naturally, by holding back the motions,
they become harder and more bulky, so that when the evil hour
cannot be put off any longer the sufferer only experiences more
pain than ever. A situation like this cannot hope to be cured unless
definite steps are taken.

Treatment. In early cases healing may be brought about by
attention to the patient's general health. Constipation is usually
the start of the hard motions which cause the crack in the anus,
so laxatives such as cascara or castor oil should be given. In order
to prevent pain when movement of the bowels takes place, special
suppositories may be used ; these will deaden the painful area
around the anus or back passage and encourage the sufferer to go
to stool whenever required. After each motion the parts around
the anus should be sponged with warm water. This treatment
will not be found sufficient for a case that has developed into an
ulcer and it will be necessary for the patient to undergo a slight
operation. It is a very simple matter for the surgeon to cure the
condition, and it is advisable, at the same time, to have the condition of the lower part of the bowel investigated in case there may

be anything present which would cause a recurrence of the mischief.

Fissure of the Nipple. Unless due precautions are taken to harden the nipples and prepare them for suckling before the baby is born, cracks or fissures may appear and cause endless pain and trouble. The best way to prevent crackling of the nipples taking place is to bathe them immediately after nursing, and then to dry them thoroughly. If they are at all tender, a little boracic acid powder and starch should be applied at intervals. If cracks have formed, then the nipples must be kept covered with a piece of lint soaked in boracic lotion until they heal. (*See also* PREGNANCY.)

FISTULA. Fistula is the name applied to any unnatural narrow channel or passage which leads from one cavity of the body to another, or which opens out from a cavity to the surface of the body. There are many varieties of fistula, but one of the commonest forms is that known as anal fistula, or fistula *in ano*.

The condition may be a simple or a very complicated affair, and the term anal fistula is usually applied to all the conditions in

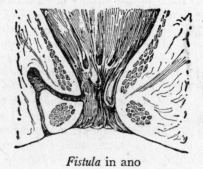

Fistula in ano

which chronic discharging openings are found near the anus or the lower end of the rectum. These channels or passages may spread in all directions and have many openings. Some may open on to the skin externally, or into the bowel internally, while others communicate both with the bowel and the outer surface of the body. There is more or less a constant discharge of pus or matter from these narrow openings, and, since the contents of the bowel usually are able to enter into the fistula, healing may be prevented.

An anal fistula is commonly due to the presence of an abscess which has been allowed to drain into the bowel or out on to the surface of the skin. The proper opening and draining of an abscess anywhere in the region of the anus would do much to prevent a fistula occurring. There is a type of abscess which appears in the neighbourhood of the lower part of the bowel which is usually a complication of tuberculosis. These abscesses if not treated properly are apt to end in the condition of fistula *in ano*.

Treatment. It is most unusual for any fistula to heal by itself without operation. Every part of the fistula must be thoroughly treated, and after the operation, complete rest will have to be taken.

FIT. The term fit is used in connection with convulsions or any other abnormal movements of the muscles.

A fit or seizure is not a disease in itself, but it may be the result of some disorder of the body. For treatment of infantile convulsions *see* under the heading INFANTS, CONVULSIONS IN; and treatment for an ordinary fit is given under EPILEPSY. (*See also* CONVULSIONS; ECLAMPSIA; EPILEPSY; FAINTING.)

FLAT-FOOT. The normal well-shaped foot has two natural arches. A larger arch extending the length of the foot from the pads of the toes to the heel, and a smaller arch extending across the foot from the ball of the big toe to the little toe. These arches of the foot may give way through weakness of the supporting muscles and flat-foot results.

To tell when flat-foot is present, wet the foot and stand on a piece of dark coloured linoleum. The outline of the foot can be plainly seen for a few minutes and can be compared with the outline of a normal foot.

Treatment. The treatment of flat-foot is by means of special exercises which are easy to perform and if persevered with will give

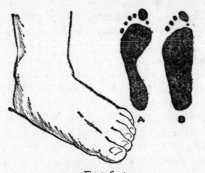

Flat-foot
A. Imprint of Normal Foot; B. Flat Foot

a very good result. Any defect in the balance of the body such as a raised shoulder, longer leg, spinal curvature should be corrected with regard to its effect on the feet as much as possible. This can usually best be done by wearing specially built-up shoes. The general health may need toning up, as some people have slacker arches when their muscles are weak through general debility. Massage to the feet may help. People with flat feet should learn to walk with the feet pointing straight ahead instead of toes turning out as so many people do. A slight degree of flat-foot is greatly improved and may be cured by simple means, but if the condition is allowed to progress it may be a more serious matter. The weight of the body will fall on parts of the foot that are not meant to support it and bad corns are the result. Also the bones of the foot press on the ground and become inflamed until it may be agony to put the foot to the ground. The muscles of the leg become strained and pain may be felt in the calves of the legs and in the thighs. In older people who have put on weight, it is very often necessary to obtain support for the arches of the feet by wearing a special supporting appliance in the shoes. These artificial arches give instant relief to the pain caused by the flat-foot, but as they are not curative to any great extent it is better for younger people to make an effort to improve the arches of the feet.

FLATULENCE. Flatulence, which is also called flatulent dyspepsia, is a condition in which there is a tendency for wind to collect in the stomach. This wind may be expelled at intervals by belching or retching, or it may be retained in the stomach causing it to be dilated and uncomfortable. Flatulence may be due to intestinal, gastric or nervous causes. Intestinal and gastric flatulence usually appear together owing to some unhealthy state of the organs of digestion, such as excessive fermentation going on in the bowel or stomach. This sort of flatulence is therefore to be treated in the same way as the indigestion which causes it, and the article on INDIGESTION should be read by those interested in it.

Nervous Flatulence. The condition known as nervous flatulence is generally due to air-swallowing, a nervous complaint in which air is continually being swallowed into the stomach. This condition is described under its medical name of *Aerophagy*.

Flatulence in Pregnancy. Flatulence is often an uncomfortable accompaniment of pregnancy, but disappears afterwards. If the discomfort is very great, retching will " bring up the wind," but pregnant women should always remember that anything in the way of straining should be avoided if possible. (*See also* PREGNANCY.)

FLOATING KIDNEY. As a general rule the kidneys are attached firmly in their normal position in the abdomen, but it sometimes happens that one or other kidney, usually the right one, is more loosely attached and is able to move from its normal position. This is called a floating kidney. Floating kidneys are fairly common and usually cause no symptoms at all, but sometimes there may be pain and discomfort to such a degree that an operation may have to be performed to anchor the kidney in its proper position. (*See also* KIDNEY.)

FLOODING. Flooding is a popular term which is commonly used to mean excessive bleeding from the womb at any time or at any age. The various causes of flooding are here outlined, and further information should be sought in the articles on the conditions mentioned in connection with flooding.

Flooding in Pregnancy. Flooding during pregnancy is always a danger signal and requires instant attention. It is usually the first sign of a threatened *miscarriage*, and if recognized and taken in time the miscarriage is sometimes prevented. This usually occurs at the end of the third month of the pregnancy, which is a time when special care should always be taken. Another condition which gives rise to flooding during pregnancy is a conception taking place in one of the tubes instead of in the womb (*ectopic gestation*). This is a very serious condition and calls for immediate operative treatment. There may be a misplaced afterbirth (*placenta prævia*), and this also is a very dangerous condition unless it is properly treated, as both the mother and the child may lose their lives at the time of the confinement owing to the afterbirth coming away before the baby, causing uncontrollable bleeding.

Accidental Hæmorrhage is a condition where there is sudden bleeding during pregnancy owing to the partial separation of the afterbirth leaving a raw bleeding surface on the side of the womb. It is not caused by an " accident " but usually by an unhealthy condition of the afterbirth. It is a serious condition and requires immediate medical attention.

Hæmorrhage due to Double Womb is a variety which has been known to occur. The bleeding in this case, which is due to an abnormality of the womb present from birth, would show itself as a continuation during pregnancy of the usual monthly periods.

Flooding after Childbirth. Flooding immediately after, or perhaps a few days after, the baby is born is usually due to a portion of the afterbirth remaining behind and preventing the womb from contracting down and sealing up the blood-vessels as it normally does.

Treatment. The treatment in these cases is to empty the womb of anything that may have been left behind as speedily as possible. Massage of the womb through the abdominal wall may help and drugs given by the doctor such as pituitrin, quinine and ergot are helpful. In some cases hot douching into the womb may be necessary. The great danger when the afterbirth is partially left behind is that it may cause blood poisoning, a very grave complication of pregnancy.

Flooding after childbirth may also be caused by *injury to the parts* caused by the passage of the baby's head or by instruments which have been used. Such cases are usually stitched by the doctor in attendance, thus controlling the bleeding and repairing the damage. Occasionally the womb becomes partially turned inside out (inversion of the uterus) when the patient has had a very bad time during labour. This condition causes severe bleeding until it has been put right again.

Flooding due to Change of Life. It is quite common to have attacks of flooding round about the age of 44 years, and it may merely mean that the patient is " on the change," but at the same time it is very important that every woman who is flooding at this age should be examined internally by a doctor, as it is the most common age for a cancer of the womb to develop and bleeding may be the first sign to draw attention to it.

Puberty. Some young girls suffer from excessive bleeding at the onset of their periods, and care must be taken of these girls to ensure that too big a strain is not put on their strength until they have become more accustomed to their periods.

Tumours. Tumours of the womb are a frequent cause of bleeding. The most common are the fibroid tumours, of which there may be many or only one present, and which may grow to a very large size or may remain very small. Their removal is usually advisable, and this may be done in several ways, for example, the application of radium, electric treatment, and removal by operation. Other tumours which cause flooding are *polypi* (tumours hanging by a stalk from the neck of the womb), ovarian tumours, and cancers.

Endometritis. This means an unhealthy condition of the womb and is usually accompanied by excessive bleeding at the periods. It is usually caused by a germ or by a misplacement of the womb.

Blood Diseases. Flooding is common in blood diseases such as *purpura* and certain sorts of *anæmia* both primary and secondary to some other disease or to an operation. The treatment in these cases is to try to cure the original disease causing the anæmia.

Gland Diseases and Debilitating Diseases. Flooding may occur in cases such as exophthalmic goitre (Graves' disease) diabetes, scurvy, heart disease, etc.

Treatment. In all the cases of bleeding the cause should be discovered and treated and, as has been said, the causes are very numerous and diagnosis is not always easy. The treatment, too, may be very lengthy. In cases of *sudden* excessive bleeding from the womb, the patient should be put in bed, lying flat without a pillow and with the bottom of the bed raised on two kitchen chairs. While awaiting the arrival of the doctor, kettles of boiling water should be prepared ready for hot douches, also clean bowls and towels should be placed ready and rolls of cotton-wool and plain white gauze and any disinfectant there may be in the house such as iodine, carbolic, Condy's fluid, or lysol. In cases where the patient is known to be pregnant a *very* tight binder round the abdomen is helpful, and so is pressure downwards with the hand placed on the upper border of the womb. Stimulants and hot drinks are likely to make the bleeding worse and should not be given until the doctor gives permission, but there is no harm in drinking as much cold water as the patient wants. In all cases of flooding, anything which comes away should be carefully kept for the inspection of the doctor.

FLUKE. Flukes are a class of worm which live in human beings or in animals. They are to be found chiefly in tropical countries. (*See also* BILHARZIASIS ; WORM.)

FLUORESCEIN. This drug is chiefly used to indicate the presence of ulcers in the cornea of the eye. A few drops composed of fluorescein, bicarbonate of soda and water, when dropped into the eye will cause the ulcer to show up by turning it bright green.

FŒTUS. Fœtus is the name given to the child after the fifth week, while it is beginning to develop within the womb of the mother.

FOMENTATION. A simple means of relieving pain can be carried out by applying hot wet flannel or lint to the part of the body which is inflamed. This is known as applying a hot fomentation. The flannel or lint should be folded so that two or more layers can be used. If a very hot fomentation is required, it will be better to use only two layers and change the application at frequent intervals, but if the fomentation need not be so hot, six or even eight layers should be used and the fomentation will retain the heat for a good long period.

In order to heat the flannel or lint, it should be cut to the desired size and laid out on a small roller towel through which a stick has been inserted at each end to make the wringing of the towel an easier matter. The towel and flannel, or whichever material is being used as the fomentation, is then placed in a basin and boiling water is poured over it until it is thoroughly soaked. The towel, with the fomentation inside it, is then wrung out as thoroughly as possible by holding a stick in each hand and twisting them in opposite directions. It is carried in the towel to the bedside in order to keep the heat in, but before applying the hot fomentation it should be opened out and shaken a little, and great care must be taken that it is not so hot that it will burn the skin of the patient. The hot wet flannel or lint must be covered as quickly as possible with a piece of mackintosh or oiled silk which has been cut a little larger than the size of the fomentation. A large pad of cotton wool should be placed over this, and the whole kept in position by a bandage or flannel binder.

A fomentation applied in this way will keep its heat for a few hours, but if the pain is intense it may be necessary to renew the fomentation every half hour. The hotter the fomentation the quicker the pain will be relieved, but again it must be advised that great care must be taken not to scald the sufferer. Sometimes the effect of the fomentation will be increased if a teaspoonful of oil of turpentine is sprinkled over the flannel or lint just before it is placed on the skin. Spongio-piline is a material which is very often used as a fomentation instead of flannel or lint. It consists of a thick pad of felt which has a backing of india-rubber and is specially manufactured for the purpose, but flannel or lint do quite as well and they are usually at hand. Wounds, ulcers, etc., are often treated by putting on boracic lint, wrung out of hot water and covered with a piece of oiled silk and a bandage.

FONTANELLE. The space between the bones of the head which is present in newly-born children is known as the fontanelle. Great care must be taken of the head until these bones join together, which usually happens by the age of eighteen months. Children who suffer from rickets or other wasting diseases do not develop as quickly as normally healthy children, and in them the closure of the fontanelle may be considerably delayed.

FOOD POISONING. Ptomaine poisoning was the name formerly used in connection with food poisoning, as it was thought to be due to putrefaction taking place and producing highly poisonous substances known as ptomaines. It is now believed that the majority of cases are due to infection with germs actually in the food, and rarely if ever to ptomaines. It must be remembered that infected foods, especially meats, are not usually altered in appearance or smell. The meat may become infected from the hands of people who store and deal with it, or it may have come in contact with infected rats, mice or flies. In cases of botulism, which is a variety of food poisoning due to a particular germ, it is only a matter of hours before very definite symptoms begin to appear. Cooking is not always a safeguard against poisoning, because although the germ itself may be destroyed, it may have produced toxins which remain unaffected by heat. Improper preservation of tinned meats, and delay in eating tinned foods once they are opened, are very common causes of poisoning. Foods may also be made poisonous by coming in contact with metals such as copper, tin or lead Very careful attention should be given to the cleaning of all metal utensils, and food should never be left standing in them for any length of time.

Another type of poisoning is known as *food allergy* in which certain persons may find certain articles of food such as fish, white of egg, certain fruits, especially strawberries, and so on, are definitely poisonous to them, and whenever they take such foods they develop various unpleasant symptoms such as nettle-rash, irritation of the bowel, erythema and eczema, or they may show symptoms of asthma.

Symptoms. The symptoms of food poisoning usually begin a few hours after the infected food has been eaten, but some cases may not become apparent for 2 or 3 days. The patient usually feels nauseated, and vomiting may take place. The bowels are loose, and later the motions may become very watery. The temperature is raised, and in severe cases the patient may show signs of collapse. In mild cases the feeling of illness may pass off in about two days, and the majority of cases recover completely after a week or so.

Treatment. The patient should be put to bed and kept warm. An emetic of mustard and water may be given, or the stomach may be washed out with a warm salt solution. Castor oil should be given, but if the diarrhœa persists, a more binding medicine, such as chlorodyne, should be substituted. Precipitated chalk, or kaolin, mixed with water, is also very helpful in soothing the stomach and bowel and stopping diarrhœa. Pain in the abdomen can be relieved by application of hot-water bottles or by hot flannels. In cases of collapse, hot coffee or other stimulants may be given. During the acute stages, the patient should only be given boiled water or whit. of egg in water, and the diet gradually increased by adding citrated milk, glucose, arrowroot, custard, eggs and fish. (*See also* BOTULISM.)

FOOT. The foot consists of the bones that lie below the long bones of the lower leg and their coverings of tissue and the muscle, with the associated tendons, blood-vessels, etc. There are 26 bones in the foot proper, 14 of these form the toes, 5 are metatarsal bones joining the toes to the heel, and the other 7 make up the heel and back part of the foot. In the part of the foot that we know as the heel the *calcaneus* rests on the ground with the *talus* above it. In front of the calcaneus is the *cuboid* on the inside of the foot, the *navicular* on the top of the foot and in front of it the *first, second* and *third cuneiforms*. It will be seen that the foot has additional bony strengthening on the inside of the foot, where the central weight of the body falls. The bones of the foot form two arches. The *lateral* arch, arching from the inside to the outside of the foot, is composed of the calcaneus, the cuboid, and the fourth and fifth metatarsal bones. The *medial* arch, arching from heel to toe of the foot, is made up of the calcaneus, the talus, the navicular, the three cuneiform, and the remaining three tarsal bones. Either of these arches of the foot may become weakened and lose its curve, thus causing the condition called flat-foot.

The foot is supplied with blood by the *plantar arteries* (internal and external) on the underneath part of the foot, and the *dorsalis*

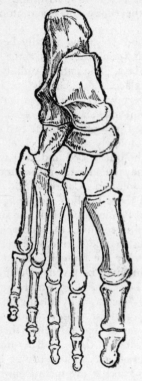
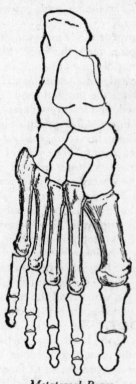

Bones of the Foot　　　　　　　*Metatarsal Bones*
(other bones of the foot in outline only)

pedis artery on the top of the foot. There are two sets of muscles which work the foot and toes, those which have their origin in the foot and those which extend from the muscles of the leg. Strong tough tissue, known as the *deep fascia*, covers the muscles of the foot. On the sole of the foot this fascia is known as the *plantar fascia* and forms a firm supporting layer stretching from the heelbone to the ball of the foot.

The foot is protected—by our habit of wearing boots and shoes—

from many cuts and injuries it might otherwise sustain, but the pressure of footwear is largely responsible for many irritating corns, callosities and blisters. The treatment of these will be found under the heading CORNS. Excessive perspiration from the feet is often a troublesome complaint for which *see* the article on SWEAT. Swollen feet are due to various causes. A fluid swelling appearing after a twist or knock to the ankle may be *synovitis*. Feet which swell in the evening may be due to weakness of the heart. Kidney diseases cause swelling of the feet. Varicose veins in the leg are a common cause of swollen feet. Many people are troubled with feet that swell when the weather becomes warm. This is merely constitutional, and the feet subside again as quickly as they swell. Chilblains in winter are another common cause of swelling of the feet. All forms of swollen feet are benefited at once by resting with the feet raised. Simple foot-rests are easily obtained and can be made at home by a handy-man. An excellent and easily made support for one leg is made of two pieces of strong thin wood about six or eight inches broad and thirty inches long, one piece being attached to the other six inches from its end and at right angles. To relieve swollen feet, they should be at a slightly higher level than the knees, so if rest is being taken on a sofa or bed, put a pillow under the feet.

FOOT DROP. When the foot cannot be raised from the ankle the condition is known as foot drop, or dropped foot. Very often the muscles of the front of the leg are paralysed, and the foot may be permanently dropped as a result. Shortening of the muscles at the back of the leg will cause the foot to drop and become fixed, but it may be possible to cure the condition by operation.

Drop foot may be due to some form of injury of a nerve controlling the muscles of the leg or ankle, or the nerves may be diseased as a result of lead-poisoning. Disease of the spinal cord may also affect the nerves and cause the foot to drop. Any symptoms should be carefully watched. (*See also* ANKLE.)

FOOT AND MOUTH DISEASE. This disease is known also as epizootic eczema, epidemic stomatitis, aphthous fever, and various other names. It chiefly affects cattle, sheep and pigs, but human beings can develop it through coming in contact with infected animals. Infection may be spread by the discharges which come from the sores, or vesicles as they are called, which appear on the feet and mouth, or it may be carried by the milk of an infected cow.

Symptoms. When a person develops foot and mouth disease, they may have a slight fever for a few days, and then sores will begin to appear in the mouth and round the lips and sometimes on the hands and feet.

Treatment. Should a case occur, the patient should be put to bed and the sores must be thoroughly treated with antiseptics. Weak solutions of carbolic acid with bicarbonate of soda are very useful as a mouth wash or for bathing the sores.

FORAMEN. Foramen is the medical term given to openings in the bones which are there for the purpose of admitting nerves and blood-vessels and such-like structures. For example, the foramen magnum is a large oval opening at the base of the skull which transmits the spinal cord and many nerves and arteries. There are many different types of openings situated all over the body and they all have their own particular name.

FORCEPS. This is an instrument which is used for grasping things which cannot be held in the fingers, or for stopping bleeding by grasping the cut end of a blood-vessel. Midwifery forceps are used in difficult cases of childbirth for extracting the child.

FORCIBLE FEEDING. Forcible or forced feeding is the conveying of nourishment to a patient who persistently refuses to feed himself or to be fed in the ordinary way, or in cases of extreme illness. It is only resorted to as an extreme measure to save life.

The method is to introduce the food by way of a soft rubber tube passed through the mouth or nose. Liquid food only is given by this means, such as milk, beaten-up egg or thin broth.

FOREARM. The forearm is the lower part of the arm between the elbow joint and the wrist. The two bones in the forearm are the radius and the ulna. (For a fuller description *see also* ARM.)

FOREHEAD. The front of the head just above the eyebrows is called the forehead, the brow or the frontal region. Wrinkling of the brow is controlled by a broad band of muscle which covers the frontal bone, the part of the skull which forms the forehead. In some people this frontal bone is very enlarged, but it is not always a sign of a large capacity for brains as so many people seem to think, but the large and bulging forehead may be due to a thickening of the frontal bone. This very often happens in children with rickets.

In many conditions such as frontal sinus disease, neurasthenia, constipation, or eye-strain, it is not unusual for pain to be felt in the region of the brow. It is quite usual to hear people say that they have a feeling as if someone was pressing a tight band across heir forehead. This very often happens after eye-strain, or neuralgia of the supra-orbital nerve which passes over the forehead. Spots on the forehead are quite common in many infectious diseases, and a seborrhœic rash may spread down from the scalp. (*See also* FRONTAL SINUS ; NEURALGIA ; SEBORRHŒA.)

FOREIGN BODY. The term foreign body is used for any

substance or article which is in a part of the body where it ought not to be. A fish-hook in the finger, or a fly in the eye, may be given as two very common examples of foreign bodies. In the following list are given a few of the more common places for foreign bodies to become lodged.

Foreign Body in the Ear. Insects or small seeds of grain, etc., often find their way into the ear and may be the cause of deafness.

Treatment. The head should be placed on one side and warm water very gently poured into the affected ear. A few drops of warm olive-oil poured into the ear and allowed to remain for a short time may dislodge the foreign body and cause it to float to the surface. If the foreign body will not move with the ordinary gentle syringing, the doctor should be called in, as it is very dangerous for an unskilled person to use instruments in the ear.

Foreign Body in the Eye. It is a very common thing for flies or small pieces of dust and grit to be blown into the eyes.

Treatment. In some cases they can be removed by merely drawing the upper eyelid over the eye, or if it can be at all clearly seen it may be removed with the corner of a clean pocket-handkerchief. If a sharp substance has become embedded such as a piece of glass or steel, castor oil should be dropped into the eye and the doctor should be sent for immediately. Very often the eye becomes so inflamed that even after the foreign body has been removed the sufferer still feels great discomfort. (*See also* EYE.)

Foreign Body in the Gullet. When a foreign body is swallowed and enters the gullet, which is the tube leading to the stomach, irritation and inflammation may be set up immediately, and a doctor must be called in ; but usually he will have to send the patient to a specialist or a hospital for its removal by means of a special kind of tube.

Treatment. In the case of a small fish-bone or any small round object, there is a possibility of dislodging it and carrying it on to the stomach by eating large quantities of brown bread and drinking a quantity of lime juice. If the foreign body fails to become dislodged, it is advisable to seek the advice of a doctor as early as possible.

Foreign Bodies in the Stomach. In many cases such things as swallowed coins, pins, etc., may reach the stomach and eventually reach the intestines without any treatment whatever.

Treatment. It is not advisable to give medicines as these may do more harm than good, but a diet of lots of new bread and fresh vegetables may assist the foreign body in its passage through the bowels. The motions should be examined to make quite certain that the foreign body is expelled.

Foreign Bodies in the Windpipe or Lung. These are sometimes inhaled when, for instance, a screw or a pin is held in the mouth and may either stick in the windpipe (trachea) or go down the bronchi into the lung. If a child gets an attack of coughing when playing on the floor, the possibility of such a foreign body must be remembered. Such foreign bodies as peas or beans are more serious than metal objects, as they set up a poisonous bronchitis, but all of them require the attention of a doctor and usually of a specialist. They are removed by an instrument called a bronchoscope, but first an X-ray examination must be done.

FORESKIN. This is a fold of skin which covers the end of the penis. In some cases this foreskin is tight and cannot be rolled back as it normally should. In such cases circumcision or removal of the foreskin is generally advised. (*See also* CIRCUMCISION.)

FORMALDEHYDE. Formaldehyde is a powerful antiseptic and disinfectant, but it is too irritating to be used on wounds and sores except in very weak solutions. There are many preparations of formaldehyde, but the best known one is formalin.

FORMIC ACID. Formic acid is found in the sting of bees and it is also present in the bodies of ants. A solution of this acid has been given inwardly in the treatment of muscular tremors and it has also been used for muscular rheumatism. The pure acid blisters the skin. (*See also* BLISTERING.)

FORMICATION. This name is derived from formica, an ant, and it is given to the sensation as of ants walking and running over the skin. This feeling and other tingling sensations felt in the skin are known as *paræsthesias*. Formication is a symptom of one sort of neuritis, or inflammation of the nerves, which is caused by alcohol and other poisons.

FOSSA. Derived from the Latin word fossa, a ditch, this term is used in connection with any depression or sunken part on the human body. There are many depressions and they each have their own particular name. For example, the ante-cubital fossa is the depression in front of the elbow and the cranial fossa is any one of the three depressions in the base of the skull which hold the lobes of the brain.

FOXGLOVE. Digitalis, a drug used in the treatment of certain diseases of the heart, is obtained from the foxglove plant. (*See also* DIGITALIS.)

FRACTURES. A fracture is the breaking of a bone, with or without damage to the surrounding tissues. Fractures are divided into various classes. If the bone is broken without any further damage it is called a *simple* fracture; if the skin is torn by the broken bone sticking through it, the fracture is a *compound* one;

if the surrounding tissues and blood-vessels are also injured, it is known as a *complicated fracture*, and there may also be a *compound complicated* type. A *comminuted* tracture is one in which the bone is smashed and splintered instead of being merely broken across. In a *multiple* fracture, the bone is broken several times ; and in an *impacted* fracture the broken ends of the bone are driven into one

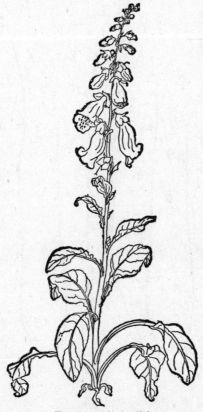

Foxglove (digitalis)

another. In children the bones do not snap easily but bend or splinter, and this variety of injury is known as a *greenstick* fracture.

The diagnosis of a fracture is a matter for medical care and skill, but in general it may be taken that a fractured limb is exceedingly painful and the patient is absolutely powerless to move the limb. Every injury where fracture is suspected should be treated as a fracture until it is proved not to be one, and in every case an X-ray examination should be carried out at the earliest possible moment. This is especially important where there may be a question of future "damages" or compensation.

Treatment. The first consideration in the treatment of fractures is to reset the bones back to a normal position. *In order to prevent any further damage, the patient must on no account be moved before*

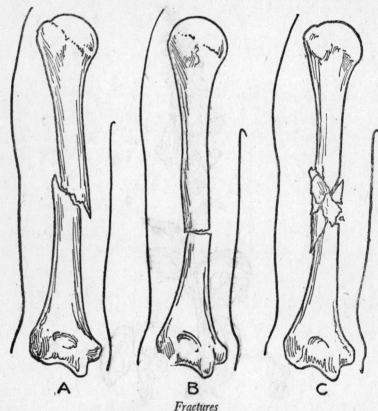

Fractures

A. Simple Oblique; B. Simple Transverse; C. Comminuted

the limb is secured in emergency splints of some kind. Before applying the splint, the limb must be straightened ; and if shortening has taken place, the limb should be pulled on with the greatest care and gentleness. There is great danger of a *compound* fracture becoming infected from contact with outside materials. The bleeding must be stopped as quickly as possible, and the wound washed and covered with a piece of lint or linen wrung out of a dilute solution of carbolic acid. This dressing should be covered with a piece of oiled silk and the whole enveloped in a thick layer of cotton wool and fixed by a bandage. It is important that the splints should be long enough to extend to the joint above and the joint below the fracture, and they must be carefully padded so as to fit the limb accurately. Where there is a fracture of the spine, pelvis, or leg,

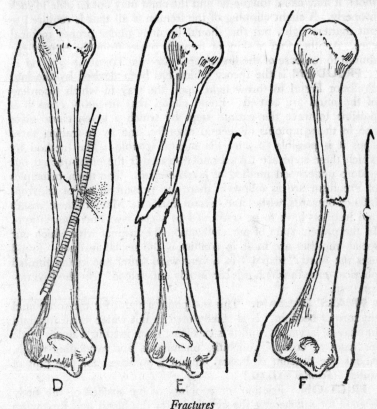

Fractures

D. Complicated; E. Compound; F. Greenstick

the patient should never be moved unless on a stretcher, as a simple fracture may become compound unless handled very carefully. As there is always a certain amount of shock associated with fractures, the patient should be kept as warm as possible until the doctor arrives. Coverings of some sort should be provided, and if possible, a hot drink of milk or broth should be given. (*See also* HÆMORRHAGE.)

FRAMBŒSIA. A tropical disease (from French *framboise*— raspberry) known also as yaws and pian. (*See also* YAWS.)

FRENUM. Frenum, or frenulum, is the term applied to any small fold of skin which restricts the movement of an organ of the body. The most common example is the short fold of mucous membrane which is found beneath the tongue. If this is unduly short, it may cause tongue-tie and the child may not be able to suck properly. A slight clipping of the frenum is all that is required to put matters right, but this should be done under proper medical care. Another fold of skin, or frenum, passes from the base of the thumb to the base of the first finger. (*See also* TONGUE.)

FREUDISM is the theory which has been devised by the late Professor Freud to throw light upon the way in which disorders of the mind are caused. Freud claims that in many cases it is possible to trace the various steps by which a given cause gives rise to the symptoms of mental disorder, and by re-tracing these steps it is possible to cure the mental trouble. The method by which these steps are traced and re-traced is the often-quoted but seldom understood method of *psycho-analysis*. The main principles of Freudism are as follows : there are present in all of us, from infancy onwards, wishes and certain instincts. Many of these wishes and instincts have to be restrained by social laws and conventions. In the present state of our civilization the instinct with which our social impulses are most in conflict is the sexual instinct. Freud uses the word " sexual " in a very wide sense, not in the limited physical sense in which it is commonly understood. (*See also* PSYCHO-ANALYSIS.)

FRIARS' BALSAM. This is a popular name for the compound tincture of benzoin. It is chiefly used in hot water as an inhalant in cases of laryngitis, and it is excellent when used in a steam kettle for cases of croup, bronchitis, pneumonia and whooping-cough. About one drachm of Friars' balsam is sufficient for one pint of water. (*See also* BALSAM.)

FRICTION. Friction, or rubbing, of the surface of the body is good for quickening the circulation of the blood and for toning up the muscles. Friction is also used as a method of rubbing in oils or such-like substances ; this method of giving medicines is known as inunction. Friction can be applied to the body by massage in various ways or by baths and douches. (*See also* DOUCHES ; INUNCTION ; MASSAGE.)

Friction Sounds. These are sounds caused by the rubbing together of two surfaces of the body. Friction sounds may be heard when two joints move over one another, but the sound is specially heard over the chest in cases of dry pleurisy.

FRIEDREICH'S ATAXIA. This is a disease of the nervous system which resembles disseminated sclerosis and locomotor ataxia, and like them, is due to a hardening of certain parts of the spinal cord and brain. It seems to affect young children and it is not unusual for several members of the same family to develop it. The chief symptoms are unsteadiness of gait which causes the patient to walk like a drunken man, and tremors of the arm and head. Later, the speech becomes slow and the eyes become affected. The feet become deformed and gradually complete paralysis may set in. The progress of the disease is very slow and may go on for as long as twenty or thirty years. No treatment is yet available for this condition.

FRONTAL SINUS. The frontal air sinuses are hollows in the frontal bone of the skull connected with the nose and filled with air ; their purpose is to give additional protection to the front part of the brain without adding to the thickness of the bone. Sometimes they are quite small and sometimes they are so large that they extend right across the eyebrows.

Treatment. Influenza and other nasal infections may cause inflammation of the frontal sinuses and may require an operation. In acute inflammation, however, operation is not usually advised, but instead hot applications to the forehead are made, and menthol inhalations are employed (from a few crystals of menthol dissolved in boiling water), being used every two or three hours. Nasal douching does more harm than good in acute inflammation, but may be useful when the acute stage is passed. (*See also* INHALATION.)

FROST-BITE. When the body has been in contact with very severe cold for any length of time, frost-bite may set in, and if the circulation is allowed to return too suddenly, the frost-bitten parts may become gangrenous, which means that they become dead. The parts of the body which seem to be attacked more than others are the fingers, the toes, the tip of the nose and the edges of the ears. These parts lie farthest away from the heart and in consequence the blood circulation is inclined to be poor. People who are in a low state of health are more inclined to suffer from frost-bite than normally healthy people, and very young children or very old people are also susceptible.

Symptoms. After long exposure to cold the circulation may become very sluggish and parts of the body may turn white and waxy-looking. There may be no pain while this is going on so that a person is sometimes quite unaware of what is happening. Blisters usually form which may gradually develop into sluggish ulcers, and if the frost-bite is very severe the affected parts may turn gangrenous and die.

Treatment. In the first place it must be mentioned that prevention is better than cure, and frost-bite may be prevented by carefully wrapping up while in intense cold, and by keeping the circulation going as much as possible by not sitting down. However, when a part of the body does become frost-bitten, the person should be kept away from all heat and the affected part should be rubbed with snow if at hand, and bathed in moderately cold water. It is important that the blood should not be allowed to get back into the frost-bitten parts too quickly as this will cause congestion of the part, and intense pain. Massage in the direction of the heart should be carried out as this will tend to keep down the congestion. If blisters appear they should be dressed with boracic ointment spread over lint and then a pad of cotton wool should be placed over them. The limbs should be raised as much as possible ; the leg may be placed on a pillow and the arm should be raised in a sling. This will help to relieve any congestion and pain. If the parts are already gangrenous, they should be kept absolutely dry, dusted with boracic powder and wrapped up in cotton wool or soft flannel. At this stage it may be necessary to undergo a surgical operation.

It must be remembered that the most important point in the treatment of frost-bite is to keep the patient away from heat as this only makes the condition worse. (*See also* CHILBLAINS ; GANGRENE.)

FRUIT LAXATIVE. The majority of fruits have the effect of stimulating the action of the bowels but some are more effective than others. Figs, prunes, apples, etc., are very excellent for this purpose and are especially good for children.

FUCUS VESICULOSUS. This is a seaweed also known as bladder wrack, which grows round the coasts of Britain. It is particularly rich in iodine, bromine and chlorine. The manufacture of iodine from this seaweed is quite an important industry, and a preparation is also manufactured which is used in the treatment of obesity. (*See also* IODINE.)

FULLER'S EARTH. This is used as a dusting powder, but it should never be used on sores or raw wounds as it is an unsterilized earth or clay which contains aluminium silicate and it may contain undesirable germs. This powder gets its name from the fact that it was used to remove grease from cloth while it was being fulled or pressed in the mill.

FULLNESS. Sufferers from indigestion often complain of a feeling of fullness which prevents them from eating a good meal. This is one of the most common symptoms of indigestion but it also may be due to other stomach disorders. (*See also* DUODENAL ULCER ; GALL-BLADDER ; INDIGESTION.)

FUNCTIONAL DISEASE. This is a vague term which one

often hears, and it is generally applied to nervous disorders or disorders of the working of the body which are not directly due to diseases of the organs of the body. (*See also* DISEASE.)

FUNGUS. One of the lowest orders of plants is known as fungus. The chief classes of fungi are the moulds, the yeasts, and the bacteria. Very often a spongy growth on the body is referred to as a fungus.

FUNNY BONE. This is a popular term used in connection with the point of the elbow, because a jar on this jars the nerve that crosses the bone near. (*See also* ELBOW.)

FUR DERMATITIS. A skin rash may appear in the region of the neck due to wearing badly dyed furs. This form of dermatitis, or inflammation of the skin, has become much more common within the last few years. (*See also* DERMATITIS.)

FURRED TONGUE. A thin white layer on the tongue may be due to a disturbance of the digestive organs, or an attack of constipation ; but on the other hand, some people seem always to have what is known as a furred tongue even though there may be no apparent reason for it. The " fur " generally consists of bacterial growth and particles of food. Sometimes drinking too much milk will cause the tongue to appear white and furred, or it may be due to too much smoking. (*See also* TONGUE, DISEASES OF.)

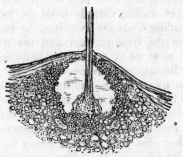

Furuncle or Boil (*beginning at hair root*)

FURUNCULUS. Furunculus is the medical name for a boil. (*See also* BOIL.)

FUSEL OIL. Small quantities of fusel oil are present in all freshly distilled spirits, but the amount gradually lessens as the spirit matures. Its effect on the body is much more powerful, and indeed rather more poisonous, than ordinary alcohol and also lasts longer. (*See also* ALCOHOL.)

GALANGAL. Galangal is a drug which is sometimes used in

the treatment of flatulence, and powdered galangal may be used as a snuff in nasal catarrh.

GALBANUM. This is a drug which is useful in cases of bronchitis. It is very often used in the form of a plaster in order to reduce inflamed swellings. It has a very unpleasant smell and taste.

GALL. Gall or nut-gall is the name given to a round growth which often appears on oak trees. It is caused by the little gall wasp when laying its eggs. These growths, or galls, contain a large percentage of tannic and gallic acids and preparations from them are used a great deal in medicine because tannic is a powerful astringent, which means that it is capable of contracting the tissues and preventing bleeding. Ointment made from galls is used in the treatment of piles.

The term gall is sometimes used in connection with bile. Gall is extremely bitter to the taste, hence the expression " bitter as gall."

GALL-BLADDER. The gall-bladder is commonly described as a pear-shaped vessel, because its shape does in fact resemble that of a pear, being broader at one end and tapering towards the other. It serves as a store for some of the bile from the liver. This bile is a very important digestive substance which is manufactured in the liver and pours from it by way of the hepatic duct, gall-bladder and common bile duct into the duodenum. Some of the bile from the liver trickles directly from the hepatic duct, which is the passage leading from the liver into the common bile duct— the passage from the hepatic duct and the gall-bladder to the duodenum—but most of it enters the gall-bladder where it is concentrated by having water removed from it, and sent on to the duodenum. The signal for the gall-bladder to begin pouring out its concentrated bile into the duodenum is the entry of the meal, eaten twenty minutes or so before, into the duodenum from the stomach. This food is mixed with the digestive juices from the stomach and when this acid mixture passes into the duodenum, which is normally alkaline, the effect is to bring the bile from the gall-bladder and liver to mix with it. (*See also* BILE ; DIGESTION.)

Gall-bladder, Diseases of. The gall-bladder is very liable to suffer from catarrh, from inflammation (cholecystitis) and from stones (cholelithiasis).

Catarrh and Inflammation of the Gall-bladder. Catarrh of the gall-bladder is fairly frequent in middle-aged persons who do not lead an active enough life and eat too much food of the stodgy starchy type. It is commoner in women than in men and especially in the " fair, fat and forty " type. It is due to infection by various germs which have found their way, either directly from the bowels, or by way of the blood-stream from some distant seat of infection such as diseased teeth or tonsils. The germs which are most frequently found in the gall-bladder are those which normally live in the intestine where they do no harm, such as the bacillus coli. It is a peculiarity of the gall-bladder that the germs of typhoid fever will linger there for many years after a person has had an attack of typhoid fever. A catarrhal state of the gall-bladder if left untreated leads in many cases to the formation of gall-stones and to inflammation.

Symptoms. Where catarrh or inflammation of the gall-bladder is present there is always a certain amount of discomfort after food. The stomach feels overloaded and there may be a definite disinclination to eat. A feeling of weight may be felt in the right side of the abdomen and pain which may be general over the right side or felt in the region just below the ribs to the right of the navel. An aching pain under the right shoulder may also be felt. Constipation is also present and there may be a slight degree of jaundice shown by a sallow skin and yellowing of the whites of the eyes.

At intervals the condition will probably become acute, and there will then be a rise in temperature with cold shivers down the spine, and a more severe pain in the region of the gall-bladder. This pain may be a steady ache or may shoot all over the abdomen and through to the back. Vomiting and nausea may be very bad.

Treatment. If gall-bladder trouble is left untreated it usually becomes gradually worse until gall-stones form and an operation may be required. Even if the complaint is not very bad it will mean persistent ill-health and a chronic feeling of being below par. Women with gall-bladder catarrh usually make their condition worse by putting on flesh, which again makes it even more difficult to obtain the necessary amount of exercise to keep the bile circulating. The first step in the treatment must be to seek out any septic focus in the body. The teeth, nose and throat must be inspected and any gynæcological conditions in women should be attended to. The diet should be light and as scanty as possible, with little fat and carbohydrate in it. More exercise should be arranged for, especially if most of the day is taken up in sedentary occupations. The increase in dancing, skating, swimming, etc., of late years has been a great boon to many people, by enabling them to " shake up their livers " in pleasant surroundings after the day's work.

The drug which is most useful for disinfecting the bile is hexamine. This should be taken with alternate doses of some alkali to counteract the irritating effect it has on the kidneys and bladder. A dose of calomel at night is a great help to some people. Epsom and Glauber salts in equal parts in the morning help to clear out the gall-bladder.

If the condition gets worse and the person becomes seriously ill it may be necessary for the doctor to drain the gall-bladder by either surgical or non-surgical means.

GALL-STONES. Gall-stones frequently form in the gall-bladder when it has suffered from catarrh for some time. Often they are present without causing any symptoms or only the symptoms of a slight catarrh, but the moment may arise when a stone becomes dislodged from the gall-bladder and begins to pass down the bile duct, on its way to the intestines. This gives rise to the condition commonly referred to as " an attack of gall-stones." Intense pain is felt, which may be so bad that the patient actually rolls about the floor or bed in agony. This is called *biliary colic*. There is often vomiting and sweating. When an attack begins the patient should be put in a hot bath. This will often be sufficient to ease the pain, but in more severe cases it may be necessary for the doctor to give morphia or a whiff of chloroform. Atropine sulphate is very useful in controlling the attacks.

Treatment. Once gall-stones have developed there is no known method of dissolving them. Some people take large doses of olive-oil under the impression that they are dissolving their gall-stones, and unscrupulous persons even undertake to treat sufferers from gall-stones by giving them something to make them sick and claiming that they have vomited up the gall-stone. Both ideas are impossible. Once the attack is over the condition must be treated medically for chronic gall-bladder catarrh or more probably surgically by the removal of the gall-stones and usually at the same time the gall-bladder.

GALVANISM. What is known as the galvanic current is made use of in medicine for the treatment of various conditions such as muscular rheumatism, etc.

GALVANO-CAUTERY. This is an electrical method used in surgery for the destruction of small growths or to shrink swollen tissues.

GAMGEE TISSUE. This is a surgical dressing made of cotton wool which has thin gauze on each side of it, called after a once famous Birmingham surgeon. (*See also* COTTON WOOL.)

GANGLION. A ganglion is a misleading term in that it is used for two separate conditions which have nothing to do with each other. The more important meaning of ganglion is a collection of nerve cells into which other nerves run and where they join together. The largest ganglion in the body is the *solar plexus,* which is situated in the middle line of the body above the navel. Another important ganglion is the *gasserian ganglion,* lying between the temple bone and the ear. The trigeminal or fifth nerve, which supplies the face and is so often the seat of facial neuralgia, passes through this ganglion.

The other meaning of ganglion is a small cyst or swelling in the sheath of a tendon which contains fluid. These ganglia are fairly common at the back of the wrist. They are small, painless and of no serious importance. Sometimes they disappear of their own accord, but if they do not do so the favourite treatment for them is to strike them hard with a book or give them a hard knock against a flat object. This will burst the swelling and disperse the fluid. The cyst will usually fill up again, however, and may have to be dissected out if it is troublesome. (*See also* GASSERIAN GANGLION.)

GANGRENE. Gangrene, or mortification, is the term used when a part of the body, usually a limb, loses all vitality and becomes dead. There are two types of this condition, " dry " and " moist." In the dry type, the dead part shrivels up, and becomes hard, dry and wrinkled, and of a dark brown colour ; while in moist gangrene the part becomes inflamed and swollen and putrefaction sets in.

Gangrene may be due to several causes, and there are certain diseases which lower the vitality of the body and make it more liable to occur. Diabetes and the disorder of the kidneys known as Bright's disease are among the chief of these. Any interference with the blood supply to a part of the body will cause that part of the body to die, and this very often happens if the main arteries have been cut or torn away as the result of an accident. Frost-bite, also, may result in dry gangrene if it has been severe. In elderly people with diseased arteries, or in *Raynaud's disease* in which the arteries are affected, or after poisoning by ergot which causes constriction of the arteries, gangrene is very liable to set in.

Treatment. Treatment of dry gangrene consists, in the first instance, of measures to prevent the part from undergoing putrefaction, or, in other words, from developing into moist gangrene. Moist dressings should never be used and dry antiseptic powder must be used in their place. When the red line appears, amputation may be performed close above it. In the moist form of gangrene boric acid and other antiseptic dressings should be applied at frequent intervals in order to keep the gangrene as dry as possible, but in rapidly spreading cases, amputation may have to be carried out at an early date. If amputation is to be successful, it must be performed high up on the limb, so as to get well beyond the infected part, otherwise a second operation may have to be performed later. Every possible care must be taken to build up the strength with nutritious food and careful nursing.

GARGLE. A gargle is a watery solution which is used to

cleanse the back of the throat. There are many drugs which may be used for this purpose but it is always advisable to use only those which can be swallowed without any unpleasant effects.

GAS POISONING. For treatment of gas poisoning *see* CARBON MONOXIDE.

GASSERIAN GANGLION. The gasserian ganglion is the collection of nerve cells where the various branches of the trigeminal or fifth cranial nerve meet. It is situated on the side of the head between the ear and the temple bone. The trigeminal nerve supplies the skin of the face and the muscles which are used in the act of

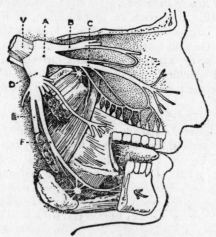

Gasserian Ganglion

A. Gasserian Ganglion.   E. Lingual Nerve.
B. Ophthalmic Nerve.   F. Inferior Alveolar Nerve.
C. Maxillary Nerve.   V. Fifth Nerve.
D. Mandibular Nerve.

eating. This fifth nerve is the nerve which is so often involved in facial neuralgia. Facial neuralgia is sometimes a very intractable and extremely painful complaint, and to ease pain which may have made a person's life miserable for years an operation has been devised by which the gasserian ganglion is entirely removed. (*See also* FACIAL NEURALGIA ; TIC DOULOUREUX.)

GASTRIC FEVER. This is an old term for typhoid fever and is never used medically nowadays.

GASTRIC or STOMACH ULCER. A gastric ulcer is an ulcer in the stomach. Gastric ulcers are also called *peptic ulcers*, in common with other ulcers which are situated in the stomach or duodenum. A stomach ulcer may be either acute or chronic, and may occur in either men or women at any age, though acute ulcerated stomachs are more common in young women than in any other class of people. Chronic ulcers of the stomach are commoner in men but are also found frequently in older women. It is not known exactly what causes gastric ulcers, but the ulcers always occur in situations where they are exposed to the action of the gastric juices which may have something to do with them, especially as ulcers appear to be more common in people who have a good flow of gastric juice. Young nervous people seem liable to develop ulcers, and the typical case is one in which a young anæmic girl suddenly has an attack of bleeding from the stomach without any definite symptoms beforehand.

Symptoms. In young persons the first warning that an ulcer has developed may be the vomiting up of blood from the stomach (hæmatemesis), an occurrence which is much more alarming than the condition warrants because these acute ulcers in young people are usually cured without much difficulty, whereas an ulcer in an older person may be a much more serious matter. There may have been preceding attacks of indigestion, pain after food, loss of appetite caused by the dread of the pain which the taking of food causes. In many cases there is vomiting of blood ; but blood may be found in the stools, which become darkened in colour as a result, a condition which is known as melæna. If there is any doubt about the presence of an ulcer an X-ray examination by means of a barium meal will usually settle the question.

Treatment. The first essential in the treatment of peptic ulcers is rest both for the body, in order that it may use all its available strength for healing purposes, and for the stomach, so that it will not be irritated more than necessary by having to deal with irritating substances in the way of food passing over the sore and ulcerated spot in its lining. To procure the necessary rest the patient is kept entirely in bed for from three weeks to six weeks, and then is only allowed to take up a strenuous life again by degrees, whilst treatment by dieting, etc., must be carried out for some months longer.

Diet is of the greatest importance in treating gastric ulcers. Milk is the most important item in the diet. Bicarbonate of soda, once a great stand-by, is now no longer recommended, but magnesia is a good substitute for it, and medicine containing atropine or belladonna is usually prescribed. Of course, any bad teeth must be attended to and any unhealthy condition in the nose or throat. (*See also* STOMACH, DISEASES OF.)

Bleeding from the Stomach (Hæmatemesis). **Treatment.** When this occurs suddenly put the patient lying flat, in bed if possible, and keep as quiet and motionless as possible. When the doctor arrives, he usually makes sure that the patient will remain still by giving an injection of morphia. Nothing must be given by the mouth until the bleeding has stopped, but if necessary the patient may be nourished by rectal injections. A simple enema will clean out the bowel, and then an injection of the salt solution called *normal saline* to which glucose has been added may be given. The mouth may be sponged out at frequent intervals with cold water, but this should not be swallowed.

GASTRITIS. Inflammation of the lining of the stomach is known as gastritis, and there are two stages of this condition, the acute and the chronic. The acute form usually develops as a result of taking some indigestible or some tainted food, or from drinking excessive amounts of alcohol. It may occur in influenza, bronchitis, pneumonia, or at the beginning of an infectious fever. In children, acute gastritis is usually present in summer diarrhœa.

Symptoms of Acute Gastritis. At the beginning of a mild attack there may be a feeling of heaviness in the region of the stomach and the tongue may be thickly coated with fur. A feeling of sickness comes on which is relieved when vomiting takes place. There may be no sign of any rise of temperature and the attack may not last longer than from 24 to 48 hours. In the more severe forms of acute gastritis, however, these symptoms become more definite, and there may be a rise in temperature to as much as 103° F. Instead of vomiting the usual stomach contents there may be a large quantity of mucus, gastric juice, and possibly some blood. The patient may suffer from collapse and faintness which may last for four or five days.

In the majority of cases, an attack of acute gastritis lasts only a short time, and apart from diarrhœa, there are rarely any complications; but in severe cases, the acute form may develop into the chronic condition, and in rare cases, ulceration of the stomach may occur.

Treatment of an Acute Attack. The patient should be put to bed and kept warm with hot-water bottles. It is necessary to clear the stomach of any irritating substance, and this may be done by encouraging vomiting. Drinks of warm water may be given for this purpose, and if vomiting is delayed, a simple emetic consisting of a tablespoonful of mustard in a glass of warm water may help matters considerably. Two grains of calomel or a good dose of castor oil will clear out the bowel, especially if it is followed by a dose of salts in the morning. Calomel should never be given to children, as it may prove too strong for them; but castor oil will be found sufficiently powerful.

No food should be given, and even after the vomiting has ceased it is better to give nothing but soda water for a time. Should vomiting still persist after the stomach has been cleared, attempts to stop it may be made by giving sips of hot water. To relieve the pain in the stomach, hot flannels or a mustard leaf may be applied to the abdomen and sips of peppermint or ginger water may be taken. If the condition does not clear up after the bowels have moved, or if the patient appears really ill, send for a doctor without further delay. For the treatment of Chronic Gastritis *see also* INDIGESTION.

GASTRODYNIA. Intense pain in the stomach is sometimes referred to as gastrodynia or gastralgia. (*See also* INDIGESTION.)

GASTRO-ENTERITIS. Inflammation of the stomach and intestines, the main symptoms of which are vomiting, diarrhœa and general weakness. (*See also* DIARRHŒA.)

GATHERING. This is a popular term applied to a boil or abscess when it comes to a head.

GAULTHERIA. Gaultheria, or wintergreen, is an American evergreen plant containing an oil, more than 90 per cent. of which is methyl salicylate. Mixed with olive-oil, it may be rubbed on the skin to relieve the pains in rheumatism or lumbago.

GAUZE. Gauze is a thin open-meshed cloth used for surgical dressings. When it has been treated with antiseptics it is referred to as antiseptic gauze. It is called gauze because it was first imported from Gaza in Syria.

GAVAGE. When a person is unable to swallow and feeding must be carried out by means of a stomach tube, this forced feeding is called gavage. By this means liquid food such as strong soups, beaten-up eggs or milk can be given. (*See also* FORCIBLE FEEDING.)

GELATIN. Gelatin is a substance which is obtained by boiling down animal tissue, bone, gristle and cartilage. It forms a colourless substance which is jelly-like when moistened, and hard and brittle when dried. It is used a great deal as a food and also in the making of pastilles, jujubes and various other chemical things. Gelatin capsules are made to hold unpleasant drugs, and gelatin of zinc is sometimes poured over ulcers in order to protect them when healing. Solutions of sterile gelatin have been injected into the body in order to raise the blood-pressure after severe hæmorrhage, and it is also capable of forming clots in the blood which is useful in the treatment of aneurysms.

GELSEMIUM. This is the root of the yellow jasmine which grows in America. It is used in the treatment of neuralgia, rheumatism and headache, but it should be used with care because in large doses it produces symptoms of poisoning. It was omitted from the new edition of the British Pharmacopœia on the ground that other drugs were more useful for the same purposes ; but many doctors think that this was a mistake and find it useful.

GENERAL PARALYSIS OF THE INSANE. This is a

disease which until lately was rightly looked upon as one of the most fatal, as well as the most horrible, diseases of the nervous system. But during the last ten years a new treatment, which will be described later, has so changed the outlook for the unfortunate sufferers from this disorder, that it is safe to say that in cases in which the disease is recognized early enough, at least one-third, and probably even more, of the cases can be so far cured that the patients can return to their ordinary work, whilst a large number, though not curable to that extent, are able to live happy, useful lives instead of dying in misery a few years after the onset of the disease, which was the only outlook for them a few years ago. But everything depends on the disease being recognized in its early stages, and only too often it is found that cure is impossible because the disease has destroyed too many of the essential nerve cells in the brain for a true recovery to take place.

It has now been proved beyond all doubt that G.P.I. is always caused by syphilis. The germ which causes syphilis can be seen in the brains of those who have died from G.P.I., and the special test for syphilis can always be found positive in the blood and spinal fluid of patients with G.P.I. The germ in the brain manufactures poisons which destroy the delicate nerve cells, and as it is the most fragile nerve cells which control our intellect, it is not surprising that mental changes are noticed fairly early in the disorder. The new treatment of G.P.I., by producing a very high temperature, kills off the germs in the brain so that they are unable any longer to produce poisons, and thereafter, as the need for the tissues to strangle the germs exists no longer, no fresh firm tissue is formed in the brain and that already present disappears in the course of time. But once nerve cells are killed they can never re-form, and so it can plainly be seen that the necessity for beginning treatment whilst as few nerve cells as possible have been damaged is vital for the cure of the condition.

G.P.I. occurs all over the world and no class or race is exempt. The infection with syphilis takes place sometimes many years before the nervous disease develops. On an average, G.P.I. occurs ten to fifteen years after the infection has taken place. It is especially likely to occur in patients in whom the syphilis has been badly or insufficiently treated. It is much more common in men than in women.

Symptoms. The first sign of the disease noticed by the relatives and friends of a patient suffering from G.P.I. is a change in his character. The affectionate husband becomes morose, depressed and neglectful, both of his own interest and of his wife. He often feels a lack of self-confidence and an apathy which is too often put down to " nerves " by his friends until more obvious changes in his personality appear. These may take one of two forms. Either the patient becomes more and more depressed, ceasing to take any interest in his hobbies and his surroundings, and obviously shows that he is incapable of work, then allowing his friends to persuade him to see a doctor, or he becomes more cheerful and lively, full of plans for doing impossible things, belittling his friends' evidence that he is " not himself " and ready with ridiculous excuses to account for his bad work and failing memory.

The latter type is much less likely to escape examination by a doctor, since the most fantastic ideas of wealth and prosperity may be possessed by an unfortunate patient with G.P.I. who has in reality " not a penny to bless himself with." Such patients will make the most absurd statements, which are to them perfectly reasonable. Thus, a man will say he possesses twenty million pounds sterling, but in the next breath will beg the doctor to give him a cigarette as he cannot afford to buy one. Or the man who claims to be the champion boxer of England will be unable even to assume a fighting attitude. But these false beliefs of wealth and fame are not so frequently met with nowadays as the depressed type of case, and it is certainly a common and sometimes excusable mistake for G.P.I. to be taken for simple neurasthenia in its early stages. The middle-aged man who becomes inattentive to his business or careless in his work, irritable, complaining of vague headache and sleeplessness is often judged to be suffering from over-work and sent for a holiday.

But certain physical accompaniments may make such a case suspect : any kind of attack, such as an epileptic fit, in a person who has not before suffered from epilepsy is suggestive of some real disease of the brain which may be G.P.I. Vision may sometimes be affected, the patient either seeing two objects instead of one for a considerable time, or he may show an obvious and not previously noticed squint. Sometimes slight seizures may occur, leaving the patient more or less paralysed down one side and the speech may alter, giving a curious slurring effect which is quite characteristic to the trained ear.

Treatment. Treatment consists in deliberately giving the patient malaria, either by letting the mosquito which carries malaria bite the patient, or by injecting into his blood the blood of another patient who has malaria. The necessary malarial mosquitoes can be obtained by a doctor from the Ministry of Health. The effect of giving malaria in G.P.I. is to produce very high temperatures in the patient's body at regular intervals, either every day, every other day or every three days, for a certain period, depending on the general health of the patient and his response to the treatment. These high temperatures kill off all, or nearly all, of the germs in the brain which are causing the disease and the patient is left, after his course of malaria, weak but much improved mentally. The improvement continues for several months, and is helped by what is called " after-treatment " with various drugs, of which arsenic, bismuth and mercury are the most commonly used. Sometimes it is considered necessary to give further injections of malaria after a suitable interval, and the prospects of cure are now so hopeful with this treatment that every patient who has improved under malarial treatment should be urged to undergo it again if the doctor thinks it wise. (*See also* MALARIA.)

GENITALS. The genitals are the organs of reproduction. (*See also* REPRODUCTIVE SYSTEM.)

GENTIAN. This is a bitter substance much used to improve the appetite and prevent indigestion, and a favourite flavouring for tonics and other medicines. (*See also* BITTERS.)

GERM. The word germ is used in two senses, first to signify any of the bacteria or microbes. In this sense it is treated under the heading GERMS. Secondly, the germ of a thing means the small kernel or nucleus which is the part of any living organism from which a similar new organism springs. We speak of the germ of a grain, but the nucleus of a cell is a germ and so is the embryo of a human being.

GERMAN MEASLES. German measles is a mild infectious disease occurring chiefly in children usually after the age of 5 years. It takes about 15 or 16 days to develop and the child is not allowed to return to school for 10 days after the appearance of the rash, or 21 days from the date of exposure to infection.

Symptoms. The child seems slightly out of sorts and develops a temperature accompanied by a slight cold, a chain of enlarged glands which feel like hard peas down the sides of the neck, and a rash which is a cross between the scarlet fever and measles rashes. The rash comes out first on the face and spreads over the body, arms and legs. It is widespread and has a red measly appearance ; it has often completely vanished in 24 hours' time.

Treatment. The treatment is simple, as the disease is not as serious as ordinary measles. The child should be kept warm in bed, and the bowels kept open with syrup of figs or milk of magnesia. The diet should consist of milk and milk puddings, such as cornflour, semolina, ground rice, Benger's food, etc. Beef-tea, fruit and any amount of water, lemonade and barley water may be given. In a day or two, when the temperature has returned to normal, and the rash has disappeared, the child will be allowed up, but should be kept isolated in the bedroom for one week after the appearance of the rash. All the usual precautions should be taken against spreading the disease, such as spreading a sheet soaked in disinfectants over the outside of the door, wearing an overall in the room, disinfecting the hands, and keeping all dishes and linens separate. No visitors or animals are to be allowed in the room. Although the disease is usually slight, it is necessary to send for the doctor when the rash appears, as it is extremely difficult sometimes to be certain that the rash is not that of scarlet fever, which is a very serious illness on account of its complications. German measles itself is a disease which usually causes no complications and is most unlikely to result in death.

GERMICIDE. Any substance which is capable of destroying germs is called a germicide. Prolonged and intense heat acts as a germicide as well as many drugs. (*See also* ANTISEPTIC ; DISINFECTANT ; GERMS.)

GERMS. Under the heading germs are included microbes, also bacilli, bacteria, yeasts—in fact, all the little living micro-organisms which cause disease in our bodies when they are growing out of place in it and in excessive numbers. Many germs, however, have their definite use in some particular part of the body, such as the *Bacillus coli*, the germ which lives normally in the colon where it helps to break up the unwanted waste materials of food in order that they may pass on and be voided. This bacillus is useful and normal in its proper place in the lower bowel and in the appropriate numbers, but when it strays into other regions such as the upper bowel and gall-bladder it becomes a source of ill-health.

Germs are the simplest form of life. They are very minute and cannot be seen without the aid of a microscope. Each germ consists of a single cell with a nucleus. It spreads and multiplies by the division of the cell and nucleus, as is explained in the article on CELLS. Some germs have no power of movement of their own, and are simply carried about in the fluids of the body, but others can move of their own accord.

The main classes of germs are the *cocci* or spherical germs, the *bacilli* or rod-shaped germs, and twisted shapes called *spirilla*. The *cocci*, the germs of which most is heard, are the *cocci* in the form of *streptococci, staphylococci*, and *pneumococci*. These cocci are the shape of a sphere when they are looked at singly, but they are more often seen in groups or strings with their sides flattened against their neighbours. The illustration commonly used to give some idea of their size is that a drop of water would contain at least 1,000 millions. The pneumococcus is the germ which causes pneumonia, the staphylococcus is the cause of boils and other skin troubles, and the streptococcus causes tonsillitis, scarlet fever, erysipelas, and various other acute infections.

Such various forms of disease as anthrax, botulism, colitis, conjunctivitis, diphtheria, meningitis, tuberculosis and typhoid fever are caused by separate and distinct varieties of rod-shaped germs or bacilli. The germs which cause syphilis are of the twisted type called spirilla.

Many diseases are due not to a single organism but to several species attacking a weakened part such as the bronchial tubes in bronchitis. Inflammation of the gall-bladder may be caused by several sorts of germs ; similarly inflammation in the stomach, the intestines, etc. Influenza is probably one of these mixed infections, though a germ called the Pfeiffer bacillus is commonly called the influenza bacillus. The germs which cause smallpox, typhus fever, hydrophobia, mumps, etc., have not been found. The name of *virus* is given to a germ which is presumed to be the cause of certain diseases, but which cannot be found, possibly because it is so small that no microscope has yet been made that will enable it to be seen. The disease, however, behaves as if there were a germ causing it, so it is presumed that there is such a germ only we are at present unable to discover it. Certainly smallpox looks very like any other infectious disease caused by germs, so it may be supposed that it is in fact caused by a particular germ, although at present this germ has not been discovered. A form of germ which is always known to cause a definite disease is called the *specific organism* of that disease, as, for instance, the tubercle bacillus which is specific for tuberculosis. Many of these specific germs, however, can be present in the body in quite large numbers without causing an attack of the disease for which they are specific, because other conditions such as the resistant power of the body are too strong for them to gain the upper hand.

Aerobes and Anaerobes.   Some germs cannot live without the presence of oxygen and these are called *aerobes*. Others die in the presence of oxygen and are called *anaerobes*. Typical aerobes are the germs of diphtheria, anthrax and cerebro-spinal fever. Anaerobes which cannot live in the presence of oxygen are the virulent germ *B. Welchii* which causes gas gangrene, and the bacillus of lockjaw. Many germs will thrive either with or without oxygen such as the coccus of pneumonia and the bacillus of typhoid fever.

Germs are killed off by solutions of carbolic acid, mercurial salts and other antiseptics, but our greatest ally in germ destruction is heat. Germs die off rapidly at a temperature of 108° F. or over, but as a general rule the exposure to heat must be kept up for twenty minutes at least. On the other hand, cold does not affect them much and in laboratories and places where it may be necessary to store germs for some time, they are often kept alive in a cooling chamber and are found to be none the worse for it. Direct sunlight is a powerful agent for killing germs, but it must fall directly on them and not through window-glass, which diminishes its power.

GESTATION. Gestation is another name for pregnancy. (*See also* ECTOPIC GESTATION ; PREGNANCY.)

GIDDINESS. Giddiness is a sensation of unsteadiness of the body which is very often accompanied by a feeling of nausea. (*See also* DIZZINESS.)

GIN. Gin is an alcoholic beverage made by distilling rye or barley, and flavoured with the juniper berry. It contains about 30 per cent. of alcohol, and in English gin only rectified spirit is used ; while in Dutch gin the spirit used is not rectified. Gin acts on the kidneys and increases the flow of urine. Gin-drinker's liver is a popular name for alcoholic cirrhosis of the liver. (*See also* ALCOHOL ; CIRRHOSIS OF THE LIVER.)

GINGER. Ginger is given in the treatment of flatulence and dyspepsia, and is used with purgatives to prevent griping pains. Half to 1 drachm of the syrup or of the tincture of ginger may be given.

GINGIVITIS. This is a condition in which the gums become inflamed. Mild types of gingivitis may be caused by lack of cleanliness of the mouth, or by the use of too hard a tooth-brush.

Treatment. Massage of the gums and the use of a mouth wash such as milk of magnesia will soon clear up the matter.

Ulcerative Gingivitis is due to an infection, and the gums become very swollen and painful and in severe cases the teeth may fall out. The infection may spread to the tonsils or the pharynx.

Treatment. In ulcerative gingivitis it is advisable to call in the aid of the doctor so that the ulcers may be painted over with an antiseptic solution, and in addition the mouth should be washed out at frequent intervals. (*See also* PYORRHŒA.)

GIRDLE SENSATION. This is a feeling of tightness around the waist which is often met with in diseases due to some disorder of the nervous system. It is generally associated with degeneration of the spinal cord and there may be symptoms of pernicious anæmia.

GLANDERS. Glanders is an infectious disease which is also known as farcy because of the " farcy buds " or nodules which appear under the skin and in the muscles. It is a disease which affects animals, especially horses, donkeys or mules, but it is contracted by people who come in contact with these animals.

Treatment. There is no specific treatment of glanders and treatment consists in dressing the ulcers with antiseptics, and in looking after the general health. The patient must be kept in bed, and the abscesses should be opened as they form.

GLANDS. The glands of the body are organs which manufacture any of the substances which are necessary to the working of the body, and which help to get rid of substances out of the system which would be harmful to it. These organs are divided into two broad classes, the ordinary glands which have a passage (duct) leading from them into which their fluids flow, and the ductless glands which, as their name implies, have no ducts. The ductless glands include many of the structures such as the thyroid gland, the adrenals, and the pituitary gland, which are now known to exercise a great influence on the health of the body by the strong action of the powerful secretions they produce. These are dealt with in a separate article called DUCTLESS GLANDS.

The ordinary glands of the body are grouped according to their use in the working of the body. There are the *lymph glands*, the *glands of elimination*, the *glands of assimilation* and a few glands for special purposes which do not come into these classes.

Lymph Glands. The lymph glands are widely scattered throughout the body. Their business is to protect the body from the action of harmful germs and substances. They are found in masses in such places as the armpits, the groins, the neck, under the knees and in the bend of the elbow, as well as amongst the deep substance of the body—the lungs, stomach, etc.

These lymph glands seem to be more active in childhood than at a later age. They act as the filters for the *lymph*—the colourless fluid which flows through the body in channels called the *lymphatic channels*, collecting the waste materials from the blood, and passing out nourishment into the tissues.

Glands of Elimination. The glands which deal with the actual passage of waste material from the tissues of the body to the outside world are called the glands of elimination. The chief of these are the sweat glands, the sebaceous glands, the kidneys, and the mucous glands which are found in the linings of all the organs of the body. The sweat glands are to be found all over the skin but are more plentiful in some places than in others. For instance, the soles of the feet and the armpits are very well provided with sweat glands. The duty of the sweat glands is to get rid of surplus water out of the tissues in the form of sweat. This water which is given off is full of poisonous material which the body must get rid of. In diseases where there is an unusual amount of poisoning of the system going on, such as rheumatism, a very useful part of the treatment is to help the sweat glands to remove these poisons by making them act as freely as possible by means of hot baths, etc. The *sebaceous* glands are situated on the hairy parts of the skin and provide an oily substance which is necessary to the health of the skin.

The *kidneys* perform the greatest part of the work by clearing the body of its waste materials. They are described under their own heading. The organs of the body are lined with mucus and in this substance are numerous glands called the *mucous* glands, which provide a clear and sticky fluid which acts as an oiling material for keeping the mucous membranes moist. It is likely that they also protect the linings of the organs from attack by germs, because when germs in excessive quantity attack a part of the mucous membrane such as the lining of the nose or bowel, a larger quantity of mucus is produced by the mucous glands which serves to wash away large quantities of the germs as in a cold in the nose.

Glands of Assimilation. The glands of assimilation are the glands which play a part in digestion of food, and absorption of the nourishment thus obtained into the body. Amongst these are all the glands of the mouth, such as the salivary glands, those of the stomach and intestinal tract, such as the glands in the duodenum, the liver and the pancreas. These are all explained under their own headings.

Glands, Diseases of. Glands are liable to be overcome by the poisons they deal with and become inflamed and may form abscesses. They are also attacked, chiefly in childhood, by tuberculosis, and may become involved in secondary growths of cancer.

When a person talks of suffering from glands they generally mean infected, swollen glands, especially in the neck. Glands in the neck, especially in children, used to be a very common disease, but the condition is fast disappearing from our midst because the infection nearly always spreads to the glands of the neck from unhealthy conditions of the nose and throat, especially tonsils and adenoids. These unhealthy conditions are now cleared up before the glands have become infected. Tuberculosis still frequently attacks the glands in the support of the intestines which is called the *mesentery*. The blood condition called *leukæmia* in which the lymph glands become greatly swollen throughout the body is discussed under its own heading.

Glandular Fever is also discussed separately, as well as *Mumps*, in which the glands of the neck (the parotid glands) become greatly swollen.

GLANDULAR EXTRACTS. In the last few years many experiments have been done to make use of extracts of some of the most important glands in the body. Many striking successes have followed the results of these experiments and probably the thyroid gland preparations are the most effective and best known. (*See also* DUCTLESS GLANDS.)

GLANDULAR FEVER. This is a condition in which the glands of the neck become swollen, and sometimes the glands under the arms and in the groin become affected. It usually occurs in epidemic form, especially in the autumn, and it may affect children living in one house, or children who are at school together. There is a moderate degree of fever which may last for a week or two.

Treatment. The child should be put to bed and the neck kept warm by rolling a flannel bandage round it. Castor oil may be given to keep the bowels open. The child should not be allowed up until a few days after the temperature has returned to normal, and convalescence may be slow as the general system may be very much depressed. Tonics and careful dieting will do much to build up the health and, if it is at all possible, a change of air would be very beneficial. This condition is very often mistaken for mumps, but though the two conditions are very similar, they are not the same, as different glands are involved. (*See also* GLANDS ; MUMPS.)

GLAUBER'S SALT. Glauber's salt, or sodium sulphate, is chiefly used as a saline purgative. It should be taken first thing in the morning in doses of a quarter of an ounce to half an ounce in a glass of water, or repeated smaller doses may be taken if desired.

GLAUCOMA. Glaucoma is an eye disease whose special sign is a tendency to increase of pressure within the eye, resulting finally in destruction of the optic nerve fibres and blindness. There are different forms of the disease, but they are considered as mainly due to the difference in rate at which the tension increases. In some of the more acute forms the pupil is greenish, and it was to these cases that the word *glaucoma*, from the Greek word meaning sea-green, was originally applied. The word is now used as a general term for all forms of the disease.

Glaucoma may occur in infants, owing to an error of development, and is then known as " ox-eye " from its appearance. It is, however, most common in people of fifty or more and may follow great anxiety or emotion.

Symptoms. An acute attack usually begins at night with severe neuralgic pains in the eye and the same side of the head, which may last for two or three days. The pain may be so acute as to cause sickness, and the patient mistakenly thinks the attack to be " only a sick headache." It is these cases that are so dangerous ; they may destroy the sight beyond repair in a day ; but an ordinarily severe case goes on for about a week, and a chronic case many months, before damage is caused.

There are all varieties between the acute and the chronic. The latter often comes on so gradually and painlessly that it is disregarded until serious damage has been done ; sometimes it comes on by steps, so to speak, the patient having a series of more or less severe " bouts," with clouding of vision. They pass away after some minutes or hours, each attack, however, leaving the sight worse than before. In chronic cases artificial lights appear to be surrounded by coloured " halos," and there are various other peculiarities of sight, such as lessening of the field of vision. The veins on the surface are distended, so that the eye is blood-shot. The pupil is wide and oval instead of being small and round, and may be greenish. The eye is harder than usual, and vision is hazy.

Treatment. The outlook in glaucoma is always serious as regards the sight, and the sooner treatment is commenced the better, especially in the acute cases. Formerly, the disease was regarded as incurable ; but, in 1857, von Graefe introduced an operation in which a small piece of the iris was removed at one point. This is still the operation for choice in acute cases ; in the less acute cases another operation is performed, where a small portion of the white of the eye is removed.

If the condition is very chronic, or if an operation is inadvisable, *eserine* drops are used. Eserine contracts the pupil and helps to open the angle of filtration. This treatment may be continued as long as desired.

GLEET. Gleet is the name given to a discharge from the urethra, generally found after an attack of gonorrhœa. (*See also* GONORRHŒA.)

GLOBUS HYSTERICUS. A common complaint in hysteria in which there is a choking sensation as if a ball were obstructing the throat. Such cases, however, should always be examined by a throat specialist, as it may or may not mean the beginning of serious disease. (*See also* HYSTERIA.)

GLOSSITIS. Glossitis means inflammation of the tongue. (*See also* TONGUE, DISEASES OF.)

GLOSSY SKIN. This abnormal condition is seen on an area of skin, the nerve supplying which is injured or diseased. The skin's functions cease, and atrophy is said to set in ; the skin becomes smooth, glossy and lifeless in appearance. The nerve of supply may be damaged in various ways, either by a direct injury, such as a gun-shot wound ; by a disease of the central nervous system, such as multiple neuritis ; or by a general disease, such as leprosy, gout, or rheumatism.

Treatment. The condition tends to disappear after a time, varying from a few weeks to a few years. No treatment beyond that of the casual disease is of any use ; but lanoline or any mild ointment may be rubbed into the affected skin to preserve its health as far as possible. If pain is present, as sometimes happens, it may be relieved by either hot or cold applications. (*See also* MULTIPLE NEURITIS.)

GLOTTIS. The narrow opening at the upper end of the larynx, or voice-box, is known as the glottis. It varies in width and shape with the movements of the vocal cords. During ordinary quiet breathing the glottis is open, but while the vocal cords are being used as in speech or singing, the opening is reduced to a mere slit. The narrow opening of the glottis is called in medical language, the rima glottidis. (*See also* LARYNX.)

GLUCOSE. Glucose is also known as dextrose and it is the form of sugar which is found in ripe fruits—especially grapes. It is also in honey and, of course, in jam made with fruits. It is an important article in the diet as it forms a very valuable food which is easily digested. Ordinary cane sugar has to undergo a chemical change before it is digested ; but glucose is what might be termed a predigested substance, so is particularly beneficial to people with weak digestions. It is also of great importance in those cases where nourishment cannot be taken by mouth and rectal feeding has to be adopted. An enema containing glucose will provide sufficient nourishment to tide a patient over a critical period, or a carefully sterilized injection may be given directly into the veins.

The body is only able to deal with a certain amount of glucose, and if this amount is exceeded, the surplus glucose is given off in the urine. This is one of the chief symptoms in the disease known as diabetes. (*See also* DIABETES ; URINE.)

GLUCOSIDE. There are many substances from which glucose —and another substance which is not sugar—can be obtained. These substances are known as glucosides. The more important ones are amygdalin, arbutin, digitalin and salicin.

GLUTEAL ARTERY. A large and important artery situated in the buttocks. This artery breaks up in various branches which supply blood to the lower limbs. (*See also* ARTERY.)

GLUTEN. Gluten is a substance found in the seed of cereals. Gluten bread is specially prepared bread made from wheat-flour from which all the starch has been removed. It is used a great deal by people who are on special diets, particularly those who cannot take a large amount of carbohydrates, as in diabetes. (*See* also DIABETES.)

GLUTEUS MAXIMUS. The chief muscle of the buttock. It helps to join the thigh-bone to the pelvis.

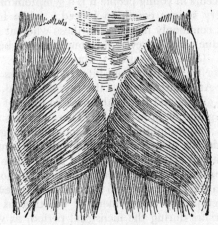

Gluteus Maximus

GLYCERINE. Glycerine is a sweet, heavy fluid which is capable of absorbing water, and for this reason it is used a great deal on the hands to keep them from getting chapped.

Glycerine has a very soothing effect on the mucous membranes, and for this reason it is used with tannic acid or iodine as a paint in cases of sore throat. Internally it has been given as a purgative in doses of 1 to 2 teaspoonsful either by mouth, but especially in the form of an enema. The result is prompt, usually occurring within less than half an hour, and there is very little pain or internal disturbance.

GLYCOSURIA. The presence of sugar in the urine is known as glycosuria. It is true that sugar in the urine is one of the chief symptoms of diabetes, but its presence does not always signify that diabetes is the cause. Special tests can be made to prove whether the glycosuria is due to true diabetes or whether the excess of sugar in the urine is merely due to some other cause.

Amongst the conditions which cause sugar to appear in the urine, probably the most common is faulty diet. If too much starchy food is taken, in other words, if the diet is over-balanced with carbohydrates, the excess sugar which the body is not able to deal with will be poured out in the urine. This condition is known as *alimentary glycosuria*, and it is met with in stout people and those who are over-fond of the good things of the table. Any disturbance of the nervous system, or of the kidneys, may also cause sugar to appear in the urine. Occasionally during pregnancy, or after a severe mental shock, glycosuria is to be found. As a general rule, if glycosuria occurs in young people it is a symptom of true diabetes, which is a very serious condition indeed ; while in people over fifty it is most commonly met with in those who eat and drink too much. With due care, however, the condition can be controlled to a large extent. (*See also* DIABETES ; URINE.)

GNAT. For treatment of gnat-bites *see also* BITES AND STINGS.

GOITRE. An enlargement of the thyroid gland, which is one of the ductless glands and lies in the neck in front of the windpipe, is known as a goitre or bronchocele. There are two main types of goitre, simple and exophthalmic. Exophthalmic goitre is dealt with fully under its own heading, and only the simple type will be discussed in this article. The thyroid gland when it is working in a normal fashion does not show in the neck, although there are occasions when the gland varies in size and activity even in healthy persons. A temporary enlargement of the thyroid gland is not unusual in females during the menstrual period, as well as during pregnancy. Such a temporary swelling is, of course, not a goitre, but at the same time it has been found that goitre is far commoner in women than in men and it is often associated with puberty, pregnancy and lactation.

Simple goitre is characterized by a very marked swelling in the front of the throat, and there is usually very little difficulty in recognizing that it is due to the thyroid gland. A simple goitre appearing at puberty or during pregnancy often disappears in a few months ; but if it is definitely associated with a district in which goitre is a common occurrence, then it is usually permanent while the person remains in that district.

Causes. There are two main theories as to the cause of goitre. It is thought that some drinking-waters lack iodine, while again it has been suggested that it may be due to a micro-organism in the water. Certainly there is no doubt that the waters of some districts are definitely goitrous, and the deep valleys in mountainous districts seem to be mostly affected. For example, it is very common in the Swiss Alps, the Italian Alps and in the mountainous parts of Germany. In India it is common among the Himalayas, and in England it occurs so often in the hilly parts of Derbyshire that the condition is known by the name of Derbyshire neck. It is also very common in parts of America where there is supposed to be a decided lack of iodine in the soil. It is important to note that people may be cured of the condition by removal to another district, just as a healthy person may develop goitre by settling in a district where it prevails.

Symptoms. Swelling of the thyroid gland may begin between the eighth and twelfth year, but as a rule its growth is at first very gradual. Later on the swelling may be very marked indeed, though there is rarely any pain. The patient is always able to swallow quite easily, and it is only when the swelling becomes very large that it interferes with breathing. During the early stages, the swelling is not hard, but in the course of time it may become firm and irregular. There are usually very definite signs of nervousness in the patient, especially if the goitre is due to over-activity of the thyroid gland (hyperthyroidism). In cases of lessened activity (hypothyroidism) there may be a tendency towards fatness and sluggishness.

Treatment. In cases where it is at all possible, a change of residence should be the first step in the cure. If this is not possible, a pure supply of drinking-water or the use of boiled water has produced very good results. Small doses of iodine are beneficial, or the swelling may be made to subside by small doses of extract of sheep's thyroid. In cases where the swelling is very unsightly, or where it is causing pressure and interfering with the breathing, a surgical operation may have to be performed. An operation is also advisable in those cases where a tumour or cyst has formed in the gland, otherwise there is the possibility that malignant changes may take place. Nowadays the surgeon never removes the whole of the gland which is the seat of the goitre, as this brings about the condition known as myxœdema, a disease due to failure of the thyroid gland. (*See also* DUCTLESS GLANDS ; EXOPHTHALMIC GOITRE ; MYXŒDEMA.)

GONORRHŒA. Gonorrhœa is a very common type of infectious venereal disease and is the cause of a great deal of ill-health and chronic invalidism, especially in women. It is caused by a germ called the gonococcus, which gains entrance to the childbearing organs and urinary tract, usually through the act of sexual intercourse, though occasionally it may be acquired through using a towel which may have been used by someone suffering from the disease.

Symptoms in Females. The patient complains of scalding pain on passing water, accompanied by a burning feeling, and irritation in the private parts, and a thick " creamy " discharge which develops in a few days' time into a thin watery discharge which is not so irritating. Later on, there may be pain in the lower part of the abdomen and warts and sore places on the private parts.

The discharge causes discomfort and soreness round the private parts and on the sides of the thighs. Sometimes the germ gets into the blood-stream and causes an " acute gonococcal rheumatism," and sometimes serious heart trouble.

Treatment (Female). It is of great importance to get medical treatment within the first few days if possible, as the earlier the treatment begins the less likelihood there is of complications. The patient should rest in bed on light fluid diet, keeping the bowels open with senna, liquorice, or salts. The drug M. & B. 693 (sulphapyridine), when used in adequate doses and for a sufficient period, is a very successful method of treatment.

Complications in Women: Bartholinian abscess, which is a tender swelling inside the private parts which may become as large as two or three inches across and often becomes very painful, is sometimes a complication of gonorrhœa. This may burst of its own accord, discharging pus, but it nearly always fills up again.

Treatment. The most satisfactory is surgical, when the abscess is entirely cut out.

Acute Cervicitis. The infection may spread into the upper parts of the vagina, setting up inflammation in the walls of the cavity and infecting the neck of the womb which is called the *cervix*. This is a difficult condition to cure as the cervix contains deep-seated glands (or pockets) in which the germs hide themselves sometimes for a number of years.

Treatment. The special treatment consists in local applications to the part of disinfectants. This can be done by inserting gelatine pessaries or plugs containing a preparation of silver such as argyrol or protargol. These pessaries have to be pushed up the cavity as far as possible to reach the cervix, and while they are being used, douching should be avoided. Adequate treatment by the drug, M. & B. 693 should, however, prevent this and many other complications.

Chronic Cervicitis. This is a condition where the disease has been going on perhaps for years and the cervix has become very unhealthy, enlarged, thickened and perhaps ulcerated. It is a continual source of infection and danger to the woman, and sometimes a cervix in this condition develops into cancer at the change of life. This is the reason why any woman who has irregular bleeding during the change of life especially, should be examined internally by a doctor.

Treatment. The treatment in these old standing cases usually presents grave difficulties. It may follow the same lines as for acute cervicitis, but each case must be considered individually and surgical operation may be necessary in some instances.

Endometritis (Inflammation of the Womb). This is a condition which has spread up from the neck of the womb to the lining of the womb. The chief symptoms are a thin watery discharge (leucorrhœa) commonly known as " the whites," excessive loss of blood at the periods accompanied by pain and a dull aching in the lower part of the back. There may also be constipation, " nerves," and general ill-health.

Treatment. In the acute stages the treatment consists of disinfecting the cavity of the womb under an anæsthetic, but where the condition has become very chronic, the whole womb may have to be removed (hysterectomy) before the patient is cured.

Salpingitis and Oophoritis. This is a condition where the germ has spread from the inside of the womb along the tubes, causing inflammation in them and in the ovaries which are attached to them. This may lead to a thickening and sealing-up of the tubes (salpingitis) causing an inability to become pregnant (sterility) and also to disease and perhaps abscess of the ovaries (Oophoritis).

Symptoms. The symptoms of an acute attack in a tube somewhat resemble those of an attack of appendicitis. The patient goes to bed with a pain in the lower part of the body, either on the right or left or perhaps on both sides. She is feverish and feels ill. The attack settles down in a day or two, but returns at intervals until the patient has developed into a state where she has always a certain amount of pain and tenderness in the pelvis and has chronic ill-health.

Treatment. The treatment of these cases is surgical or by diathermy (electrical heat), but a good deal can be done towards relieving the symptoms by giving large, hot vaginal douches (115° F.), very slowly twice a day, and by using glycerine and ichthyol pessaries (10 per cent.) at night inserted as high as possible. A good tonic such as Easton's syrup (a small teaspoonful three times a day after meals) and a daily dose of salts to relieve constipation are very helpful.

Urethritis and Cystitis. In these conditions the germ has attacked the bladder and the opening into the bladder. The patient complains of pain on passing water and also of having to do so very often. When this condition occurs, there is usually another germ to blame as well as the gonococcus.

Treatment. The treatment is rest in bed during the acute stages on low diet, drinking lots of barley water and plain water, and taking salts to keep the bowels open and medicine to disinfect the urine. Treatment by M. & B. 693 must be continued and pushed.

Gonorrhœa in Men: Symptoms. The disease comes on

suddenly with irritation at the outlet of the pipe, combined in a few days with scalding during the passing of water and also with a thick creamy discharge which tends to persist and become worse if the condition is left untreated. There may also be pain in the groin and a painful little lump on one side or the other.

Treatment (Men). Rest in bed, with light nourishing diet, large quantities of bland fluids and no alcohol, attention to the bowels and adequate drug treatment by a doctor. The introduction of the new sulphonamide drug, M. & B. 693 (sulphapyridine), has revolutionized the treatment of gonorrhœa, but it must be given by the doctor and in sufficient doses, otherwise relapses are not unknown. The patient should on no account carry out the irritation himself unless shown how to do it by a doctor, as wash-outs improperly done push the disease back still further down the pipe. If the patient is out of bed a suspensory bandage should be worn. Great care must be taken to avoid infecting the eyes with the hands.

Complications in the Male: Urethritis and infection of the bladder, and possibly also the kidneys, are the chief complications in men. If the inflammation of the urethra is allowed to become chronic, it leads to thickening of the tissues and narrowing of the passage into the bladder. This is sometimes so troublesome that the patient cannot pass water at all and instruments (bougies) have to be passed to make the passage wider. Such complications are rare nowadays if the drug treatment has been efficient. In all cases it is a good thing to flush the organs out by drinking large quantities of water and by taking medicine to disinfect the urine.

Prostatitis. Inflammation of the prostate from the urethra may be a complication of gonorrhœa and will need treatment such as rest, massage, or perhaps surgical treatment.

Epididymitis. This condition is caused by inflammation of the duct known as the epididymis, which lies to the back of the testicles. Where the condition is due to gonorrhœa, rest should be obtained for the part by wearing a suspensory bandage and the treatment for gonorrhœa should be carried out efficiently.

Periurethral Abscess. When an abscess occurs in the region of the urethra the treatment is surgical.

Conclusion. In all cases of gonorrhœa, whether male or female, there is a risk of an attack of acute infection of the joints (acute gonococcal rheumatism). The treatment for this is rest in bed—with the joints kept at rest—followed by gentle massage, opening medicine, tonics, light diet, and treatment by vaccines or serum.

In any case of gonorrhœa, great care should be taken not to spread the infection to the eyes through getting the germ on the fingers, thus causing the very serious condition called gonorrhœal conjunctivitis. This condition is the most common cause of blindness from birth. The baby's eyes become infected from the vaginal discharge of the mother, and unless treated immediately with a strong silver preparation such as protargol or argyrol, the sight is permanently damaged.

In *all* cases of gonorrhœa it is *urgent* that the patient should receive medical treatment immediately, the alternative being more or less chronic invalidism for life, as well as the possible infection of others.

GOOSEFLESH. This is a very common condition which is brought on by cold, fright, etc. Acne also causes a goosefleshy appearance on the legs and arms in which there are little acne pustules.

Treatment. For gooseflesh which appears to be fairly chronic, improve the general health, apply friction to the arms and legs by vigorous rubbing with a loofah every day, and use a sulphur soap which may be adapted to use instead of sulphur ointment by rubbing on fairly dry at night and leaving on until the morning. If the goosefleshy appearance does not clear up see a skin specialist, as the condition must be one of some definite skin trouble such as acne, dermatitis, or some form of lichen.

GOUT. Gout is a painful disease in which there is an excess of the substance called uric acid in the blood. It has a marked tendency to be hereditary. This tendency to inherit the liability to gouty troubles is called the gouty *diathesis*. Gout is no longer the scourge it was, although the "gouty diathesis" is still present in a large proportion of the population.

Causes of Gout. The gouty diathesis or hereditary predisposition to gout is important and men are more often attacked than women. Alcohol plays a large part in causing gout and it is noticeable that the fermented liquors are more dangerous than the distilled spirits. Poisoning by lead may also cause gouty symptoms. Rich food in excess combined with lack of exercise and indulgence in liquor may be said to be the root evils in causing gout. On the other hand, poor feeding combined with faulty hygiene and overindulgence in malted liquors also causes gout.

Symptoms. In a typical attack of gout the patient may be awakened in the morning with a severe pain in a joint, usually the joint of the big toe or a thumb. The joint swells and becomes intensely hot and painful so that the victim cannot bear to have it touched or to move it. Any jarring of the foot will cause him to cry out with pain. A feeling of illness may also be present, such as headache, vomiting and feverishness. If treatment is begun the swelling and pain in the joint will subside in a few days and the

joint will return to its former state ; but the attack will almost
certainly return perhaps in a few months' time or perhaps after a
couple of years. The next attack will be identical with the first or
a new joint may be affected. As time goes on the attacks become
more frequent ; or after a few attacks the condition may become
more or less chronic. Chalky deposits called *tophi* are found in the
proximity of joints and tendons, most frequently round the joints of
the large toes and fingers, and often in the outer rim of the ear.
The presence of these tophi makes the diagnosis of gout a certainty.
The affected joints lose a good deal of their power. Gouty people
are subject to skin diseases and frequently are asthmatical.

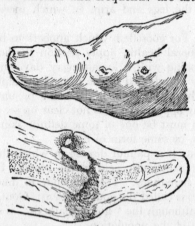

Gouty Big Toe : The Section shows **Tophi**

Treatment. Treatment must be aimed at keeping the gout at
bay, and avoiding acute attacks which need never occur where a
reasonable endeavour is made to counteract the gout. The rule
should be to live temperately, eating moderately and restricting the
diet as far as meat, liver, coffee are concerned. White bread, butter,
milk puddings, green vegetables and fruit are good. Alcohol
must be avoided and salt should be left out of the food. It is well
to take large quantities of water or mineral water between meals.
Spa treatment is a valuable beginning to the treatment of gout,
because it gives the patient an opportunity of breaking completely
with the old bad habits of diet and hygiene which surround him
at home. There used to be a saying " once gouty, always gouty,"
but this need not be so. With care it is not necessary to have acute
attacks of gout such as were taken as a matter of course fifty years
ago and, in fact, these are becoming a rarity owing to the advance-
ment of knowledge of hygiene and health matters.

G.P.I. The medical abbreviation for General Paralysis of the Insane, *which see*.

GRAFTING. By grafting we mean the operation of removing a small piece of human skin, bone or nerve from one part of the body in order to transplant it to another part. This operation has to be done when a vital piece of bone or muscle has been destroyed and can be replaced by a piece from a less vital part of the body. Skin from another part is grafted to cover unsightly injuries on the face, for instance.

GRANULATION TISSUE. When a wound or a cut is healing, new large, round cells form to connect the surfaces together. These new cells are called granulation tissue because the surface appears to be studded with little grains. It sometimes happens that there is an overgrowth of granulation tissue ; this is called exuberant granulation, or the slight swelling which takes place round the wound is often popularly referred to as proud flesh. (*See also* IN-FLAMMATION ; PROUD FLESH.)

GRANULOMA. This term means a tumour which has formed on granulation tissue. This is caused by various forms of inflammation such as occur in tuberculosis, syphilis, leprosy, yaws and glanders.

GRAPE SUGAR. This is another name for glucose and dextrose. This name grape sugar is used because of the large quantity of glucose found in ripe grapes. (*See also* GLUCOSE.)

GRAVEL. Under certain conditions, stones may form in the kidneys owing to deposits of uric acid. In some cases these stones may be quite large in size and only one may form, or there may be a large collection of very tiny ones. Gravel is the name given to the collection of very fine stones which are so small that they are able to pass into the bladder and then through the urethra along with the urine. Gravel can be detected as a sediment in the urine as soon as it is passed. (*See also* BLADDER ; CALCULUS ; URINE).

GRAVES' DISEASE. Exophthalmic goitre is associated with the name of Dr. Graves, the Irish physician who was the first to give a full description of the disease in 1835. (*See also* EXOPHTHALMIC GOITRE.)

GRAVID. Gravid means pregnant. It is most commonly used in connection with the pregnant womb, which is described as a gravid uterus. It is not customary to talk of a gravid woman, but a pregnant woman.

GREEN BLINDNESS. This is a form of colour blindness which also goes under the name of red-green blindness. (*See also* COLOUR BLINDNESS.)

GREEN SICKNESS. This is a form of anæmia which has the medical name of chlorosis. (*See also* ANÆMIA.)

GREENSTICK FRACTURE. In a young child the bones, like the young green branches of a tree, are not so brittle as when they are fully matured, so that they are more inclined to bend than to snap in two when they receive a violent blow. This bending is known as a *greenstick fracture*. (*See also* FRACTURES.)

GREGORY'S MIXTURE or POWDER. This is a popular and useful purgative for small children which is made up of rhubarb, heavy magnesium carbonate, light magnesium carbonate and ginger.

GREY MATTER. The grey matter of the brain is the brain tissue in which most of the nerve cells are situated, and is therefore of the greatest importance in the working of the body. (*See also* BRAIN.)

GRIPING. Griping is a type of pain set up by the presence of some irritating substance in the bowel. (*See also* COLIC ; FLATULENCE ; INTESTINES.)

GRIPPE. This is a French term for influenza. English people often refer to it as the grip. (*See also* INFLUENZA.)

GRISTLE. Gristle is the popular name for cartilage. Cartilage in the human body is very similar in composition and appearance to the gristle of animals which is easily recognized in meat. (*See also* CARTILAGE.)

GROCER'S ITCH. A skin disease which appears on the hands and wrists of grocers and is caused by the handling of sugar or other substances. (*See also* DERMATITIS.)

GROIN. The groin is that part of the body where the abdomen and the front of the thigh meet. It is marked by a slight groove or furrow, and in very stout people, friction may occur if absolute cleanliness is not observed. This is particularly so in fat babies, and careful attention should be given to see that the parts are washed, dried and powdered after each napkin is changed.

The groin is important because of the large blood-vessels which lie just under the skin, and also because of the lymph glands which are grouped there. These glands frequently become enlarged in diseased conditions and are then sometimes referred to as buboes. Bubonic plague gets its name from the enlargement of these glands. Pain, and enlargement of the glands in the groin, may occur through some other part of the body being diseased. The nerves which come from the spinal cord may carry pain to the groin ; such a situation may arise when the spinal cord is diseased or when the kidneys or reproductive organs are diseased.

GROWING PAINS. Many children complain of dull aching

pains in the arms or legs which the mother simply puts down to growing pains. The vague term of " growing pains " has been used for years without any real basis for its use, because the progress of growth should cause no pain to a child. It is generally believed that these pains are actually a mild form of rheumatism, and it has been found that the majority of children who suffer from these pains show other symptoms of the presence of rheumatism. (*See also* RHEUMATISM.)

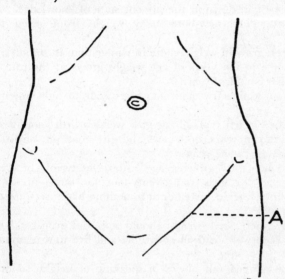

Diagram illustrating Position of Groin

GROWTH. The following points give a fair estimate of children's height at different ages as set down by authorities in this matter ; it must not, however, be taken as an infallible guide :

Height. The new-born baby's height—or length—is about twenty inches.

Children grow more in the summer-time than in winter, probably because of the sun.

Up to the age of five years growth is said to be faster than at other periods of life.

From five to ten years, boys grow faster than girls.

From ten to fifteen years, girls grow faster than boys.

From fifteen to twenty, boys grow faster than girls.

Up to fourteen, two and a half inches a year may be added by both boys and girls.

At twenty, girls reach their full height.

At twenty-four, boys reach their full height.

Some authorities say that soon after the age of two years the child is half as tall as it will be when fully grown. If this is so, we ought to be able to calculate the adult height of children at a tender age. But so much depends on food, on family characteristics, on conditions bodily and mental, on health or sickness, to say nothing of those mysterious little organs of the body known as ductless glands, to which scientists are paying great attention, that no rule can be laid down at the present state of knowledge.

Weight. The new-born baby weighs from seven to eight pounds.

Children grow in weight more in winter than in summer.

From five to ten years of age weight grows at the rate of from four to five pounds a year.

From ten to fifteen years it may increase from eight to ten pounds a year.

From five to ten years of age girls weigh a little more than boys.

Up to fifteen years, both boys and girls may put on from eight to ten pounds in one year.

From when the " growing age " stops—at twenty or even some years earlier for girls and twenty-four for boys—up to middle age, say fifty, weight increases at something like three-quarters of a pound a year.

At fifty, increase in weight should stop and even get less, if we want to keep well, lead an active life and live to a reasonably old age.

But, as pointed out above in speaking of height, so many influences must be taken into account that these figures can only be considered as rough calculations.

(*See also* ACHONDROPLASIA ; DUCTLESS GLANDS ; PITUITARY.)

GROWTHS. By growths we mean any abnormal formation occurring in the body and continuing to grow there. The most common growths are tumours and cysts, but corns and any sort of lumps are also growths. Growths are divided into two classes, benign and malignant. *Benign* growths are those which do not seriously interfere with the functioning of the body, whereas *malignant* growths are those such as cancer which shorten life.

GUAIACOL. Guaiacol is a colourless liquid which is used in the treatment of tuberculosis.

GUAIACUM. A resin which is used in the treatment of chronic rheumatism and lumbago. It also acts as a laxative and is useful for stimulating sluggish livers. For dysmenorrhœa (painful menstruation) it may be taken three times daily for a week before the period commences.

GUINEA-WORM. The adult worms are found in man and cause a condition which is known as *dracontiasis*. (*See also* FILARIA ; WORM.)

GULLET. The gullet is the popular name for the ŒSOPHAGUS, and a full account will be found under that heading.

GUM. Gum is a heavy sticky substance which is obtained from the trunks and branches of various trees. The two best-known gums used in medicine are gum acacia and gum tragacanth. Gums are used for throat lozenges as they are very soothing to inflamed surfaces. Gum acacia is most useful in cases of hæmorrhage, and it is given in the form of an injection in order to stop further bleeding.

GUMBOIL. Gumboil or alveolar abscess is a condition in which the gum becomes very inflamed and swollen, usually as the result of an abscess at the root of a decayed tooth. If the health is in a very low state, a chill may cause inflammation and swelling to occur.

Symptoms. Pain may be felt in the region of a decayed tooth, and matter usually collects at the root which gives rise to an abscess. The gum gradually thickens and is very painful, and in about two or three days' time the abscess may burst into the mouth, or it may even burst through on to the cheek.

Treatment. It is better to have the abscess lanced or treated before it bursts of its own accord, and if the abscess is due to a decayed tooth or root, this matter should be attended to as soon as possible. Relief to the inflammation may be gained by the application of hot fomentations, or by painting the gum with tincture of iodine in the early stages. (*See also* ALVEOLAR ABSCESS ; TEETH.)

GUMMA. Gumma is the name given to a tumour which may appear on any part of the body as a result of syphilis. The tumour may cause no pain, but it may cause dangerous interference and pressure on some vital organ of the body. (*See also* SYPHILIS.)

GUMS, DISEASES OF. Diseases of the gums usually occur through infection or as a result of irritation. Too vigorous and too frequent use of a hard tooth-brush may cause the gums to recede, especially on the canine and more prominent teeth. Ulcers may form on the gums as a result of a badly fitting dental plate. This matter can be quickly cleared up by a visit to the dentist in order to have the plate adjusted. Small ulcers or sore spots may appear on the gums or surrounding tissues owing to some disturbance of the digestion. These usually clear up in a day or two, but the mouth should be kept clean with an antiseptic mouth-wash. Gingivitis is a state of inflammation of the gums which is due to infection or irritation. Pyorrhœa is one of the most important diseases of the gums and it is a condition in which large quantities of pus are found in the sockets of the teeth. The general health should be attended to and a visit to the dentist must be made. Antiseptic mouth-washes should be used frequently. If the gums are soft and spongy, a daily massage with the fingers will encourage the circulation and improve their condition. (*See also* GINGIVITIS ; GUMBOIL ; PYORRHŒA.)

GYNÆCOLOGY. The study of the diseases of women, especially those affecting the sexual organs, is known as gynæcology, from a Greek word *guné* meaning a woman.

HABIT SPASMS. Many people, especially young children, have irregular muscular movements which affect different parts of the body, such as jerking the head about, twitching the shoulders, flickerings of the eyelids, grimacing, frowning, etc. These movements are performed unconsciously, but are under the control of the person since they can be immediately stopped if the person's attention is drawn to them, and they never take place during sleep. The cure for these spasms, which are really only bad habits, is for the person himself to be on the lookout for them and avoid them, or in the case of a child, careful and kindly training by the parents or teachers. It is not the slightest use using harsh measures and scolding—because the movements invariably become worse when the person is in an emotional state.

(*See also* FIDGETS ; ST. VITUS's DANCE ; TIC.)

HÆMATEMESIS. Hæmatemesis literally means vomiting of blood. Bleeding may occur in the stomach as a result of acute gastritis, cancer, or as a symptom of ulcer of the stomach. It may also occur in certain diseases of the blood such as hæmophilia, purpura and severe anæmia. If the hæmatemesis is severe, the patient usually has a feeling of faintness and nausea, and then vomits up the blood. Blood brought up in this way is generally dark in colour and may have the actual appearance of coffee grounds. It should be remembered that blood may be swallowed from the nose or throat, and there is also the possibility of blood being swallowed from the lungs. (*See also* HÆMORRHAGE.)

HÆMATINURIA. The presence of blood in the urine is known as hæmatinuria and it is an indication of disease of the blood, or of the kidneys, or bladder. (*See also* BLADDER ; BLOOD ; KIDNEY ; URINE.)

HÆMATOCELE. The collection of blood in a cavity of the body, especially in the pelvic cavity in females or in the testicle in males, is known as hæmatocele.

HÆMATOMA. A tumour or swelling containing blood is known as a hæmatoma. It may be the result of some injury, and it is very commonly found on the head of a new-born child after a long and difficult labour.

HÆMATURIA. This term signifies the passing of red blood corpuscles in the urine. *Nephritis* (Bright's disease) is one of the commonest causes of this condition, but it may result from stones, inflammation, or growths in the bladder. In tropical countries the passing of blood in the urine may be a symptom of *bilharziasis*, a disease caused by worms. If the blood is thoroughly mixed with the urine on passing, it is probably coming from the kidneys ; if the blood appears only at the beginning of the flow it probably comes from the urethra, and if it is noticed at the end, the site of the bleeding may be the bladder. The colour of the urine depends on how much blood is passed. In some cases, if there is a large amount of blood present, the urine may be almost black or may present a smoky appearance. With small amounts it may be only faintly tinged, or may present no change at all to the naked eye. In certain cases the presence of the blood cells can only be recognized under a microscope, or by having the urine tested with chemicals. (*See also* BLADDER ; KIDNEY ; URINE.)

HÆMOCYTOMETER. This is an instrument for counting the number of corpuscles present in the blood. This information is very valuable to the doctor as it gives him an indication whether or not his patient is suffering from anæmia. (*See also* ANÆMIA ; BLOOD ; CORPUSCLES.)

HÆMOGLOBIN. Hæmoglobin is the colouring matter in the red corpuscles which produces the red colour of blood. People who suffer from anæmia are pale because of the absence of hæmoglobin in the blood. (*See also* ANÆMIA ; BLOOD.)

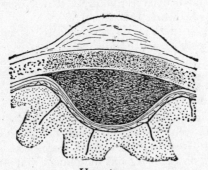

Hæmatoma

HÆMOPHILIA. This is the medical term for bleeder's disease. It is a condition in which the blood does not clot in the normal time, and the patient may bleed to death unless special precautions are taken. (*See also* BLEEDER'S DISEASE.)

HÆMOPTYSIS. Hæmoptysis, or the spitting of blood, is a condition which may be due to various causes ; but the most frequent cause, by far, is tuberculosis of the lungs, especially when the blood is in any quantity. Another fairly frequent cause is disease of the mitral valve of the heart, which causes the lungs to be " waterlogged " with blood. Any other causes (growths in the lung, severe anæmia, etc.) are very rare. While the nose may bleed into the throat, and the blood be coughed up, it is usually a mistake to blame blood-vessels in the throat for bleeding ; the blood is much more likely to have come from the lung. Bleeding which comes from the throat, mouth or nose is termed spurious hæmoptysis, whereas blood which comes from anywhere below the larynx is termed true hæmoptysis. (*See also* TUBERCULOSIS.)

HÆMORRHAGE. By hæmorrhage is meant bleeding of any description from any part of the body, but for general purposes most people use the word bleeding for small losses of blood such as that from a cut finger, and hæmorrhage for a larger flow. In external bleeding the blood penetrates through the skin, or gathers visibly just under the skin and is plain to see with the naked eye. In internal bleeding, however, there may be nothing showing which an unskilled person would recognize as blood. The blood will be coming from some part of the interior of the body and will eventually be given off in the stool or urine, but in such an altered form that it bears no resemblance to the bright red fluid we call blood. This is called *occult blood*, meaning hidden blood. It is common in ulcerated conditions of the stomach or intestines, and if it is present in such large quantities that it darkens the colour of the stools it is known as *melæna*.

Treatment. In the case of very small cuts and scratches, the pressure of a bandage will usually be all that is required to stop the bleeding. All profuse bleeding rapidly becomes a serious matter, so the subject is dealt with in First Aid.

Internal hæmorrhage will be recognized by the condition of the patient before the blood appears in the stools. A person bleeding internally becomes cold with clammy skin, pale lips and finger nails, quick and feeble pulse, quickened breathing and sometimes breathlessness. There is usually great restlessness, a very anxious and drawn look on the face, and the patient may say that he feels his life ebbing away from him. Obviously the condition is dangerous and the bleeding must be stopped by skilled attention as soon as possible, and after the bleeding has been stopped means must be taken to restore the vitality of the patient. It is now considered that death from bleeding is most often due to the fact that the heart cannot work properly without a certain amount of fluid in

the blood-vessels, so the first thing to be done after a bad hæmorrhage is to restore the proper amount of fluid to the blood-vessels,
so that the heart will be able to continue its rhythmical pumping.
In a very urgent case, the doctor may inject a quantity of the salt
solution *normal saline* straight into a vein, or it may be injected into
the tissues under the skin in some fleshy part of the body. In less
urgent cases the saline may be injected into the bowel to be retained
there, or the patient may be given large quantities of warm fluids
to drink.

Bleeding from the lungs is bright red, frothy, and is coughed up.
Blood from the stomach is darker in colour and is usually compared
to coffee-grounds. It is vomited up. In both cases the patient
must lie down and be kept quiet until a doctor is fetched.

HÆMORRHOIDS. The name commonly used for hæmor-
rhoids is *piles*, and the condition is fully described under that heading.

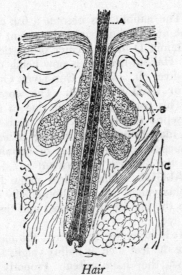

Hair

A. Hair; B. Sebaceous Glands; C. Muscle (erector pile)

HAIR, THE. A hair is formed from elongated horny cells
arising from the epidermis or outer layer of the skin, and grows
from a tube in the skin called a hair follicle. It has a root and a
shaft, which is rounded in straight hair, oval in curly hair, and
varies greatly in thickness. The surface of each hair is covered
with scales, arranged in overlapping fashion like tiles on a roof.
The colour of the hair is due to the varying amount of colouring
matter in its substance. White hair occurs when numerous air-

spaces form in its cells. The root of the hair ends in a dented knob ; into this dent fits the papilla, which is a little knot of blood-vessels. This nourishes the hair, and without it the hair dies. The root is the growing point of the hair, the rate of growth being about six inches in a year. The hair is kept glossy by the oil from the sebaceous glands, which open into the follicle.

HAIR, SUPERFLUOUS, or HIRSUTIES. This condition, also known as Hypertrichosis, occurs when an abnormal growth of hair is present. It is present in both sexes, varying from a downy moustache in a lady to—in a few cases—a shaggy pelt of hair covering the whole body. The cause of the condition is unknown ; repeated greasy applications, and a naturally greasy skin, strengthen the growth.

The " home " methods of removal are by shaving, depilatories, singeing. The medical methods are electrolysis, X-rays, and " punching."

HALIBUT. The halibut has become a fish of primary importance in medicine and dietetics since the recent discovery that its liver contains Vitamin D in far greater proportions than does the liver of the cod. Halibut-liver oil is now being used for the same conditions as cod-liver oil. (*See also* COD-LIVER OIL ; VITAMINS.)

HALITOSIS or BAD BREATH. The word halitosis means a foul breath. This condition may be due to numerous causes, most commonly septic tonsils or decaying teeth. Diseases in the nose and throat may bring about a state of foul breath ; also constipation, dyspepsia, or the eating of certain foods may be responsible. (*See also* BREATH, OFFENSIVE.)

HALLUX VALGUS. The medical name for the great toe is hallux, and hallux valgus is a condition chiefly found in growing children in which the big toe is displaced and lies either above or below the second toe.

Treatment. It is far better to prevent the formation of avoidable deformities of the feet such as hallux valgus than to rely upon treating them when they have arisen. Properly shaped shoes in childhood and youth are the very best preventive for such conditions. When it is noticed that the child's toe is bending inwards place a wad of cotton-wool, or a little spool-shaped plug made of rubber which is sold for the purpose, between the big toe and the second toe inside the stocking. Continued wearing of this will do much to straighten out the toes provided that the shoes are roomy enough at the toes.

In adults operation is the only real cure, but separating the toes and massage and exercises will help a lot to keep the condition from getting worse. Walking on tiptoes with bare feet and the toes turned in is a useful exercise that can be practised for a short time daily whilst dressing and undressing or at any odd moment, or place the pad between the toes and rise to the tiptoes a dozen times in succession, increasing the number as it becomes easier.

HAMMER TOE. Hammer toe is a condition in which one or more of the toes is bent into the shape of an inverted V. This deformity is usually caused by wearing badly-shaped shoes.

In some cases the toe may be straightened by the use of a splint, but this form of treatment is uncomfortable and may take a long

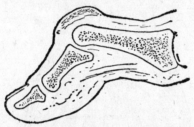

Hammer Toe in Section

time. A slight operation on the toe may be necessary to bring it down into line with the other toes.

HAMSTRINGS. The tendons situated at the back of the knee on the outer and inner sides are termed the hamstrings. (*See* also KNEE.)

HAND. The hand in the human being is a very highly specialized tool, and therein lies one of the greatest differences between human beings and animals. Even the cleverest ape has not the delicate sense of touch and the ability to control the movements of the hand that the human being, even the child, has. The difference lies in the brain which has for innumerable generations supervised the training of our fingers and hands until they are now the means by which the vast majority of us earn our daily bread. It will be realized, therefore, that we must take great care of our hands. Any sign of inflammation must be attended to at once and it is especially necessary to take measures to keep dirt and germs away by means of a small bandage, fingerstall, etc.

Structure of the Hand. The hand is hinged on to the fore-arm by the joint called the wrist joint, by means of which it can move up and down, and from side to side. The normal hand turns easily from the position in which it is palm upwards to the position in which the palm faces downwards ; it should also bend either up or down to the position of a right angle.

Skeleton of the hand. The main bones of the hand are the five metacarpal bones situated in the palm of the hand and connecting the wrist bones with the finger bones. Each metacarpal bone is jointed on to a finger which consists of three small bones called the *phalanges*, except the thumb which has only two phalanges. Three principal nerves, the ulnar, median and radial, supply the hand and divide into a network of small branches radiating to the

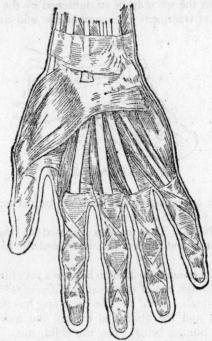

Hand : Tendons and Muscles of the Fingers

fingers. The veins on the back of the hand, which are so superficially placed that they can often be easily seen, are tributaries of the basilic and cephalic veins. The hand is well supplied with muscles and tendons which carry out the various movements of the hand.

HANGNAIL. This unsightly and somewhat painful condition is caused by neglect. If the cuticle (the fine skin at the base of the nails) is not pushed back regularly, and in consequence overgrows, the skin will tear and in places become detached, forming hangnails.

If hangnails form, they should be cut off with fine scissors, the small wound touched with a caustic stick, and covered with court plaster.

HARE-LIP. It sometimes happens that a baby is born with the two halves of its upper lip not joined together, and this is called a hare-lip from its resemblance to the split lip of a hare. In the embryo the upper lip develops in three pieces : two side flaps and a middle strip, and the join in these parts—which normally takes

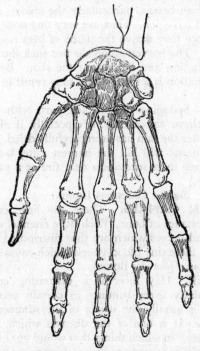

Bones of the Right Hand—Palmar aspect

place before birth—is represented in our faces by the two raised lines on each side of the furrow in the middle of the upper lip. When hare-lip occurs it is usual to leave it alone for the first few weeks until the baby has learnt to suck, then an operation is performed to join the two parts of the lip. In the great majority of cases the operation is completely successful and very little trace of the defect can be seen in after life.

HARTSHORN. A liniment known as oil of hartshorn is made up of a solution of ammonia and almond oil. It is used in the treatment of bronchitis and cold in the chest.

The name hartshorn is really an old term for ammonia, as ammonia was, at one time, extracted from the horns or antlers of harts or stags. (*See also* AMMONIA.)

HARVEST MITE. These little mites have many names, but the most popular ones are the harvest bug, the mower's mite, and the bête rouge. They have eight legs, while their young have only six. The adult mites are vegetarians and are to be found on gooseberry bushes, grass and other vegetation. The young burrow into the skin of human beings, particularly the ankles, arms and neck, and set up great irritation. They are very tiny creatures, bright red in colour, whence they derive the name of bête rouge.

Symptoms. The harvest mites do not suck the blood but they cause great irritation and itching on the skin. By scratching the skin further irritation is set up, which may result in a severe attack of dermatitis.

Treatment. Sponging the affected parts with weak ammonia will help to relieve the irritation, especially if zinc ointment is applied freely after the skin has been carefully dried. An application of petrol or benzene will kill the harvest mite, but care must be taken not to place these substances near fire or a naked light. (*See also* DERMATITIS.)

HASHISH. *See also* CANNABIS INDICA.

HAVERSIAN CANALS. These are little canals that run through the substance of bone. Each little channel contains minute blood-vessels and nerves which are thus distributed throughout the bones, and it is these tiny blood-vessels which cause a bone to bleed when it is broken. (*See also* BONE.)

HAY FEVER. Hay fever is a distressing condition which comes on regularly every summer in certain people and whilst it lasts, which is usually the whole of the summer, renders their lives miserable. It is one of the diseases which are now called " allergic diseases " in which things that would not hurt the ordinary person act as poisons to some people and bring on severe symptoms. The other allergic diseases are asthma and urticaria.

Symptoms. The symptoms of hay fever come on with great regularity in the early summer each year. They resemble a cold in the head of varying severity, sometimes there is just itching of the eyes and running of the nose but often there are severe attacks of sneezing, great swelling of the eyes and severe nasal catarrh, asthma or breathlessness and the patient may become quite ill, even running a temperature. Hay fever is always worse in the country than in town-dwellers, and it has been found that the pollen of several sorts of grass cause it in susceptible people, the most serious one being Timothy grass.

Treatment. A great deal can now be done in the way of treatment for people with hay fever. The first step is to discover what pollen is to blame and this is done by a simple test. A small amount of an extract of the suspected pollen is dropped into the patient's eye, or extracts of various pollens are rubbed into little scratches on the arm. The pollen which is harmful to the patient will cause a little inflammation. Having discovered which pollen is causing the hay fever it is necessary to try to render the patient less susceptible to it by injecting an extract of it in small doses into his blood-stream. This injection treatment must be begun well in advance of the hay-fever season or it will not be able to protect the patient. The usual month to begin is March or April. These courses of injections will have to be continued each year, but usually the patient grows out of the tendency to a great extent.

When an attack occurs there are various remedies that may be used to settle it down. A spray containing a mixture of adrenaline and chloretone may be used, or a soothing ointment may be used inside the nose. Some people are benefited by taking glucose or calcium, or both. Ephedrine locally or internally is a useful new remedy, and some people obtain benefit by slight cauterization or by ionization of the nasal passages.

HEAD. The head consists of the skull, or cranium, and the face. The skull contains the brain, which controls the nervous activity of the body. The face contains the organs of sight (eye), smell (nose), taste (tongue), hearing (ear). In animals the sense of touch is also largely situated in the face, but in human beings it has been almost entirely transferred to the hands.

Certain of the bones in the head contain air cavities which are called sinuses. These communicate with the nose and are the means by which resonance is given to the voice. They can be the seat of infection which has spread from the nose and which gives rise to a painful and dangerous condition called sinusitis.

HEADACHE. The causes of headache are very numerous, and vary from slight indispositions in some part of the body to severe mental or physical disease. Almost any upset in any part of the body can have headache for a symptom, and people use many different terms, words to describe their headaches, such as stabbing, aching, nagging, throbbing, boring, nails being driven into the head, or tight bands being tied round the head.

Headaches in Children. When a child complains of headache it is as well to take his temperature at once, because headache is usually the first symptom of any of the infectious fevers such as measles, scarlet fever or influenza. If there is no temperature the most likely causes are costiveness or eye strain. If the headache is very severe the child should be taken at once to a doctor to be examined in case it is the beginning of some severe trouble such as meningitis or mastoiditis.

Headaches in Adults are very common. Some people get a headache in heavy muggy weather and can always foretell the approach of a thunderstorm by the appearance of a headache. Many women have a severe headache of the variety known as a " sick headache " each month. Other people get a severe headache when they go too long without food. The severe attacks of sick headache known as migraine appear to be constitutional and hereditary. They are described in a separate article. A very common cause of persistent headaches is a fault in the eyesight which is not being corrected by wearing the proper glasses. Defective teeth, and nose and throat troubles are also very frequent causes of headache. Stomach, liver, heart and kidney diseases all give rise to severe headaches. Headache is usually a troublesome symptom in nervous diseases such as hysteria, neurasthenia, etc. Any feverish attack such as influenza, malaria, etc., usually starts with severe headache. The type of headache which might be described as a severe pain in the head rather than ache may be the result of some injury or disease of the brain itself. Neuralgia and rheumatism sometimes cause pain which is definitely felt in the head.

Treatment. Many of the simple passing headaches to which people are subject will disappear with quite simple treatment. An aperient pill at night with a drink of health salts in the morning will usually clear up a " bilious " headache. There are many excellent remedies to be bought for the simple headache, such as phenacetin, aspirin, antifebrin, antikamnia, phenazon, pyramidon and others. Some suit one person and some another ; but when such a drug is taken it will always act better if the person lies down in a darkened room and tries to sleep while the drug is taking its effect. It is often useful to combine caffein with one of the above drugs because of the depressing effect they often have on the patient. If the headache is combined with excitability a tablet of the three bromides may be useful. (*See also* MIGRAINE.)

HEAD LOUSE or PEDICULUS CAPITIS. Head lice are little grey creatures with a black line at the outer edge of the body. They are found chiefly in the heads of dirty people. The eggs of the louse are known as *nits*, and these are white in colour and cling firmly to the hair.

The lice cause considerable irritation to the scalp which is called *pediculosis* and the scratching which follows very often sets up unpleasant skin troubles.

Absolute cleanliness is the only way to keep free of these creatures once they have been found in the head. The hair should be washed at least twice a week and careful inspection should be carried out. Children at school should be given particular attention to see if lice or nits are present. Applying paraffin oil to the head is the simplest way of killing the lice. This should be well rubbed into the head at night and left on for about ten hours. A bathing-cap worn over the head will avoid soiling the pillows. This operation should be carried out the following morning and evening, then the morning after that the hair should be thoroughly washed with soap and water. Soaking the hair in equal parts of vinegar and water is an excellent way of loosening the nits which then can be removed by means of a small-toothed comb. Another remedy is oil of sassafras which is used extensively for the destruction of lice and their nits. This should be applied to the hair and left on for about twenty-four hours. Any irritation on the scalp should be treated with olive oil or some soothing ointment. All combs, brushes, and caps should be disinfected before using again. This can be done by putting about a teaspoonful of lysol to each pint of water and soaking everything well before washing with soapy water.

HEARING. The sense by which the sound vibrations of the air are conveyed to our brains is known as hearing. The ear is the organ of hearing, whence the vibrations are carried by the auditory nerve to our brains. (*See also* DEAFNESS ; EAR.)

HEART. The heart is the mainspring of the human machinery. If it stops, death must follow. As it is therefore the most important single organ in the body, the heart is not only well protected by Nature against injury by its position, but it is so constructed that although it never stops working whilst we are alive, yet a certain amount of rest is obtained for it between each beat. It is roughly the shape of a pear turned upside down with the lowermost part called the apex, corresponding to the stalk-end, pointing downwards and to the left, whilst the thicker portion, called the base, points backwards and to the right. About two-thirds of the heart lies to the left of the middle of the breast-bone, whilst the other third lies to the right. The size of the heart in an average adult is about five inches long, three and a half inches broad and two and a half inches thick. It weighs about nine ounces. The most important part of the heart as far as its work is concerned is the muscle of which it is chiefly made. As long as the muscle is able to act properly and to pump the blood through the various parts of the heart into the blood-vessels and so into all the organs of the body, the heart will do its work well. Once the muscle is damaged the heart is no longer a hundred per cent. efficient. The walls of the heart, which are all made of muscle, enclose four separate spaces or cavities, two auricles, the right and the left, and two ventricles, the right and the left. The right auricle and ventricle open into each other, whilst the left auricle and ventricle also open into each other ; but there is no communication between the right and left auricles or the right and left ventricles.

The right auricle receives its blood from all the veins of the body through two large veins, the superior and inferior vena cava (*see* Diagram in Photographic Supplement). From the right auricle the blood passes into the right ventricle, whence it is pumped through a large blood-vessel, the pulmonary artery, to the lungs. In the lungs the blood takes up the oxygen which is necessary for the nourishment of the tissues of the body and is returned to the heart into the left auricle by four large veins, the pulmonary veins.

From the left auricle the blood passes into the left ventricle, and from there it is pumped into the biggest blood-vessel of all, the aorta, which distributes the blood all over the body. Both the ventricles have more work to do than the auricles, because they have to pump the blood farther, but whereas the right ventricle has only to send the blood through the lungs, the left ventricle has to send it all over the body. It is not surprising, therefore, that the muscles forming the wall of the left ventricle is nearly three times as thick as the muscle forming the wall of the right ventricle, whilst the muscle of the auricles is very much thinner than that of either ventricle. Nature has very cleverly provided a method to ensure that the blood goes the right way in the heart, that is, always from auricle to ventricle, and not the reverse way, from ventricle to auricle. This method acts on the valve system and there are a series of valves, like doors, at the entrance to each of the cavities of the heart, which shut immediately the blood has passed through them and thus prevent any falling back into the cavity it has left. There are also valves at the junction between the right ventricle and the blood-vessel which arises from it (the pulmonary artery), and between the left ventricle and the aorta. (*See* Diagram in Photographic Supplement.)

On an average, the heart beats seventy-two times a minute. It beats more quickly when we are standing up than when we are sitting down, and slowest of all when we are lying in bed. Hence the importance of rest in bed in the treatment of serious heart disease.

Diseases of the Heart. There are some diseases of the heart which may occur at any age ; but, generally speaking, various types of disease attack the heart at certain ages and it is convenient to discuss disorders of the heart as they occur in childhood and adolescence, in adult life and in old age. Before these are dealt with, however, it must be said that many symptoms which the average person thinks are due to heart trouble have, in fact, nothing whatever to do with that hard-worked and much abused organ. It is merely protesting as a result of some condition in another organ. For example, an over-loaded stomach will, in a person who is foolish enough to go straight to bed on top of a heavy meal, give rise to a very severe attack of palpitation and pain round the heart. Similarly, a person who is suffering from anæmia will often be short of breath and have palpitation, but these symptoms are only the expression of the poor quality of the blood which is sent to the heart ; when the heart is supplied with a richer blood, or in other words, when the anæmia is cured, the symptoms of heart trouble disappear.

Fear, or a sudden fright, will also, in a nervous person, give rise to what may appear to be a quite alarming attack of palpitation of the heart, but this is a symptom only of the nervous control of the heart getting temporarily upset and is of no consequence. The heart itself is healthy. This is the explanation of what was called " Soldiers' heart " during the war, or D.A.H. Unable to give expression to their fear in any other way, the natural fear of the soldiers at the front was translated, quite unconsciously, into a symptom of heart disease. It is possible to tell by careful examination exactly how much the heart is capable of doing, and it was found that in these " irritable hearts " the working capacity was as good as that of a normal heart.

Heart Disease in Childhood and Adolescence. In some children the communication between the right and left sides of the heart, which is present before birth, does not close at the proper time and so there is a mixture of venous blood (which has not been sent to the lungs to pick up oxygen) with the oxygenated blood which is sent to all the other tissues of the body, and this causes one form of heart disease in children. Fortunately, this is a rare condition, like another condition from birth in which the artery which takes blood to the lungs is narrower than normal, so that less blood than usual can be oxygenated at a time. The children who suffer from these failures in development are " blue " children, physically and mentally. They are small, dainty people, but have bluish faces and are always short of breath, getting tired easily. They need much more care and attention than normal children to rear them, as they are liable to lung troubles besides the usual childish illnesses.

It is in childhood and early adolescence that acute rheumatism attacks, and unless the greatest precautions are taken, the heart is affected, never to be perfectly healthy again. It cannot be too strongly brought home to parents that a child who complains of pains in the joints (often called " growing pains "), or a sore throat, or who is " jumpy " with St. Vitus's Dance, is threatened with permanent heart disease if these complaints are not taken seriously and treated.

Heart Disease in Adult Life. Apart from the sequels to rheumatic infection in childhood and the same infection in early adult life, the most crippling cause of heart trouble in early middle life is syphilis. This disorder especially attacks the great blood-vessel, the aorta, which supplies the smaller arteries.

In early middle life also, the conducting apparatus of the heart may become diseased, in some cases the cause being unknown, in others being due to the results of syphilis. Whatever the cause, the result is the same : the ventricles no longer respond to every contraction of the auricles, since the conducting apparatus either conducts only every second, third, or fourth beat, or it fails to conduct at all, and the ventricles contract at their own rate, which is about 40 beats per minute, instead of the normal 72. This very slow beating of the ventricles sometimes produces attacks of unconsciousness with convulsions. These attacks are of serious import as they signify that insufficient blood is being supplied to the brain.

Heart Disease in Old Age. Heart disease in old age is either the result of arterio-sclerosis, or of degeneration of the muscle of the heart. Sometimes there is a combination of these two conditions, as the arteries which supply the heart itself, the coronary arteries, become narrowed through arterio-sclerosis and the heart-muscle degenerates because the blood supply is not sufficient for its needs. The pumping action of the heart is thus affected and gradually it fails to be able to maintain the circulation. Occasionally, a large part of the heart-muscle is suddenly deprived of its blood supply by a coronary artery getting blocked up ; it becomes so narrowed that only a small quantity of blood can pass, and then one day it gets blocked altogether. If a main coronary artery is affected in this way, death is almost sure to follow immediately.

In simple gradual degeneration of the heart-muscle, failure of the power to do much without getting short of breath and over-tired is the usual complaint. Pain round the heart is not common. This condition may continue for years with but few symptoms and signs, provided that reasonable care is taken of the limited capacity of the heart for work.

The Treatment of Heart Disease. In any form of heart disease the essential treatment is to limit the patient's output of energy to that which the heart is capable of sustaining without further damage. Every case of heart trouble must be under the care of a doctor. All that can be said here is to indicate a few simple rules which will serve merely to emphasize the general line of treatment in heart disease. Rest for the heart is, above all, the most important measure, and rest it must be, and the patient must on no account get up out of bed to wash or to go to the lavatory.

This is especially important in the case of children with rheumatic heart disease, as a lengthy period spent in bed when the heart is first attacked may save it from serious damage. It is advisable for anyone with a damaged heart to rest in bed at least one day a week if this is at all possible, and over-exertion must at all costs be avoided. Occupations should be chosen in which manual labour is reduced to a minimum. On the other hand, a certain amount of exercise should, unless ordered to the contrary, be taken. Easy walking, or games which do not involve a deal of exertion, such as bowls, for example, should be enjoyed ; but any noticeable shortness of breath after exertion is a warning to "go slow." Personal hygiene is very important ; the mouth should be kept scrupulously clean and the teeth must be kept free from sepsis as septic teeth harbour germs which will attack a heart already damaged and give rise to a very serious and often rapidly fatal disease of the lining membrane of the heart. The use of alcohol and tobacco must be regulated by the patient's medical attendant, as each individual case has to be considered separately ; but generally speaking, it is possible to allow a patient who has been a heavy smoker and drinker a small amount of liquor or tobacco, though any increase in his symptoms or signs may necessitate their withdrawal.

Treatment of heart disease has been almost revolutionized since the introduction of certain drugs. The salicylates have already been mentioned in connection with rheumatic heart disease. The use of digitalis in a stronger form and in large doses has saved many a person's life which would have been thrown away twenty years ago, whilst the onset of dropsy, formerly a dreaded sign, can now be combated with success by new mercury preparations. Another drug, quinidine, has been very successful in expert hands in restoring the normal rhythm of the heart where this has been upset. (*See also* ANEURYSM ; ANGINA PECTORIS ; ARTERIO-SCLEROSIS ; ENDOCARDITIS ; MYOCARDITIS ; PERICARDITIS ; etc.)

HEARTBURN. This is the name given to a burning feeling extending up from the stomach through the chest to the mouth. It is due to the flowing back of acid fluid from the stomach—it sometimes happens that a quantity of this fluid may actually reach the mouth—accompanied by a gush of saliva. It is due to indigestion, and it is also one of the symptoms of various disorders of the stomach. During pregnancy heartburn may frequently occur and cause considerable discomfort.

HEAT. The usefulness of heat is well shown by the way we rush to the hot-water bottle in all sorts of emergencies. Placing a hot-water bottle on a particular spot, such as an earache or a pain in the stomach, is a local application of heat, and the pain is relieved by the action of the heat which calls a larger supply of blood and the fluid called lymph to the spot. By this means more of the antidotes to disease which the blood and lymph contain are brought to the spot where they are needed, and the heat also eases pain by causing relaxation in muscles and nerves of the affected part.

Heat applied to the body as a whole in the form of baths increases the activity of the skin, and thus rids the body of the poisons which cause such diseases as rheumatism.

HEAT-STROKE. An illness resulting from exposure to the sun. (*See also* SUNSTROKE.)

HEEL. The heel is the hinder part of the foot and it is formed by a bone called the os calcis or calcaneum. This bone bears most of our weight when we are standing, but the heel is raised with every step we take by the muscles of the calf, which are attached to the bone by the tendon of Achilles.

Apart from the usual diseases which may attack bones, the heel is not subject to disease. Severe pain may be a symptom of rheumatism. (*See also* ACHILLES TENDON.)

HELIOTHERAPY. Heliotherapy is the term given to the treatment of disease by exposure to the rays of the sun. (*See also* SUNLIGHT.)

HEMICRANIA. See HEADACHE.

HEMIPLEGIA. Paralysis of one half of the body is known as hemiplegia. It is caused by diseases affecting the central part of the brain. (*See also* BRAIN ; PARALYSIS.)

HEMP. Extracts of Indian hemp produce a powerful drug known as cannabis indica, hashish, or bhang. (*See also* CANNABIS INDICA.)

HENBANE. The henbane plant gives us a drug known as hyoscyamine as well as other preparations, especially the alkaloid hyoscine. (*See also* ATROPINE ; HYOSCINE.)

HEPATIC. Hepatic means anything associated with the liver. A *hepatic abscess* is an abscess of the liver. The *hepatic artery* is the artery which supplies the liver with blood, and the *hepatic ducts* are the passages by which the bile flows away from the liver. The hepatic ducts join with the cystic duct leading from the gall-bladder to form the common bile duct which leads into the duodenum.

HEPATITIS. Hepatitis means inflammation of the liver. (*See also* LIVER.)

HERBALIST. A person who deals in medicinal herbs is known

as a herbalist. As a rule these people are not qualified druggists
or chemists.

HERNIA. The popular name for hernia is " rupture " and
it is a common condition amongst men and boys and not so common
amongst women. By hernia is meant the protruding through its
covering of any organ of the body. The way hernia arises is well
seen in the abdomen, where all the organs are contained in a
covering called the abdominal wall. For one reason or another
there may be a weak spot in this abdominal wall through which
a piece of bowel or any of the organs contained in the abdomen
may protrude. This protrusion will be seen as a lump under
the skin which covers the abdomen. Similarly a coil of brain may

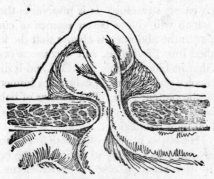

Hernia (Umbilical)

be pushed through the covering of the brain, which is also called
a hernia.

Inguinal Hernia. The most common hernia is that called
inguinal hernia. It occurs in both men and women. The wall
of the abdomen is composed of a sheath of muscles in which there
is an opening to permit of the passage of a cord. In men it is the
cord that suspends the testicle, and in women there is a cord passing
from the womb to the tissues in the groin. The opening for the
passage of these cords forms a weak spot in the abdominal wall and
a loop of intestine can readily protrude through it, forming an
inguinal hernia.

Femoral Hernia. Another common hernia is the *femoral
hernia*, which occurs at the weak spot where the great blood-vessels
of the abdomen pass into the thigh. The lump in this case is felt
in the groin, at a spot lower down than the lump formed by the
inguinal hernia.

Umbilical Hernia. Hernias are also apt to occur at the

umbilicus or navel. This hernia may occur at any age, but is most often found in small babies. It is also found in middle-aged women who have had several children and have grown stout.

Ventral Hernia. A ventral hernia is a hernia that occurs at the site of a former operation. The abdominal wall is often left in a weak state after an operation, especially one in which there has been a tube for drainage purposes, and a hernia may occur here.

Treatment. Often a hernia does not cause very much inconvenience and it is sufficient to wear a properly fitting support, called a *truss*, after the hernia has been replaced in position, or reduced as it is called ; but at any moment there may be further trouble especially if heavy weights have to be lifted or there is any condition which causes straining. It is preferable therefore to have an operation, which will give a better chance of cure. The great danger of hernias in the abdomen is always that the loop of intestine which has pushed into the hernia will become *strangulated*, that is, so compressed that its blood-supply is cut off and it dies. A strangulated hernia is a very serious matter, calling for immediate operation in order to save the patient's life. The hernias of babies and young children can nearly always be cured by wearing a small pad over the navel held on by a bandage.

HEROIN. Heroin is a drug obtained from morphine, which it resembles very much in its general action on the body. It is used a great deal to give relief in cases of troublesome and incessant cough. Unfortunately, as with morphine, there is a great liability to develop the drug habit, which when once formed is quite as difficult to break as the morphine habit. (*See also* OPIUM.)

HERPES. Herpes of the face occurs commonly on or near the lips. The symptoms are itching and " tightness " of the skin, followed by swollen reddish patches, which in a few hours are covered with little blisters. If uninfected, they dry up in about 7-10 days. In those subject to herpes, any little "upset" to the health may bring on an attack. If cases occur persistently on the same area, infection from the teeth, nose, etc., should be suspected.

Treatment. Those who recognize the early signs may limit an attack considerably by bathing the part with very hot water, or by applying collodion. Four per cent. silver nitrate in spirit of nitrous ether is also recommended. The blisters should be protected by a mild antiseptic powder.

Herpes Zoster, which is a ring of herpes encircling the body, is more usually called Shingles, and is described under that title.

HEXAMINE. Hexamine, a drug which was formerly known as urotropine, is manufactured from formalin and ammonia. It is given as an antiseptic in the treatment chiefly of infections of the bladder.

HICCOUGH. Hiccough is caused by a sudden contraction of the diaphragm due to some irritation of the nerves.

Hiccough may occur as a symptom of a more serious condition than a slight attack of indigestion. In nervous disorders it may be one of the symptoms of epilepsy, encephalitis lethargica or hysteria. It often occurs in nephritis or uræmia, or it may be due to tetanus, hydrophobia or strychnine poisoning.

Treatment. If the hiccoughing is due to indigestion, it is often relieved by drinking a glassful of water with a little bicarbonate of soda or bismuth carbonate. Holding the breath for as long as possible is an old remedy; also stooping forward and drinking out of the far side of a glass. When the hiccoughing is due to some complicating condition it may be necessary to give soothing drugs such as chloretone or luminal.

HIP. By the hip we mean the whole region of the hip-joint where the lower limb joins on to the main trunk of the body. As human beings are dependent on the hip-joint for their means of moving themselves from place to place and for the support of the body in the upright position, it is, as might be expected, the largest and strongest joint in the body.

The hip-joint is a ball and socket joint, the ball being the well-rounded head of the femur (thigh-bone), while the socket is a cup-shaped hollow in the haunch-bone (pelvis), called the *acetabulum*.

Hip Disease. This is usually a tuberculous condition which is more popularly known as "hip-joint disease" and it is almost confined to delicate children. The symptoms start quite early in life and become more noticeable as time goes on.

Symptoms. The child generally complains of tiredness, and is noticed to walk with a slight limp. He may complain of pain in the leg or the knee, and movement of the limb is usually limited in all directions. When standing or walking, the patient will make every effort to save putting weight on the affected side, and as the condition advances this limp will become more pronounced. Gradually the muscles begin to waste about the hip and the limb alters in appearance. The thigh is bent upwards, while the foot is bent outwards, and there is usually a great deal of pain and some swelling.

Treatment. The general treatment of hip-joint disease is the same as for other tuberculous conditions. The child should be kept in bed and some form of splint should be used to keep the limb in position. He should also live in the open air as much as possible and once the limb is straightened he may go about, preferably in the country. (*See also* TUBERCULOSIS.)

Hip, Dislocation of. Dislocation of the hip at birth is by no means rare, and it is due to the imperfect formation of the acetabulum, the cup-shaped hollow in the haunch-bone into which the head of the thigh-bone fits. It is not usually noticed until the child begins to walk, and then it will be seen that the child walks in a curious waddling sort of way. In all cases it is desirable that an X-ray photograph should be taken to find out the exact type of the dislocation.

Treatment. The treatment of this condition is purely surgical and convalescence may be quite a lengthy matter. When dislocation happens as the result of an accident the patient should never be moved until the arrival of a medical man. (*See also* DISLOCATION.)

HIRSUTIES. This is the medical name for the condition commonly known as superfluous hair.

HIVES. This is a name which is applied to many eruptions of the skin especially urticarial rashes. (*See also* URTICARIA.)

HOARSENESS. Hoarseness or huskiness of the voice is generally the result of catarrh or inflammation of the vocal cords, but it may also result from pressure on the nerves that control the movements of the cords. Disease in the region of the glottis will affect the voice, or sore throat may arise from over-use of the voice and cause a certain amount of hoarseness. Diseases which affect the vocal cords are tuberculosis, cancer and syphilis. No person should have chronic hoarseness for a month without having the larynx examined by a specialist in case any serious disease may be beginning.

HOBNAIL LIVER. *See* CIRRHOSIS.

HODGKIN'S DISEASE. Hodgkin's disease, otherwise known as lymphadenoma or lymphogranuloma, is a disease in which the lymph-glands and the spleen become enlarged. The condition is named after Thomas Hodgkin (1798–1866), an English physician who was the first to make records of several cases of this disease.

Symptoms. The disease usually comes on very gradually and men are more often affected than women. The first symptom is enlargement of the glands of the neck and there may be a great feeling of weakness accompanied by breathlessness. The glands in the groin and under the armpits may swell up, and the glands in the chest and abdomen may also become affected. These enlarged glands may cause pressure on the nerves of the various parts affected and much pain may result. Pressure on the spinal cord may cause paralysis to take place. A slight degree of fever is generally present and it is not unusual for the skin to turn a bronzed colour. At this stage there may be definite symptoms of anæmia and the patient usually complains of weakness and loss of weight. The cause of the complaint is thought to be tuberculosis, but although there are several theories as to the actual cause, nothing, as yet, has been definitely proved.

Treatment. There is no known cure for Hodgkin's disease, but treatment with arsenic usually causes a temporary improvement. Plenty of rest, fresh air and nourishing food should be given. X-ray treatment has also been known to cause a temporary improvement. (*See also* LYMPHATICS.)

HOMICIDAL MANIA. Homicidal mania is the state of insanity in which there is the unrestrained impulse to kill human beings. (*See* INSANITY ; MANIA ; MELANCHOLIA.)

HOMŒOPATHY. A system of treatment of disease by drugs which, if given during health, would produce the same symptoms as the disease. These drugs are given over a long period in very small doses.

HOOKWORM DISEASE. Hookworm disease, or ankylostomiasis as it is medically termed, is produced by the presence in the human body of a worm known as the hookworm. Another name for this condition is " miner's anæmia." The worms produce thousands of eggs which are discharged from the intestine of the infected person. When these come in contact with damp soil or water, they hatch out into embryos which enter the skin of someone else and then pass by means of blood to the heart and lungs, and finally into the intestine. They usually enter the human body through the soles of the feet, producing what is known as " ground itch." The disease is to be found particularly in warm climates such as Egypt, India, China, Ceylon and the Southern States of North America.

Symptoms. Small sores and swellings may occur in the feet, but these usually heal up within a week or so. Several months may pass before the patient becomes aware of any other symptoms. Later on he may complain of shortness of breath, palpitations, and general weakness. There may also be flatulence and constipation, or diarrhœa. The appetite is usually good, but pica (dirt eating) is a characteristic of the disease. The complexion may appear pale and sallow, and the temperature may be slightly raised. The stools usually are stained with blood. The disease may go on for many months if untreated, but under treatment the chance of recovery is usually good.

Treatment. In the treatment of this disease various anthelmintic drugs are used (anthelmintic is the name given to any drug which is used in the treatment of worms). Oil of chenopodium and carbon tetrachloride are very largely used, but they should not be taken unless under medical attention. Prevention of the disease consists in giving careful attention to the disposal of fæces or excreted matter ; the water supply must be pure, and shoes and stockings should be worn, especially by children.

HORDEOLUM. *See* STYE.

HORMONES. By hormones we mean substances which are produced by various glands of the body and poured by them directly into the blood-stream of the body. In other words they are the *secretions* of the *ductless glands*. (*See* DUCTLESS GLANDS.)

HOSPITAL. A hospital is a building for the treatment of sick or injured persons, and in this country may be either a *voluntary hospital*, a *municipal hospital*, a *state hospital*, or a *private hospital* or nursing home ; a voluntary hospital with less than 50 beds in the country and small towns is termed a *cottage hospital*. The oldest of the voluntary hospitals is St. Bartholomew's, founded in London in the twelfth century, and the largest is Edinburgh Royal Infirmary, which has over a thousand beds and will have several hundreds more when its extensions are completed.

HOUSEMAID'S KNEE. Frequent kneeling may cause a swelling to appear on the knee which usually becomes inflamed. (*See also* BURSA.)

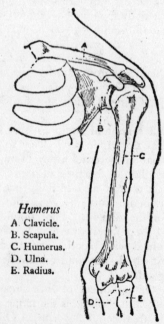

Humerus

A Clavicle.
B. Scapula.
C. Humerus.
D. Ulna.
E. Radius.

HUMERUS. The humerus is the bone of the upper arm, extending from the shoulder-blade (scapula) to the elbow joint. It fits into the hollow of the scapula called the *glenoid fossa* and forms a ball and socket joint. At the elbow it is jointed with a hinge joint to the lower or fore-arm.

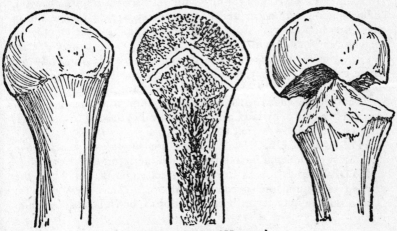

Epiphyseal Line (Humerus)

HUMPBACK. Humpback, or hunchback, is caused by curvature of the spine and the typical case is usually due to tuberculous disease of the spinal column (Pott's disease). Old people often become slightly humpbacked because of their inability to stand up straight, or rheumatoid arthritis may cause changes to take place in the spine. (*See also* POTT'S DISEASE ; SPINE.)

HUNTINGTON'S CHOREA. This is a hereditary disease of the nervous system in which the use of the muscles is lost gradually until the patient dies of exhaustion through being unable to swallow. The earliest symptoms are irregular muscular movements like those of the ordinary chorea (St. Vitus's Dance), which become worse until the patient can no longer use his hands or limbs. His mentality deteriorates and he slowly sinks into inertia and dies after a period of anything up to twenty years from the first signs of the disease. The cause and cure are unknown and it is definitely of a hereditary nature.

HYDATID DISEASE. This is a disease in which cysts form in various parts of the body owing to the presence of immature tapeworms. The eggs of these tapeworms are almost always conveyed to human beings by dogs ; usually through the dog licking the skin, or perhaps through licking the dishes from which food is eaten. The custom of kissing pet dogs cannot be too strongly guarded against.

Symptoms. A hydatid cyst produces no symptoms while it is small, but as it grows larger, which it does very rapidly, it may cause a great deal of damage by pressing on some organ of the body. In some cases a cyst may rupture with quite serious results, or again, inflammation may occur and a deep abscess appear on the site of the cyst. In a few rare instances the cyst, which is largely made up of clear fluid along with the head of the tiny worm, may dry up and gradually disappear. The commonest sites in the body for these cysts are the liver, the lungs, the brain, the kidneys, or the heart, but they may be found in any part of the body.

Treatment. There is no medical treatment which can be of any use in a case of hydatid cyst, but removal of the cyst by operation may be successfully carried out.

HYDRAGOGUE. Hydragogues are substances which have the ability of inducing the body to expel water. (*See also* DIURETIC.)

HYDROCELE. A hydrocele is a collection of fluid near the testicle, or around the spermatic cord which comes away from it. This condition may occur in infants at birth, but it is most common

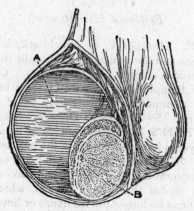

Hydrocele
A. Hydrocele; B. Testis

in middle-aged men. In the majority of cases, there is no apparent reason for this accumulation of fluid, although some cases may be due to injury, or disease of the testicle.

Symptoms. A swelling is slowly seen to form on one side of the scrotum, the bag which holds the testicles. The swelling may be rounded in shape, or pear-like, and the size depends on how much fluid is present.

Treatment. There are two courses of treatment open to a

person with this condition. Either he can have the fluid drawn off by tapping, or he can have the condition cured by an operation. Tapping is done by means of a hollow needle, and as a rule, this method of treatment has to be repeated every few months. By having a surgical operation performed, the condition can be cured so that no further fluid is able to collect and form a swelling. Any person with a tendency to hydrocele should wear a special belt which keeps the scrotum supported in a small bag, and by this means the accumulation of fluid may be lessened.

HYDROCEPHALUS. The condition of hydrocephalus, or water on the brain, occurs most frequently in children. Some cases are due to malformation before birth.

Treatment. Treatment, either medical or surgical, is usually of little avail. In some cases, small doses of thyroid extract appear to be helpful. Deep X-ray treatment has also been tried. Much depends on the cause of the condition. In some cases the condition may become arrested and the children grow up and are quite intelligent.

HYDROCHLORIC ACID. Hydrochloric acid is a strong corrosive acid produced by the gas given off when sulphuric acid is added to salt and passed through water. This acid is present in the gastric juice in small quantities. It is, therefore, of great value in the treatment of cases of indigestion due to the deficiency of gastric juice. It is also given in small quantities to increase the flow of bile in cases where dyspepsia is due to disorders of the liver.

HYDROCYANIC ACID. *See* Prussic Acid.

HYDROGEN PEROXIDE. Hydrogen peroxide when it comes in contact with the tissues of the body gives off oxygen, which accounts for its antiseptic action. Because of this action it is greatly used in the treatment of sores and inflamed wounds. When sprayed on the wound, many little gas bubbles are formed which help to remove the pus which is present. Equal parts of hydrogen peroxide and water may be dropped into discharging ears, or into an ear which has become blocked up with wax, as it helps to soften the wax and to bring away any other matter present in the ear.

Diluted with about three parts of water, it makes an excellent mouth-wash, and is very soothing to painful ulcers of the mouth.

Hydrogen peroxide has also bleaching properties which are made use of for bleaching the hair. A few drops on the tooth-brush will help to whiten the teeth, and is particularly good for removing the yellow stains which appear from too much smoking.

It is of great value in aiding the removal of dressings which have become stuck to a wound, and it is also useful in helping to stop bleeding. It can be used on the skin with perfect safety as it does not set up any irritation.

HYDRONEPHROSIS. This condition is due to a blocking in the urinary passages below the kidney which causes swelling to take place in the kidney. (*See also* DROPSY ; KIDNEY.)

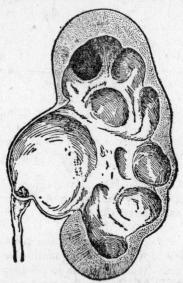

Hydronephrosis, with stone in the Ureter

HYDROPHOBIA. Hydrophobia is a very dangerous disease due to the bite of an infected or rabid dog, but other infected animals, especially wolves, may cause it. Since the enforcement of the Muzzling Order in 1897, hydrophobia has vanished from this country, although previous to that it was not uncommon. The disease is due to a germ which is present in the saliva of infected animals, and it is by means of this saliva, which is carried into the wound made by the teeth, that the disease is given to human beings.

Symptoms. The symptoms do not arise for some considerable time after the bite—usually about six weeks ; but the time may vary from ten days to six months. The wound, which has usually healed up, begins to look red and irritable, and the patient becomes very depressed and restless. In a few days the restlessness may give way to excitement and wildness. The patient finds pain and difficulty in swallowing, and the sight of water may cause violent spasms and contractions of the muscles of the throat ; hence the name hydrophobia (" fear of water "). This stage lasts about three days and the patient is usually in a very distressed condition. Finally, complete collapse and unconsciousness takes place, and death may occur within a few hours.

Treatment. When a person is bitten by a dog, no efforts should be spared thoroughly to disinfect the wound. If the dog is suspected to be rabid the police should be at once notified so that the animal may be looked after by the proper authorities. The authorities will then arrange for the bitten person to have the Pasteur treatment, or rather, a modification of the original treatment carried out by that great scientist in 1885. This treatment consists in inoculating the person daily over a period of at least fourteen days, with gradually increasing doses of the germ which causes hydrophobia until he becomes immune to the full strength of the germ. This treatment has been the means of saving thousands of lives, and there are now Pasteur Institutes in most countries of the world where treatment can be carried out.

HYDROTHERAPY. The method of treating diseases by employing the waters at a spa or " hydro " is known as hydrotherapy.

HYDROTHORAX is a condition in which clear fluid is found in the pleural cavity. (*See also* DROPSY ; PLEURISY.)

HYMEN. The hymen is a delicate membrane which partly closes the entrance to the vagina in women. The hymen is usually broken through at the first sexual intercourse, but this cannot be taken as an infallible sign that such intercourse has taken place, since in some women comparatively slight strain such as might arise in athletic pursuits will cause it to rupture.

HYOID BONE. The hyoid bone is a U-shaped bone situated in the neck above the larynx. The important muscles of the throat and tongue are attached to it and it serves as their support.

HYOSCINE. Hyoscine, or scopolamine, is a drug which resembles atropine in its action on the nerves of the body, but it is more rapid and twice as strong. It is a powerful sleep-inducing drug and it is often used to quieten persons suffering from acute mania, or delirium tremens. (*See also* ATROPINE ; HENBANE.)

HYPERACIDITY. An excess of acidity in the gastric juice is medically known as hyperacidity and hyperchlorhydria. (*See also* ACIDITY.)

HYPERÆMIA. The excessive flow of blood to, or congestion of, a part of the body is known as hyperæmia. (*See also* BLISTERING ; COUNTER-IRRITANTS.)

HYPERÆSTHESIA. When the skin is highly aware of the slightest touch, the condition is known as hyperæsthesia. This is a common symptom in many nervous diseases and in hysterical patients there are frequently patches of skin that are more sensitive than others.

HYPERCHLORHYDRIA. *See* HYPERACIDITY.

HYPERIDROSIS. Excessive sweating is technically known as hyperidrosis. In tuberculosis, night sweats are very common, or sweating may occur after the use of certain drugs. (*See also* SWEAT.)

HYPERMETROPIA. This is the technical term for what is more commonly known as long sight. (*See also* ACCOMMODATION ; ASTIGMATISM ; EYE.)

HYPERPIESIA. The condition medically termed hyperpiesia is more commonly spoken of as high blood-pressure, and is described under the heading BLOOD-PRESSURE.

HYPERPYREXIA. When the temperature reaches 105·8° F., the word hyperpyrexia is used to describe the state of excessive fever. (*See also* FEVER.)

HYPERTRICHOSIS. The growth of hair on unusual parts of the body is known as hypertrichosis. (*See also* DEPILATORY ; HAIR, SUPERFLUOUS.)

HYPERTROPHY. This word comes to us from Greek words meaning over-nourished, and the term is used to describe parts of the body which have become greatly enlarged. The muscles of an athlete generally become greatly enlarged as the result of strenuous exercise, and it is quite common for the right arm of a tennis player to be larger than the left, owing to hypertrophy of the muscles. In diseases of the kidneys it may be necessary to remove one of them, and the other usually becomes greatly enlarged because of the double amount of work which falls to its lot. Hypertrophy of the prostate gland occurs in a large percentage of men over the age of sixty, and its increase in size may obstruct the outflow of urine. Hypertrophy of the muscles of the heart may cause great enlargement of that organ. This condition occurs in the hearts of athletes, but the heart may become flabby and unhealthy if exercise is suddenly stopped, so that athletes should " tail off " with less violent pursuits. (*See also* HEART.)

HYPNOTIC. Any drug or measure which causes sleep is known as a hypnotic or soporific. An anodyne is a drug which relieves pain, whereas a hypnotic merely induces sleep. Of the drugs which act as true hypnotics the chief are chloral hydrate, chloralamide, bromides, sulphonal, trional, veronal, paraldehyde and hyoscine. Nowadays, mixtures of these with other drugs are commonly used. The narcotic drugs morphia, opium, alcohol, etc., also act as hypnotics, but they cause a feeling of excitement first.

HYPNOTISM is a condition of sleep which is artificially produced, or a trance-like state, in which the will of the person hypnotized is open to suggestions which may be made to him by the person who has produced the hypnotic state. (*See also* AUTO-SUGGESTION ; HYSTERIA.)

HYPOCHONDRIASIS is a condition of misery in which the sufferer believes that there is something wrong with his health, whereas he is, as far as medical science can discover, perfectly sound in " wind and limb." (*See also* MELANCHOLIA.)

HYPODERMIC INJECTION. The method of giving certain drugs by means of a hypodermic syringe is now largely used because of the rapidity with which the drugs are absorbed into the system, and also because the dosage can be judged with the greatest accuracy. (*See also* INJECTION.)

HYPOGASTRIUM. For convenience of description it is usual to divide the abdomen into regions. The hypogastrium or hypogastric region is the lowest part of the abdomen, lying in the middle line of the abdomen, below the umbilicus and above the private parts. It contains coils of small intestine and the beginning of the rectum. When distended the bladder may protrude into the hypogastrium, also the womb in pregnancy.

HYPOGLOSSAL NERVE. The hypoglossal nerves or twelfth cranial nerves are the nerves which work the muscles of the tongue. There are two of them and each serves one side of the tongue.

HYSTERECTOMY. The operation for the removal of the womb, which is done for various conditions, especially such as cause prolonged bleeding from the womb, and more particularly for large fibroid tumours and for cancer. (*See also* FIBROIDS ; WOMB.)

HYSTERIA is a disease, mainly of young, physically healthy women, in which there is a lack of control over acts and feelings, often accompanied by certain bodily complaints. It is important to insist that although the disease exists only in the imagination of the person affected by hysteria and although various extraordinary bodily illnesses may be imitated, yet to the sufferer these illnesses and symptoms are very real ; she is no malingerer. This point cannot be too, strongly insisted upon, because to treat a person suffering from hysteria as a malingerer, and to tell her to " pull herself together," is not only useless but harmful. The patient has no inkling of the nature of her trouble, and it is only by very careful and wise treatment by a doctor who has had special experience in dealing with hysteria that such patients can be permanently cured.

The symptoms of hysteria may be either mental or physical. The physical ones are so striking that they nearly always call attention to themselves. Sudden loss of power in one or more limbs is a very common symptom of hysteria. The patient is apparently quite helpless to walk or to feed herself. Yet the most careful examination fails to reveal any signs of disease of the structures of the nervous or muscular systems which could possibly account for such a complete paralysis.

All symptoms of hysteria are dramatic ; they ensure that attention shall be paid to the sufferer. And there is always something to be gained from the presence of a physical symptom : the unconscious memories may choose to disguise themselves by physical symptoms, but once these show themselves the patient appears perfectly happy. It might be expected that a person who had to lie in bed all day because she was unable to walk would be depressed, to say the least of it. Not so the victim of hysteria. She has gained her object in two ways and is therefore happy : her unconscious memories have translated themselves into something which the world can see and sympathize with, and she cannot be expected to face the battle and realities of life whilst she is physically incapacitated. It must be repeated that this knowledge is not possessed consciously by the hysteric ; one of the main problems of the treatment of hysteria is to get the patients to understand how their paralysis or loss of voice (another very common symptom) has come about. It is of little use to cure the symptom by suggesting that it will get well—the underlying cause for the symptom must be threshed out with the patient. A most distressing, as well as a most difficult symptom to prove that it is truly hysterical, is the fit, or convulsion indulged in frequently by the unfortunate hysteric. These convulsions mimic those of epilepsy very closely, and no one except a doctor should attempt to distinguish between the two types of fit. The body may be bent backwards and forwards and the most peculiar positions may be taken up ; the movements of the arms and legs get more and more violent, and the patient may foam at the mouth, scream, or sob. She is never really unconscious, although she will not answer when spoken to and will deny all knowledge of what has happened during the fit. But these fits never occur when the patient is alone, or when she is in any position of danger, as do true epileptic fits. They always cease on admission to hospital if curtains are placed round the bed so that there is no audience.

One of the most puzzling of all the physical symptoms of hysteria is the loss of feeling to pain, which is almost always found in this condition. The loss of feeling is either on one side of the body, and on the corresponding arm and leg, or it is found on both arms and hands, usually to the level of the elbows. The extraordinary thing about this loss of feeling is, that a patient who suffers from it will allow a large pin to be stuck right through her arm, and even to be left sticking in, whilst she declares she feels nothing at all—and to all intents and purposes she does not feel that sensation we call pain. But the most amazing feature of this loss of feeling is that it can be produced at any place on the patient's body by suggesting that she will not feel any pain if a pin is inserted in her flesh at a certain spot. And it can also be removed by suggesting that feeling has returned to that spot after a certain amount of stroking or patting, or whatever aid to his suggestion the doctor cares to use.

But hysteria may imitate in its symptoms almost any physical disease and before the diagnosis of hysteria is even thought of, the most careful examinations are necessary to prove that no disease which can be responsible for the physical symptoms of the patient is present. There is one nervous disorder which occurs in young people with which hysteria is often confused, because this disorder can, and often does, cause loss of power in one or other limb for a short time. This disorder is disseminated sclerosis, and it is specially important to avoid such a mistake occurring because the type of young person who is attacked by disseminated sclerosis is often the same type, good-looking, charming and usually plump, as shows the physical symptoms of hysteria.

It is interesting that the form of " escape " from reality which results in failures of memory with the development of a " second personality " capable of carrying on a patient's affairs is much more common in men who suffer from hysteria than in women. It must not be thought that hysteria is only seen in women : it may be present in men, especially in those who have a family history of nervous or mental trouble, and it may also occur in children, in whom isolation in a hospital ward is almost essential for any hopes of cure. In adults, the frank discussion of their mental troubles with a doctor almost invariably reveals the underlying cause of the hysterical symptoms and should result in cure. (*See also* DISSEMINATED SCLEROSIS.)

HYSTERICAL or SELF-PRODUCED DERMATITIS. This occurs in two classes of persons : malingerers, who are generally men, and hysterical patients, who are often girls in their teens or early twenties.

ICE AND ICE-BAG. In cases of fever it is sometimes necessary to give cold applications, and these can be carried out most conveniently by placing chopped ice in what is known as an *ice-bag*. The bag is made of rubber and is closed by a screw cap. As a rule a piece of flannel is placed between the bag and the skin, and in cases of emergency an ice-bag could be manufactured out of a rubber sponge-bag so long as the top was tied together with a piece of string. When there is any internal bleeding from the stomach or throat, or in cases of inflammation of the throat or mouth, small pieces of ice should be given to the patient to suck, a fresh piece being given as each bit melts. Ice sucked in this way may help to relieve vomiting, and sipping iced soda water is equally as good. Severe headache and delirium are often relieved by placing an ice-bag over the forehead. Pain is usually relieved in the abdomen or elsewhere by a cold application, and in cases where the patient is unable to bear the weight of an ice-bag on the body, the bag should be suspended from a bed-cradle. (*See also* HÆMORRHAGE.)

ICHTHYOL. Ichthyol is a brownish substance with a disagreeable smell which is obtained by distillation from a deposit of fossilized fish, in the same way that tar is obtained from fossilized trees (coal). It is used chiefly in the treatment of certain chronic skin diseases, such as dermatitis and acne. Used in conjunction with glycerine it is applied in cases of erysipelas, and also in' the treatment of inflammation of the womb. (*See also* ACNE ; DERMATITIS.)

ICHTHYOSIS. Ichthyosis, or the fish-skin disease, is so called because those suffering from it have a dry scaly skin somewhat resembling that of a fish. All varieties may be seen (the mildest fortunately being the commonest), from a mere dryness of the skin to cases where the patient is covered with " large horny masses, and the skin resembles rather that of a reptile."

Treatment. The treatment consists in supplying to the skin the fat which it so sadly lacks ; the patient should take a daily bath, and afterwards grease himself thoroughly with lanolin, almond oil, etc. A diet rich in fats is also recommended.

ICTERUS. The word icterus is just another name for jaundice, the yellow colouring of the skin and " whites " of the eye caused by the presence of bile in the blood. *Icterus neonatorum* is a form of jaundice found in newly-born babies. (*See also* JAUNDICE.)

IDIOCY is a condition of imperfect development of the brain which exists from birth, and which is so marked that the sufferers therefrom are unable to protect themselves from the common dangers of life. As long as they live they have to be looked after and protected like young children. It is difficult to train such beings to be clean in their habits, and this is one of the great trials in dealing with these unfortunates. There are many different types of idiocy, of which only two need special mention here. One is the Mongolian type, so called because they have the slanting " almond-eyes " like a Chinese. The children with this form of idiocy are often the last of a large family. These children differ from the ordinary idiots in being trainable to a certain extent. They are very fond of music, and will beat time to a rhythm and can be taught to play the simpler musical instruments. They are also very quick to imitate any actions they see, and therefore do well in institutions where they can copy those whose sole duties are to train them to make the best of their limited brain power. Mongolian idiots do not often reach adult life because they are very liable to chest troubles and have little power of resistance.

The other form of idiocy is of great interest, because it is the one form which, if taken in time, is capable of great improvement, if not of complete cure. This form is cretinism, and is now known to be due to lack of the thyroid gland. The effect of giving these children the correct treatment, which is large doses of thyroid gland by mouth, is often little short of miraculous. They lose their fatness in a remarkably short time ; they grow quickly and cease to have a dwarf-like appearance, and their mental state improves also, though the amount of improvement can never be prophesied in any particular case. In some cases the mental state becomes almost normal ; this applies particularly to those cases in which the condition has been recognized and treated at an early age. In others, the brain power never develops above that of a feeble-minded child. (*See also* CRETINISM ; MENTAL DEFICIENCY ; THYROID GLAND.)

IDIOPATHIC. Idiopathic is a word used in medicine to mean a disease or symptom, for which no cause can be recognized. It is peculiar to the disease, or to the person.

IDIOSYNCRASY. By idiosyncrasies we mean individual peculiarities of constitution or temperament. Some people are more or less violently upset by contact with ordinary substances which do no harm to the majority of their fellow human beings, as for instance, people to whom such common articles of food as milk or eggs act as a poison, bringing on one of the diseases which are now known as *allergic* diseases, i.e. hay fever, asthma, migraine and urticaria (nettle-rash), etc. These people are said to have an idiosyncrasy for the substance which harms them. It is very common for patients to have an idiosyncrasy in connection with some particular drug, as for instance, a violent headache may follow the taking of quinine, etc. (*See also* ALLERGY ; ANAPHYLAXIS.)

ILEO-CÆCAL VALVE. The last part of the small intestine before it joins on to the large intestine (colon) is called the *ileum*. The blind end of intestine called the cæcum joins on at this point, and the ileum acts as a valve at the entrance to the cæcum in so much as it allows the contents of the small intestine to flow in one direction, i.e. into the cæcum only. This is called the ileo-cæcal valve.

ILEUM. This is the name given to the lowest part of the small intestine or bowel. (*See also* INTESTINE.)

ILIAC REGION. The abdomen is spoken of as if it were divided up into compartments to simplify descriptions of symptoms, etc. The two iliac regions are the two lowest parts of the abdomen on the right and left and are so called because they lie in front of the *iliac bones*, or iliac crests as they are also called. These iliac bones are the two wing-like crests at the back of the haunch-bones. The cæcum and the appendix lie in the right *iliac fossa*, and pain is felt there when they are inflamed. Pain in the iliac fossæ in women is often due to some derangement of the female reproductive system. (*See also* ABDOMEN ; GROIN.)

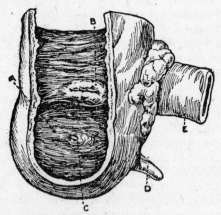

Ileo-Cæcal Valve
A. Cæcum; B. Valve; C. Opening into Appendix;
D. Appendix; E. Ileum.

ILIUM. The ilium is the haunch-bone. It is also called the innominate bone and is described fully under the heading INNOMINATE.

ILLUSION. Illusions, hallucinations and delusions are all states in which a person misinterprets facts, and believes in his misinterpretation. The three misinterpretations differ in form. Take the case of ghosts. To see a man crossing the garden path in the twilight and mistake him for a ghost is an *illusion*. To think you see a man crossing the path when there is no one there is a *hallucination*. To see a man crossing the path and *believe* that he is a ghost is a *delusion*. Illusions are harmless mentally. They are in fact merely mistakes. Hallucinations are often harmless but are sometimes signs of mental disorder, and delusions are definitely signs of mental abnormality.

IMBECILITY. A form of feeble-mindedness similar to that of idiocy, but as a rule an imbecile shows a greater degree of intelligence. (*See also* IDIOCY ; MIND.)

IMMUNITY. In the medical sense, immunity refers to the powers that certain animals and men have which make them insusceptible to various germ diseases. Animals vary in their immunity to different germ infections : the dog and the domestic fowl, for example, are quite immune to anthrax and lockjaw, that is, they never have these diseases. Even amongst different races of mankind there are great variations in disease-resisting powers : the negro races are relatively insusceptible to malaria and yellow fever, while, on the other hand, smallpox is an exceedingly fatal disease amongst them.

The normal blood contains substances which are hostile to germ life and so tend to protect against disease. Everyone knows that certain people when exposed to infection do not contract the disease. This is due to those protective qualities which constitute " natural " immunity. It is also well known that one attack of an infectious disease protects against another attack of the same disease. In such cases, an " acquired " immunity has been developed. This response on the part of the blood can be artificially produced and used to prevent possible infection. In the case of " vaccination," a mild attack of smallpox is induced and the protective powers of the blood are so stimulated by it, that immunity to smallpox is obtained. Such an acquired immunity is not permanent, hence the need for re-vaccination. Vaccine treatment is simply the injection into the blood-stream of dead germs with the object of increasing the resistive powers of the blood to these special germ infections. Vaccines are commonly used to prevent typhoid, paratyphoid and cholera.

In the body, germs produce their harmful effects by manufacturing poisons (toxins), but the blood counteracts this by producing an antidote or antibody. It is the formation of such substances which enable a person to recover from an attack of a certain disease, and it is their persistence in the blood in some quantity which gives immunity against further attacks of the same disease. It is possible to produce anti-poisons, or, as they are called, antitoxins, for diseases such as diphtheria and lockjaw and, by injecting the antitoxins into the blood of a sufferer, the disease is greatly diminished in severity. This is termed *passive* immunization as opposed to the *active* immunization of vaccine treatment. (*See also* ANTITOXIN ; BLOOD ; GERMS ; LEUCOCYTES ; SERUM.)

IMPERFORATE. The word imperforate means without an opening, and in medicine this term is most commonly used in connection with the anus. It sometimes happens that a child is born with no opening through which the contents of the bowel can be discharged, and if no action of the bowel occurs within twenty-four hours of birth, the anus should be examined and the matter can usually be put right by a simple operation. (*See also* ANUS.)

·IMPETIGO. Impetigo is a common and very easily spread skin disease, in which pustules (festering spots) appear on the face and scalp and sometimes on the other parts of the body. It is extremely catching and may run rapidly through a family or school.

Symptoms. Little red patches appear first on the skin of the face or head, which turn into watery blisters. The fluid in these blisters turns yellowish and they break, leaving yellowish scabs, surrounded by a reddish ring. As these rings may run into each other and cover large tracts of the face the condition can be most unsightly, but fortunately the scabs do not leave permanent scars.

Treatment. Impetigo is a very simple disease to treat, but the most important thing is to get treatment started quickly. Washing and shaving, or hair combing or brushing must be forbidden as the infection is so rapidly spread by these means. The only thing that can be done is to facilitate the drying up of the crusts, which is best done by the use of a good drying powder, or a lead and spirit lotion. Powders that can be used are boracic, zinc, or talcum. A preparation that combines both the lotion and powder treatment and is easy to use is a thick calamine lotion. Paint on and leave to dry, renewing at intervals. See that the child does not pick the scabs, but that they are allowed to drop off when they are ready.

Impetigo on the Scalp. Impetigo on the head is much more difficult to deal with. If the condition is very bad it may be necessary to cut off the hair in the case of a girl. If, however, there are only a few spots widely separated this will not be necessary. It will be sufficient to clip the hair short in the region of the spots. Powders and calamine lotions are not suitable for the head so a spirit lotion must be used ; one with mercury being the best. When the crusts are dry on both the face and the head they can be softened by the use of a mercury ointment and this will make them ready to come off sooner. (*See also* DERMATITIS.)

IMPOTENCE in the medical sense is used to denote lack of sexual power in the male.

INCISION. This is a term which is used in surgery. It is applied to a cut or a wound.

INCISOR. The four front teeth of each jaw are called the incisors. (*See also* TEETH.)

INCOMPATIBILITY. When substances do not mix together they are said to be incompatible.

INCONTINENCE means inability to control the passage of urine from the bladder, or fæces from the rectum (back passage). It is sometimes used to denote sexual intercourse outside marriage (the opposite of continence). Very young children up to about twelve months cannot control the bladder and rectum at will, but gradually from that time a voluntary control is established. In children and some nervous adults, a sudden fright or shock may induce the urine to be passed involuntarily, and in certain diseased states, notably those affecting the spinal cord, these symptoms may arise. The passing of urine is a reflex controlled by the mind and is dependent upon the healthy state of the nervous system.

Incontinence of fæces may occasionally occur in nervous children under strain, but in adults it may arise as a result of injury or disease of the brain or spinal cord or as a sequence to injuries or operations on the rectum. (*See also* BED-WETTING ; BLADDER, DISEASES OF ; DIARRHŒA ; ENURESIS.)

INCUBATION. The incubation period of any disease is the time which passes between the actual infection and the first appearance of its symptoms. The average incubation periods of the more important infectious diseases are as follow :

Disease		Incubation Period
Chicken-pox		10 to 16 days
Diphtheria		2 to 4 ,,
Erysipelas		1 to 3 ,,
German Measles		14 to 17 ,,
Influenza		1 to 5 ,,
Measles		10 to 14 ,,
Mumps		18 to 21 ,,
Scarlet Fever		2 to 3 ,,
Smallpox		12 to 14 ,,
Typhoid		10 to 21 ,,
Whooping Cough		10 to 14 ,,

INDIAN HEMP. *See* CANNABIS INDICA.

INDICAN. This is a substance which is present in the urine in normal people, but is increased in amount when putrefaction is going on in the bowel. Its presence in the urine in large amounts therefore means that there is marked constipation or even intestinal obstruction.

INDIGESTION. This condition may be defined as one in which discomfort, distress or pain is felt in the abdomen (belly) during or after a meal. It is also referred to as dyspepsia and it is distinguished as the commonest of all the ailments of civilization. Most commonly, indigestion is associated with actual disorder of the stomach or bowels, but dyspeptic symptoms may arise during the course of many other diseases.

Causes. Overworking of the digestive organs is one of the most frequent sources of indigestion. Constipation is inevitably associated with indigestion, and this further induces mechanical changes which handicap the whole digestive apparatus. Pain in the pit of the stomach is the familiar symptom which arises from the dyspepsia of constipation.

The food is often eaten too hastily, with the result that it is imperfectly chewed and mixed with saliva so that additional work is thus thrown upon the stomach. Upsetting the natural rhythm of the stomach by taking meals at irregular times is harmful to good digestion, as is also the bad habit of eating between meals. Tea or coffee when too strong, and when taken to excess, have an astringent and irritating effect upon the lining of the stomach, diminishing the flow of juice and causing digestive trouble. Abuse of alcoholic liquids acts in the same way. Any sepsis (or poisoning) arising from the gums, teeth, tonsils or nose, is apt to cause indigestion owing to the constant swallowing of poisonous matter. Worry and anxiety by preventing the free flow of the stomach juice readily lead to dyspepsia. One type of indigestion is associated with a functional disturbance of the stomach, i.e. there is some breakdown in the digestive mechanism without any structural defects. Too much acid or too little acid may be secreted by the stomach glands (hyperchlorhydria and hypochlorhydria.)

Another type is associated with actual disease of the stomach or duodenum, such as dilation, inflammation (gastritis), and ulceration and cancer.

Indigestion may also arise in connection with liver, gall-bladder, heart, kidney, appendix and lung disease. The diagnosis in this type is often difficult, as is also the case where mental causes, neurasthenia and hysteria, are the underlying factors.

INFANTILE CONVULSIONS. Convulsions in infants, that is, in children under the age of 2 years, must be looked upon in quite a different light from convulsions or fits in adults. They may not mean very much, or they may be of serious importance, and in any case they require the advice of a doctor. Many fevers in children, such as whooping-cough or measles, may begin with a convulsion, or they may be due to such minor ailments as teething, over-feeding, indigestion, constipation, or intestinal worms. On the other hand, convulsions may be a symptom of rickets or of some serious venous disorder. These convulsions are generally caused by some weakness of the nerve cells which may be inherited from the parents, or which may develop after birth. The children of parents who suffer from some nervous disorder such as hysteria, alcoholism, insanity, etc., are very liable to be subject to convulsions. In cases where the system becomes poisoned, for example, in diseases of the kidney, convulsions may follow as a result of the poisoning.

Excessive or unsuitable diet may induce convulsions in a healthy child. Other common causes of irritation are an adherent foreskin or obstruction to the air-way by tonsils and adenoids.

Asphyxia or severe hæmorrhage may cause such a loss of oxygen in the body that the nerve cells become weakened, and the result is seen in convulsions.

Symptoms. Typical convulsions begin with a dazed look, followed immediately by momentary pallor and dilatation of the pupils of the eyes. The head falls forward, or the child sinks to the ground and becomes unconscious. Breathing is irregular ; there is frothing at the mouth, and the contents of the bladder and bowel may be passed. The attack may be over in a few seconds, or last for hours with intermissions. They are nearly always followed by a period of more or less profound sleep.

In early infancy frequent attacks of petit mal (minor epilepsy) consisting of momentary pallor, dilatation of the pupils, drooping of the head and loss of consciousness, suggest " fainting " or heart disease rather than epilepsy. There is no difference between the symptoms of infantile convulsions and epilepsy.

The outlook, as far as life is concerned, is usually good. Convulsions themselves are rarely fatal. With regard to recurrences if there is an obvious cause, such as gross overfeeding, or intestinal inflammation, the probability is that the fits will cease if these causes are attended to. Where there is no real cause, e.g. all that can be found is a tooth which has or has not cut through the gum when expected, the probability is that the fits will recur on very slight provocation.

Treatment. As the most common cause is improper feeding, a grain of calomel or a teaspoonful of castor-oil should be given. The lower bowel should be irrigated with salt solution, or at any rate an ordinary enema given with soap and water. Hot baths, so frequently advised, are of little use, but may be soothing and relieve colic when present. Ice should be applied to the head if the temperature is raised above the normal. Rectal injections of chloral with double the amount of bromide in 2 oz. of water, for an infant of six months, are sometimes advised by the doctor ; but such drugs are, of course, only given under medical advice.

Children who suffer from fits only in consequence of emotional excitement or physical fatigue should be treated by careful attention to their mode of up-bringing, education and environment. Bromides may have to be given for two or three months, but not indefinitely. A bromide medicine is liable to bring the child out in spots. To lessen the chance of this a few drops of an arsenical solution are often added to the bromide mixture. Luminal is even more useful in controlling a convulsion which is not due to obvious over-feeding, etc. It can be given by itself as a powder, or in solution as the sodium salt. It does not produce any skin rash or spots, and does not tend to dull the mentality to the same extent that the bromides do. This drug must never be discontinued suddenly after prolonged administration, as there is the possibility of a series of successive fits intervening.

INFANTILE DIARRHŒA. This is a serious type of diarrhœa which affects young infants and which may leave them very pinched and ill. Flies play a very important part in carrying the germs of the disease, and particular care should be taken to see that the milk of hand-fed babies is stored in a cool and safe place. The condition is discussed fully under the heading DIARRHŒA.

INFANTILE PARALYSIS   (Acute Anterior Poliomyelitis). This is an acute infection of the spinal cord by a germ which causes destruction, or partial destruction, of parts of the spinal cord which helps to control the power of movement, thus causing loss of movement in a limb or limbs or other part of the body, according to which part of the spinal cord has been damaged. The disease most commonly attacks children between 1 and 3 years of age and occurs usually in August and September. It is spread by " carriers," that is to say, people who have the germ in their noses and although perfectly healthy themselves, are able to infect other people. It may occur in epidemics or in isolated cases, and it is interesting to note that when it occurs in epidemics the disease takes a much milder form and 50 per cent. of the cases make a complete recovery.

The child should be isolated for 14 days after exposure to infection.

Symptoms. The illness always comes on suddenly, after an incubation period of 4–7 days, with a slight feverish attack and vomiting and perhaps stiffness of the neck. A few hours, or perhaps a few days later it is discovered that the child is unable to move one of its limbs.

Infantile paralysis is sometimes confused with acute rheumatism, but an examination of the fluid from the spinal column during the acute stages will practically always reveal to the expert the presence of the germ.

Whether the patient will recover or not depends upon what part of the spinal cord has been damaged and to what extent. During an epidemic about one in every ten cases dies, and of the remaining nine children four are left crippled, of which some have weakness of both legs and arms, some are mentally defective, while others have a squint or perhaps permanent blindness. In those cases where the onset is most sudden the recovery is usually more complete than those cases where it is not noticed for some time that the child has partly lost the power of movement.

The greatest amount of improvement in the limb occurs within the first six months, after which it becomes very slow or ceases altogether.

Treatment. During the acute stage the child is kept in bed, lying still, as any movement of the child or the limb may make the condition much worse.

The affected limb should be supported comfortably, in order to prevent deformity such as wrist-drop or foot-drop occurring, and as soon as the pain has eased off it should be put in splints and a cradle should be rigged up over the limb to take the weight of the bed-clothes. A curved fire-guard or a three-legged stool may be used for this purpose.

Injections of serum may be given. Hexamine in small doses is useful as a disinfectant for the spinal fluid.

The nursing in these cases is of the utmost importance. The bowels should be kept freely open with mild aperients such as milk of magnesia or syrup of figs and the child should be kept on milk diet with a large amount of fluid such as water, lemonade, and barley water. When the acute stage has subsided and there is no more pain, usually three or four weeks from the beginning of the illness, the limb should be gently massaged to keep up the tone of the muscles, thus increasing the chance of recovery of the power of movement.

Electrical treatment is very helpful at this stage and the child should be encouraged to try to move the limb itself. Later on light non-inflammable celluloid splints can be applied to the limb to keep it in good position, but these must be frequently removed so that the massage and electrical treatment can be continued. Operative treatment may be necessary in the later stages from time to time to divide the contracted tissues and correct deformity in the limb. At all times during the illness the limb should be kept extra warmly covered.

INFANTILISM. This is an abnormality of development which results in a failure to grow up. The individual bears into adult life many of the physical and mental characteristics of a child. (*See also* BRAIN ; CRETIN ; DWARF.)

INFARCTION. If a part of an organ in the body is deprived of its blood supply *infarction* may occur. Each organ is supplied with blood by an artery which in the tissue subdivides or branches into numerous small vessels each controlling the nutrition of a cone-shaped piece of the organ. Should one of these branches be blocked by a small clot of blood, or a fragment of a growth on a heart valve (embolus), the conical part is deprived of blood and is called an *infarct*. This portion of tissue may die and, as it is bloodless, it is known as a *white* infarct. This is often seen in the spleen and kidney. It may happen, as in the case of the lung, that blood from neighbouring veins passes into the empty vessels and engorges them. In such instances, the term *red infarct* is applied, and if the blood is squeezed into the surrounding tissues, it is called hæmorrhagic.

INFECTIOUS DISEASES. Diseases which are capable of being transferred from one person to another are termed *infectious*. If actual contact with a diseased person is required to convey it to another, the disease may be called *contagious*. Some diseases such as anthrax, glanders and tuberculosis may be conveyed to man from infected lower animals. The infectious diseases are very numerous and include those which are popularly termed " the fevers."

Certain infectious diseases must be " notified " to the Medical Officer of Health for the district. This is usually undertaken by the doctor attending the case. The chief notifiable diseases include : scarlet fever, diphtheria, smallpox, erysipelas, typhoid, dysentery, typhus, acute lobar pneumonia, tuberculosis, cerebro-spinal fever and encephalitis lethargica. From time to time diseases such as mumps, measles and chicken-pox may be made notifiable in a particular locality.

The duration of the incubation and quarantine periods for the different infectious diseases are given under the heading INCUBA-TION. (*See also* SERUMS.)

INFLAMMATION. The reaction of animal tissues to any irritant is described as inflammation. There are four characteristic signs, viz. redness, heat, swelling and pain. Inflammation is of the nature of a defensive mechanism against injury from any cause, germ infection, chemical irritants and heat as in a burn. The lymph of the blood contains substances which are harmful to germ life, while the white cells wage warfare on the germs eating them up when possible. Sometimes, however, the fight between the germs and the white cells results in the latter being killed and in this way *pus* cells are formed and if this takes place on a large scale an *abscess* results.

Treatment. In the treatment of inflammation three points must be observed : (1) removal of the cause ; (2) rest for the inflamed part ; (3) removal of the products of inflammation. Rest will lessen pain and reduce the work of the part, so permitting it to concentrate against the enemy. Occasionally it may be possible to get rid of the offending agent at once, as when a foreign particle gets into the eye, or by washing and cleaning a dirty wound. It is possible to assist Nature by applying hot dressings (fomentations) which increase the blood supply to the part and so increase the available amount of lymph and white blood-cells. Also, hot applications tend to relieve the pain. If pus should form, it should be permitted to escape. This may necessitate incision with a knife. Chronic inflammation may follow in an acute form, or the intensity of the initial inflammation may be very slight and the resistance of the tissues low so that the inflammation process is long drawn out. (*See also* ABSCESS ; BOIL.)

INFLUENZA. This is an infectious disease, occurring in epidemic form, and from time to time ravaging the whole world. A very serious one broke out in 1918, and prior to that date, in 1889-90. It may occur at almost any time of the year, but is generally most prevalent in the colder months. It is caused by a germ or microbe, but the specific nature of this germ is still undecided. Recent research points to a filterable virus, i.e. a germ so minute that it cannot be seen by a microscope, but able to pass through a fine porcelain filter. Infection takes place when a sufferer coughs, sneezes or speaks loudly, emitting droplets of expectoration which are laden with germs. It is possible that handkerchiefs and clothes harbour the germs and act as distributing agents.

The symptoms of this disease are many and varied, and may show themselves in all the systems of the body. After invasion with the germs, there is a short incubation period of from one to four days and the onset is sudden and marked by shivering, rise of temperature, headache, sickness, vague muscular pains and a feeling of exhaustion. The throat may be sore and there is often a dry irritating cough. Three main types of influenza occur : respiratory, gastro-intestinal, and nervous. In the first, bronchitis, pleurisy and pneumonia may arise ; in the second, there is catarrh or inflammation of the stomach and intestine, with sickness and diarrhœa, pain in the belly and sometimes jaundice ; in the third and nervous type, headache is very severe ; there may be an excessively high temperature and occasionally meningitis may arise. Influenza thus shows considerable variation in type, and in different epidemics one or other of the types tends to predominate.

As a rule, the course of the disease is short, lasting from three to five days, but complications are very apt to arise and delay con-valescence. Bronchitis may persist for some weeks and not infre-quently develops into broncho-pneumonia (a patchy inflammation of the lungs). In all forms of the disease, heart symptoms are common and constitute one of the major dangers of influenza. Inflamma-tion of the middle ear is not uncommon as a sequel to influenza and occasionally the infection may spread to the brain and spinal cord. One of the most troublesome symptoms of the aftermath of influenza is mental depression which may even amount to an attack of melancholia. Even in mild cases of influenza a degree of prostration occurs which seems to be out of proportion to the severity of the symptoms and may leave behind an enfeeblement of the general health which may take some months or even years to overcome.

Treatment and Prevention. The patient should be isolated and precautions taken to avoid spread of infection. Even the mildest cases should be treated in bed, as this lessens the chances of com-plications arising. The room should be very airy—as fresh air is the best preventive against spreading influenza throughout a house-hold. The diet should be light : milk, beaten-up eggs, beef tea and fruit juices. If the throat is sore, an inhalation of Friar's balsam will be of benefit, and if there is tightness of the chest a linseed poultice will relieve the discomfort. Aspirin is the drug generally used in the treatment of influenza. It is given in ten-grain doses, every four hours, during the acute stage of the illness. During convalescence, a tonic such as Easton's syrup is helpful in restoring appetite and energy, and if possible a change of air to the hills or seaside is very desirable. To avoid influenza during an epidemic endeavour to live as much as possible in the open air. Keep away from warm crowded rooms, theatres, etc. The diet should be generous, containing plenty of raw fruit, green vegetables and dairy produce. Every effort must be made to prevent any tendency to constipation. It may lessen the risk if the throat is sprayed or gargled every morning with a weak solution of Condy's fluid. Mixed vaccines to stimulate immunity against influenza are now available and in many cases have proved of value.

INGROWING TOE-NAIL. This is a condition in which the outer edge of the big toe-nail presses into the flesh and causes a very tender spot to appear. Badly-fitting shoes are very often the cause of this painful condition, but probably the chief cause is cutting the nail in the wrong fashion. The nail of the big toe should be flat and should never be cut too short. The outer edges should never be trimmed down at the sides as this induces the nail to curve instead of remaining perfectly flat ; in fact, it is better to cut the nail lower at the centre. Trimming the nail in this way will help to avoid the condition.

INHALATION. Inhalation is a method of treatment in which drugs can be taken into the body by the breath. In this way general anæsthesia is usually carried out by means of a special inhaling apparatus. Steam inhalation is perhaps the most popular form of this type of treatment. It is used especially in cases of bronchitis and in inflammatory conditions of the nose and throat. A very simple way of carrying out this treatment is to fill a jug with boiling water into which has been placed a teaspoonful of Friar's balsam or any other soothing volatile oil. The head is covered with a towel and held over the jug so that the fumes from the jug are not allowed to escape. The patient should breathe through the mouth as well as the nose in order to allow the soothing fumes to reach the mucous membranes of these parts. (*See also* ASTHMA ; ATOMIZER ; BRON-CHITIS.)

INJECTION. Medicinal remedies in solution are sometimes administered by forcing them into the tissues of the body from a syringe fitted with a hollow needle.

An injection may be intradermal, i.e. into the skin, this method being used for producing local anæsthesia or insensitiveness to pain. The most usual way for administration of drugs is hypodermically, i.e. under the skin. Some drugs are liable to irritate the skin (mercury and quinine), and these are given intramuscularly, i.e. deeply into a muscle usually of the thigh. Intravenous injection, directly into the blood-stream, can be accomplished through a vein, usually one of the surface veins of the arm at the elbow. This is the most rapid way of obtaining the action of a drug. Injections may be made into the spinal canal in order to secure insensitiveness to pain for operation purposes. An injection into the bowel is called an enema, while injections into the nose or vagina are termed douches. (*See also* DOUCHE ; ENEMA ; HYPO-DERMIC INJECTION.)

INNOMINATE. This word means unnamed, and it is strange that it should be applied to a number of important structures, the innominate bone, the innominate artery and innominate veins.

The innominate *bone* or haunch-bone is large and irregular in shape and really consists of three bones : the ilium above, the ischium behind and the pubis in front.

The innominate *artery* is one of the largest in the body. It comes directly from the main arterial stem (the aorta) on the right side and it breaks up into two branches, the right common carotid and the right subclavian arteries which supply with blood the right

side of the head and the right upper limb respectively. The innominate artery lies close behind the highest part of the breastbone,
behind, it is closely related to the windpipe and the right lung
comes in contact with it.

The innominate *veins* are two in number, the right and the left,
each receiving the blood from its own side of the head and neck,
and the corresponding upper limb. They are short wide vessels
which soon unite to form the superior vena cava which carries
the blood to the right auricle of the heart.

INOCULATION. This is the operation by which disease
germs, dead or greatly reduced in virulence, are introduced into
the body through injection under the skin. A considerable number
of diseases are prevented and treated by this method of inoculation.
The most important of these are smallpox, typhoid, para-typhoid,
rabies, dysentery, tuberculosis, and common septic infections such
as boils, acne and catarrh of the nose. (*See also* Antibody ; Antitoxin ; Serums.)

INQUEST. If there is any reason to suspect that a person has
died a violent or unnatural death, the circumstances must be investigated and the matter made the subject of a formal inquiry.
The inquest, as it is called, is conducted by the coroner, with or
without a jury, this being left to his discretion.

INSANITY. Strictly speaking, this is a legal term denoting
the civil state in which an individual is unable to look after himself
or others, and is a menace to society. It signifies that liberty must
be restricted and a certain degree of legalized control must be
exercised. In such a state of mind a person requires to be " certi-
fied," and this implies detention for the purposes of care and treatment in a mental hospital.

There are a great many types of insanity and a great many
causes. In about 40 to 50 per cent. of cases, an unstable mind is
inherited, but in a very considerable proportion of cases external
factors, such as alcohol, syphilis, childbirth, physical exhaustion,
hardened arteries, severe fevers, brain tumours and injury, diabetes
and prolonged mental stress, are the direct causes of the mental
symptoms. Some forms of insanity are associated with great depression and impulses to suicide, others with excitement and violence.
In one type, there is tendency to a gradual breaking up of the
mind (schizophrenia or dementia præcox), while in another, delusions of persecution are the chief symptom. Confusional mental
disorders, or insanity, are generally due to some variety of brain
poisoning.

Contrary to popular opinion, a great deal can be done for the
insane by scientific methods of treatment. The modern mental

hospital is very different from the asylums of last century. It is no longer merely a place of detention : its organization promotes the alleviation and, in many cases, the cure of the mentally sick. (*See also* MENTAL DEFICIENCY ; MENTAL DISEASE.)

INSECT BITES. This subject is dealt with fully under the heading BITES AND STINGS.

INSECTS. *See* BED-BUGS ; MOSQUITO.

INSOMNIA. Sleeplessness or insomnia is a symptom of disturbed working of the mind or body. It is, in itself, very dangerous to health, particularly in the case of growing children who suffer stunting in mind and body as a result. Among the common causes which may initiate sleeplessness are lack of fresh air from bad ventilation of the bedroom, insufficient exercise, heavy meals before retiring, late hours and mental work carried beyond the stage of weariness. With sensitive people, a strange bedroom, unaccustomed sounds or lights, a pillow of unusual height, an uncomfortable mattress or too heavy bed-clothes are liable to make falling asleep difficult. Bodily ill-health, particularly when associated with pain, and notably in heart or chest complaints, frequently hinders sleep, while mental ill-health ranks as a chief cause of insomnia. Worry or apprehension are formidable enemies of sleep for they tend to reach their highest pitch at bedtime.

Sufferers from persistent insomnia are apt quickly to reach the stage when they despair of ever again enjoying a good night's sleep. This hopeless attitude is very natural, but it must be fought against. The first step is to convince the mind that the disability is remediable. That accomplished, the sufferer should examine his habits of life and try to discover the cause or causes of the insomnia. Provided there is no physical disease requiring medical attention, there are certain measures which if persevered in will eventually restore the sleep rhythm.

Sufferers from insomnia should spend the hours before retirement in some unexciting pastime and go to bed at approximately the same time every night, as habit plays a large part in the function of sleep. Late meals are taboo, as also strong coffee or tea, but a glass of warm milk is soothing and promotes drowsiness. The bedroom must be well ventilated without being cold, and the bed comfortable with light but warm bed-clothing. The body should be warm before retiring. Cold feet are a common cause of sleeplessness, therefore a hot-water bottle may be necessary. A warm bath is often valuable as it promotes relaxation of the muscles.

When in bed, it is best not to anticipate a bad night or think deliberately about getting off to sleep. The sufferer should concern himself only in making himself thoroughly comfortable and should try to *stop* thinking. A word of warning. It is most inadvisable for anyone to have recourse to sleep-producing medicines except under the personal direction of the doctor. Such drugs are dangerous when wrongly used and are seldom necessary if natural means to sleep are fully tried. (*See also* SLEEP.)

INSUFFLATION. The introduction of powdered drugs into the nose, throat or ear is called insufflation and the apparatus, which simply consists of a rubber ball attached to a vulcanite tube, is termed an insufflator.

INSULIN. In the pancreas, one of the digestive glands in the abdomen, are groups of cells called the islets of Langerhans which produce an internal secretion (i.e. passed directly into the blood-stream), called insulin. This substance is necessary for the utilization of sugar by the body and its absence or deficiency leads to diabetes mellitus. Insulin was only discovered in 1922 by Banting of Toronto, and it is now prepared commercially and used extensively in the treatment of diabetes. Since its introduction the mortality caused by diabetes has lessened by one-half. It is generally given by injection under the skin and the doses must be carefully controlled according to the amount of sugar in the blood. Insulin is particularly valuable in the treatment of diabetic coma. (*See also* DIABETES ; DUCTLESS GLANDS ; PANCREAS.)

INTERCOSTAL. This name is applied to the nerves, muscles and vessels which lie between the ribs. The space between each rib is also known as the intercostal space.

INTERMITTENT CLAUDICATION. This condition, sometimes called intermittent limp, consists of numbness, tingling, pain and cramp in the muscles of the leg. It comes on after walking and leads to a limping gait or it may cause complete inability to walk. As a rule the condition subsides rapidly, but tends to return after further walking. This affection is often associated with hardening and thickening of the arteries (arterio-sclerosis) and is caused by a spasm of the narrowed arteries depriving the muscles of their blood supply. (*See also* ARTERIO-SCLEROSIS ; DEGENERATION.)

INTERMITTENT FEVER. There are many diseases in which periods of fever are present, for example, in cases of malaria, or in the later stages of tuberculosis ; on the other hand, the fever may be more or less continuous with short periods in which the temperature returns to normal. Such a condition is referred to as intermittent fever.

INTESTINAL STASIS. This term is applied to the stagnation of the contents of the bowel and is most commonly used in connection with constipation. (*See also* AUTO-INTOXICATION ; CONSTIPATION.)

INTESTINE. The intestine or bowel is that part of the digestive system which extends from the outlet of the stomach to the anus and it is approximately twenty-five feet in length. It is suspended in the cavity of the abdomen, or belly, by folds of tissue called the mesentery. The intestine is divided into two parts, the small and the large. The former extends from the stomach to the junction with the latter at the cæcum, a pouched portion of the large intestine to which the appendix is attached.

INTOXICATION. This term is applied to any form of body poisoning. The poisons may be taken by the mouth, e.g. alcohol, morphia, cocaine or hashish, or the poisons may be derived from the body as in the case of intestinal intoxication from constipation, or thyroid intoxication from excessive activity of the thyroid gland.

Alcoholic intoxication produces well-known symptoms and if very intense may lead to coma (unconsciousness). The respiratory and heart centres are depressed and this may lead to fatal results in some cases.

Treatment. Treatment should aim at emptying the stomach either by an emetic (mustard and water) or by the use of the stomach tube. Then, a hot stimulating drink of coffee should be given and the patient kept warm with hot blankets and bottles.

INTUSSUSCEPTION. This condition consists of the passage of a part of the bowel into the adjoining part : it is as if one part was telescoped into the adjacent part. Most often this takes place at the junction of the small intestine (bowel) with the cæcum.

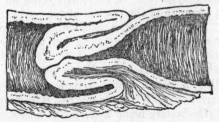

Intussusception

The end of the small intestine normally projects into the beginning of the cæcum, and, in the state of intussusception, this portion travels along the interior of the large bowel—sometimes for a considerable distance, occasionally as far as the anus.

Intussusception occurs most commonly in young children under twelve months. It arises most probably from the presence of some irritant in the food. This calls forth violent expulsive movements of the bowel and so carries the end of the small intestine into the cæcum. The outstanding symptoms are vomiting, prostration and the passage from the bowel of a little blood-stained jelly-like substance.

Treatment. An immediate operation is necessary to save the life of the child, but if medical aid is not immediately forthcoming, an enema of warm water will be beneficial.

A chronic form of intussusception occurs in adults, often associated with a bowel tumour. The symptoms are not so urgent but there is some danger of obstruction of the bowels. Treatment is by surgical operation. (*See also* INTESTINES.)

IODINE. Weak tincture of iodine is most often used as an antiseptic in cases of wounds of the skin when it is painted on. It is sometimes used to prepare the skin prior to a surgical operation. The strong tincture is used as a counter-irritant, i.e. to produce a surface irritation. on some deep-seated inflammatory process. If the skin is at all sensitive it will produce blistering, so that it must be used with caution. It should be remembered that the use of iodine for the treatment of cuts and abrasions does not exclude the need for thorough cleansing of the wound first of all with clean water.

Iodine is sometimes used in ointment form for the treatment of skin affections—and for rubbing over rheumatic joints and muscles. The weak tincture in very small doses, 2 to 5 minims, may be used internally to relieve vomiting and nausea. It is also used in the treatment of rheumatoid arthritis.

Iodine is normally present in the body, being an essential constituent of the secretion of the thyroid gland.

Poisoning. If the tincture is accidentally swallowed, give an emetic (salt or mustard and water), and then thin starch, arrowroot or bread freely.

Iodized Salt. At table, salt containing a small amount of potassium iodide, a salt of iodide, is now available, and it is of benefit in a certain type of simple goitre. It is believed that this form of goitre (Derbyshire neck) is related to a deficiency of iodine in the drinking water.

Iodism. If iodine or iodides are given in excess they may produce symptoms known as iodism. The eyes and nose run freely, the saliva is increased ; there is dull headache and sometimes depression. Treatment is obvious : stop the administration of the iodine preparation.

IODOFORM. This substance, made from alcohol, iodine and carbonate of potassium, is generally available as a lemon-yellow crystalline powder. It has a distinctive odour not unlike strong seaweed and it is nearly insoluble in water but dissolves in ether. It contains

90% of iodine. Iodoform is used as a local antiseptic, for it liberates iodine on contact with the tissues. It is used for dusting septic wounds and sores, ulcers and abscess cavities. Care has to be taken not to apply iodoform to large raw surfaces or poisonous symptoms may arise. It is often employed as a surgical dressing when it is applied to gauze. A paste made up of bismuth, iodoform and liquid paraffin is used for packing abscess cavities : this is commonly referred to as B.I.P.P.

IONIZATION. Ionization or ionic medication is an electric treatment from which great things were hoped when it was introduced first. It aims at depositing curative drugs in the tissues by means of an electric current. This method of treatment has proved valuable in many cases, but has not proved the cure-all it was thought it might.

IPECACUANHA. This is the dried root of a Brazilian plant. The drug stimulates expectoration, but in large doses is emetic, i.e. causes vomiting. Ipecacuanha has also some action in producing sweating. The drug, in various preparations, is largely used in the treatment of bronchitis and other diseases of the respiratory system. It may be used as tincture of ipecacuanha, or as compound ipecacuanha powder (Dover's Powder). Ipecacuanha is very useful when the bronchial tubes are filled with secretion. It stimulates coughing and rids the tubes of the accumulated secretion.

Emetine, the alkaloid of ipecacuanha, is used in the treatment of amœbic dysentery. A considerable care has to be exercised in treatment with emetine as it has a harmful effect upon the liver and kidneys. Emetine is also used as an emetic in the treatment of poisoning when it becomes necessary to empty the stomach rapidly.

IRIS. The coloured part of the eye is known as the iris and it surrounds the black centre part of the eye known as the pupil. Its purpose is to regulate the amount of light which enters the eye. (*See also* EYE.)

IRON. This metallic element is normally found in the body, chiefly in the red pigment or hæmoglobin of the blood. It is the iron pigment which enables the blood to absorb and carry oxygen to the cells of the body. Iron is primarily obtained by the body from the vegetable kingdom and, as there is a small but constant destruction and excretion of this element, it is essential that the stock should be replenished regularly by eating iron-containing food.

Iron deficiency may lead to a form of anæmia, most often observed in young girls living under unhygienic conditions, which is called chlorosis. In such cases prolonged administration of iron in medicinal form (as well as by eating foods rich in iron) is necessary, as all the tissues have been disorganized by its lack.

Iron can be given in a great variety of ways medicinally. One of the most popular and useful is in the form of Blaud's Pills, which are not proprietary articles, but the name given to an old formula. These are given in 5–15 grain doses twice or thrice daily after meals. As iron is astringent, it may be necessary to give some aperient at the same time. Iron preparations may not agree with certain people, causing upset of digestion, and occasionally it may be necessary to give the iron by hypodermic injection. Apart from anæmia, states of exhaustion, or convalescence after feverish diseases, or nervous break-downs, will benefit from iron combined with some stimulating drug such as strychnine.

Certain natural mineral waters contain iron, notably those from Buxton, Trefriw and Marienbad. They are termed *chalybeate* waters.

IRRIGATION. Irrigation of the bowel, more popularly known as the *Plombières douche*, is carried out in the treatment of mild types of dysentery and colitis (inflammation of the colon). A rubber tube is inserted into the rectum and several pints of fluid are slowly allowed to run in. Various types of antiseptics may be given, but as a rule, what is known as a normal saline solution is used for this purpose. *Irrigation of the stomach* is carried out in the treatment of duodenal or gastric ulcers. Irrigation is also a valuable means of cleansing cavities such as the vagina, etc. This is done by means of a douche ; but irrigation of the womb, which is a much more serious affair, can only be carried out by a doctor. Irrigation is also a valuable way of removing pus, etc., from a septic wound. (*See also* DOUCHE ; ENEMA.)

"ITCH, THE " (Scabies). The itch, or scabies, is an infectious disease of the skin produced by the Acarus scabiei, an insect just visible to the naked eye. It lives upon the skin, and the female burrows into it to deposit her eggs. At the point of entrance is a tiny blister, and from this a greyish line or burrow is seen. The parts generally affected are the skin between the fingers, the front of the fore-arms and elbows, the arm-pits, the nipples, the lower part of the abdomen, the genitals, and the buttocks. The face seldom suffers. In infants, the whole body, including the scalp, may be affected.

In adults, the eruption is very varied, according to the degree of personal cleanliness. If a person who has contracted the disease accidentally, baths daily, and has frequent changes of clothing, a few pimples only will be seen, and the sole complaint will be the itching. On the other hand, in the uncleanly, on whose skin not only the acarus, but other parasites find a happy undisturbed home, the eruption may be very widespread, with boils, dermatitis, etc.

Treatment. Sulphur is the great stand-by in treatment. A usual method of treatment is for the patient to have a hot bath, in which he soaks for 30 minutes, meanwhile scrubbing himself vigorously with a nail-brush and soap. Then he should dry himself and anoint the whole of his body from the neck downwards with sulphur ointment. For effectual treatment, an adult needs 1 lb. of ointment ; it is a very common mistake to find too little being used. He should finish by " washing " the hands well with the ointment. He then puts on old clean night-clothes, gloves, and socks, and goes to bed in an uninfected bedroom. This procedure is repeated 5 times at intervals of 12 hours ; in the meantime the patient's clothes, bedding, etc., are thoroughly disinfected. At the end of this time the patient will be cured.

In the cleanly, a hot bath every night, and the use of sulphur soap will generally cure in 3 or 4 days.

In severe cases, and especially in children, sulphur must be used with caution, or B-naphthal ointment substituted. Stavesacre, styrax, and Balsam of Peru are also employed in special cases.

ITCHING. For itching symptoms due to general causes *see* PRURITUS, *also* PRURIGO.

JACKSONIAN EPILEPSY. Described by John Hughlings Jackson, an English physician who was born in 1834 and died in 1911, this is a form of epilepsy in which the spasm is limited to a single group of muscles in the face, arm, or leg, but may also involve other groups of muscles. (*See also* EPILEPSY.)

JAIL FEVER. The outbreaks of typhus fever were at one time so common in jails that it became known as jail fever. (*See also* TYPHUS.)

JAUNDICE. Jaundice is due to the presence of bile in the blood which causes the skin to turn yellowish in colour. There are many different causes of this condition, and naturally the symptoms vary in accordance with the cause. The commonest form is that known as *catarrhal jaundice*, due to an inflammation or catarrh of the bile-duct which prevents the flow of bile from the liver and gall-bladder into the intestine. This inflammation, it has been found, usually begins in the duodenum, or first part of the small intestine, then spreads to the bile-duct where it causes an obstruction. Jaundice may also occur in almost any general fever, or it may result from obstruction caused by the passage down the bile-duct of gall-stones.

Symptoms. Catarrhal jaundice may result from exposure to chill, or possibly as a result of overwork and strain. There may be a feeling of nausea and depression for a few days and the skin may feel irritable and itchy. The whites of the eyes are yellow, and the skin also is bright yellow. The tongue is furred and the temperature may be raised to 99° or 100° F. The part of the body over the liver and gall-bladder may feel very tender to the touch. The urine is dark in colour, and the motions are rather offensive, large, and pale, or putty-coloured. The jaundice generally takes about two or three weeks to disappear and as a rule the skin gradually regains its normal colour.

Treatment. The patient should be kept in bed until the colouring matter has disappeared from the urine. The bowels should be kept open with salts and, if necessary, an enema should be given. The diet should have very little fat in it, in fact, it would be better to exclude fat altogether. Liquid, or semi-solid, food should be given, such as barley-water, meat extracts, toast and rusks, and about half-a-pint of milk daily. If the skin is very irritable it should be bathed with a weak solution of carbolic acid or bicarbonate of soda.

Obstructive Jaundice. Obstructions which may bring on symptoms of jaundice include gall-stones, a tumour or cancer arising in the gall-bladder, the presence of round worms, or a hydatid cyst. Obstruction may also be caused by pressure on the bile-duct owing to enlarged glands or a growth in any of the surrounding organs.

Infantile Jaundice. Jaundice is very often seen in new-born infants, appearing during the first two days of life. Mild cases may be regarded as a practically normal occurrence, and it clears up after a week or two without any treatment whatever. More severe types may be due to absence of the bile-duct, or some other form of obstruction, and the outlook may be very serious indeed. (*See also* GALL-BLADDER, DISEASES OF.)

JAW. The jaws or jawbones are two sturdy bones of the face into which the teeth are fitted. Of the two jaws the lower is by far the stronger—and it is a much harder task to extract the teeth from it. The lower jawbone is angular in shape and fits into the temporal bone at a point in front of the ear, forming a hinge joint. The upper jaw is altogether a slighter one, and is composed of two bones which are firmly attached to the other bones of the upper part of the face. The teeth fit firmly into sockets in the two jaws which are called *alveoli*.

Dislocations of the jaw are of fairly frequent occurrence but can be easily replaced. Between the ends of the two jaws are little pads of cartilage each of which is called a meniscus. These serve as shock absorbers and to relieve the wear and tear of friction between the two jaws. These menisci sometimes get jerked out of place, causing great pain until they are replaced.

JEJUNUM. This is the name given to the middle portion of the small intestine.

JIGGER. The jigger-flea is also known as the chigoe, or sand-flea, and it is found chiefly in tropical countries. The female burrows under the skin, especially between the toes and under the soles of the feet, to lay her eggs. When the eggs become hatched out, they produce a severe irritation which may proceed to serious ulceration and inflammation.

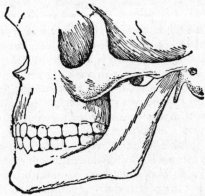

Upper and Lower Jaws

JOINTS. Joints or articulations in the body are formed when two bones or cartilages meet. The joints of the body are divided into two groups : the fixed joints which have no power of movement, and the movable joints.

Fixed joints are those like the joints between the bones of the skull and the vertebræ of the spine, where there is a layer of cartilage between the two bones, binding them together, but not permitting movement to any noticeable extent. In the spine the result of a long series of little bones with flexible cartilage joints between them is to make the whole spine slightly flexible, but this is not true movement.

Movable Joints. To make up a movable joint four different structures are necessary : the two bones, the layer of cartilage which covers the end of each bone, a capsule of fibrous tissue which holds the bones together and, lastly, the lubricating fluid—called *synovial fluid*—which oils the movements of the joint.

Varieties of Joints. Movable joints are divided into groups according to their range of movement. The most freely movable joint is the *ball and socket*, like the hip or shoulder in which one bone has a rounded head like a ball which fits snugly into a cup-shaped socket in the other bone, and allows movement in every direction. Joints in which the movement is mainly in one direction, as in the wrist and ankle, are called *gliding joints*. *Hinge joints*, which include the knee and the elbow, move chiefly round one axis like a hinge.

JUGULAR VEIN. There are three large veins on each side of the neck, known as the anterior, external and internal jugular veins.

JUICE. Any of the fluids produced by organs of the body may be referred to as juice. For example, gastric juice is made by the stomach and it contains ferments which are necessary to the proper digestion of protein food and the clotting of milk. Intestinal juice contains ferments which deal with the digestion of carbohydrate foods ; while pancreatic juice, by means of its ferments, assists in the digestion of starches and fats. The three types of foodstuffs, carbohydrates, proteins, and fats, are all dealt with and digested in the course of their journey from the mouth. (*See also* DIGESTION ; FERMENTS.)

JUNKET. Junket is milk which has been acted upon by rennet so that it forms a soft curd which is much more easily digested than plain milk. It also lends itself to delicate flavouring so that an invalid does not tire of it as easily as of milk. It is thus an excellent food for invalids and patients who are on a milk diet as, for example, after a gastric ulcer. (*See also* CASEIN ; CURDS.)

KALA-AZAR. Kala-azar is a disease in which the chief symptoms are enlargement of the spleen, wasting, and intermittent fever. The infection is due to a very tiny parasite which is transmitted to human beings by the bite of a sand-fly. The condition seems to flourish in warm, moist climates, especially in parts of India, China and West Africa. Infantile kala-azar is found along the shores of the Mediterranean.

Treatment. The death-rate has been greatly lowered by injections of sodium antimony tartrate solution in freshly prepared sterile water. An untreated case may go on for as long as two years, when death usually takes place from wasting and weakness, or some septic complication.

KAOLIN. Kaolin is also known as china-clay or white clay. It consists mainly of a natural silicate of aluminium which is powdered and freed from gritty particles. It is sometimes used as a protective application in cases of eczema or other skin diseases and it is also used as an ingredient of the modern type of poultice like antiphlogistine. Internally it is an excellent remedy, mixed with water, for diarrhœa, food poisoning and dysentery, one or two tablespoonfuls taken every hour until the symptoms abate.

KELOID. An overgrowth of tissue, usually occurring at the site of a scar, is known as a keloid. The scar does not shrink in the ordinary way but tends to remain raised up, and the surrounding tissue becomes wrinkled.

KERATITIS. Inflammation of the part of the eye known as the cornea is termed keratitis or interstitial keratitis. (*See also* CORNEA.)

KERATOSIS. The term keratosis is used to denote any overgrowth of the horny layer of the skin. Ordinary corns or callosities may be looked upon as an exaggerated example of this condition. Keratosis senilis is the term applied to the roughening of the skin which occurs in elderly people. (*See also* CALLUS; CORN; SKIN.)

KIDNEYS. The kidneys are a pair of glands placed in the back of the abdomen just below the waist-line on either side. Their function is to collect certain waste materials from the blood and the spare water from the tissues in the form of urine. The urine is then passed by the kidneys by way of the two tubes called the ureters to the bladder and thence by the urethra to the exterior. It is obvious, therefore, that the kidneys must be kept in good working order if the body is not to be poisoned with waste materials.

The kidneys are usually described as bean-shaped, being slightly narrower in the middle with bulging ends, much the same shape as a bean. At the upper portion of each kidney a small gland called the *suprarenal* gland or *adrenal* is attached. These are ductless glands and are of great importance in the correct working of the body. (*See also* DUCTLESS GLANDS.)

Displaced and Floating Kidney. One or both kidneys may become displaced from their normal position, usually as a result of general laxness of the front wall of the abdomen in women who have had several pregnancies. As a general rule the condition causes no inconvenience. Sometimes there is a kidney which is insecurely attached to the neighbouring organs and sudden acute pain with perhaps sickness and faintness may occur from time to time owing to its sudden displacement.

Treatment. Often it is sufficient to change the position and the pain passes off; or, if it is very troublesome, an operation may be performed to fix it. A great deal of unnecessary fuss is made by young nervous people about these so-called floating kidneys. The best cure for them is to fatten up, so that the pads of fat may keep the kidneys more securely anchored.

Kidney Diseases. Perhaps the most common disease of the kidneys is the chronic inflammation known as Bright's Disease or Nephritis. This is described under its own heading. The kidneys

are very subject to *stones* or calculi. The presence of a stone may
pass unnoticed until it begins to move and pass towards the bladder,
when there may be attacks of excruciating pain as it passes down
the narrow ureter. The remedy is to have the stone removed by
operation if it does not pass naturally. Where there is any tendency
to kidney troubles the kidneys should be kept well flushed by means
of drinking copious draughts of water between meals ; but it should
be ascertained, as well, whether the water of the district is suitable
for kidney cases. In some neighbourhoods kidney trouble is much
more common than in others and it is customary to blame the water
for the increased number of people who suffer from " stone."

Tuberculosis may affect the kidneys and if one only is affected
it may be removed with benefit to the patient. Tumours and
cancer also affect the kidneys. (*See also* CALCULUS ; NEPHRITIS.)

KING'S EVIL. This term was used a great deal in the olden
days in connection with the disease known as scrofula, in which
the lymphatic glands of the neck became enlarged. It is now considered to be a form of tuberculosis. The term king's evil arose

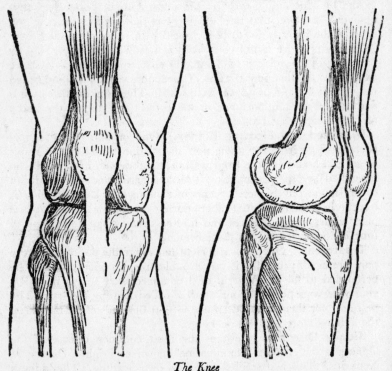

The Knee

from a superstition that the disease was supposed to be curable by the touch of the king's hand.

KLEPTOMANIA. This is the name given to a mental state in which the patient is unable to resist the temptation of stealing things. Very often the articles which are stolen are of very little value and in this way the condition differs from the mental state which drives some people, especially collectors, to possess certain objects.

The treatment of kleptomania lies in a mental analysis of the individual; and the modern treatment by psycho-analysis may do much to bring to light the underlying motives which cause the impulse to steal. (*See also* PSYCHO-ANALYSIS.)

KNEE. The knee-joint is the joint between the upper and lower bones of the leg, that is, the thigh-bone or femur, and the shin-bone or tibia. The other and smaller bone of the leg, the fibula, does

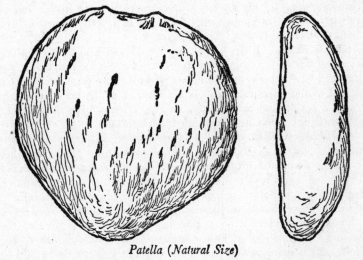

Patella (Natural Size)

not come into the joint but becomes associated with the shin-bone at a point lower than the knee.

Unlike other joints the bones that are connected by the knee-joint are not fitted into each other. The thigh-bone has two knobs which rest on flat places on the end of the shin-bone. Cartilage covers the ends of the bones and there is a large pad of fat in front of the joint and a small plate of bone called the knee-cap or *patella*. Between the knee and the smaller leg bone, the tibia, there are two pads of cartilage called, from their shape, the *semilunar cartilages*. The strength of the joint depends very largely upon the firm binding of muscular tissues and the strong ligaments. Behind the knee the muscles of the leg, coming down the thigh and up the leg, leave a small diamond-shaped space between them called the *popliteal* space.

Diseases and injuries of the knee. The knee is the most complicated joint in the body and it is very difficult to get at it for treatment purposes. As the knee is essential in our movements of walking and sitting it is obvious that a small injury to it may cause a large amount of disability. The joint may become infected with germs whose rapid spread may cause very serious illness. The diseases that affect other joints of the body also affect the knee joint. These are found under their own headings, such as ARTHRITIS ; SYNOVITIS ; TUBERCULOUS SWELLING.

Injury to the semi-lunar cartilage causes a great deal of pain and temporary disablement. It is a very common thing for the semi-lunar cartilages to be dislocated in games such as football. The knee-cap, too, is readily dislocated, but total dislocation of the knee is very rare and is only the result of great violence.

Housemaid's Knee. *See* BURSITIS.

KNEE JERK. If the knees are crossed and a light tap is given with the tips of the fingers on the front of the knee just below the knee-cap, the leg is seen to make a sudden jump forward. This is known as the knee jerk. In certain diseases of the nervous system this action does not occur, and it is very often of great importance to the doctor when he is making his diagnosis.

KNOCK KNEE. This is a deformity of the lower limbs medically known as *genu valgum*. When the feet are placed together it will be found that the space separating the ankles is abnormally wide, and as a result the knees knock together when walking. Sometimes the inner part of one knee may be more prominent than the other, but as a rule both knees are affected.

Treatment. In young children the treatment is, firstly, the general treatment for rickets. Massage and manipulation of the limbs will help to straighten them out, but this is only helpful in very young children whose bones have not yet hardened. In more advanced cases splints may be worn, or a special boot with walking irons may be found beneficial. In very severe advanced cases, operative treatment is the only means of straightening out the limbs. (*See also* KNEE.)

KNUCKLE. The knuckles of the hands are the joints which connect the hand with the fingers. When the fist is closed, the knuckles of the four fingers can be seen to stand out very prominently, but the knuckle of the thumb never shows up to any great extent. In babies, a row of dimples usually replaces the knuckles. (*See also* FINGERS ; HAND.)

KOCH'S BACILLUS. Robert Koch, a German bacteriologist (1843–1910), was the first to discover the germ which causes tuberculosis. After years of patient research work he found that tiny rod-like organisms were present in every case of consumption, and as a result of his discovery many diseases which were then unnamed were able to be classed as definite cases of tuberculosis. The term Koch's bacillus is now applied to the tuberculosis germ. (*See also* TUBERCULOSIS.)

KYPHOSIS. Kyphosis means humpback or curvature of the spine with the prominent part of the hump directed upwards. A slight form of this condition is more commonly known as round shoulders. This condition is usually due to faulty habits of standing and can easily be corrected by the mother or teacher. It may also be found in rickety children or in children afflicted with adenoids ; or sometimes bad eyesight will cause a child to stoop forward in a peering attitude.

In adults, round shoulders may result in those who have to stoop constantly over their work. Rheumatism, especially rheumatoid arthritis, is a very common cause of this condition. When children are born, the spine is shaped in a very definite curve which disappears as growth proceeds, but in old age it is seen that the spine again reverts to its curved position.

Treatment. In young children the defect can be prevented by insisting on correct posture, and by seeing that stooping is avoided when the child is sitting down. Any underlying condition such as rickets, adenoids, or bad eyesight should be given attention, and the general tone of the system should be stimulated by plenty of fresh air, good food, plenty of sleep, and sufficient exercise of the right sort. Once the condition of curvature of the spine has become established it must be treated by special remedial exercises.

LABOUR. Labour is the name given to the act of childbirth, and is usually looked upon as divided into three stages. The *first stage* begins with the onset of " labour pains," due to the regular, rhythmic contractions of the muscular walls dilating gradually the mouth of the womb ; at first the pains come on about every quarter of an hour or twenty minutes, but the interval gets shorter and shorter and the pains become stronger and stronger ; this stage may last for 24 hours or more in a woman who is having her first child, but usually lasts a much shorter time in a woman who has borne children. The *second stage* is one in which the mouth of the womb has become fully dilated and the child is being expelled from the womb to the exterior ; this stage usually lasts about three or four hours in a first childbirth, but lasts a much shorter time—sometimes only a minute or two—in a woman who has previously had a child ;

during this stage the pains become more and more severe, and it is at this stage that chloroform or another anæsthetic is usually administered to ease the pains, which are worst just as the head of the child is being born. After the child is born the doctor or nurse cuts and ties off the umbilical cord, which connects the navel of the child to the afterbirth or placenta, the structure which is attached to the mother's womb and supplies the infant with nourishing blood while it is still in the womb. The *third stage* of labour consists in the delivery of the afterbirth or placenta, which usually comes away, accompanied by a few slight pains and some bleeding, within half an hour of the birth of the child.

LABYRINTH. The labyrinth comprises not only an essential part of the organ of hearing, the internal ear or cochlea, but also the sense organ of balancing, in the three delicate semicircular canals. The labyrinth consists of two parts : the *osseous labyrinth* and the *membranous labyrinth*, which lies within the former.

LACTATION. Lactation is the period during which the child is suckled at the mother's breast.

LACTIC ACID. Lactic acid, or soured milk, is very often of use in the treatment of disorders of the intestine, such as summer diarrhœa and colitis. Tuberculous ulcers may be treated with good results by applying pure lactic acid with a brush. Certain skin diseases may be treated in the same way.

LACTOSE. Lactose is the technical name for the sugar of milk.

LAMENESS. Lameness may be due to many causes, ranging from pain caused by a corn on the toe to the more serious conditions, such as paralysis and so on. Many people have a slight limp owing to stiffness in the joints caused by rheumatism. In children, one of the conditions which causes serious lameness, and which may not improve in adult age, is hip-joint disease ; infantile paralysis is also responsible for lameness and deformity. (*See also* HIP-JOINT DISEASE ; RHEUMATISM.)

LANGERHANS' CELLS. Little masses of cells which are scattered throughout the pancreas and which are responsible for pouring out a substance which enables the body to use up its carbohydrate food, are known as the islands of Langerhans, so called after Ernst Robert Langerhans, a German, who was the first to describe them. In the condition known as diabetes, these cells become diseased and are no longer able to carry out their work ; thus the body becomes overloaded with carbohydrates (sugar, etc.). Insulin is an extract of the islands of Langerhans taken from the pancreas of the ox, and it is used in the treatment of diabetes. (*See also* DIABETES ; INSULIN.)

LANOLIN. A fat obtained from the wool of the sheep is known as lanolin, and it is a useful and soothing ointment. When rubbed on the skin it is believed to be more quickly absorbed than most fats, and because of this, it forms a basis for other substances such as mercury, etc.

LAPAROTOMY. The operation of cutting through the abdomen for the purpose of dealing with any of the internal organs, is known as laparotomy.

LARYNGISMUS STRIDULUS. A spasmodic condition of the larynx in which the breath is suddenly caught, followed by a loud crowing noise as the breath comes back. It is most common in children with rickets, but may also occur as a symptom of laryn-geal catarrh. (*See also* CROUP.)

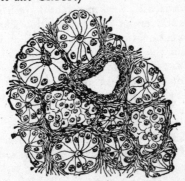

Pancreas
Arrow shows islands of Langerhans

LARYNX. The larynx is the organ of speech. The position of the larynx is at the Adam's apple in front of the neck ; it consists of a large *thyroid cartilage* (the part which projects as the Adam's apple), a ring cartilage, or *cricoid* below it, a pair of tiny *arytenoid* cartilages placed on the edge of the cricoid, at the back, and the *epiglottis*, which sticks out above the larynx and protects it. The *vocal cords* are tense ligaments attached to the arytenoid cartilages, and as they move to and fro and vibrate, the voice is produced by air passing through the chink between them.

Larynx, Diseases of. Disease of the larynx usually shows itself first by hoarseness, which may be so marked that the voice is completely lost. The usual cause of *acute laryngitis* is the extension downwards of a cold or influenza, and it may be accompanied by severe pain deep in the throat ; it is best treated by keeping the patient in bed (if the temperature is raised) and giving him ten grains (two tablets) of aspirin every four hours, also inhalations of Friar's balsam (one teaspoonful in a pint of boiling water, the steam being inhaled), or menthol, and cold applications (towels wrung out of cold water, or else an ice-bag) to the neck. *Chronic laryngitis* is usually caused by over-use or bad production of the voice, and happens most often in professional singers, actors or actresses, clergymen or school-teachers. The essential in treating *chronic laryngitis* is to rest the voice—if necessary by keeping silent altogether for a time. A nasal douche (bicarbonate of soda and common salt, half-and-half, use half a teaspoonful of this powder in a half-pint of cool water and sniff it *gently* through the nose) often helps chronic laryngitis by keeping the nose clear ; smoking is bad for this condition and alcohol is worse. A throat specialist can spray the larynx with weak cocaine or with adrenaline, and paint the vocal cords with weak perchloride of iron solution, weak silver nitrate solution or an oily preparation like gomenol ; but such methods of treatment require special skill and experience.

If a person loses the voice for more than a month the larynx should *always* be examined by a throat specialist ; it may only be a simple chronic laryngitis, but it may be something more serious, for the larynx is sometimes affected by tuberculosis or by cancer, which can only be treated successfully at an early stage of the disease. (*See also* BRONCHITIS ; INFLUENZA.)

LASSAR'S PASTE. A paste used in the treatment of eczema, etc., consisting of salicylic acid, zinc oxide, powdered starch and vaseline.

LAUDANUM. This is a popular name for tincture of opium.

LAUGHING GAS. Nitrous oxide which is given as an anæsthetic before undergoing a slight operation is commonly referred to as laughing gas.

LAXATIVES. *See* APERIENT ; CONSTIPATION ; PURGATIVE.

LAYETTE. The full outfit of garments, bedding, etc., for the new-born infant is called a layette.

LEAD. The salts of lead are used a great deal in medicine because they have a powerfully astringent (drawing together) action on the skin. The most important salts are the acetate, the iodide and the oxide ; the acetate is the only one given internally.

Lead Poisoning. At one time, lead poisoning was very common in industry among people who came in contact with the metal, but nowadays Government regulations have been introduced which afford a great deal of protection. Nevertheless, chronic poisoning is very liable to affect those who deal with lead, such as lead-smelters, painters, glaziers, plumbers, and so on. On the other hand, lead may be introduced into the system by means of our food or our drinking-water. For example, a water supply may become contaminated by lead which has been dissolved from the pipes through which the water passes, or tinned foods may become contaminated by lead from the solder which seals the tins. Both these occurrences are, in fact, quite rare ; but danger does exist as regards a water supply in cases where the water is of a peaty nature, or where it is contaminated by impurities, as both these instances give the water an added power of dissolving out lead from the pipes.

Poisoning may also occur through breathing particles of lead dust in the air ; formerly it was thought that the only way the lead was introduced into the body was with the food, because the workers did not wash their hands before meals. Certainly washing the hands, which is one of the compulsory measures introduced by the Government, forms a very important part in the preventive treatment of lead poisoning. Other measures which give protection include the changing of clothes, the use of respirators, the provision of suitable exhaust flues and electric fans, and the use of Epsom salts, milk, lemonade or sulphuric acid.

Symptoms. In cases of acute lead poisoning where a large dose of lead has been taken either accidentally or with suicidal intent, the patient suffers from burning in the mouth, vomiting, cramps in the legs, severe pains in the intestine, and convulsions. Cases of acute poisoning are rare, but cases of chronic lead poisoning such as occur amongst workers are so common that a full description is necessary.

In chronic cases, the earliest symptoms are constipation and intestinal colic. The worker complains of lassitude and tiredness, and of vague pains in the arms and shoulders. Cramps may occur in the legs, and he may lose his power of concentration. The lead circulates through the blood and produces a state of anæmia which leaves the patient very pale, and the skin takes on a greyish tinge. A blue line may be seen on the gums at the base of the teeth which is due to lead sulphide being formed by putrefaction in the mouth. Lead very often produces chronic inflammation of the nerves which control the muscles, and any part of the body may be paralysed. It is very common for the muscles of the hand to be affected in this way, producing a condition known as wrist-drop. Inflammation of the nerves of the eye, or optic neuritis, may be present, and gout is a very common symptom.

Treatment. In the treatment of lead poisoning the stomach should be emptied by an emetic such as mustard and water. Salts should be taken every four hours until the bowels are thoroughly cleared out. Potassium iodide was the drug which was formerly given in every case, but it has now been replaced by the parathormone or ammonium chloride treatment. The diet should be regulated by a medical man, as it is necessary to regulate the calcium in the system. The anæmia which results from the poisoning should be treated with an iron tonic. The intestinal colic is treated by hot fomentations, and if necessary the doctor may give an injection of morphia or some other drug. After the patient has been cured, he should, if possible, seek employment in some other type of work, especially if there is any sign of a recurrence of the symptoms. In cases of poisoning from contaminated drinking-water, every effort must be made to remove the source of the poisoning.

LEECH. In the old days leeches were extensively used in the treatment of the sick ; in fact, it may be safely stated that at one time leeches were applied to the patient as a matter of routine

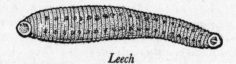

Leech

no matter what his ailment. They are very rarely used nowadays for bleeding a patient, though the method may be used on certain occasions. (*See also* BLEEDING.)

LEG. The leg extends from the knee to the ankle, the upper part of the limb being the thigh. (*See also* ACHILLES TENDON ; BONES ; BOW LEG.)

LEISHMANIASIS. A group of diseases due to infection with certain parasites known as protozoa of the Leishman-Donovan type is known as leishmaniasis. The group includes kala-azar and oriental sore (Aleppo button). In South America the oriental sore is known as espundia, and it is a condition in which ulcers may form inside the mouth and nose as well as on the skin. (*See also* ALEPPO BUTTON ; KALA-AZAR.)

LEMON. The juice of the lemon contains a large percentage of citric acid and other acids which are very valuable in preserving the alkalinity of the blood. It will be found that many people who suffer from indigestion obtain great relief after taking the unsweetened juice of a fresh lemon. The lemon also contains vitamin C, which is known as the antiscorbutic vitamin, and it is greatly used in the prevention and cure of scurvy.

LENS. The lens of the eye, which is situated behind the pupil, acts, by the bulging or flattening brought about by the ciliary muscle, by focusing objects at varying distances upon the retina. Over the age of about 40 it begins to lose its power of focusing and spectacles may be needed to help this. The disease called cataract is due to the lens becoming hardened and opaque. (*See also* EYE.)

LEPROSY. Leprosy is a wasting disease caused by a germ, which especially affects the skin and nerves, and results in mutilations and deformities. It is infectious, and though nowadays very rare in Great Britain, is still found in many other countries.

Symptoms. The patient may have intermittent attacks of fever, with aching of the bones, headache, and sometimes nose-bleeding. Finally, the spots on the skin, by which the disease can be recognized, appear.

The nodular form appears as little yellowish-brown lumps or nodes, generally on the face, the backs of the hands and wrists, and the feet and legs, until the face assumes a hideous, lion-like appearance. The mucous membranes of the mouth, nose, and throat are also affected, and the eyes. The voice becomes hoarse, and breathing may be difficult. The fingers and toes are first deformed and later drop off. This form generally lasts about 8 or 9 years, and ends fatally.

The masculo-anæsthetic type is much milder. It appears as reddish-brown spots, usually on the back and the limbs. At first there is increased sensitiveness and neuralgic pains, but as the disease progresses, anæsthesia of the affected skin develops. The hair and nails come off, the fingers and toes come off, and the muscles shrink. This form may last 10, 20, or 30 years, and may pass into the nodular form and end fatally, or, quite commonly, recover, though the patient may be " only a miserable remnant of a human being."

Treatment. The treatment is still on the whole unsatisfactory. Many remedies have been tried, the most useful being chaulmoogra oil, salicylate of soda, gold and silver salts and vaccines. Remedies may be given to relieve such symptoms as ulceration, but surgical methods are often required. The most important thing, however, is to *prevent* the spread of the disease by raising the standard of personal and household hygiene, and to recognize early cases as soon as possible.

LESION. A lesion is a wound, injury, or sore which causes changes to take place in the tissues of the skin.

LETHARGY. A condition of drowsiness or stupor which may be due to disease or physical fatigue. The most prominent disease which induces this feeling of drowsiness is encephalitis lethargica. (*See also* COMA ; FATIGUE.)

LEUCOCYTE. The colourless or white cells of the blood are known as leucocytes. All leucocytes are able to move about, and they are formed in the lymphatic tissues (lymphocytes) and in bone-marrow. The normal number of leucocytes in a healthy person is from 7,000 to 8,000 per cubic millimetre of blood (i.e. in a space the size of a pin's head) and very important information can be gained by noticing changes in the proportions either one way or the other. An increase in the number of white cells in the blood is called leucocytosis, and a lessening of the number is referred to as leucopenia.

LEUCOCYTHÆMIA. A permanent increase of the white cells of the blood. (*See also* LEUKÆMIA.)

LEUCOCYTOSIS. This term means an increase in the number of white cells in the blood. Leucocytosis is not a disease, but it is an indication that the blood is in a state of defence, ready to do battle and attack any invading germs of disease. During many acute infective diseases the number is largely increased. For example, in cases of pneumonia the number of white cells may be doubled, and the patient is very well equipped to fight the infection, but if the infection has proved too strong and poisoned the bone-marrow so that it can no longer respond and carry out its work, the outlook may be very serious indeed.

LEUCODERMA. A condition of the skin in which whitish patches appear is known as leucoderma. If a patch of leucoderma develops on the scalp, the hair growing on that area loses its colour, and the same applies to the hair on any part of the body where these whitish patches appear. The condition is incurable and treatment is not very satisfactory, but much can be done to hide the white patches with the aid of cosmetics. (*See also* ALBINISM.)

LEUCOPENIA. A decrease in the number of white cells in the blood is known as leucopenia.

LEUCORRHŒA. Any discharge which comes from the female genital passage which is not blood is termed leucorrhœa. It is usually of a whitish colour and is more commonly referred to as " the whites." The condition may occur in females of all ages and may vary a great deal in each individual.

In children, there may be inflammation and redness around the opening of the front passage as well as a discharge. The condition is usually caused by want of cleanliness, or irritation from thread-worms. Fortunately the condition is easily cleared up. The parts must be thoroughly washed several times a day for a few days with some antiseptic lotion. Boracic acid will be found very soothing, or a solution containing enough potassium permanganate to colour the water a faint red, may be used with good results.

In grown-ups, unless the discharge is excessive, no special treatment is necessary, but the general health should receive attention.

The condition may be caused by rheumatism or anæmia, and once these conditions are attended to, the discharge may completely clear up. The bowels must be kept open, as constipation tends to aggravate the condition. If the discharge is thick and milky in consistency and is in excess of the normal secretions which lubricate the genital passage, the condition may be due to inflammation of the womb following on childbirth. If the discharge is mixed with pus, it is an indication of the presence of an acute inflammation. This type of discharge may be due to gonorrhœa, or it may be due to irritation set up by the presence of a pessary which has been left in too long. An occasional watery discharge, apart from pregnancy, may be due to growths of a cancerous nature. It is always advisable for anyone suffering from a distressing discharge to consult a doctor as soon as possible and have a local examination carried out so that the right sort of treatment and cure can be assured.

Treatment. When the discharge is due to weakness and debility much can be done by bracing up the system with the proper diet and fresh air. It is important that the bowels should be regulated, and a really hot douche every day to cleanse the parts will be found very beneficial. At least a quart of water should be used to each douche, and antiseptic substances such as potassium permanganate (sufficient to tint the water a pink colour), boracic acid, hydrogen peroxide or tannic acid may be added to the water. If the condition is very severe or due to some definite disease, these measures will not effect a cure, and some special form of treatment may have to be carried out under the doctor's orders.

LEUKÆMIA. This is a disease in which there is a persistent increase in the white cells of the blood. There are many other symptoms which accompany this condition, such as enlargement of the spleen and changes in the marrow of the bones, or enlargement of the lymph glands all over the body. The cause of the disease is not known and the diagnosis depends on a microscopic examination of the blood.

There is no cure for this condition and the disease may go on for about three years.

LEUKOPLAKIA. A condition in which there are whitish patches on the surface of the tongue and inside the cheek is known as leukoplakia. Antiseptic mouth washes should be used, and some cases have been satisfactorily treated with radium.

LICHEN PLANUS. Lichen planus is an inflammation of the skin and mucous membranes characterized by papules or pimples. On the skin these favour the flexures or "bends," especially the wrists, the thighs above the knee, and the back of the neck. They are grouped into irregular, ringed, or linear patches. The pimples are flat, small, shiny, and mauve in colour. Older patches are brownish and scaly, except at the margins, where the characteristic pimples are seen.

The patient often feels very ill, though feverish symptoms are rare. His chief complaint is itching, which may be so severe as (literally) to drive him nearly mad. At times this seems to be out of all proportion to the small area of skin affected.

Sometimes the spots come and go rapidly, at other times they persist for months. The long-standing ones often cause a permanent brown discoloration of the skin, especially of the legs. The papules or spots in some cases tend to form along the lines of the veins, or along scratch-marks. The older scaly patches often resemble a skin disease known as psoriasis. In some cases warty growths appear.

The cause of the disease is unknown. The outlook varies, some cases recovering rapidly, others, more commonly, are prolonged. A widespread case may take six months ; the patchy variety, especially on the legs, may persist for years.

Treatment. The internal treatment is principally by arsenic and mercury, in the former cases with great care as to dosage. These cure successfully in many cases. An ointment containing carbolic acid and mercury perchloride is often very helpful ; it tends to prevent the severe itching. X-rays in careful hands give good results. The diet should be simple, and alcohol and tobacco avoided.

LIENTERIC DIARRHŒA. This is a nervous form of diarrhœa in which the food passes quickly through the bowel without undergoing digestion. (*See also* DIARRHŒA.)

LIGAMENT. A ligament is a structure which serves to bind together the bones at the joints. If undue strain is put upon the muscles, the ligaments then come in for their share of the strain, which often causes them to be torn or ruptured. (*See also* JOINT.)

LIGATURE. When a blood-vessel is cut, the thread-like material which the surgeon uses to tie it together is called a ligature. The material used for ligatures is usually catgut, but for very fine vessels linen thread or silk may be employed. (*See also* CATGUT.)

LIGHT TREATMENT; ARTIFICIAL SUNLIGHT. The sun is not only the source of all light, but also maintains all animal and vegetable life.

Scientists discovered that as well as its *visible* rays the sun gave off *invisible* rays at either end of the spectrum. Those at the lower end were termed *infra-red* ; those at the higher end, *ultra-violet*. Owing to the density of, and impurities in, the atmosphere, however, many of these rays do not reach us.

A Danish doctor, Niels Finsen, gave to the world the first artificial source of ultra-violet rays. In November, 1895, he began to treat his first patient by means of his electric carbon arc lamp. The case was one of long-standing lupus (tuberculosis) of the face, and in four months was completely cured.

Eight years later Finsen died at the early age of forty-three, but on the foundation laid by him great progress has since been made, and light treatment now holds an increasingly important place in preventive and remedial medicine.

In 1903 Dr. Rollier started work at Leysin, 5,000 feet up in the Alps in Switzerland. There the clear atmosphere, the light reflected from the snow, and the dependable climate permit of treatment by natural sunlight with excellent results amid stimulating surroundings.

Since Finsen's epoch-making discovery much progress has been made. Modern *mercury-vapour*, *tungsten*, and other lamps are richer in ultra-violet rays than actual sunlight.

Effects of Light upon the Human Body. *General Effects.* It is not certain *how* the invisible rays act upon the body; it is only certain that they *do* act.

One theory is that the healing process is brought about through the nervous system; another, that the rays are absorbed by the blood. Whatever the explanation, the ultra-violet rays have a powerful action and all forms of animal life are stimulated by light treatment. Appetite, vitality, and general tone are improved, and most patients undergoing treatment experience a feeling of well-being.

Local Effects. Ultra-violet rays have been used locally for many conditions, with varying results; probably their effects are more marked in general than in local treatment.

LINIMENT. Liniments, or embrocations, are preparations intended for application to the skin by rubbing. They are usually of an oily nature, which enables them to be absorbed, thus helping to remove pain and stiffness. The most important liniments for relieving pain are made up with aconite, belladonna and chloroform. When mixed together in equal parts, this is known as A.B.C. liniment, and it is a very popular mixture for neuralgia, rheumatism, etc. Iodine liniment is applied to swollen joints, and opium liniment may be used to relieve various painful conditions. Liniment of ammonia, more popularly known as oil of hartshorn, is also good for painful conditions, and turpentine and the acetic liniment of turpentine, along with camphor, croton oil, ammoniated camphor, soap, are all excellent liniments for stimulating the skin.

LINT. Lint is made from linen cloth which has been scraped on one side so that one side presents a fluffy appearance while the other is smooth. When applied to wounds, the smooth surface should always be next to the skin as it is less likely to stick. Boracic lint is most commonly used for dressing cuts or sores of any sort, and it should be wrung out of some antiseptic lotion or hot water before it is applied. Lint is also a useful way of applying ointments to the skin, and here again, the smooth side should be undermost.

LIPOMA. Lipoma is the name given to tumours which are largely composed of fat. (*See also* TUMOURS.)

LIQUOR AMNII. More commonly known as "the waters," liquor amnii is the fluid which surrounds the child in the womb. The average amount of this fluid is about a quart, and it serves to protect the child from injury. (*See also* LABOUR.)

LIQUORICE. Liquorice powder is a popular laxative, and it is very suitable for children or for women during pregnancy. Liquorice also disguises the taste of other preparations, especially that of aloes, cascara, Epsom salts, and other bitter substances. It is very soothing for cases of sore throat, and many sweets are made containing liquorice which are useful for stopping a cough.

LITMUS. Litmus is a blue vegetable dye which is obtained from various species of lichen, and it is employed for determining the presence of acids and alkalies. Litmus paper when steeped in an alkaline solution becomes blue, and when in contact with acid fluids, becomes red.

LIVER. The liver is the largest gland in the body. It lies on the right side of the abdominal cavity and is dark-brown in colour and solid to the touch. The liver is looked upon as the great store-house of the body and many chemical substances are dealt with and given off when the occasion arises. For example, when an increase of energy is required, the liver gets busy and manufactures energy-giving substances out of the digested food, especially sugary or starchy foods. But if the diet is excessive or ill-balanced, the storage power of the liver may become over-taxed, especially if no exercise is taken to allow the liver to use up the extra sugar, etc. The liver also manufactures bile, which is an important substance in aiding digestion. Disturbance of the workings of the bile ducts causes the condition known as jaundice, which is dealt with under its own heading. (*See also* CIRRHOSIS OF THE LIVER ; DIGESTION; GALL-BLADDER.)

LIVER FLUKE. A parasitic flat worm which infests the bile ducts and liver of sheep and is responsible for the disease known as sheep rot. Occasionally these liver flukes are found in man.

LOBE. A rounded part of an organ which is subdivided from the neighbouring parts is termed a lobe, such as the lobes of the liver or of the brain. The lower part of the ear which is soft and rounded is known as the lobe or lobule of the ear.

LOCHIA. The discharge which takes place from the womb during the first week or two after childbirth is known as lochia. (*See also* LABOUR.)

LOCKJAW. *See* TETANUS.

LOCOMOTOR ATAXIA is a chronic disease of the nervous system which is one of the late results of syphilis. It is found in men at least ten times as commonly as in women, and the symptoms may first appear as long as twenty years after the infection.

Symptoms. One of the features of the disorder is a loss of the sense of position in space. If a person with locomotor ataxia is asked to stand with his feet together and is then asked to shut his eyes, he sways from one side to the other, and may even fall. Similarly, if asked to point with his index finger to his nose, keeping his eyes shut, he will be unable to do so, but aided by his eyesight, he can do this perfectly. Changes in the coverings of the spinal cord (the meninges) produce pains, the character of which is peculiar to the disease.

These are called " lightning " pains, and they occur in bouts. They are especially liable to be felt at any spot where a bone comes to the surface, as at the ankle or wrist. This symptom of " lightning " pains may be present for many years before any other symptoms are complained of. In fact, it is not out of place to say here that locomotor ataxia, though it used to be a very severe, crippling, and in the end fatal disease, has now, through modern methods of treatment, so altered its nature that twenty or more years may pass before a patient with this disorder suffers any more inconvenience from his trouble than occasional bouts of these pains.

But much depends on the early treatment of the disease, and a patient in early middle life who suffers from what he thinks are bouts of " rheumatic " pains should at all events be examined to make sure that his pains are not the " lightning " pains of locomotor ataxia.

Treatment. The usual treatment of the general disorder consists in a course of injections with salvarsan or similar preparations, which have a remarkable effect on the cause of the disease. General tonics also help to keep these patients healthy, for it has been noticed that patients with locomotor ataxia particularly need to be kept " up to par," for if they get such mild infections as colds or bronchitis, the disease seems to progress more quickly. But in those patients who come under observation late in the course of the disorder, their most distressing symptom is their difficulty in walking straight. Certain exercises have been devised by Frenkel to help these people to re-educate their muscles, so to speak.

E.F.D.

14

LOIN. The loin is the part of the back which lies between the last rib and the top of the pelvis. Pain is felt in this part of the body during an attack of lumbago and in some forms of backache.

LONG SIGHT. Medically known as hypermetropia, this condition is discussed under that heading.

LORDOSIS. When the spine is unnaturally curved forward the condition is known as lordosis. (*See also* SPINAL CURVATURE.)

LOUSE. *See* HEAD LOUSE.

LUMBAGO. In this affection, pain and stiffness are felt in the muscles of the small of the back. Any bending or turning may be extremely painful ; in fact, some patients may find that to sneeze or cough is a very disastrous experience. Lumbago may also be caused by strain or injury or it may be associated with rheumatism.

Treatment. If the pain is at all severe, the patient should remain in bed and be kept as warm as possible with hot-water bottles placed near the back. Massage or vigorous rubbing with a liniment will help to relieve the pain. Turkish baths are good in slight cases, and aspirin tablets, not more than two at a time, will be found very soothing. The bowels should be kept open with suitable medicine.

LUMBAR REGION. The part of the body which is most commonly called the small of the back is medically known as the lumbar region.

LUMINAL. A soothing drug which is very closely allied to veronal. Luminal sodium is used a great deal in the treatment of epilepsy and in other conditions where a quietening effect is required. (*See also* EPILEPSY.)

LUNATIC. This term is applied to people who are mentally unsound. The name lunatic is derived from luna, the moon, because at one time an insane person was supposed to be influenced by the moon. (*See also* INSANITY ; MENTAL DISEASE.)

LUNGS. The lungs are structures which are among the most essential to life in the body. There is a left lung and a right lung, situated in the thorax with the heart between them, and they are protected by the ribs. The function of the lungs is breathing or respiration, which means the interchange of the gases of the body with the gases of the atmosphere in which the body lives. Air passes down the throat to the trachea or windpipe into the lungs, along the tubes called bronchi ; these divide and subdivide into little bronchioles, the smallest of which are tiny little tubes less than a hundredth of an inch wide, and ending in little air sacs called " alveoli " ; these alveoli are made of a delicate membrane covered by blood capillaries (the smallest blood-vessels) and so delicate are the microscopic walls of the alveoli and the capillaries that the blood can take up oxygen from the air in the alveoli and the air can take up carbonic acid gas and other impurities from the blood.

The right lung is in three divisions, or lobes, and the left one (which is smaller, because of the heart being more on the left side) in two lobes. Both lungs are covered with a delicate moist membrane, the pleura, and the cavity in which they lie is also covered with a similar membrane, so that when the lung expands or contracts it moves freely within this cavity.

Diseases of the Lungs. Inflammation of the lung itself, which is caused by two or three different kinds of germs, is called *pneumonia* ; inflammation of the lining of the lung is called *pleurisy* ; *bronchitis* is inflammation of the lining of the air tubes or bronchi ; *bronchopneumonia* is a kind of pneumonia which has spread from a bronchitis and is of a more " patchy " type than a *lobar* pneumonia, which is an inflammation of the lung tissue affecting a whole lobe or more than one lobe ; *bronchiectasis* is a chronic abscess cavity, usually at the base of a lung, which has developed in a bronchial tube— it is said to be often due to inhalation of some foreign body into the lung. *Phthisis* or pulmonary consumption is due to infection with tuberculosis.

LUPUS (Tuberculosis of the Skin). Tuberculosis may attack the skin in various ways, producing several distinct varieties of the disease.

Lupus vulgaris is the most common type. It is characterized by reddish-brown patches, composed of tiny nodules embedded in inflamed skin. The disease is destructive, causing ulceration and scarring. It tends to heal at one place and spread at another.

Later, ulceration takes place, with underlying infection of the lymph-glands, bones, and other parts. The ulcers are irregular, deep and do not heal. The nose and the lobes of the ears are commonly attacked by the disease and gradually " nibbled away." The tip of the nose may be beak-like, or in bad cases the whole of the soft parts destroyed. The upper lip becomes swollen, thickened, and ulcerated. On the hands and feet, and about the genitals, deformities are likewise caused. The mucous membranes are also attacked in very many cases.

This type, when neglected, produces the most terrible disfigurement. Nowadays, badly disfigured patients are comparatively seldom seen.

Treatment. Preliminary treatment varies somewhat in the different varieties. Crusted discharging ulcers are scraped with a " sharp spoon," followed by the constant use of an antiseptic ointment. After this, the aim of treatment is to destroy the tubercle

organism. This is done by surgical removal, which must be thorough;
or by burning with strong caustics, which, though effective, are
painful and cause unsightly scars; or by milder caustics.

Ultra-violet ray treatment by " sunlight lamps," the Finsen and
Kromayer light methods, and radium and carbon dioxide snow for
small areas, are all excellent, the first especially so.

Remarkable benefit has recently been obtained by the Gerson
diet, in combination with irradiated ergosterol, which contains
vitamin D. The essentials of the Gerson diet are the exclusion of
salt, fresh uncooked vegetables in large proportion, restriction of
meats and of water, rich fat and protein but low carbohydrate foods.

LYMPH. The fluid which circulates through the lymphatic
vessels of the body is known as lymph. This fluid is the watery
portion of the blood which is filtered through the walls of the
capillaries. The term lymph is also used to describe the serum
obtained from the blood of calves which is used for vaccination.
(*See also* DUCTLESS GLANDS; SERUM; VACCINATION.)

LYSIS. The gradual ending of a disease, especially a fever.

LYSOL. Lysol is obtained from coal-tar and it is a powerful
antiseptic. Lotions made up with lysol are used for cleansing the
skin or for vaginal douches. The usual strength is about a teaspoonful of lysol to a pint of warm water.

M. & B. 693. The trade name of the drug called also sulphapyridine, used successfully in the treatment of pneumonia,
meningitis, gonorrhœa, etc.

McBURNEY'S POINT. This is a spot on the abdominal
wall midway between the navel and the point of the haunch-bone.
(*See also* APPENDICITIS.)

MACULA. A term meaning a spot. A freckle, port-wine stain
or any such spot may be called a macula. The *macula lutea* is the
yellow spot of the eye. (*See also* BIRTHMARKS; EYE; FRECKLE.)

MADNESS. *See* HYDROPHOBIA; INSANITY; MENTAL DISEASE.

MADURA FOOT. Madura foot or fungus foot is a tropical
disease, found in India and other hot countries, in which the foot
swells and cracks form in it which discharge matter containing little
black or white granules, which are really a species of fungus. The
fungus probably gains an entrance into the foot through a sore or
scratch.

MAGNESIUM. Magnesium sulphate is the popular and
powerful purgative known as *Epsom Salts.* Magnesium oxide, which
is commonly called magnesia, is very useful in cases of stomach
trouble where there is too much acidity. Milk of magnesia and
magnesia cream are pleasant ways of taking it. A very favourite
and useful mixture is the mixture of magnesium sulphate and

magnesium carbonate called mistura alba or *white mixture*. Magnesium citrate or effervescing citrate of magnesia forms a very pleasant and cooling summer drink.

MALAISE. By malaise is meant a feeling of illness or physical discomfort.

MALAR. The malar bone is the cheek bone. (*See also* BONE.)

MALARIA. Malaria is a very common disease. It is also known as marsh fever, jungle fever, or just " fever." In this country it is contracted only in a very few cases, but there are many people who have acquired the disease abroad and are still subject to attacks of it.

Malaria is a recurrent disease and is commonly divided into three groups according to the periods at which the bouts of fever return. (1) *Quotidian*, or daily ; (2) *tertian*, or recurring every three days ; and (3) *quartan*, recurring every fourth day.

History of Malaria. In 1880 a French scientist, Laveran, was able to show that there was a parasite which was always found in the blood of patients with malaria. Later on, in 1894, the late Sir Patrick Manson and the late Sir Ronald Ross were able to prove that the same parasite could be found in the blood of a certain group of mosquitoes called the *anopheles*. From this they worked out that the anophele mosquito in the act of biting a person transferred the disease to that person. Similarly, by biting a person who has already contracted malaria the anophele mosquito can acquire the disease, and may later on bite a healthy person and give him malaria. After the parasite has been conveyed into the blood of a healthy person by the bite of the mosquito it grows and eventually splits up into a host of little bodies or off-springs, and at this point the attack of malaria begins. This explains the different periodicity of the disease, because some parasites take only one day, some three and some four to hatch out a brood and let them loose in the bloodstream of the bitten person.

Symptoms. The first stage is one of shivering and general malaise. The patient feels tired, with aching head and limbs, and a cold feeling with bouts of shivering. The second stage is the hot and feverish stage. The temperature rises very suddenly to great heights and the pulse and breathing become rapid. The aches continue and there is great restlessness and often delirium. Vomiting and diarrhœa are common. The third stage is in the nature of a crisis. Sweating is profuse, the temperature comes down rapidly and the patient becomes much more comfortable. The trouble is not over, however, because unless it is energetically treated the attack will return in exactly the same way, after one, three or four days, according to the type, and each attack will leave the patient weaker.

Treatment. Malaria is one of the diseases for which there is a very definite line of treatment and for which a drug is specific —that is, particularly curative for that disease. This drug is *quinine*. Quinine is so generally used for malaria that no household in tropical countries would dream of being without it. Before giving the initial dose of quinine, however, it is best to give a large dose of calomel, followed by salts. This is important. During an attack of malaria as much as 30 grains of quinine sulphate should be taken daily, except in the case of a pregnant woman, who should take it in smaller doses at shorter intervals. It is as well to continue a daily dose of 10 grains for three or four months after an attack of malaria, and some people take a small dose such as five grains as a daily routine while they are in a malaria-infested neighbourhood, or if they have been exposed to the infection. Quite recently other effective drugs have been introduced, namely, *plasmoquine* and *atebrin*.

Wise persons will take precautions against contracting malaria if their lives should bring them into tropical regions. These precautionary measures include excluding mosquitoes from dwellings by the use of fine mesh wire gauze over windows and doors, and netting round beds. Gloves and high boots should be worn by those who are out at nightfall when the mosquito is about and at its busiest. Strong smelling oils such as oil of lavender and citronella may be freely sprinkled over the clothing, or mixed with the face powder, etc. (*See also* MOSQUITO ; QUININE.)

MALE FERN. The oily extract of the root of male fern (*filix mas*) is the chief remedy for destroying tapeworms. (*See also* FERN ; TAPEWORM.)

MALIGNANT. By malignant is meant dangerous to life. A malignant growth usually means a cancer. The opposite of malignant in medicine is benign.

MALINGERING. Malingering is a deliberate attempt to appear to have a disease or disability for the purpose of evading a duty or gaining some financial or other advantage.

MALNUTRITION. Malnutrition is the state of being undernourished owing to insufficiency of food, the wrong sort of food or some constitutional reason which prevents the food eaten from being turned into the requisite nourishment for the body.

MALT contains a ferment or digestive substance called *diastase* which works on starch and turns it into malt sugar. In the form of extract of malt it is a valuable aid to a weak digestion, and is also nourishing and strengthening because of the malt sugar (maltose) it contains. It is therefore often prescribed for people suffering from wasting and weakening diseases.

MALTA or UNDULANT FEVER. Malta fever, which is

also called undulant fever or Rock fever, is a very common complaint around the Mediterranean Sea and in other warm countries where goats' milk is used. It is now recognized as being not uncommon in this country too. In Malta, where it is a serious problem, the Government takes important steps to deal with it.

Malta fever is due to a germ called the Brucella abortus, and it is believed to be spread through the medium of goats' and cows' milk.

Symptoms. The illness is not a very severe one, although it may continue in a long drawn-out form over even a period of years and wear the patient out. There is loss of appetite, headache, sleeplessness, and slight fever ; in the evenings neuralgic pains and swellings in the joints appear. The patient may become very much emaciated and exhausted.

Treatment. Unlike malaria there is no absolutely effective treatment for this fever. The feverishness may be relieved by cold sponging if the temperature is very high. It can be prevented by thorough pasteurization of milk. When convalescent, tonics must be taken to build up the strength. (*See* UNDULANT FEVER.)

MANDIBLE. The lower jaw is called the mandible. (*See also* JAW.)

MANGANESE. In medicine it is chiefly used in the form of potassium permanganate, which is a powerful antiseptic, disinfectant and deodorant. Condy's fluid is an easily obtainable form in which to use permanganate. Manganese preparations are also used as injections for the treatment of boils and other infections.

MANIA. Insanity in which the patient becomes dangerously excited is called mania. (*See also* INSANITY ; MEGALOMANIA ; MENTAL DISEASE ; MONOMANIA.)

MARASMUS. Wasting in a small child is called marasmus.

MARROW. Bone-marrow is a substance found in the inner channels of the long bones of the body. It has to do with keeping up the supply of red blood corpuscles in the blood and is, therefore, a very valuable substance. The marrow from the bones of oxen, sheep and calves can be eaten as an ordinary article of diet or in larger quantities by those suffering from anæmia and similar blood diseases, especially children with rickets, wasting and debility.

MASSETER. The masseters are a pair of muscles passing over the ends of the jaws in front of the ears. They are the chief muscles used in chewing.

MASTICATION. By mastication we mean the act of chewing. Good mastication is necessary in order to turn the food into the pulpy well-salivated mass which is suitable for swallowing into the stomach.

MASTITIS. Mastitis is another name for inflammation of the breast. (*See also* BREAST.)

MASTODYNIA. Any pain in the breast may be called masto-dynia, though it is often used to refer to a neuralgic ache for which there is no apparent organic cause. Very heavy and pendulous breasts often ache, and a loose support such as a well fitted bust-bodice will give relief. Some women feel neuralgic pains in the breasts at special times or when they are tired and run down. It must never be forgotten, however, that a woman who is not used to having pain in the region of the breast, should have herself examined by a doctor when such a pain appears, because it may be the beginning of some more serious condition. For fleeting attacks of mastodynia warmth over the breast or a belladonna plaster will usually give relief. (*See also* BREAST.)

MASTOID. The mastoid process is part of the temporal bone of the skull ; it is the rounded part that projects behind the ear and contains numerous air cells, the purpose of which is to protect the delicate structures of the ear.

MASTOIDITIS, or inflammation of the mastoid, is a serious disease, which may spread to the brain and cause meningitis, or may cause blood-poisoning by pouring the poisons of the inflamma-tion direct into the blood-stream. The *simple mastoid operation*, however, is very effective when performed early and leaves no ill-effects. The *radical mastoid operation* is done in chronic cases and in brain complications ; it brings about deafness, as the whole middle ear has to be cleared out in this operation, but sometimes a certain degree of hearing remains.

MASTURBATION, or self-abuse, is a bad habit which is common among adolescents. It is less important than used to be believed, as it is usually a temporary matter and leaves no per-manent ill-effects. (*See also* SEX HYGIENE ; PSYCHOTHERAPY.)

MATERIA MEDICA. Materia medica is the old name for the science of drugs. This is now called *pharmacology*, which includes the action of drugs upon the body.

MATERNITY BENEFIT. A woman who is insured under the National Health Insurance Act, or who is the wife of an insured man, is entitled to a maternity benefit on the birth of a child. For details see the article on NATIONAL HEALTH INSURANCE ACT.

MAXILLARY BONES. The maxillary bones are the pair of bones which form the upper jaw. (*See also* ANTRUM ; JAW.)

MEASLES. This is a very infectious disease which is common amongst children in springtime. In most places it is now notifiable to the Public Health authorities. The incubation period, or time it takes to develop after exposure to infection, is three weeks. It is worthy of note that measles is much more serious in children of under five years of age than in older children. Placental extract is given successfully as a preventive, especially in epidemics.

Symptoms. The first sign the mother notices is that the child is off colour for four or five days, and seems to have a bad cold in the head with running eyes and nose. If the mother looks inside the child's mouth at this period she may notice some little white patches the size of a pin head on the inner side of the cheek which are typical of measles, and the child will by this time have developed a hard ticklish cough. On the fourth day of the illness the child becomes very feverish and a rash appears first behind the ears and round the mouth and spreads rapidly all over the body. The rash is red and blotchy and may last from three to five days.

Mothers do not, as a rule, realise the seriousness of measles, and sometimes allow the rest of the children to sleep in the same room, so that " they may all get it while they are at it." This is a wicked thing to do, because more children die from the complications of measles than from any other infectious complaint.

Complications. *See* Pneumonia; Eye and Ear, Diseases of.

Treatment. The doctor should be in attendance on all cases and, wherever possible, the child should be isolated and treated at home. The injection of convalescent serum (i.e. the blood serum of healthy convalescents from measles) into contacts brings protection which lasts about a month ; and similar injections during the first few days of the incubation period will lessen the severity of an attack. The treatment is simply to make the patient sweat and keep the bowels freely open. A dose of opening medicine, preferably castor-oil (one tablespoonful for a child of seven and two teaspoonfuls under that age), should be given, followed by a daily dose of milk of magnesia, unless there are signs of diarrhœa.

All through the illness it is advisable to give the child as much fluid to drink as possible in the form of ordinary cold water, lemonade and orangeade made from fresh fruit, barley water (made by boiling and straining pearl barley) or imperial drink, made by mixing the lemonade and barley water together. If the child is restless and hot it should be sponged down frequently with lukewarm water with a drop of disinfectant in it. The room should be kept darkened, as the light is irritating to the child's eyes. The window should be kept open, but care must be taken that the bed in not in a draught.

The *eyes* should be bathed hourly with a soft piece of cotton-wool dipped in weak boracic lotion, each piece being burned as soon as it has been used once. The *mouth* should be swabbed three times a day in the same way with glycerine and borax or hydrogen peroxide or glycothymoline. If the *ear* discharges or if there is

14*

pain behind the ear the doctor should be informed at once. The *cough*, which is the most troublesome feature, is treated by medicine to loosen and soothe it. It is a help to rub the chest with goose grease or camphorated oil and cover it back and front with a little plain cotton-wool. In cases where the cough remains hard and troublesome, antiphlogistine (obtained from any chemist, with directions for use on the jar) should be applied on the back and front of the chest morning and evening. Pyramidon has recently been recommended for the treatment of measles, and when given early it has been found in some cases to stop short an attack.

The child should not be allowed to return to school under four-teen days from the date of the first signs of the appearance of the rash, and a child who has been exposed to infection should not return until sixteen days have elapsed. (*See also* DISINFECTION ; GERMAN MEASLES ; INFECTIOUS DISEASES.)

MEATUS. The word meatus refers to a passage or tunnel in the body. The passage in connection with which it is most generally used is the external auditory meatus or ear-hole. (*See also* EAR.)

MECKEL'S DIVERTICULUM. *See* DIVERTICULITIS.

MECONIUM. For the first two days of an infant's life it frequently passes motions of a dark greenish-black sticky fluid. This substance is called meconium. After the first forty-eight hours of life the meconium disappears and the normal baby stools appear. (*See also* STOOLS.)

MEDIASTINUM. The space lying between the two lungs is called the mediastinum. It contains the heart, the windpipe and gullet, and the aorta and other great blood-vessels of the chest.

Inflammation occurring in this region is known as *mediastinitis*.

MEDITERRANEAN FEVER. *See* MALTA FEVER.

MEDULLA or BULB is that part of the nervous system which lies at the back of the head, occupying the lowest part of the skull, and which joins the brain above to the spinal cord below. It contains all the means by which we are able to move our limbs ; to feel such things as pain and temperature in every part of the body ; and, most important of all, by which we are able to breathe.

MEGALOMANIA is an exaggerated belief in one's own power or ability. It may perhaps best be described as an *insane conceit*. Simple megalomania is fairly common in a mild form, but as a symptom of more serious mental trouble it is very common. One of the first symptoms of *general paralysis of the insane* (q.v.) is often megalomania.

MEGRIM. *See* MIGRAINE.

MELÆNA. The dark-coloured, almost black, stools which

contain blood and are passed in conditions like ulceration of the bowels or stomach. The bleeding when the stools are black is usually from the lower part of the stomach, the duodenum or the higher parts of the small intestine. Many mixtures which are taken as medicine will darken the stool, notably those containing iron and bismuth. (See also STOOLS.)

MELANCHOLIA is a type of disorder of the mind in which the outstanding symptom is depression, which may be so marked that the patient seeks refuge in suicide. The bodily health is also affected in this disorder, and the patient looks and feels physically ill as well as being mentally sick. The mental picture in melancholia is one of utter misery.

It is advisable to have these patients under supervision in a mental hospital. The chief dangers in melancholia are lack of nourishment and suicide. It is often necessary to guard against suicide by strict observation both day and night, and the refusal to take food may have to be met by forcible feeding.

MEMBRANE. A membrane is a thin sheet of tissue covering or lining any organ of the body. Membranes such as those lining the intestines, the nose, etc., which are moistened by the sticky fluid substance called mucus, are called the *mucous membranes*. In a state of ill-health these mucous membranes are apt to develop an additional amount of mucus and catarrh is produced.

The largest single membrane of the body is the *peritoneum* or lining of the abdomen. The membrane which lines the chest and covers the lungs is called the *pleura*. There are many smaller membranes throughout the body, such as the small membranes which lie between bones. The coverings of muscles called *fascia* are fibrous membranes.

MEMORY. Most of us find that it is easier to remember by " association." That is, we form " links " in our minds between new impressions and those which we have experienced before: one thing reminds us of another, and so a chain of thought is created which lays down a new impression to be stored and reproduced when required.

MENIÈRE'S DISEASE or SYNDROME. Menière's disease is a chronic progressive disease in which there are attacks of giddiness, deafness on one side of the head only and noises in the head (tinnitus) and vomiting. The cause of Menière's disease is not known.

Treatment. If the condition is due to blocking up one of the eustachian tubes this is cleared up by the use of the eustachian catheter. In persistent cases restriction of fluids and a salt-free diet is advised nowadays. In very severe cases alcohol is injected into one of the semicircular canals of the ear, or the auditory nerve may be severed by operation. (See also EAR ; TINNITUS.)

MENINGES are the coverings of the brain and spinal cord which protect the delicate nervous structures from injury and also serve to carry the blood away from the brain when all its oxygen has been used up by the tissues. There are three layers to these coverings : the *dura mater* (the outermost one), the *arachnoid,* and the *pia mater.* In between the arachnoid and the pia mater there is a small space, filled with a fluid produced in a gland-like structure in the brain. This fluid, called cerebro-spinal fluid, circulates all over the brain substance and the spinal cord, and is the fluid that actually nourishes the brain, the gland-like structure extracting from the blood just those things which are required to nourish the brain and rejecting the remainder.

MENINGITIS is inflammation of the meninges (*see* MENINGES), and it may occur as a result of some general disease of the body, as tuberculosis, or it may be caused by the spread of some disease in the ear or nose through the skull into the meninges. One particular form of meningitis is called CEREBRO-SPINAL FEVER and has already been dealt with under that heading.

Signs of irritation of the meninges begin to appear : severe headache is complained of, the child may develop an obvious squint and may have a fit. By this time the child will be unwilling to be examined or questioned, but will lie curled up in bed, probably with its head buried in the pillow to avoid looking at the light. There may be some rise of temperature, and the temperature as a rule goes on rising until just before death. Pain is a most distressing feature of the disease and the child often gives rise to a plaintive cry which once heard is never forgotten. The head is held back with the chin tilted into the air. A certain sign, called " Kernig's sign," is nearly always present in these cases : if a child is placed on its back in bed so that one leg is resting on the bed and the other one is bent at the hip and knee, it is found that it is not possible to straighten out the bent leg at the knee joint without causing pain to the patient and pulling up the leg which rests on the bed. The course of the disease may be weeks, or it may end quite quickly, within a week, following a few days of merciful unconsciousness. It is impossible to tell how long the patient will live. The condition is recognized and the type of germ causing the meningitis is determined by withdrawing some of the cerebro-spinal (*see* MENINGES) fluid from the spinal canal with a needle.

Treatment up to the present has been hopeless in cases of meningitis caused by the germ of tuberculosis. All that can be done is to keep the patient as comfortable as possible by ice-bags to the head and cold sponging. Withdrawal of cerebro-spinal fluid relieves the headache for a time in all cases of meningitis. In those forms in which the germ has come from either the ear or the air spaces connected with the nose, usually the streptococcus or the pneumococcus, sulphonamide drugs, such as prontosil or M. & B. 693, are now being used successfully.

MENINGOCELE is a lump which may appear in the mid line of the back of a newly-born child at any place from the bottom of the skull to the lowermost part of the spine. When the baby coughs or cries, the lump gets larger and can be felt to be soft, with fluid contents. Meningocele may sometimes be treated by surgery, and the lump taken away without damage to the spinal cord underneath; but many cases are best left untouched, since the condition gives rise to little or no trouble, and the lump should then be protected by a suitable shield.

MENOPAUSE. See CHANGE OF LIFE ; MENSTRUATION.

MENORRHAGIA. This is the name given to excessive loss of blood during the menstrual period. (See also FLOODING ; MENSTRUATION.)

MENSES. The monthly periods in a woman. (See also MENSTRUATION.)

MENSTRUATION. Menstruation is the medical name for the monthly loss of blood which occurs normally in adult women, and which is popularly called by such names as " the courses," " the periods," " being unwell," etc. It consists of a periodic discharge from the womb. Every woman differs both as regards the duration of the periods and the length of time between them ; for example, bleeding may occur at intervals of three to five weeks and may last for as short a time as two days or as long a time as ten days. But each woman should be regular in the type to which she belongs. If she has a three or four days' flow every twenty-eight days, which is the most usual period, she should be able to count on the period appearing every four weeks with great regularity and lasting the same number of days each time. Menstruation usually begins between twelve and fourteen years of age and lasts until the woman is forty-five to fifty-five years of age. The late forties are the most usual age for its cessation, which is called the menopause or climacteric, or more popularly is referred to as the change of life.

During the menstrual period a tiny egg, or ovum as it is called, which is so small that it can only be seen with the aid of a microscope, is set free from the ovary and passes down the *fallopian tubes* to the womb. If it meets the male fertilizing agent (spermatozoön) the menstrual flow does not take place and pregnancy begins, otherwise it is discharged from the womb with the menstrual flow.

In addition to the inconvenience caused by the periods, most women experience slight feelings of discomfort before the period begins. They may feel languid, nervy and irritable, and have pains in the abdomen or in the back. Some women are always constipated during a period, whilst others start the period with an attack of diarrhœa ; but unless there is some definite reason for it, menstruation must not be regarded as a period of ill-health. It is a perfectly normal function, and for most women entails no stopping of their usual activities. It may be as well to take a little extra care to avoid chills and over-tiredness, but otherwise life should go on much as usual. Some women do not take a bath during the period, but for those who are used to a daily bath it may be safely continued so long as it is restricted to a short warm bath. Cold baths are better done without and sea-bathing should be missed for a few days.

Abnormalities of Menstruation. Amenorrhœa, Menorrhagia and Metrorrhagia.

Amenorrhœa. This term is applied to the absence of the menstrual period. In some cases menstruation never begins owing to imperfect development of the womb or other internal organs. This may be rectified by a surgical operation, but not always. It is much more common for the menses to stop after having made an appearance. Chlorosis, or anæmia, accounts for many cases of amenorrhœa in young girls. There may be other causes, such as excitement, shock, mental strain, change of climate, or exposure to cold before or during the menstrual period. It is usual for the menses to make their reappearance after the cause has been removed, even in the case of amenorrhœa resulting from disease. The natural causes of amenorrhœa are pregnancy, the onset of the menopause or change of life, and usually lactation or nursing.

Menorrhagia and Metrorrhagia. Excessive bleeding at the menstrual period is called *Menorrhagia*, whilst irregular bleeding at times between the periods is called *Metrorrhagia*. Anything over a week is excessive for a period, but many women have periods as long as a week, quite normally, and it is quite common in young girls who usually grow out of the tendency when the periods become established. Certain blood diseases such as anæmia may cause profuse periods. The cause of metrorrhagia or irregular bleeding should always be investigated by a doctor, especially if it comes on in a woman whose periods have previously been regular. All the causes of profuse and irregular bleeding are discussed in the article on FLOODING, which is a general name for the condition. (*See also* CHANGE OF LIFE.)

MENTAL DEFICIENCY is a condition in which the mind has failed to reach a normal stage of development. It is one of the three groups into which all cases of abnormal minds can be divided, the other two being mental disease and mental decay or dementia.

Mental deficiency has been made the subject of an Act of Parliament, which states that it is the condition in which an individual is so undeveloped mentally from birth that he is unable to adapt himself to the ordinary requirements of society except under care, supervision and control. There are three grades of mental deficiency : idiocy, imbecility and feeblemindedness, of which the first and the last, being of most importance, are treated under their separate headings. Imbecility is laid down by the Act of Parliament already referred to as the state of those persons in whom there exists from birth or from an early age mental defectiveness not amounting to idiocy, yet so pronounced that they are incapable of managing their affairs or themselves, or, in the case of children, of being taught to do so.

MENTAL DISEASE. The causes of mental disease may be divided into those which arise in the mind itself and those which may be traced to some disturbance of a physical nature, either in the brain or elsewhere in the body.

Physical Causes of Mental Disease. Poisons produced by germs which live in the digestive organs, or in the throat or sometimes at the roots of the teeth, constantly get into the blood and are carried to the brain, and in some people whose nervous systems are not as strong as they might be severe mental break-downs are caused in this way. The killing-off of the germs and getting rid of their accumulated poisons will cure these patients. Other bodily conditions which may cause mental disease are syphilis, alcoholism and disease of the blood-vessels that occurs in old age. Epilepsy too (q.v.) may cause mental disease. In people in whom there is a family history of mental trouble, the two great crises of life, namely puberty and the change of life, sometimes prove too much for the individuals and they escape, as it were, by developing mental troubles. Childbirth also can affect women in this way ; but it is exceedingly rare for grave mental trouble to follow childbirth unless there is some definite history of it in the family.

Mental Disease which has its origin in the Mind. These disorders are described under the heading HYPOCHONDRIASIS. We do not yet know the way in which mental disease arises from the mind itself, but in many cases there can be little doubt that the mental trouble is a form of escape from an unconscious grievance, which once was conscious, and which has made ordinary life unbearable to the patient.

MENTHOL. Menthol is very useful as a local anæsthetic and is put up in convenient forms for rubbing on such neuralgic surfaces, especially in cases such as facial neuralgia where the nerves involved are near the surface. For toothache, menthol may be rubbed on the gums or placed in the socket of the tooth. The crystals themselves are a very favourite inhalation for colds in the head, sore throats, etc.

MERCURIAL POISONING. In cases where substances containing mercury have been swallowed the mouth will be burnt and the patient will be in great pain ; there will also be vomiting and collapse. An ordinary emetic such as salt in water may be given, and restoratives in the shape of brandy in milk to treat the collapse. A doctor will have to be sent for at once.

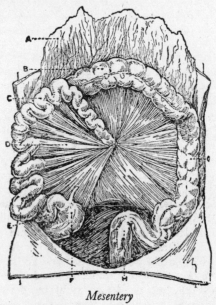

Mesentery

A. Omentum; B. Transverse Colon; C. Jejunum; D. Mesentery; E. Ileum;
F. Cæcum with Appendix; G. Descending Colon; H. Rectum.

MERCURY. Mercury, or hydrargyrum, is a liquid metal substance and is very useful in medicine. It is very easily expanded by heat and this property is used to measure temperatures. A small amount is placed in a bulb in an enclosed tube to form the instrument called the thermometer.

It is a very useful remedy in the treatment of syphilis. Many useful ointments are made from it. The favourite powder for infants known as grey powder is a mercury preparation, and so is calomel which has such a powerful effect on the liver.

Mercury is a very powerful antiseptic (perchloride of mercury), and it forms the basis of many lotions, such as black wash.

MESENTERY. The organs of the stomach are enclosed in a large bag of membrane called the peritoneum. In the peritoneum there are folds called mesenteries which attach the various parts of the tube conveying the food to the stomach to the back wall of the abdomen. (*See also* ABDOMEN ; INTESTINES.)

MESMERISM. *See* HYPNOTISM.

METABOLISM. By metabolism we mean the various processes by which our food is transformed into substances which are absorbed into the blood-stream and lymph glands for the purpose of nourishing and building up the body, and the waste materials are abstracted from the food ready to be discarded from the body. In this process the various organs of the digestive tract play a large part together with the ductless glands. Certain diseases are called disorders of metabolism, such as diabetes, gout, myxœdema and obesity. (*See also* BLOOD ; DIGESTION ; DUCTLESS GLANDS.)

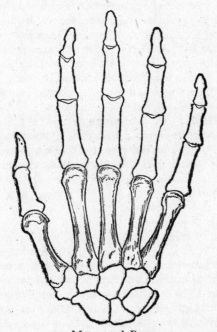

Metacarpal Bones
(other bones of hand in outline only)

METACARPUS. The metacarpal bones are the five bones in the palm of each hand to which the fingers are attached. (*See also* FINGER ; HAND.)

METASTASIS. By metastasis is meant the spread of disease from one organ to another. Cancer spreads by metastasis.

METATARSUS. The metatarsus is composed of the five metatarsal bones of the foot. (*See also* FOOT.)

METHYL SALICYLATE. Methyl Salicylate, or artificially made oil of wintergreen, is of the greatest use for the treatment of rheumatic and other pains.

METHYLATED SPIRIT. Methylated spirit is a mixture of nearly pure alcohol and wood-naphtha. In the form known as surgical spirit it is of the greatest use in surgery for the disinfection of instruments, avoidance of bed-sores, etc.

METRITIS. Inflammation of the wall of the womb is known as metritis.

METRORRHAGIA. Irregular bleeding from the womb. (*See also* FLOODING; MENSTRUATION.)

MICROBE. A microbe is a germ. The word microbe literally means a small living thing. Micro-organisms, bacteria and bacilli are other names for microbes. (*See also* GERMS.)

MICROSCOPE. A microscope is an instrument which magnifies small objects very greatly. Without the microscope we would know nothing about the germs of disease, blood cells and many other minute things which are of the utmost importance to our health.

MICTURITION. By micturition is meant the act of passing urine. (*See also* BED-WETTING ; BLADDER, DISEASES OF.)

MIDDLE EAR. The inner part of the ear between the drum and the passages leading to the nose is called the middle ear. Inflammation of the middle ear is called *otitis media*. For a full description of the ear *see* EAR.

MIDRIFF. An old-fashioned name for the Diaphragm and it is described under that name.

MIDWIFE. A midwife is a woman who attends upon another woman in her confinement. Since 1908 it is compulsory for any woman who practises midwifery for gain and as a profession to be trained to pass an examination and be subject to inspection. She puts the letters C.M.B. after her name, signifying that she has received a certificate from the Central Midwives Board. An untrained woman may of course assist at a confinement in an emergency when there is no trained help to be had.

MIGRAINE is a form of nervous headache which occurs periodically. There is some evidence that it runs in families, and if a mother is subject to these headaches then it is very likely that her children will also suffer from them.

Odd things seem to happen : bright lights which jump about

and then form weird patterns are seen, or the patient may suddenly only see half of everything he looks at, or he may see coloured flashes. Another queer thing may happen ; he may get " pins and needles " all up one side of his body and face. Then the head-ache usually starts, and it may vary in different attacks from a dull ache at the back of the head to such a severe throbbing that the patient is unable to lie down, sit up, or find any position which relieves his pain.

After a period, which may vary from half an hour to a day or more, the headache stops, either after the patient has been sick, or after he has slept. Most people who suffer in this way find that if they can sleep they awake free from headache, though feeling weak and " washed out," as though they had had a sleepless night. Not all the things that have been described will happen in any one attack of migraine ; but any of them may be the only sign of the condition. Of all the symptoms, the headache which occurs at intervals is the most constant. Most cases of true migraine start at a very early age ; the subjects of it are liable to " bilious attacks " in childhood and after puberty the headaches seem to take their place.

No one cause has been found for this disorder. Many things are known which will bring on an attack in anyone who is subject to the attacks. Excessive tiredness, either bodily or mental, is a well-known cause. Certain articles of diet such as too many sweets, or rich pastry, or fruit will bring on an attack in others. Eye-strain, infection of the back of the nose and of the tonsils has been known to produce frequent attacks which were lessened on removal of these causes. Certain emotions, especially rage or humiliation which the subject could not at the time express for fear of the con-sequences, have often been shown to bring on attacks.

Treatment. Prevention of the attacks amounts to discovery of the particular cause in a particular case and the treatment thereof. In the attack itself little can be done for the victim except to leave him, or her, in a darkened room which has been selected for its quietness and to let him lie or sit in whichever position gives the most relief until sickness or sleep relieves his pain. No one drug has been found to suit every case of migraine. It may be necessary to try several before one is found which will ward off or shorten an attack. In general, it is easier to ward off the attacks by means of drugs than to shorten or relieve an attack once it has started. (*See also* HEADACHE.)

MILIARIA. (*See* SWEAT RASH.)

MILIARY TUBERCULOSIS. This is a severe form of the disease in which the tuberculosis spreads rapidly throughout one or more organs of the body and tiny hard lumps which are said to resemble millet seed (whence comes the name) are found in the various organs affected, most commonly the lungs. (*See also* Tuberculosis.)

MILK FEVER. Milk Fever is the popular name for an attack of feverishness coming on in the mother about the second or third day after the birth of a child. Milk fever has become much rarer since more aseptic methods have been used at the time of labour and since women have been taught to prepare and harden the breasts beforehand so that they will not become cracked and sore when they are first used. (*See also* Pregnancy.)

MINER'S ANÆMIA. *See* Hookworm Disease.

MINER'S ELBOW. *See* Bursitis.

MINER'S NYSTAGMUS. A condition sometimes found in miners in which the eyeballs turn from side to side. This causes poor sight and often nervous troubles. It is thought that the dim light in which the miner works may be the cause. (*See also* Nystagmus.)

MISCARRIAGE. If a pregnancy terminates before the baby is old enough to have a separate life, that is before the 27th week of the pregnancy, there is said to have been a miscarriage. (*See also* Abortion ; Childbirth ; Pregnancy.)

MOLAR. The molars are the back teeth with which we grind our food. (*See also* Teeth.)

MOLE. A mole is a birthmark in which there is a tumour in the skin containing the brown colouring matter of the skin in excessive quantity. Sometimes the mole will be covered with hair as well. (*See also* Birthmark ; Skin.)

MONGOLISM. This is an unfortunate severe type of mental deficiency with which a child is occasionally born. It is called Mongolism because the child has the square face and upward slanting eyes which are characteristic of the Mongolian race. It is not known what causes mongolism ; but the child is usually the last of a large family, and it is surmised that the mother's powers of reproduction have become impaired. It is important to distinguish Mongols from cretins, because the cretinous child can be turned into a practically normal human being by suitable medical treatment, whereas there is nothing much to be done for the little Mongol child beyond caring for it in as kindly and sympathetic manner as possible. Their mentality remains that of a young child ; but they are usually happy, cheerful and affectionate people and easy to get on with. (*See also* Mental Deficiency.)

MONOMANIA is a form of insanity in which the patient's whole interest is centred round one delusion, or false belief. (*See also* Delusion ; Insanity ; Mental Disease.)

MORNING SICKNESS. One of the very earliest signs of pregnancy is morning sickness which is a slight attack of nausea or actual sickness on first rising from bed in the morning. In most women it is nothing more than the bringing up of a mouthful of clear fluid, but in different women it differs very much. (*See also* CHILDBIRTH ; PREGNANCY.)

MORON. A moron is a person of little sense. It is equivalent to our use of the word feeble-minded. (*See also* IDIOCY ; MENTAL DEFICIENCY.)

MORPHIA. The name morphia is applied popularly to morphine and the drugs derived from it. It is an alkaloid obtained from opium and its effects are much the same.

MORPHINISM. Chronic poisoning by morphia and the development of a craving for morphia are known as morphinism. (*See* POISON.)

MORTIFICATION. The mortification of a part of the body means the death of that part by gangrene. (*See also* GANGRENE.)

MOSQUITO. There are more than a thousand different species of mosquitoes, but only a certain number of these are responsible for carrying the germs of malaria. Several species of mosquitoes convey dengue and yellow fever, and others have been proved to carry the small worms called filaria bancrofti, which cause the condition known as filariasis. The female mosquito lays her eggs in stagnant water, and great masses of eggs may float together until the hatching process commences. It takes two to three days for the larvæ to appear, and they are very small and transparent and are popularly known as wrigglers. The larvæ lie just below the water and they have a tail-like breathing apparatus which penetrates the surface.

When the importance of the mosquito in relation to disease was fully realized, steps were taken to abolish their breeding grounds. The permanent cure of killing the larvæ is carried out by pouring oil on the surface of the water, thus choking up their breathing tubes. Stagnant pools may be drained, or the mosquito can be prevented from breeding on its surface by creating a flow of water or making a tidal wave.

In the matter of warding off insects, oil of citronella, oil of bergamot, cloves, thymol or cassia may be smeared over the exposed parts of the skin, which seems to have a certain amount of success. In the tropics, certain precautions must be taken to guard against their bite. It is important to see that all possible inlets to a house are adequately covered with netting. (*See* MALARIA.)

MOTIONS. It is usual to talk of the evacuations of the bowels as motions. (*See also* STOOLS.)

MOTOR AREAS. Our movements which we perform deliberately are caused by discharges of energy from cells in a region of the brain which is known as the motor area, meaning the area which deals with movement.

MOUNTAIN SICKNESS. People who go from a lower altitude into the mountains are liable at first to be overcome by attacks which are called mountain sickness. There may be a feeling of great muscular weakness, bad headache and a necessity to gasp for air. Sickness or nausea are also frequently present. Mountain sickness is caused by the diminution of the quantity of oxygen in the air at higher altitudes, and it is therefore common amongst aviators who go up to great heights. People who go to live in the ordinary inhabited mountainous regions such as Switzerland often feel the mountain sickness at first but they become acclimatized after two or three weeks. In the case of the attempts to climb the highest mountains in the world, such as Everest, it is the question of the lack of air suitable for human beings to breathe that has hitherto made it impossible to reach the summits. Special respirators have been invented to make breathing possible at great heights.

MOUTH. The mouth is generally considered in two parts. The *vestibule* or space between the lips and cheeks and the teeth and gums, and the mouth proper, which is the large cavity between the teeth and the throat. The tongue lies on the floor of the mouth, which contains the blood-vessels and glands which produce saliva.

Inflammation of the mouth is called *stomatitis* ; inflammation of the tongue is *glossitis*, and inflammation of the gums is *gingivitis*.

MUCOUS MEMBRANE. The linings of various organs of the body are moistened with the sticky substance called mucus and are called mucous membranes. Any inflammation of a mucous membrane increases the flow of mucus and causes the condition known as catarrh. (*See also* CATARRH ; MEMBRANE.)

MUCUS. Mucus is a sticky, slimy substance which is poured out over the mucous membranes which line various organs of the body. It serves as a protection from friction and also protects the delicate membrane from too easy attack by germs. Thus when anything irritates the mucous membrane a greater flow of mucus than usual is poured forth.

MULTIPARA. A woman who has had more than one child is called a multipara.

MULTIPLE NEURITIS. Neuritis occurring in more than one nerve at the same time is called multiple neuritis. It is of course an extremely painful condition, and is usually the result of some poison which is circulating in the blood, or of a chronic disease such as diabetes. Chronic alcoholism is often accompanied by multiple neuritis. People who work with lead or arsenic also get it frequently. (*See also* NEURITIS.)

MUMPS. Mumps is one of the commonest of the acute infectious diseases. It is very infectious, and the danger of infection is not over for a fortnight to three weeks after the symptoms appear ; then the *incubation period* is also up to three weeks, so no household that has had a case of mumps is safe from it until nearly six weeks have elapsed. As it is extremely difficult to get people, especially children, to remain in isolation for that length of time, it is often found that a second case occurs in the same household when it has been thought that all danger was over for some weeks.

Symptoms. The usual fever symptoms are present, raised temperature, up to 100° F. or higher, being the rule. The most characteristic symptom, however, is the swelling of the glands of the neck under the ear and perhaps under the chin. These are the parotid glands and the submaxillary glands. The swelling and soreness begin on one side and after a few days usually spread to the other side of the face as well. The worst points of tenderness are about the ear and under the edge of the jaw. The swelling may be immense and there may be a great deal of pain, though as a rule the patient does not become as sick and feverish as in some of the other fevers.

Treatment. The patient must of course be put to bed and isolated with all the usual precautions against the spread of infectious disease. Fluid diet and sponging will keep the fever in check. The mouth must be rinsed at intervals with an antiseptic mouthwash such as potassium permanganate, and hot or sometimes cold fomentation should be applied over the swollen glands. It may be necessary for a doctor to prescribe something for the relief of the pain.

Complications. The worst of these complications is inflammation of the pancreas, called *pancreatitis*. This requires careful treatment, as in some cases diabetes has followed upon inflammation of the pancreas during an attack of mumps. In males the testicle sometimes becomes inflamed, a condition which is known as *orchitis*, and requires immediate treatment lest the gland should become weakened. Inflammation of the kidney (nephritis) may also arise after mumps.

MURMUR. Any unusual sound, other than the ordinary heart sounds, which is heard when listening to the heart is called a murmur, or a bruit, which is a French word meaning a noise. Some murmurs are evidence of heart disease, but some have no especial significance. (*See also* HEART.)

MUSCÆ VOLITANTES. These are the floating specks which sometimes appear before the eyes when the liver is upset.

MUSCLE. The muscles of the body are composed of cells which have the power of changing their shape, and it is by this power of the muscular tissue to change its shape that the movements of the body are able to be carried out.

Muscles are divided into three classes : *Striped muscle* is so-called because when it is examined under a microscope its fibres show

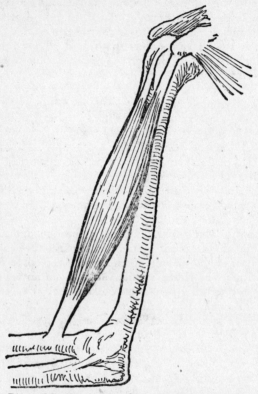

The Biceps Muscle of the arm, showing the two heads from which it arises and the tendon in which it ends

cross-striping. *Voluntary* muscle is one which can be controlled by the will of the individual, whereas involuntary muscle works without the conscious knowledge of the individual. The muscles of the arm are voluntary muscles, but the muscles of the stomach are involuntary. *Skeletal* muscle is the muscle tissue which covers our bones or skeleton.

In order to keep a muscle healthy and in good working trim it must be kept in constant use, or it will waste and become feeble.

It is for this reason that the entire body needs exercising if the daily occupation is such that some sets of muscles do not get their share of use. Muscles can be increased in strength and bulk to a remarkable degree, as is shown by the enormously developed muscles of professional gymnasts, etc. The danger of over-developing the muscles is, however, that unless the exercise is kept up the muscles suffer from fatty degeneration, and the middle-aged athlete is, therefore, as often as not fatter and puffier than the individual who did not build up so much muscle when young.

Diseases and Injuries of the Muscles. When a muscle has been overstretched it is said to be *strained*.

Inflammation of the Muscles is called myositis and may occur in any situation in the body. It may be due to infection by germs, or to a chronic disease such as tuberculosis or syphilis. Fibrosis or thickening of a muscle may result from long-continued irritation, such as the condition known as rider's muscle. The muscles may be invaded by certain species of worms or by hydatids in countries where these parasites are found. Tumours sometimes arise in a muscle and are called *myomas*. Muscular rheumatism is called *myalgia* or *fibrositis*. Painful spasms in the muscles are called *cramps*. *Atrophy* or shrinking and wasting of the muscle may be the result of the cutting off of the nerve supply of the muscle, as in the case where the nerve has been severed, or it may be due to a rare and somewhat mysterious disease called progressive muscular atrophy. (*See also* CRAMP ; FIBROSITIS.)

MUTISM. This is simply another name for dumbness.

MYALGIA. This is another name for muscular rheumatism. (*See also* FIBROSITIS ; RHEUMATISM.)

MYASTHENIA. Myasthenia or Myasthenia gravis, as it is more frequently called, is a rare disease of the muscles, the cause of which is unknown and for which no certain cure has yet been found. It usually comes on in young adults of either sex. There is a gradually increasing weakness of certain muscles. The first muscles to be affected are usually those of the head, eyes and mouth, then those of the chest, until breathing becomes difficult. The patient feels tired very easily and can only use the muscles after rest has restored them to a slight degree. There is great difficulty in keeping the eyes open or the mouth closed, and eating becomes almost impossible through great weakness. This state of weakness is gradually progressive.

It has recently been found that the injection of prostigmine relieves the symptoms of this disease completely, but the condition reverts to that before injection in a few hours, when another injection will again cause recovery.

MYCOSIS. By mycosis we mean infection of the body by some form of fungus. Ringworm is a mycosis ; thrush and actinomycosis are other diseases caused by fungi.

MYDRIATIC. When the pupil of the eye is excessively enlarged it is called mydriasis. Drugs such as atropine, which are used to increase the size of the pupil, are called mydriatics. (*See also* ATROPINE ; EYE ; PUPIL.)

MYELITIS. Inflammation of the spinal cord or softening of the cord is called myelitis. The condition is a serious and fatal one if it is due to disease, when paralysis and wasting occur, but if it is due to pressure on the spinal cord there is a possibility that the pressure may be removed and recovery effected. (*See also* PARAPLEGIA ; POLIOMYELITIS ; SPINAL CORD.)

MYELOMA. A tumour in a bone which is found sometimes in young people. It is usually harmless but should be removed by operation.

MYOCARDIAL DEGENERATION. Degeneration of the myocardium or heart muscle may be due to different causes, but the result is the same, namely heart weakness and heart failure. A common cause of myocardial degeneration is fibrosis, where the muscle is impeded in its working by an overgrowth of the fibres which surround it. Fatty degeneration is another common cause of myocardial failure. In obese people the fat is deposited in and around the heart muscle causing it to become weak and degenerated. (*See also* HEART.)

MYOCARDIUM. The muscle of the heart is called the myocardium, and inflammation of the heart muscle is called *myocarditis*.

MYOPATHY. Myopathy is a hereditary condition in which there is shrinking of the muscles without any apparent cause. It attacks young people in families which suffer from it, and males are more often the victims than females.

Treatment. No special treatment has been devised, but the general health must be kept as good as possible and the patient should be on a building-up régime. Massage and electrical treatment may do some good. Occasionally the disease is arrested.

MYOPIA. Myopia is the technical name for short sight. (*See also* ASTIGMATISM ; EYE.)

MYOSITIS. Myositis is the medical name for inflammation of a muscle. (*See also* MUSCLE.)

MYXŒDEMA. This is a condition which is fairly common in middle-aged women though it occurs in men and children also. It is due to deficiency in the juice which is produced by the thyroid gland.

Symptoms. The typical patient is a middle-aged woman who becomes fat and puffy, with coarse skin and bloated features. She has pudgy hands, muddy complexion with a slight flush over the cheekbones, and a loss of hair from the scalp, eyebrows, etc. The intellect usually becomes duller, the patient being heavier and slower in her speech and understanding than she used to be. Fat deposits occur in such regions as the shoulders, the abdominal wall and the breasts. A well-developed case of myxœdema is easy to distinguish, but the condition may creep on gradually without the woman noticing it until it is well established.

Treatment. As the disease is due to thyroid insufficiency the results of administering thyroid extract appear almost miraculous. In a very short time the woman regains her health and will retain it as long as she takes the thyroid extract. A word of warning is due here. Thyroid extract has a marked effect on the heart and must never be taken except on a doctor's advice, and whilst the patient is on it she should be kept under observation from time to time, and should report at once any untoward symptoms such as palpitations or breathlessness, which means too much is being taken. (*See also* DUCTLESS GLANDS ; THYROID GLAND.)

NÆVUS. *See* BIRTHMARKS.

NAILS, DISEASES OF. *Abscess* of the nail is very often the result of a splinter, or some such material, being run in below the nail. In order to allow the pus to discharge the nail may have to be cut or split, otherwise the pain may be almost unendurable. As soon as there is any hint of inflammation occurring in the nail, hot fomentations or Antiphlogistine should be applied. (*See also* WHITLOW.)

Ingrowing nail is a condition which occurs frequently in the nail of the big toe and it can cause a great deal of misery and unhappiness. (*See also* INGROWING TOE-NAIL.)

Injuries to the nails cause them to turn black owing to the pressure of blood beneath them. If the injury has been severe, the nail is almost sure to come off ; but a new one should grow in unless the injury has damaged the nail-bed very severely.

The appearance of the nails very often indicates the general state of health ; for example, white spots usually make their appearance when the health is a bit below par and grooves indicate the presence of rheumatism.

NAPKIN RASH. This occurs in children with sensitive skins, or in those who have not been properly cared for. The treatment of this condition will be found under ERYTHEMA.

NARCOSIS. A state of unconsciousness which closely resembles deep sleep. The drugs which produce this condition are known as narcotics. (*See also* ANÆSTHETICS.)

NARCOTICS. *See* HYPNOTICS ; ANÆSTHETICS.

NASAL CATARRH. *See* CATARRH, NASAL.

NASAL FEEDING. *See* FORCIBLE FEEDING.

NASO-PHARYNX. The naso-pharynx is the part of the throat which lies between the nasal passages and the back of the mouth.

NATIONAL HEALTH INSURANCE ACT, THE. This Act, passed in 1911, has two main objects : (1) to secure for the insured person any necessary medical attendance ; (2) to compensate him while sick, for the loss of his wages. The cost of this is shared between the worker, the employer, and the State. All wage-earners over 16 (unless their income exceeds £420) must be insured ; juvenile contributors are boys and girls between school-leaving age and 16, and they are eligible for free medical attendance, treatment, and medicines if employed under conditions in which they would be compulsorily insurable if over 16. The weekly contribution is 2s. 0d. for men and 1s. 7d. for women, the employer paying 1s. 0d. and 9d. respectively ; for juvenile contributors it is 4d., payable half by employer and half by worker. The contribution is paid by special stamps sold at any post office, and it is the duty of the employee to see that his card is kept stamped up to date. For contributors employed in the mercantile marine on foreign-going ships the weekly contribution is 1s. 9d. for men, 1s. 4d. for women, and 2d. for juveniles, the employer paying 9d., 6d., and 1d.

The benefits of the Act are : (1) Medical benefit ; (2) Sickness benefit ; (3) Disablement benefit ; (4) Maternity benefit ; (5) Additional benefits (such as dental and ophthalmic benefits).

By an additional Act of 1928, an insured person is credited with contributions not only for every week during which he is employed, but also for those in which he is ill or genuinely unemployed. If, however, he falls into arrears, his benefits are reduced in proportion.

By an Act passed in December, 1937, juveniles between the ages of 14 and 16 became insured for medical benefits only, to bridge the gap between the school medical service and the National Health Insurance panel system ; this continues until the contributor's sixteenth birthday, when the ordinary scheme comes in. Persons aged 65 and over are subject to special rates of 10d. and 7d. for men and women respectively, whilst in employment, the employer paying the whole amount.

The medical benefit arrangements are made by local Insurance Committees. Any registered medical practitioner may have his or her name on the " panel." An insured person has free choice of doctor and can obtain medicines, etc., from any chemist who does National Insurance Act dispensing. The doctor gives such certificates as are required for sickness, disablement and other claims.

NAVEL. *See* UMBILICUS.

NEAR-SIGHTEDNESS. This condition is medically known as myopia. (*See also* SIGHT.)

NECK. The neck is the column which supports the head, and it also contains the passages through which air and food are conveyed to the rest of the body. The painful condition known as stiff neck is due to a rheumatic inflammation of these muscles, and wry-neck is usually caused by strain on either one side or the other.

Many other important structures of the neck are closely related to the sternomastoid muscles, such as the carotid artery, the jugular vein, the larynx, the pharynx, the thyroid gland, and the vagus nerve—an important nerve of the heart, etc. The larynx can be felt to move up and down in the front of the neck, especially during the act of swallowing. In men, the Adam's apple is a very prominent feature.

Swelling of the neck is almost always due to enlarged glands which may be infected from the teeth, the tonsils or the ear. Tuberculosis is a disease which frequently attacks the glands of the neck ; *see also* article on GLANDULAR FEVER. The swelling of the thyroid gland, which lies low down in the front of the neck, is fully dealt with under the heading GOITRE.

Several large important veins run down the neck, the chief of these being the external jugular vein. Wounds in this part of the neck are liable to cause very severe bleeding and unless immediate measures are taken to arrest the hæmorrhage, death may result. A broken neck is almost always fatal owing to the inevitable damage done to the nerves connected with the brain. (*See also* GLANDS ; JUGULAR VEIN ; TUBERCULOSIS.)

NECROSIS. Necrosis means the death of a part of the body, but the word is used with special reference to the death of bone.

When the blood-supply is cut off from a part of a bone it becomes necrosed. (*See also* BONE ; EROSION ; GANGRENE.)

NEPHRITIS. Nephritis, or Bright's disease, is a condition in which there is inflammation of the kidneys or there may be degenerative changes in the kidneys. There are several forms of this condition, but the chief varieties may be classified as acute and chronic.

Acute nephritis is frequently caused by exposure to cold or wet, or it may arise as a complication of some other disease such as scarlet fever, erysipelas or diphtheria. Inflammation of the kidneys may also occur as a result of poisoning by irritating substances such as turpentine or corrosive sublimate, etc. The disease mainly affects children and young adults.

Symptoms. In some cases the onset of the disease may be

insidious and the first symptoms to be noticed are redness of the urine and a certain amount of puffiness around the eyes. Other cases may develop quite suddenly, showing all the characteristic symptoms of acute nephritis within a day or two. Dropsy, or swelling of the body, with puffiness of the eyes, face and ankles, is almost always present in varying degrees. Vomiting and nausea frequently occur early on in the condition, and this leads to loss of appetite and disturbance of the digestive system. The temperature is commonly raised to about 100° or 101° F., though in adults there may be no fever present. The skin is dry and the tongue furred, and the patient may be very troubled with headache. There is frequently pain in the back and loins, and diarrhœa may develop. Changes take place in the urine from the very beginning of the disease. It is greatly reduced in quantity and the colour becomes dark and smoky from the presence of blood. When tested, a large amount of albumin is found to be present and it also contains enormous numbers of blood-cells. The course of this disease is very serious, but even extreme cases may recover completely with the proper treatment.

Treatment. As soon as a patient shows the slightest sign of nephritis he must be put to bed and kept as warm as possible. Blankets should be used instead of sheets, and flannel should be worn next to the skin. The temperature of the bedroom should be moderately warm and all draughts avoided. The doctor should be called in at once, as some cases quickly develop into the chronic stage, which, in many cases, proves fatal. If there is much swelling present, sweating may be induced by hot packs and hot-water bottles. The bowels must be kept open daily in order to help the elimination of waste matters from the body and so ease the work of the kidneys. There has recently been an almost complete change in the diet advised in acute nephritis. Instead of giving lots of fluids, and especially milk, to " wash out " the kidneys, it is now realized that so much fluid during the early stages only increases the œdema, and, in addition, milk contains salt and protein which are retained in the body while the function of this organ is impaired. In order to spare the kidney as much as possible, no salt and protein (milk) should be given and the intake of water should not be greater than the output of urine. For the first three or five days, therefore, only a little weak tea or lemonade or half an orange two or three times a day should be given. Then the diet may be increased by giving cooked fruit, sugar, cooked vegetables and rice, butter and cream. In about a week or ten days a certain amount of protein should be given—to keep up the needs of the body—in the form of milk, eggs, chicken, fish, with bread. There is no doubt that abstinence from food and drink in the early stages of acute nephritis is good treatment, but the thirst may be troublesome. No·salt should be added in cooking as long as there is any swelling present in the body. The patient must be kept in bed until all traces of blood have disappeared from the urine, the swelling has gone, and the temperature is normal. Large doses of alkalies, such as bicarbonate of soda and citrate of potash, are nowadays often advised with benefit. Iron tonics should be given during convalescence to deal with the anæmia which usually makes its appearance in connection with nephritis ; these tonics will help to improve the appetite.

Chronic Nephritis may follow an attack of acute nephritis, but in some cases the acute attack may have passed unnoticed. Here again there are varying degrees of the condition, but the outlook is serious because of the degeneration which takes place in the kidneys. The swelling and dropsy tend to spread and may even affect the lungs.

Treatment. Special care must be taken to avoid chills and the diet must be regulated by a doctor. The bowels should be kept open and no alcohol should be taken. It is now recognized that restriction of protein may be harmful in chronic nephritis, but the high protein diet now advised should not be given when the activity of the kidney is impaired. Such a diet consists of lean meats, whites of eggs, skimmed milk, gelatine, beans, peas, and oatmeal. (*See also* DROPSY ; KIDNEY.)

NERVOUS HEADACHE. *See* MIGRAINE.

NERVOUS SYSTEM is the means by which each part of our body is made aware of what is the condition at any particular moment of every other part, and also is the means by which we communicate with the outside world.

In man, the nervous system is generally divided into the central nervous system, which consists of the brain and the spinal cord, and the peripheral nervous system, which consists of all the nerves in the body other than those attached to the brain itself.

The internal organs, such as the heart, digestive organs and lungs, not only have the ordinary nerve supply which controls their action, but they have a special nerve supply called the *sympathetic* nervous system. The sympathetic nervous system is situated in the spinal cord and the lowest part of the brain, from which tiny nerves are given off to all the organs of the body. We are never conscious of the sympathetic system and we have no control over it, because it is an " emergency system " which is always ready to act and is therefore not to be used at will. Nevertheless, in some people the sympathetic system is more irritable than in others, and in them, a very slight fright will produce all the symptoms which we associate with a state of terror. (*See also* BRAIN ; NEURITIS.)

NETTLE-RASH. *See* URTICARIA.

NEURALGIA is pain felt along a nerve. There are very many different causes for neuralgia as well as many different positions where the pain may be felt, but the character of the pain is nearly always the same. The pain of neuralgia is of a severe shooting or throbbing nature and the skin, along which tiny branches of the nerves run, is often very tender to the touch. Another curious feature of the pain of neuralgia is that it is not continuous but occurs in little bouts, which are made worse by exposing the skin to the cold.

Tic douloureux. This is felt on the face, usually on one side only, all over the one side, or round the eye only, or rarely, round the nose and chin only. The pain is exceedingly sharp and is always felt worst in a draught or in cold weather. The skin of the part of the face on which the pain is felt is so tender that patients dread washing their faces, and if asked to show where the pain is situated they do not touch the face, but carefully keep their pointing finger a half an inch away from the painful area when indicating its extent. The lightest touch in severe cases will bring on an attack of this tic douloureux, and the pain may become so bad that these unhappy patients will even think of suicide rather than endure it. Fortunately, we can relieve this pain by means of an injection of alcohol into a nerve of the face. The result is that the patient loses the pain, but is left with a numb feeling on that side of the face. It may be necessary to repeat this injection in a year or eighteen months, but the relief afforded by the injection can really only be appreciated by those who have suffered from this pain of tic douloureux.

Much more often is neuralgia of the face caused by decaying teeth, the nerves of which are connected with those of the face. And even a plug of wax in the ear has been known to give rise to very bad neuralgia of the temple. Neuralgia of the back of the head is very common after sitting in a draught, and this is due to a slight thickening of the covering of the muscles of the back of the neck which presses on the sensitive nerves.

One form of neuralgia may puzzle many doctors before the spots of " shingles " appear. Perhaps four or five days before a crop of " shingles " shows itself, a patient may complain of neuralgia on one side of the chest, abdomen or face. Nothing can be found to account for this pain until the spots appear.

Other causes of neuralgia may be such general diseases as diabetes or arterio-sclerosis, whilst the early pains of locomotor ataxia are often taken for a simple neuralgia. *Sciatica*, which is one of the forms of neuritis and is described under that heading, always starts as a neuralgia.

Treatment. The cure of any type of neuralgia depends entirely on the cause, but the pain itself is dealt with in three main ways. These are by means of heat, warmth, and the use of drugs which make the whole nervous system less sensitive to pain. The drugs which " damp down " the sensitiveness of the nervous system to pain are many. The coal tar group of drugs such as aspirin, phenacetin and pyramidon are often helpful, whilst in other instances the bromides or tincture of gelsemium afford relief. (*See also* ARTERIO-SCLEROSIS ; LOCOMOTOR ATAXIA ; NEURITIS.)

NEURITIS means inflammation of a nerve, and the changes in the nerve are those of swelling and redness which are associated with that process. According as to which particular bundles of nerve units are damaged in a neuritis, so will the main symptoms be either those of loss of power in the limbs, or of pain, but usually some bundles of both systems of units are damaged, and so although the chief symptoms may be those of loss of power, yet the patient will also have some pain in the part of the limb controlled by the particular nerve, and he will be unable to feel things as well as usual in the limb : it will be numbed.

The causes of neuritis are many ; but, generally speaking, the chief causes are poisons, whether simple chemical poisons, or the poisons produced by disease in the body, or by such germs as that which gives people diphtheria. The chief chemical poisons which may give rise to neuritis are lead, arsenic and alcohol. *Lead poisoning* is rarer now than it was, as lead paint is not used so much. *Arsenic neuritis* is seen sometimes as the result of taking arsenic over a long period of time, but one outbreak of arsenic poisoning with neuritis took place in 1906 as the result of accidental contamination of beer with arsenic. This form of neuritis chiefly affects the legs and loss of power with intense pain occurs.

Alcoholic neuritis is the result of drinking spirits in large quantities over a long period of time. It is one of the most painful forms of neuritis known, and attacks both the arms and the legs.

In diphtheria, neuritis of a particular type occurs : the nerves which control the movements of the eyes and of the palate are damaged by the poison made by the germ of diphtheria and so the patient is unable to read, as he cannot fix his eyes on the print ; and food, instead of going down the gullet, is brought back through the nose. The outlook for this form of neuritis is good, as it nearly always gets better within a few weeks.

Treatment. The first thing is to discover the cause and to remove it at once. In the first stage of treatment, after the cause has been removed, the patient must rest in bed. When the pains are severe, application of heat and liniments containing belladonna often give relief. Massage, at first very gentle and then more energetic, is very helpful. (*See also* NERVOUS SYSTEM ; SCIATICA.)

NEUROLOGY. This name is applied to the branch of medicine which deals with the nervous system and its diseases.

NEUROMA. Neuroma means a tumour connected with a nerve. They are usually composed of nerve tissue and may be exceedingly painful. (*See also* TUMOUR.)

NEUROSIS is a mild form of mental disorder in which the troubled mind draws attention to itself by causing some bodily symptoms. There are many different kinds of neurosis, and the more important ones are discussed under the headings of ANXIETY and HYSTERIA.

NEUROTIC. Anyone of a very temperamental nature whose actions are influenced by the emotions is said to be neurotic.

NIPPLE, DISEASE OF (Paget's Disease). This is a serious disease of the nipple which begins with a peculiar hardness of the skin and goes on to intractable ulceration. It is a form of cancer which commences in the milk-ducts or tubes at their endings on the surface of the nipple. Slight itching is generally present, and this alternates with attacks of pain, which is sometimes very severe.

The disease nearly always attacks women of middle age. Pain in the breast should always have the opinion of a doctor, even if it does turn out to be only a neuralgia.

Treatment. This consists in the removal of the whole breast. The complete operation has to be performed later in any case, if the patient's life is to be preserved. (*See also* CANCER ; DERMATITIS ; PAGET'S DISEASE.)

NITRIC ACID. Nitric acid is greatly used to destroy warts because of its powerful caustic action on the tissues. Like all acids it is an antiseptic, but it is too irritating to be used for ordinary purposes even in weak solutions.

NITRITE. *See* AMYL NITRITE.

NITROGEN. About two-thirds of the atmosphere is made up of nitrogen, a colourless, odourless gas necessary to all animal and plant life. (*See also* AIR ; OXYGEN.)

NITROGLYCERINE. This oil, which is well known in other circumstances as an explosive, has the same action as amyl nitrite and it is frequently taken by people who suffer from severe pain in the heart. (*See also* AMYL NITRITE ; ASTHMA.)

NITROUS OXIDE. This is also known as laughing gas and it is given as an anæsthetic for short operations. (*See also* ANÆSTHETICS.)

NODE.   A node is a lump or swelling usually upon the surface of a bone. The term nodule is applied to small swellings.

NOSE.   The organ which supplies us with a sense of smell is situated in the nose, but the nose has a much more important function, in that it forms the upper end of the air passages which lead to the lungs and so provides us with a means of breathing.

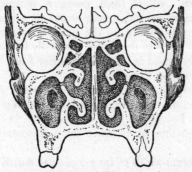

Coronal section through Nose, showing nasal passages and maxillary antra

The interior of the nose is divided into two narrow cavities by a thin partition known as the septum, and these cavities run directly backwards about two inches. The septum is covered with the general mucous membrane which lines the nose. On each side

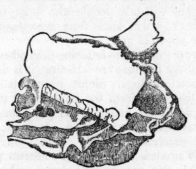

Ethmoid Bone

three delicate bones, the turbinals, project into the nasal passage ; they come from the ethmoid bone, which has air cells in it connected with the nose, similar to the frontal sinus and the maxillary sinus or antrum. For diseases of the nose *see also* ADENOIDS ; ANTRUM ; CATARRH, NASAL ; FOREIGN BODY ; POLYPUS ; SINUS.

NOTIFICATION OF DISEASE. The diseases a medical practitioner is compelled by law to notify are the following : Small-pox, scarlet fever, typhus fever, typhoid fever, relapsing fever, continued fever, puerperal fever, puerperal pyrexia, diphtheria, erysipelas and tuberculosis. Certain other diseases may be made notifiable at the option of the local sanitary authority.

NUMBNESS. Apart from being a symptom of a disease, numbness or loss of sensation may occur in a limb by pressure on a nerve. In many diseases of the nervous system, numbness may occur in various parts of the body, especially in the hands and feet ; this is frequently found in those who suffer from hysteria. (*See also* HYSTERIA ; NERVOUS SYSTEM.)

NUX VOMICA. Nux vomica, in small doses, is a bitter tonic which stimulates gastric digestion. (*See also* STRYCHNINE.)

OBESITY. People who are too fat have become so either by reason of over-eating or because there is something wrong with them.

The two different kinds of fat people are called *exogenous*, that is, coming from outside ; and *endogenous*, that is, coming from inside. This means that in the one case too much is taken in, which is simple over-eating, and in the other case the control of what is taken in, whether too much or too little, is out of gear and deals with the intake in an unusual way.

Exogenous Obesity. Too much fat, whether from one reason or another, is a very serious and real danger, so much so that no insurance company will take people who weigh much outside the average limit, because they know from experience that fat people seldom live to a good old age.

Certain foods are much more fattening than others. But, curiously enough, it is not the fats that are fattening, it is the starchy foods ; bread, cakes, potatoes, sugar, plums, prunes, bananas, puddings. And it is just these that form the staple of all meals and are so convenient at odd times. Sugar, bread and potatoes are the chief offenders. These should be restricted. It is the purpose of the sugars and the starches to provide physical energy ; when they are not actually needed, as in lack of sufficient physical exercise and fresh air, then they are carefully stored up by the body in the form of fat.

Although it is true that thyroid extract can bring about fat reduction, and more recently dinitro-o-cresol has had similar results, all such drugs must be taken with caution and only under medical advice, as serious and indeed fatal results have occurred.

Endogenous Obesity. This type of obesity is due to certain diseases involving the internal glands of the body : the thyroid, the pituitary, the ovaries, the testicles, the suprarenal, etc. Disturbance of the ovarian function at the menopause or change of life often leads to abnormal deposits of fat in women. Most young people who get fat do so by reason of some defect of the glands. There are, of course, many types and conditions, but it is important to observe that such cases are due to ill-health and disease. No such case should be allowed to experiment with diets or medicines or drugs ; they require very careful and very serious treatment, as they are the unfortunate sufferers of a serious and unsightly illness.

The hereditary tendency to fat so often seen in families is usually associated with a glandular error.

OBSTETRICS. The branch of medicine which deals with pregnancy and childbirth is known as midwifery or obstetrics.

ŒDEMA. The swelling which occurs in dropsy is known as œdema. There is an accumulation of watery fluid beneath the skin, and indentations or pits can be made in the flesh by pressing with the finger. (*See also* DROPSY.)

ŒSOPHAGUS. The œsophagus is the tube by which food is conveyed down the throat to the stomach. It begins at the level of the lower end of the larynx (Adam's apple) and lies immediately behind the windpipe. Any trouble in the œsophagus usually shows itself first by some slight difficulty in swallowing, which is very often put down to nerves. If this is persistent, however, an X-ray examination should always be done and if anything abnormal is noticed, an examination by the special tube called an œsophagoscope carried out. Curious pouches of the œsophagus, due to straining, are not uncommon, and strictures and growths of the œsophagus may be very serious and fatal. (*See also* GULLET.)

OMENTUM. A long fold of the peritoneum which hangs down over the intestine is known as the omentum. (*See also* OBESITY.)

ONYCHIA. A disease of the nails in which inflammation takes place is known as onychia. The nail usually becomes discoloured and is thrown off, but is replaced by the growth of a new one. (*See also* NAILS.)

OPHTHALMIA. Inflammation of the eye. (*See also* CONJUNCTIVITIS ; EYE.)

OPIUM. Opium is perhaps the best known of all the narcotic (sleep-producing) drugs and it is the oldest and most certain remedy for pain. It is the dried juice of the unripe seed-capsules of the white poppy and it contains a large number of alkaloid substances, at least eighteen in number, of which the following are the most important : morphine, codeine, narcotine, and thebaine.

OPTIC NERVE. The second pair of cranial nerves are called the optic nerves and they connect the eye with the brain. (*See also* EYE.)

ORBIT. The bony cavity which contains the eye is called the orbit. (*See also* EYE.)

ORCHITIS. Inflammation of the testicle is known as orchitis. When the infection spreads along the cord it is known as epididymitis. (*See also* EPIDIDYMITIS ; TESTICLE.)

ORGANIC DISEASE. Disease of an organ which causes an alteration in the workings of the body is said to be an organic disease. A disease in which no such changes can be found is said to be functional.

ORGANO-THERAPY. Treatment of disease by the administration of animal organs or extracts of them, such as thyroid gland, insulin, adrenalin, pituitrin, etc., is known as organo-therapy. (*See also* DUCTLESS GLANDS.)

ORTHOPÆDICS. This is the term given to a branch of surgery which deals with the treatment of fractures and joint affections and the correction of deformities.

OSSIFICATION. The formation of bone is called ossification.

OSTEITIS. A chronic disease of the bones which does not commence until late in life is known as osteitis, or Paget's disease of the bones. The bones usually show signs of softening which alters their shape to a certain extent, but subsequently they harden, leaving them in a deformed state such as curvature of the spine, curvature of the bones of the leg, and enlargement of the head. The cause of the disease is not known, but a patient may live for twenty or thirty years after onset of the condition. There is no specialized treatment, but aspirin will be found helpful in relieving any pains. (*See also* BONE ; OSTEOMYELITIS.)

OSTEO-ARTHRITIS. A disease in which there is inflammation in the joints and in which changes take place in the bones. (*See also* RHEUMATOID ARTHRITIS.)

OSTEOMALACIA. This is a condition of the bones in which, owing to a lack of calcium, they become softened and are liable to break. It may be due to a lack of the proper vitamins in the diet, especially vitamin D, or to a lack of sunshine and a deficiency of calcium in the blood.

Treatment. The patient should be given cod-liver oil and put on a diet rich in calcium and phosphorus obtained from eggs, milk, fish and vegetables. As much sunshine as possible should be obtained and unhygienic surroundings should be avoided. (*See also* BONE.)

OSTEOMYELITIS. This condition is most commonly met with in children between the ages of three and fourteen, but it may also occur in adults. The term osteomyelitis means inflammation in the marrow of a bone and it is caused by infection either in the blood itself or from an injury to the skin through which the germs have penetrated.

Symptoms. Severe pain is usually felt in the bone (usually a leg bone) and the neighbouring joints may feel painful and tender. Very shortly after the first symptom of pain, the patient begins to feel ill, and there may be high temperature and swelling of the affected limb. If an operation is not carried out immediately, pus will collect and a large abscess will form, which will gradually make its way through the tissues to the skin. In some cases the abscess may burst or spread into a neighbouring large joint, and a severe state of poisoning may be set up.

Treatment. Operation must be carried out as soon as possible, otherwise there is the possibility that the child may die from septicæmia, or blood-poisoning, or the bone of the leg may be permanently damaged. The operation consists of boring through to the bone in order to allow the pus to discharge freely. (*See also* BONE.)

OTORRHŒA. A discharge from the ear is known as otorrhœa. (*See also* EAR ; MASTOID.)

OTOSCLEROSIS. A type of deafness in which changes occur in the bony walls of the labyrinth or internal ear is known as otosclerosis. There are usually noises in the ears and deafness gradually becomes worse as time goes on, though it seldom goes on to stone deafness. The treatment is not very satisfactory, and a specialist's advice should be sought early on. (*See also* EAR.)

OVARIES. There are two ovaries in the female, one on each side within the pelvis, each about an inch in length and oval in shape. Each ovary is joined to the womb (uterus) by a broad band which contains within its folds a tube known as the Fallopian tube along which the tiny ovum (the microscopic egg, or female sexual element) is conveyed from the ovary to the womb. The period of menstruation takes place when an ovum is set free (at regular intervals of about four weeks) from the ovary and travels down to the womb ; if it is not impregnated it escapes from the womb with the blood which comes away. Each menstruation resembles a slight pregnancy which has not been made complete through the ovum not having been impregnated. (*See also* MENSTRUATION.)

OVUM. An ovum is the single cell which comes from the ovary of the female, and after it has become impregnated by the male, it is capable of developing into an individual. (*See also* EMBRYO.)

OXALIC ACID POISONING. Oxalic acid poisoning is usually the result of taking salts of lemon in mistake for Epsom salts or a like substance. It is a very corrosive poison, and it destroys any tissue it comes in contact with. It causes intense burning pain in the mouth, throat and stomach, followed by vomiting and collapse.

Treatment. On no account should an emetic be given as this will only cause further irritation to the throat and stomach. Lime chalk or whiting mixed with a little water is the best remedy and if these substances are not at hand, strip some whitewash off a wall or ceiling. Follow with a dose of castor oil, and keep the patient for three or four days on nothing but milk and lime water and give as little water as possible.

OXYGEN. A colourless gas, odourless and tasteless, oxygen forms rather more than one-fifth of the bulk of the atmosphere. It is necessary to life, and every time we breathe we give the blood a fresh supply.

Oxygen is prepared in large quantities for commercial purposes and it is stored in steel cylinders from which it can be obtained at any desired rate by turning a stop-cock. In many conditions the blood is not capable of carrying its normal amount of oxygen and in such cases the administration of the gas gives great relief. Pure oxygen is supplied by means of inhalation in cases of asphyxia, especially in pneumonia, valvular disease of the heart, anæmia and poisoning.

OZÆNA. The unpleasant smell from the nose due to crusts forming in the interior is known as ozæna. The condition arises where there is a lack of mucous secretion and is probably due to an infection. It is usually treated by nasal douches followed by a paint containing glycerine and glucose, half and half; treatment has to be continued for months. (*See also* NOSE.)

PAGET'S DISEASE. Paget's disease of the nipple is a serious condition and is discussed under the heading NIPPLE. Paget's disease of bone is a chronic disease described under OSTEITIS.

PALATE. The arch which forms the roof of the mouth is known as the hard palate. In some people this arch is higher than in others. At the back of the mouth the fleshy part which hangs down is called the soft palate, and from the middle of the soft palate hangs the narrow projection known as the uvula. (*See also* CLEFT PALATE ; MOUTH.)

PALPITATION. This is the name given to the condition where a person becomes aware of the heart beating against the chest-wall and usually beating more quickly than normal. The condition may be due to real disease of the heart muscle or valves, but is much more commonly due to some less important cause where there is no actual disease. *Excessive indulgence* in tobacco, tea, coffee or alcohol is very bad for the heart as these substances act as poisons in some people.

PALSY. This is another name for Paralysis.

PANCREAS. (*See also* DIABETES ; DIGESTION ; DUCTLESS GLANDS ; INSULIN.)

PAPILLOMA. A growth on the skin or mucous membrane of which a wart is a common example. (*See also* WART.)

PARACENTESIS. The operation in which the wall of a cavity is punctured in order to allow fluid to be discharged. The term is commonly used for the incision of an inflamed ear drum. (*See also* EAR ; MASTOIDITIS.)

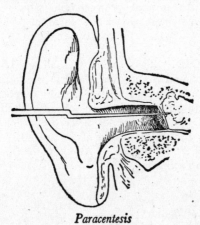

Paracentesis

PARALYSIS means loss of power of movement in a part of the body and is due to some injury to, or disease of, the nervous system. The extent of any paralysis depends entirely on which part of the nervous system is damaged and to what the damage is due. In infantile paralysis, which is caused by a germ attacking the central nervous system, there is usually much more paralysis in the stage of the attack itself than there is after the attack is over.

Birth paralysis is due to injury to the brain at birth and may take many forms. The most common is weakness of one side of the body and of the corresponding arm and leg.

In adults, paralysis of one side of the body and the corresponding arm and leg is about the most common paralysis, and is known as Hemiplegia. Paralysis of both legs may occur in many diseases of the nervous system, such as disseminated sclerosis and locomotor ataxia. One of the diseases of old age is paralysis agitans, or the " shaking palsy," in which there is a stiffness of the

15*

muscles of the limbs, especially of the arms with tremor first of the fingers, and later, of the whole arm.

This " shaking palsy " also occurs in young adults as a sequel to encephalitis lethargica and it is one of the most distressing results which follow " sleepy sickness."

Certain forms of paralysis are due to hysteria in which bodily weakness and paralysis of the limbs is caused by mental trouble. Only when the mental trouble is dealt with can the " paralysis " be cured. (*See also* DISSEMINATED SCLEROSIS ; ENCEPHALITIS LETHARGICA ; HYSTERIA ; LOCOMOTOR ATAXIA ; NEURITIS ; ST. VITUS'S DANCE.)

PARASITE. An animal or vegetable which lives upon or within another creature is known as a parasite. (*See also* BED BUG ; FILARIA ; GUINEA WORM ; HEAD LOUSE ; ITCH ; JIGGER ; LIVER FLUKE ; WORM.)

PARATHYROID. Two pairs of small glands which lie to the side of and behind the thyroid gland in the neck are known as the parathyroids. When these glands become damaged or removed the nervous system appears to suffer. (*See also* TETANY.)

PARATYPHOID. A type of fever which closely resembles typhoid fever, though milder. (*See also* TYPHOID.)

PARKINSON'S DISEASE. Another name for paralysis agitans. (*See also* PARALYSIS.)

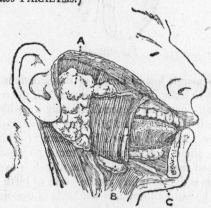

Parotid Gland
A. Parotid Gland; B. Submaxillary Gland; C. Sublingual Gland

PAROTID GLAND. One of the most important glands which supply the mouth with saliva. (*See* MUMPS.)

PARTURITION. The act of giving birth to a child is known as parturition. (*See also* LABOUR.)

PATELLA. The small rounded bone projecting from the knee-joint is known as the patella or knee-cap. (*See also* KNEE.)

PATHOLOGY. Pathology is the science which deals with the causes of and the changes produced in the body by disease.

PEDICULOSIS. *See* HEAD LOUSE.

PELLAGRA. A curious disease which occurs in tropical and sub-tropical countries, pellagra is characterized by eruptions on the skin accompanied by disorders of the digestive and nervous systems.

PELVIS. The pelvis is the space contained within the haunch bones which join together in front, with the bone known as the sacrum behind. It contains the lower part of the large intestine, that is, the pelvic colon, and rectum and also the urinary bladder, and in the female, the womb and ovaries. Close to the brim of

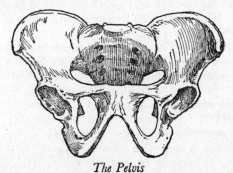

The Pelvis

the pelvis are the great blood-vessels which run from the abdomen to the lower limbs.

PENIS. The penis is the male organ of generation. It is through the urethra, or tube of the penis, that the contents of the urinary bladder as well as those of the seminal vesicles escape.

PERFORATION. A hole made through the wall of an organ is known as a perforation, but the term is usually used in connection with the stomach or intestines. (*See also* APPENDICITIS ; DUODENAL ULCER ; EAR ; GASTRIC ULCER ; PARACENTESIS.)

PERIMETRITIS. Inflammation of the membrane that lines the pelvis or womb is known as perimetritis or pelvic peritonitis. It is a very serious and painful condition and there is great danger of the inflammation spreading upwards into the abdominal cavity. (*See also* PERITONITIS.)

PERINEUM. The area situated between the opening of the bowel behind and the genital organs in front is termed the perineum. During labour it is quite common for this area to become torn owing to the progress and force of the child, and the defect, if not properly repaired at the time of the birth, may lead to prolapse of the womb and other disorders. (*See also* Womb.)

PERIOD. *See* Menstruation.

PERIOSTEUM. The membrane covering the surfaces of bones is known as the periosteum. (*See also* Bone ; Necrosis.)

PERIOSTITIS. Inflammation on the surface of a bone which affects the periosteum is known as periostitis.

Treatment. The mild cases require only rest and hot fomentations or other soothing applications. Severe cases require immediate operation so that the pus can be removed from the bone otherwise the inflammation may spread and cause the whole limb to be affected. (*See also* Bone ; Necrosis ; Osteitis.)

PERISTALSIS. The peculiar wave-like movement by which the contents of the stomach and bowels are moved forward is known as peristalsis. This movement is caused by a series of contractions of the muscles. (*See also* Colic.)

PERITONEUM. The membrane which lines the abdominal cavity is known as the peritoneum. It also forms a covering for most of the organs contained within the abdominal cavity and as it passes from one organ to another the peritoneum forms numerous folds. (*See also* Abdomen ; Mesentery ; Omentum.)

PERITONITIS. Peritonitis means inflammation of the peritoneum or membrane lining the abdominal cavity and organs. The inflammation is very often started as a result of a gastric ulcer, typhoid fever, gall-stones, or any condition which leads to perforation of the stomach, bowels, bile-ducts or bladder. Abscesses or cysts may burst and so start up inflammation, and appendicitis is a very common cause of peritonitis.

Symptoms. The symptoms usually begin with severe pain in the abdomen accompanied by vomiting. The temperature may rise as high as 104° or 105° F. There may be a certain amount of diarrhœa at first, but the bowels soon become constipated. The patient is found to lie on his back with the knees drawn up and the breathing is very shallow. The abdomen becomes distended and is very tender to the lightest touch. The tongue becomes furred and dry and the facial expression is drawn and anxious. The outlook is very serious, especially in the puerperal form which sometimes comes on a few days after childbirth. Acute tuberculous peritonitis may follow tuberculosis of the abdominal glands, the intestines, or the genital organs.

Treatment. Immediately the diagnosis is made the question of operation must be considered. In cases due to perforation, operation is usually carried out immediately, because it is necessary to remove any septic material from the abdomen as soon as possible.

Peritonitis due to tuberculosis is usually treated medically and not surgically. The patient should be kept in bed, preferably in the open air, and the diet should be good and nourishing. (*See also* PERITONEUM.)

PERNICIOUS ANÆMIA is a serious disease of the blood most commonly affecting men in middle life and usually manifesting itself in a gradually increasing weakness and a yellow colour of the skin. The diagnosis can only be made precisely by a microscopic examination of the blood, and this should always be carried out by the doctor (or a consulting physician) at an early stage of the disease, both to differentiate it from other serious diseases which may resemble it and to get treatment begun as soon as possible. For, while a few years ago everyone who contracted pernicious anæmia died of it in a comparatively short time, nowadays it is easily controlled (and sometimes completely cured) by a special diet and treatment instituted by Drs. Minot and Murphy of Boston, U.S.A.

Treatment. To-day pernicious anæmia is usually treated by giving the patients liver extracts made up in various palatable forms, or it may be given by injection ; the only thing against this is the expense, and because they are comparatively expensive patients are apt to take less than the dose they ought to take. Hog's stomach and stomach powder are cheaper than liver and liver extract, and as they are just as effective as liver, patients would do well to take them instead of it. Fresh liver in effective amounts costs about 8d. to 1s. 10d. per day, while fresh stomach in an equal dose costs only about ½d. to 1d. An active desiccated stomach powder should be mixed and taken in cold fluids or foods ; pepsac and gastrexo are potent stomach preparations and are cheap and cost less than 2d. a day in an effective daily dosage, once the patient has got his blood back to approximately normal ; during the period of treatment while this is being done about four times the amount is necessary. It is important to look at the point of view of expense in the treatment of this disease, because the treatment—whether by liver or stomach—usually has to be kept up for life.

Intramuscular extracts are now available that bring the cost down lower than previously by enabling the patient to have injections at intervals of two to six weeks, once the blood has been got back to an approximately normal standard.

PEROXIDE OF HYDROGEN. A solution of oxygen in water, commonly used as an antiseptic. (*See also* HYDROGEN PEROXIDE.)

PERSPIRATION. Moisture which is given off from the skin is known as perspiration or sweat. (*See also* SWEATING.)

PESSARIES. An instrument for supporting the womb when it is displaced is called a pessary. The term is also used for medicated suppositories which are introduced into the vagina.

PETIT MAL. This term is used in connection with a very mild epileptic fit. (*See also* EPILEPSY.)

PHAGOCYTE. A cell which is able to destroy germs and other harmful particles in the blood is termed a phagocyte. (*See also* LEUCOCYTE.)

PHALANGES. The bones in the fingers and toes are known as the phalanges. There are three of these, in each finger and toe, the proximal, the middle and the distal ; but the thumb and the big toe have each only two.

PHARMACOLOGY. The part of medical science dealing with the knowledge of the action of drugs about the body. It used to be known as materia medica.

PHARYNGITIS. This condition is an inflammation of the part of the throat immediately beyond the mouth. (*See also* LARYNGITIS ; TONSILLITIS.)

PHARYNX. The pharynx can be seen at the very back of the mouth when it is wide open. The term throat is popularly applied to this part, but strictly speaking the pharynx is the cavity into which the nose opens above and from which the larynx and gullet open below. The part which lies behind the nose is called the naso-pharynx. (*See also* PHARYNGITIS.)

PHENACETIN. This drug is commonly used to give relief in headaches and neuralgia as it is particularly good for deadening pain, but it should not be taken in quantity as it has a very depressing effect.

PHENOL. *See* CARBOLIC ACID.

PHIMOSIS. A condition in which the foreskin cannot be drawn back to uncover the penis is called phimosis. The only satisfactory treatment is by circumcision, which consists in removing a part of the foreskin so that it can be easily drawn back. The operation should be carried out as early as possible, because in very young children it is a slight affair, while the longer it is postponed the more troublesome it becomes. (*See also* BALANITIS ; PENIS.)

PHLEBITIS. Inflammation of the veins, usually accompanied by clotting of the blood in the veins, is known as phlebitis. It may occur after childbirth, typhoid fever, or a surgical operation and is frequently a complication of varicose veins. The affected limb is tender and subject to aching and shooting pains. The part surrounding the vein becomes swollen and there may be bad cramps in the limb. It is treated by rest and soothing applications, such as belladonna in glycerine. The patient must be kept in bed until all signs of inflammation have disappeared, and the diet should be very light. It may be necessary to wear an elastic bandage for support if the limb is inclined to swell. A very useful drug in cases of phlebitis is extract of horse chestnut, a French preparation, which usually eases the pain and even seems to have a curative action sometimes. (*See also* THROMBOSIS.)

PHLEGM. The material which is brought up after coughing is popularly called phlegm. It is also medically known as sputum or expectoration. (*See also* EXPECTORATION.)

PHLEGMASIA. This term applies to a condition which may occur during the lying-in period of childbirth in which the leg or legs become swollen. (*See also* PHLEBITIS ; WHITE LEG.)

PHTHISIS. *See* TUBERCULOSIS.

PHYSICIAN. A physician is a doctor who treats diseases by drugs and other methods than that of surgery.

PHYSIOLOGY. The branch of medicine in which the normal workings of the body are studied is known as physiology.

PHYSOSTIGMINE. This drug is obtained from the calabar bean and is used in eye work and in Myasthenia gravis, q.v. (*See also* CALABAR BEAN.)

PIA MATER. This name is given to one of the three membranes surrounding the brain and spinal cord. (*See also* BRAIN.)

PIGMENTATION. Pigment is the term applied to the colouring matter of various substances in the body, particularly in the blood. (*See also* ALBINO ; JAUNDICE.)

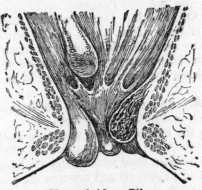

Hæmorrhoids or Piles

PILES. Medically known as hæmorrhoids, piles is a varicose condition of the veins of the lower part of the rectum.

Piles may be external or internal. External piles appear as tags of skin outside the opening of the rectum and do not cause much irritation unless they become chafed or infected, when they cause great pain and discomfort for several days. Internal piles have no very marked symptoms until they begin to bleed, but they may protrude from the opening and if not pushed back, they may become bruised and acutely painful.

Chronic constipation, sitting about too much, lack of exercise, alcoholic excess and pregnancy are the most usual causes of piles. To cure them, the constipation must be treated by diet and drugs if necessary. The parts around the opening should be kept scrupulously clean, using cottonwool instead of the ordinary paper, and a soothing ointment containing gall may be applied at intervals. If the piles do not disappear with improved habits and hygiene, they should be injected with a sclerosing solution by a doctor. Operation is only advised in the more severe cases. (*See also* FISSURE.)

PIMPLES. Small raised and inflamed spots on the skin are called pimples or papules. (*See also* ACNE ; DERMATITIS.)

PITYRIASIS. Various types of skin diseases of which scaliness is the chief feature are described as pityriasis. (*See also* DANDRUFF ; DERMATITIS ; LICHEN ; PSORIASIS.)

PLACENTA. The placenta is a structure planted on the wall of the pregnant womb which connects the blood supply of the mother with the circulation of the developing baby (or fœtus) by means of the umbilical cord containing important blood-vessels. (*See also* AFTER-BIRTH.)

PLAGUE. (*See* BUBONIC PLAGUE.)

PLASTER OF PARIS. Dried calcium sulphate is used to make plaster of Paris splints. One pint of water is used to two pounds of plaster and this sets rapidly and firmly. Bandages impregnated with the powder are called plaster of Paris bandages, and are used when the limbs must be kept in position, such as in fracture, etc.

PLETHORA. An excess of blood which causes a fullness of the blood-vessels is described as plethora.

PLEURA is the membrane that covers the lungs and also lines the cavity—in which the lungs lie—called the pleural cavity. The pleura secretes a serous fluid which helps the lung when expanding or contracting to slide up and down in the pleural cavity with equal ease, although the lung lies close against its wall. (*See also* LUNG.)

PLEURISY is inflammation of the pleura, or covering membrane of the lung. Usually only one lung is affected, and often only part of its surface. It is generally caused by exposure to cold and wet ; but it may be a manifestation of tuberculosis or a complication of various diseases, such as pneumonia, or even Bright's disease (of the kidney).

The temperature is usually a little raised, 99° F. or 100° F., the breathing is shallow (to avoid expanding the lung over-much), the pulse quickened and the patient complains chiefly of a severe " stitch in his side," worse on breathing.

Treatment. The treatment of pleurisy includes rest in bed, fluid diet, the application of tincture of iodine or of antiphlogistine to the affected side ; strapping the ribs firmly with sticking-plaster almost right round. If the iodine or antiphlogistine is not enough to relieve the pain, a sedative cough mixture and ten grains of aspirin or something similar may be given at bedtime. After an attack of pleurisy the chest should always be X-rayed to make sure that the lung is healthy.

Wet Pleurisy or Pleurisy with effusion. This is a second type of pleurisy, when the inflammation of the pleural membrane is followed by an outpouring of fluid between the wall of the chest and the surface of the lung.

Treatment. The doctor, when he examines the chest, finds marked dullness over the affected lung, and may have to draw off the fluid with a syringe, especially when it shows signs of pressing on the heart. Sometimes tincture of iodine or antiphlogistine applied to the chest is enough to dry up the fluid, when it is present in small amount only. Convalescence must be prolonged, the chest X-rayed, and breathing exercises carried out regularly, as it is in this type of pleurisy that tuberculosis most frequently develops afterwards.

PLEURODYNIA. Sharp pain in the nerves and muscles that lie between the ribs is called pleurodynia. It may be due to rheumatism or to neuralgia. Drugs of the salicylate group such as aspirin, etc., are very useful. (*See also* FIBROSITIS ; RHEUMATISM.)

PLOMBIÈRES DOUCHE. Washing out of the lower bowel by means of a soft rubber tube through which several pints of water are slowly allowed to run is known as the Plombières douche. (*See* DOUCHE ; IRRIGATION.)

PNEUMONIA or inflammation of the lungs, is of two types called broncho-pneumonia and lobar pneumonia.

Broncho-pneumonia, sometimes called catarrhal pneumonia, is an extension of bronchitis (inflammation of the lining of the little tubes that lead air into the lungs) into the tissue of the lung and affects little patches in the lungs here and there.

Treatment. The treatment is similar to that of bronchitis.

Lobar Pneumonia is the variety commonly meant when the term " pneumonia " is used, and it is so called because an entire lobe or division of the lung is affected by the inflammation and may be " solid " with the thick secretion that is poured into the air vesicles of the lung.

Symptoms. Pain in the side of the chest, shivering, a high temperature—from 101° F. up to 104° F. or more, a quick pulse, rapid breathing (sometimes difficult breathing), " rusty " sputum, and a flushed face are the easily recognized symptoms that denote pneumonia.

Treatment. The treatment of pneumonia has recently been revolutionized by the introduction of M. & B. 693 (sulphapyridine), which, given in adequate doses, reduces the temperature to normal in a few days, in most cases, and has saved many lives. It sometimes causes severe reactions, from which a slow recovery may be made.

PNEUMONIC PLAGUE. (*See* BUBONIC PLAGUE.)

PODOPHYLLUM. (*See also* PURGATIVE.)

POISONS AND POISONING. (*See* opposite page.)

POLYPUS, NASAL. Growths which occur on one or both sides of the nose are called polypi (plural of polypus). Removal of the polypi, which is a simple matter, may make a great difference to the patient's health and mental outlook. If they recur,

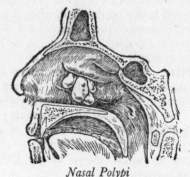

Nasal Polypi

a more radical operation may be necessary. A polypus may also occur in the ear or in the womb. (*See also* EAR ; NOSE ; WOMB.)

POLYURIA. The passing of an excessive amount of urine is known as polyuria. The normal amount passed in one day is about two and a half pints. Excess may be due to nervous causes when no treatment is required, or to some serious disease such as diabetes or inflammation of the kidney. There may be a temporary state of polyuria after fever. (*See also* DIABETES ; NEPHRITIS ; URINE.)

Table of Principal Poisons and their Antidotes

Poison.	Signs.	Treatment.
Corrosive Acids		
Acetic Burnett's fluid Hydrochloric }	Lips and mouth burnt and stained.	*NO EMETIC.* Give water at once to dilute the poison. If possible add chalk, magnesia, or ceiling plaster. For the pain give oil, milk, or beaten-up eggs.
Nitric (Aqua Fortis) Sulphuric Tartaric }	Pain from mouth to stomach.	
Carbolic acid Creosote Lysol }	ditto ditto ditto	As above, but use Epsom or Glauber salts.
Oxalic acid }	ditto	An emetic *may* be given, then chalk, magnesia, or plaster.
Corrosive Alkalis		
Ammonia Lime Potash Soda }	Lips and mouth burnt raw. ditto ditto ditto	*NO EMETIC.* Give water at once to dilute the poison. If possible add vinegar, lemon or lime-juice.
Irritants		
Antimony Arsenic	Vomiting, retching, faintness, purging, cramps.	*EMETIC.* Water, tea, or milk; beaten-up eggs, salad oil. Keep patient warm.
Cantharides Copper Food, bad Iodine Lead Lunar caustic Mercury Paraffin Petrol	ditto ditto ditto ditto ditto ditto ditto ditto ditto	ditto ditto ditto (starch and ditto water.) ditto ditto ditto ditto
Phosphorus	ditto	As above, but *NO* oil.
Narcotics		
Opium Morphia Laudanum Chloral	Sleepiness, pallor, slow pulse, slow, stertorous breathing, " pinpoint " pupils, musty breath.	*EMETIC.* Condy's fluid or potassium permanganate. Combat sleepiness. Hot coffee. Artificial respiration if breathing fails.
Chlorodyne Conium (Hemlock) Dover powder Headache powders Paregoric Paraldehyde Sulphonal Veronal	ditto ditto ditto ditto ditto ditto ditto ditto	ditto ditto ditto ditto ditto ditto ditto ditto
Cocaine }	Giddiness, pallor, rapid, feeble pulse.	*EMETIC.* Warmth, stimulants, artificial respiration.
Deliriants or Narcotic Irritants		
Atropine Belladonna Hyoscyamus }	Excitement, dry mouth, thirst, dilated pupils.	*EMETIC.* Combat drowsiness. Strong coffee.
Nux Vomica Strychnine }	Bitter taste, dilated pupils, spasms, difficult breathing.	*EMETIC.* Charcoal, wood cinders, tincture of iodine, " stewed tea." Large doses of potassium bromide.
Aconite	Tingling in mouth and throat. Dulled sight and hearing, difficult breathing.	*EMETIC.* Stimulants, warmth, rest. Tincture of belladonna 30 drops, or tincture of digitalis 20 drops.
Prussic acid Cyanides }	Giddiness, staggering, coma. Staring eyes, clammy skin.	*EMETIC.* Instant cold water, douches on face and back of neck, brandy, ammonia to the nostrils.
Digitalis }	Green vomit, heart failure.	Stimulants, repose for some hours.
Alcohol }	Drowsiness, deep sleep, collapse.	*EMETIC.* Strong coffee, keep moving. Later put into a warm bed.

POST MORTEM. This term, meaning after death, is used in connection with an examination of the body following death, of which the cause is uncertain or unknown.

POTT'S DISEASE. This term is frequently applied to curvature of the spine which results from tuberculous disease. Percival Pott (1713—1788), a Famous English surgeon, was the first to describe the condition. (*See also* SPINAL CURVATURE ; TUBERCULOSIS.)

POULTICES. Poultices are not so much used now as they were formerly, because antiphlogistine and similar preparations are so much easier and safer to work with. But as this is not always at hand when it is wanted, poultices have still frequently to be made. The commonest in use are made of bread, linseed, and mustard.

PREGNANCY. Pregnancy is the state of being with child. The earliest symptom is the stoppage of the monthly periods, and the child's birth may be expected nine months and a fortnight from the first day of the last period. Some women, however, have reduced periods for three months after conception has taken place, and if they have not noticed the scantiness of the period, they may miscalculate when the birth is due. There is usually no doubt, however, after quickening has been observed. Quickening is when the movements of the child in the womb become so strong

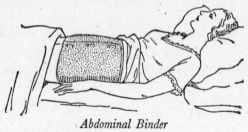

Abdominal Binder

that the mother feels them ; this usually occurs at four and a half months. After the stopping of the periods, the next symptom to be noticed is " morning sickness." A small quantity of clear tasteless fluid is vomited each morning on rising. There may be no feeling of nausea, the fluid being simply brought up. Sometimes this happens in the evening instead of in the morning ; but once a day is the rule, and if there is a persistent vomiting during the day, or if the condition continues after the fourth month, a doctor's advice should be sought. The next symptom of pregnancy occurs in the breasts, which swell and may be painful. The veins are fuller and may show up blue on the chest. The nipples become more prominent and the area around them becomes darker in colour with raised pimple-like bodies on the brown part. During the first three months there may be a frequent desire to pass water, but this feeling disappears for a few months. When it returns, it usually signifies that the end of the pregnancy is very near. In the later stages of pregnancy there is a brown line running downwards from the navel, and there are lines of stretching on the abdominal wall which may remain as faint white scars after childbirth. These are called striæ. They may also be caused by any disease with great distension of the abdomen. During pregnancy there may be either constipation or diarrhœa, the digestion may be troublesome, and there may be heartburn or water-brash. There may be a dislike for certain articles of food and a longing for others. The weight of the abdomen may cause swollen legs with varicose veins. There may be great trouble with itching of the genital organs and some women have a heavy white discharge. All these symptoms should be treated in a common-sense fashion as they arise and a little care will help to lighten any inconveniences. The danger signals which must be referred to a doctor at the earliest possible moment are bleeding, fits, albuminuria (the presence of albumin in the urine), and the stopping of the movements of the child in the womb. Bleeding may be the sign of a miscarriage, and albumin in the urine, or a sudden fit, may be the symptoms of the condition known as eclampsia. (*See also* CHILDBIRTH ; ECLAMPSIA ; LABOUR ; PUERPERIUM.)

PRESBYOPIA. A condition of the sight which occurs as a natural outcome of old age is known as presbyopia. The structures of the eye lose their power of focusing properly, and near work becomes increasingly difficult. The use of spectacles is necessary to deal with the condition. (*See also* ACCOMMODATION ; EYE ; VISION, ERRORS IN.)

PRESENTATION. The part of the child in the womb which is in the position to appear first during childbirth is referred to as the presentation. In the most favourable cases the child presents the head, with its back directed towards the mother's front ; this is known as the vertex presentation. Other presentations are described as brow, breech, shoulder, foot, or transverse and so on. In a breech presentation, the child present the buttocks, and a transverse presentation means that the body of the child lies across the opening of the womb. (*See also* CHILDBIRTH ; LABOUR.)

PROCTITIS. Inflammation of the rectum or anus is known as proctitis. (*See also* ANUS ; RECTUM.)

PROGNOSIS. An opinion or forecast of the course, duration and ending of a disease is described as a prognosis. (*See also* DIAGNOSIS.)

PROGRESSIVE MUSCULAR ATROPHY is a disease of the nervous system which occurs in middle life and which is much more common in men than in women.

Patients attacked by this disease succumb to lung trouble, as the muscles which control breathing waste away and the patients are unable to breathe properly, or they may choke if unable to cough.

The disease most commonly shows itself first by a wasting away of the muscles of the hand. The patient notices that he is not able to " make a fist " as easily as he could and it becomes difficult to separate the fingers. Later, the hand becomes drawn into a claw-like shape. Wasting of the muscles of the legs may be the next sign of the disease, and very often there is not only weakness of the legs, but they become very stiff. Difficulty in swallowing, in speaking and in moving the tongue are late symptoms and these cause the patient much distress. The muscles which move the lips are also attacked late in the disease, and so the lips cannot meet and the saliva drips from the mouth.

Treatment. When this disease has been recognized, unless the cause can be shown to be due to syphilis, the only treatment is to help the weakened muscles to keep as much of their strength as possible by massage and electrical treatment, carefully given so as not to tire the muscles. When the muscles of the throat and chest are attacked, great care must be taken to prevent food getting into the throat instead of into the gullet, and so reaching the lungs. It is usually found that patients are able to take semi-solid food with more comfort and less risk than either liquids or completely solid food.

PROLAPSE. The falling downward of some organ of the body from its normal position is called prolapse. Falling of the womb is perhaps one of the commonest forms of prolapse in women and it can be the cause of a great deal of suffering and unhappiness. Satisfactory results can be obtained by operation, but if for some reason or another an operation is not advisable, the condition can be remedied by wearing a suitably shaped pessary. Wearing a pessary does not cure the condition but only holds the parts together as long as it is worn. (*See also* WOMB ; ANUS.)

PROPHYLAXIS. The prevention of disease is known as prophylaxis, and any measures taken to prevent disease are known as prophylactic measures. (*See also* INOCULATION.)

PROSTATE GLAND. The organ surrounding the neck of the bladder and the beginning of the urethra in the male is known as the prostate gland. It is rather like a chestnut in shape and can be felt from the rectum behind. So far as is known its only purpose is to secrete a fluid that lubricates the urethra and is ex-

creted with the semen. This gland is of importance, because in
old age it is liable to increase greatly in size, thus causing obstruction between the urethra and the bladder. There is difficulty in
passing water, which can only be overcome by inserting an
instrument known as a catheter to draw off the water from the
bladder. An operation known as prostatectomy can be carried out,
in which all or most of the enlarged prostate can be removed, so
leaving a free passage for the urine. Inflammation of the prostate
gland is known as prostatitis and it is usually the result of gonorrhœa,
but it may also occur as a result of infection from the kidneys or

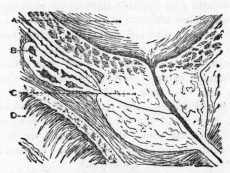

Prostate Gland
A. Bladder; B. Seminal Vesicle; C. Prostate; D. Rectum

bladder. The condition is a very painful one and the patient
should consult a doctor as soon as possible. (*See also* GLEET ;
GONORRHŒA.)

PROTEIN. Protein is an organic substance found in various
forms in vegetable and animal life. Albumin, or white of egg, and
gelatine are typical examples of a protein substance.

PROUD FLESH. This is a popular name given to granulation tissue, which often arises in an ulcer which has become septic
and inflamed. (*See also* GRANULATION TISSUE.)

PRURIGO. Prurigo is a chronic skin disease, characterized by
small rounded, reddish papules or pimples, which are intensely itchy.

Symptoms. It chiefly affects the lower part of the abdomen,
the buttocks, the back of the arms, and the front of the legs, but
may spread over the whole body. It has some relation to urticaria
(nettlerash), as it often begins as urticaria in early childhood,
gradually changes to prurigo, and lasts indefinitely.

Treatment. The treatment of the first two forms is especially
directed towards finding the underlying cause, which is thought
(like urticaria) to be a chronic poisoning. The patient is very

thoroughly examined. Some experts restrict the diet considerably, others allow generous meals, and cod-liver oils, etc. Iron tonics, thyroid extract, and iodine are helpful. Anti-itching ointment containing carbolic acid is very comforting, and seems also to have some curative value. Ultra-violet ray treatment also relieves the itching, and X-rays are even more successful.

Prurigo nodularis is treated by removal of the nodules followed by X-ray treatment until the itching has entirely ceased. (*See also* SKIN.)

PRURITUS. The term pruritus is used for all forms of itching, and this unpleasant and irritable state of the skin can be brought about in a great many different ways. Itching may be a symptom of many skin diseases, such as dermatitis, lichen planus, prurigo and urticaria, etc., and the scratching which naturally follows may set up a serious state of affairs. Contact with rough or woollen clothes is a common cause of itching, especially in children. Parasites, such as lice, etc., may bring about the condition, and the bites and stings of insects are also liable to prove troublesome. The skin condition known as " the itch," or scabies, is caused by a tiny parasite which burrows under the skin, but once the mite is destroyed the condition very quickly clears up. (*See also* DERMATITIS ; LICHEN PLANUS ; PRURIGO ; PSORIASIS.)

PRUSSIC ACID. Also known as hydrocyanic acid, prussic acid is contained in the oil of bitter almonds, but it can be manufactured by distillation of potassium ferrocyanide with dilute sulphuric acid. It is a strong poison undiluted, but is given dilute in small doses in dyspepsia, to quieten gastric pains, and to stop vomiting. It is commonly included in cough mixtures. (*See also* HYDROCYANIC ACID POISON.)

PRUSSIC ACID POISONING. If a large dose has been taken, symptoms usually make their appearance almost immediately. The patient becomes insensible, the eyes are fixed and glistening, and the skin is cold and clammy. Treatment consists of giving an emetic immediately or washing out the stomach with a tube. Artificial respiration must be carried out and ammonia may be applied to the nose, but treatment is not usually of much avail. (*See also* POISONS.)

PSITTACOSIS. A contagious disease of parrots, which is sometimes communicated to man, is known as psittacosis.

PSOAS. This name is given to a powerful muscle which arises from the spinal column in the back. It passes down and round the pelvis, and through the groin and joins the inner side of the thigh bone. Disease of the spine is very liable to lead to an abscess within the sheath of this muscle and the pus may travel down the fibres, and finally work its way into the upper part of the thigh. Such an abscess is known as a psoas abscess and it is usually the result of tubercular infection of the spine. (*See also* ABSCESS; TUBERCU-LOSIS.)

PSORIASIS. Symptoms. Psoriasis is a common chronic inflammation of the skin, characterized by rounded reddened patches of various sizes, which are covered with dry silvery scales.

Treatment. Arsenic used cautiously is very useful in chronic cases, and sodium salicylate in acute. Potassium iodide, green iodide of mercury, and thyroid substance are sometimes successful.

Externally, chrysarobin in vaseline is by far the best treatment. It is rubbed in twice daily, baths being taken regularly to remove the scales. (The face and eyes are protected, as chrysarobin is irritating.) About a fortnight suffices for a cure. (*See also* DERMA-TITIS.)

PSYCHO-ANALYSIS. A method of treating nervous disorders, in which the patient talks freely of every thought that comes into his mind to the analyst, until a link is found which is causing the upset. (*See* FREUDISM.)

PSYCHOSIS means a disorder of the mind, but in actual practice the term is restricted to the more severe forms of mental disorders, which will be found discussed under INSANITY.

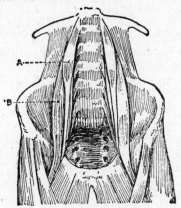

Psoas Muscle
A. Psoas Minor; B. Psoas Major

PTOMAINE. A form of poisoning due to eating decomposed food is known as ptomaine poisoning. (*See also* BOTULISM ; FOOD POISONING.)

PTOSIS. Drooping of the upper eyelid is known as ptosis. If this condition is present at birth it is usually due to maldevelopment of the muscle that lifts the eyelid ; if it occurs later on in life, it may be due to paralysis of the muscle. (*See also* EYE ; EYELID.)

PTYALIN. Ptyalin is the name of the ferment contained in the saliva by which starchy foods are turned into sugar in order to aid digestion. (*See also* FERMENTS.)

PUBERTY. The period in which the child gradually passes into manhood or womanhood is called puberty. (*See also* ADOLESCENCE.)

PUBIS. The bone that forms the front part of the pelvis is called the pubis or pubic bone. (*See also* BONE.)

PUERPERIUM is the time between the birth of a child and the restoration of the mother to perfect health, and usually lasts about a month. During this time the womb, from being big enough to hold an infant, has to regain its normal size of a pear, and the discharge from it, blood-stained at first, gradually becomes clear and then stops altogether. The breasts, which are of course enlarged in pregnancy, begin to secrete milk in quantity during the puerperium, generally beginning two or three days after the child has been born. It is usual for a mother to remain in bed for the first ten days of the puerperium, though some specialists nowadays say that this is quite unnecessary and allow the patient up almost at once. For the first two or three days the mother should have a milk diet only, but after that should return to ordinary food, with plenty of fluids.

PULEX. Pulex irritans is the scientific name for the common flea. (*See also* JIGGER.)

PULMONARY. Anything pertaining to or affecting the lungs is described as pulmonary. (*See also* LUNGS.)

PULSE. The pumping of the blood through the heart causes changes to take place in the blood-vessels, and each time blood is pumped through, the arteries swell and then contract again ; this is known as the pulse. The pulse can be felt in any artery that lies near the surface ; but the artery which runs over the bones of the wrist is chosen for this purpose. The examination of the pulse affords valuable information to the doctor. The pulse rate is usually about 72 beats per minute, but it varies a great deal in different people. Some people may have a normally quick pulse, while others are habitually slow without affecting the health in any way. The quality of the pulse is marked, whether it is full and bounding, rapid and thin, or feeble and soft. A rapid pulse occurs in fevers, certain diseases of the heart, and nervous disorders. In typhoid fever, the pulse becomes very slow, and this is recognized as one of the symptoms of the disease. An irregular pulse is one where some beats are felt more strongly than others. It may be present in heart disease, but it may also be due to indigestion or anything which upsets the nervous system such as over-indulgence in alcohol, coffee or tobacco. There is a type of irregular pulse common in young people, and also people recovering from infectious diseases, in which the pulse rate is affected by the breathing, but it is not a harmful condition. (*See also* BRADYCARDIA ; HEART.)

P.U.O. These letters stand for pyrexia of unknown origin, and they are used as a convenient term for cases of fever the nature of which is still in doubt. (*See also* FEVER.)

PUPIL. The pupil is simply a hole in the iris of the eye, which is composed of two layers of muscle. One layer is arranged in circular fashion, and on contracting diminishes the size of the pupil ; the other radially, which on contracting increases the size of the pupil. (*See also* EYE.)

PURGATIVE. Drugs or other methods which are used to produce strong action of the bowels are known as cathartics or purgatives. (*See also* APERIENT ; CATHARTIC ; CHOLAGOGUE ; CONSTIPATION ; DIARRHŒA ; HYDRAGOGUES ;)

PURPURA. Purpura consists in an eruption of reddish-purple spots, due to escape of the blood from the vessels into the skin or mucous membranes. (*See also* ERYTHEMA.)

PUS. Pus, or matter, is a thick fluid which is found in abscesses, ulcers, and on any inflamed and discharging surfaces generally, consisting of bacteria and broken-down tissues. The colour may vary from white to greenish-yellow according to the type of germ causing the condition. (*See also* ABSCESS ; BOIL ; CARBUNCLE.)

PUSTULE. A small abscess appearing on the skin or mucous membranes is called a pustule. (*See also* ACNE ; ANTHRAX ; SMALL-POX.)

PYÆMIA. A form of blood-poisoning in which abscesses appear in various parts of the body, to which infection has been carried, is known as pyæmia. The symptoms of the disease resemble those of septicæmia. (*See also* SEPTICÆMIA.)

PYELITIS. Inflammation of the part of the kidney known as the pelvis, the upper end which is connected with the ureter, is described as pyelitis. (*See also* BACILLURIA ; KIDNEY ; NEPHRITIS.)

PYORRHŒA. Pyorrhœa is a disease of the gums which may cause serious upset to the general health by the absorption of poisons by the blood-stream and by the constant swallowing of the poisons discharged into the mouth. It is due to a germ (or, more accurately, an amœba) infection and it attacks all ages and conditions of people, but those in good general health with carefully tended mouths will not be so liable as others. The teeth should be put in order by a dentist and antiseptic paints, tooth-pastes, or mouth-washes used freely. If this is not sufficient to clear up the condition, vaccines may be tried, and if they fail, if may be necessary to remove the teeth, but this should only be the very last resort. (*See also* DENTAL DRILL ; GINGIVITIS ; GUMS, DISEASES OF.)

PYURIA. This term is used to describe any condition in which there is pus in the urine. (*See also* URINE.)

QUARTAN FEVER. This is a particular type of malaria which comes on every fourth day. (*See also* MALARIA.)

QUICKENING. This term is used to describe the feeling of movement inside the womb caused by the unborn child. (*See also* CHILDBIRTH ; LABOUR ; PREGNANCY.)

QUININE. Quinine is a very important alkaloid drug obtained from several species of cinchona bark. The best-known use of the drug is in the treatment of malaria, and it is usually taken by the mouth unless ordered to be injected by the doctor. Quinine will not only cut short an attack of malaria, but it is capable of preventing one if taken about three hours before the attack is due.

Quinine is a powerful antiseptic, and it is capable of destroying germs and preventing fermentation and putrefaction ; but, unfortunately, it is far too expensive for ordinary use. It is often given in small doses for cases of neuralgia, and it is sometimes useful in the early stages of cold in the head and bronchitis. In fevers, sulphate of quinine may be given to lower the temperature, though it should never be given when the heart's action is feeble. As a tonic, small doses may be taken after meals either liquid or in tablets, or it is more commonly taken with other tonic substances such as iron and strychnine. (*See also* MALARIA.)

QUINSY. An abscess in or around the tonsil. (*See also* TONSIL ; TONSILLITIS.)

RABIES. (*See* HYDROPHOBIA.)

RADIUM. Radium is becoming more and more used in the treatment of cancer, whether by the insertion of radium and radon " seeds " into and around a growth, or whether by radium at a distance, as in a " bomb " containing several grams.

RANULA. A cystic swelling under the tongue. It is generally due to the blocking up of one of the ducts of one of the two sublingual salivary glands. The obstruction is usually due to a stone or calculus. (*See also* CALCULUS ; SALIVARY GLANDS.)

RAYNAUD'S DISEASE. The disorder described by the famous French physician, Raynaud, is characterized by disturbances of the circulation in various parts, especially the fingers and toes. There is apparently no organic disease of the arteries, and the interference with the blood supply is due to the nerves controlling the size of the blood-vessels. It is more common in damp and in cold weather, and is practically unknown in warm climates.

There is a widespread spasm of the arteries and smaller blood-vessels so that not a drop of blood enters the part affected. Some-time later the blood-vessels open out widely and the dead white finger becomes bright pink. There is often a stage in which the part is blue between the white and the pink stages.

Curiously enough in frost-bite the order of events is reversed. In frost-bite the part becomes pink, then blue, and finally white ; whereas in Raynaud's disease the part becomes white, blue, and then pink. In moderate grades of the blue stage some little blood trickles through the sluice gates ; but in the deep purple skin of a typical example the circulation has ceased and death of the part is imminent.

A more severe form may also affect the fingers, toes, tip of the nose and ears. The pain is very severe. Both feet may be swollen to the ankles and the toes may be quite black.

Treatment. The tendency of this disease should be countered, if possible, by warm clothing in the winter. The gloves, shoes, etc., must be sufficiently loose not to cause any constriction of the cir-culation. The mild attacks require no treatment. In the more severe forms the parts affected should be wrapped in cotton-wool and kept at rest. The use of calcium lactate, nitroglycerine, etc., prove useful in some cases. Galvanism and ultra-violet light are additional forms of treatment. If gangrene occurs, the parts affected must be kept covered with antiseptic dressings.

RECTAL FEEDING. A certain amount of fluid is absorbed from the large bowel under normal conditions. Solutions of glucose undergo some absorption, as the glucose is the sugar which is normally the end product of all starchy food and is absorbed as such into the blood-stream. Other ingredients may include milk which has been peptonized or digested for 24 hours ; if peptonized for a shorter time it is quite useless from the point of view of absorption.

RECTOCELE. A weakness of the wall of the rectum which shows itself as a protrusion in a woman, of the front wall of the rectum through the back wall of the vagina which lies immediately in front.

RECTUM. Is the end part of the bowel. It extends from an S-shaped bend, known as the sigmoid flexure, down to the anus and opens at the exterior by means of the anal orifice. It is over six inches in length. The anal portion is surrounded by two sets of muscle ; the inner one is a thickening of the normal circular muscle fibres of the bowel and is under involuntary control. It is known as the internal sphincter. Outside this is a voluntary muscle under the direct control of the conscious mind and it is known as the external sphincter.

Diseases of the Rectum. Foreign bodies include solid accumu-
lations of fæcal matter. Sometimes there is a core consisting of a
stone, fruit stone or intestinal worm. These foreign bodies produce
a sensation of discomfort and heaviness, and colic and pains in the
loins and legs. There is also a constant and frequent desire to go
to stool, usually without any result except a few drops of mucus
due to the straining. The treatment is to give a rectal douche to
soften the mass and then a suitable aperient.

Cancer of the Rectum. *See* CANCER.

A polyp is a simple, non-malignant growth which grows from
the wall of the rectum and is attached to it by means of a stalk or

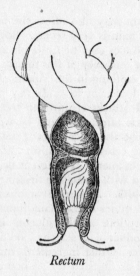

Rectum

pedicle. It is more common in children and grows very slowly.
Its presence is indicated by the passage of blood from the rectum,
straining at stool without effect, and the presence of a tumour
inside. This simple growth is readily removed by the simple operation of burning or cutting through the stalk.

Rectal prolapse means the passage through the anus of some
portion of the wall of the intestine. It is common in infants when
the external muscles are weak. It is aggravated by constipation.

Inflammation of the rectum, or *proctitis*, usually follows inflammation of the large intestine. If it is due to local trouble, the cause
is usually inflamed piles, venereal infections, eczema, foreign bodies,
immoral practices, drastic purgatives, etc. There is much pain
and agonizing straining. The condition may heal up, or become

chronic. Abscess formation, ulceration, the development of a fistula and stricture formation are all possible complications.

A stricture of the rectum may result, apart from a new growth, from any previous inflammation. Chronic obstruction gives rise to a similar train of symptoms. The original cause of the condition must be treated and dilatation of the stricture by the passage of instruments, or even a cutting operation, will be needed. (*See also* COLITIS ; INTESTINE ; PILES ; ANAL FISSURE.)

REFLEX ACTION. An unconscious act which is controlled by the spinal cord without the intervention of the will. (*See also* KNEE-JERK.)

RELAPSING FEVER. This is an infectious illness due to a germ of the spirochætal type, that is, it has a long wavy outline when seen under the microscope. It lives in the blood, and is transmitted by lice through scratch marks in the skin. This disorder is characterized by recurring bouts of fever lasting for several days and separated by periods of normal temperature of about the same duration.

Symptoms. The illness begins suddenly with a chill, extreme weakness, violent pains in the head and marked backache. There may be vomiting. Jaundice may occur, but the stools retain their normal colour.

These symptoms last from 3 to 10 days, usually 6, and then suddenly disappear with marked sweating and the copious passage of urine, and the temperature becomes normal and the patient wants to get up. This normal state lasts from 3 to 15 days, and then a new attack begins. This usually lasts a slightly shorter time than the first. The second attack ends in the same sudden way. This relapse may occur three times, sometimes more, and ultimately a cure is the rule.

Treatment. Preventive measures include the destruction of lice and other animals liable to convey the parasite. Organic arsenic compounds, such as sulpharsan, etc., are of value against all the spirochætal type of germs. A special serum has been made. General treatment for the fever and heart stimulants are also indicated.

RELAXED THROAT. *See* PHARYNGITIS ; TONSILLITIS.

RENAL. Something belonging to the kidney.

REPRODUCTIVE SYSTEM. In the *male* the reproductive system consists of the testicles, which secrete the seminal fluid containing spermatozoa, the vas deferens or duct of the testicle, the seminal vesicles, in which the fluid is stored, the prostate gland, the urethra, and the penis. In the *female* the reproductive system consists of the ovaries, which give rise to the ova, the Fallopian tubes, which convey them to the womb, the womb or uterus, the vagina or passage up to the womb, and the external genitals.

RESPIRATION. Respiration is the act of breathing by which the living organism, whether human being or animal, exchanges the gases which it manufactures in itself for the gases in the air around it in which it lives. This exchange of gases is absolutely necessary to the maintenance of life, since the gases breathed out carry poisonous waste materials out of the body, and the gases breathed in bring oxygen which is food for the tissues of the body.

RETINA. The innermost coat of the eye-ball, which is sensitive to light, is called the retina. If the retina becomes inflamed the condition is called *retinitis*. (*See also* EYE.)

RHEUMATIC FEVER. *See* RHEUMATISM, ACUTE.

RHEUMATISM is a generalized or localized infection of the system, caused by germs and the poisons they produce in the blood, and the symptoms are usually made worse by exposure to cold, damp and fatigue. It takes various forms which must be described separately. Acute Rheumatism is more often known as rheumatic fever. Chronic Rheumatism is commonly called rheumatism quite simply. Muscular Rheumatism or Myalgia and Rheumatoid Arthritis are other forms.

Rheumatism, Acute. Acute Rheumatism, commonly called rheumatic fever, is a severe attack of rheumatism accompanied by fever which may have serious complications and should be treated with great care. Children and young people are the most usual victims and females have it more often than males.

Symptoms. A child may slip into an attack of rheumatic fever gradually without the beginnings of the attack being noticed. The child may be out of sorts, complaining of pains in the limbs, and if the temperature is taken it will be found to be slightly raised. One day the child will become acutely ill, with a temperature of 100° F. or over, and there is acute pain and swelling in a joint, or several joints. Sometimes as one joint subsides another may swell. In most cases there is a good deal of sweating and the sweat has a characteristic sour smell. There may be sore throat. Sometimes rheumatic nodules or little lumps are found under the skin in such places as the back of the hands, chest, over the knees, at the elbows and so on. These nodules or swellings may come and go quite quickly. The temperature, with proper treatment, will usually return to normal in about a week or ten days, and the pain will fade out of the joints, although it may go from joint to joint.

Treatment. Rheumatic children should have their throats and teeth well cared for and any unhealthy teeth or tonsils should be removed as they seem to render the child more liable to an attack of rheumatic fever. When the attack occurs it is of the greatest importance to put the child to bed and keep it there, not allowing it to get up at all, or even to have more than one pillow. The bed-pan should be brought to it. A doctor will be necessary, as the child is in danger if rheumatic fever is neglected. The salicylate drugs are of the greatest use in the treatment of all forms of rheumatism. The affected joints should be rubbed with gualtherium or some such ointment and should be kept wrapped up in cotton-wool. The bowels must be kept open with calomel at night and salts in the morning. The diet must be bland and fluid until the fever subsides. Later on it will have to be increased very gradually to semi-solids. Leave meat out entirely until the patient is well recovered. A long convalescence will be required. The danger in all cases of rheumatic fever is that the heart rarely escapes damage in some degree or other unless the greatest care is taken and there is very prolonged rest. Other complications which occur are St. Vitus's dance and cerebral rheumatism, in which there is a very high temperature.

Chronic Rheumatism. Chronic rheumatism or ordinary rheumatism is a very common disease in the British Isles, and causes a great deal of pain and disability. The temperature may be slightly raised and there is a great deal of stiffness in the joints, but the condition generally responds very quickly to treatment by heat and salicylate of soda. Bluish-red swellings sometimes make their appearance in long-standing cases, especially on the front of the legs. (*See also* BATHS.)

Muscular Rheumatism. This form of rheumatism usually attacks middle-aged people, and it is very common among outdoor workers who have to face all weathers. The symptoms are pain and stiffness in the joints and they are increased by changes in the weather or by changes in the temperature of the body. Warm clothing should always be worn during cold weather and damp clothes must be changed immediately. Muscular rheumatism is also known as fibrositis, or myalgia, and when it occurs in the side it is known as pleurodynia ; lumbago is muscular rheumatism in the small of the back or loins, and torticolis is the term used when it occurs in the neck. (*See also* FIBROSITIS ; LUMBAGO.)

RHEUMATOID ARTHRITIS is a disease of the joints which occurs in two quite different forms. The one form is particularly common in women during the child-bearing period of life and the cause of the condition is quite unknown. Because the cause of this form of rheumatoid arthritis is unknown, it is called " primary " rheumatoid arthritis, to distinguish it from the other form, which occurs with equal frequency in men and women ; the other form is due to long-continued infection, and is therefore called " secondary " rheumatoid arthritis.

"**Primary**" **rheumatoid arthritis** may begin by attacks of cramp or weakness in the muscles of the hand, or the hands may become unnaturally cold in mild weather. Sometimes the onset may be acute, with a rise of temperature, accompanied by a swelling of the joints of the fingers. It is characteristic of this form of rheumatoid arthritis that the muscles and joints of the fingers are first, and most severely affected. Both sides are attacked and gradually the disease spreads to the wrist joints, so that the wrists become very stiff. Wasting of the muscles of the hands is very marked, and in advanced stages, not only are the wrists and fingers stiff, but the hands become deformed, the fingers being drawn up, and the whole hand twisted towards the little finger. In association with the changes in the joints, the patient's general health declines, and such symptoms as anæmia, palpitation of the heart with a quick pulse, sweating, and extreme coldness of the hands and feet may arise.

Treatment. To secure any improvement, the general health must be kept at a high level, and so the patient must be prepared for a long course of treatment. First, any unnecessary mental and physical strain must be avoided. The diet must be a generous one, with plenty of fresh fruit and vegetables ; it is not necessary to avoid meat. General tonics such as arsenic, iron and cod-liver oil, are often of benefit. Iodine and thyroid extract are often valuable in certain cases, but the response to these drugs is rapid if they are going to be of any value, and of course, they must only be taken under medical advice. Massage is useful to the affected joints ; these joints should be gently moved each day and supported in the best position for recovery by light splints, if necessary.

"**Secondary**" **rheumatoid arthritis** may come on either acutely, with a high temperature, when it may be mistaken for rheumatic fever, or it may arise fairly rapidly without any signs of fever. The disease attacks both large and small joints, the fingers, wrists, elbows, toes, ankles and knees, being commonly attacked on both sides of the body. The usual signs of inflammation of a joint are present : the affected joints are swollen, " doughy " to the touch, tender on pressure, and very painful when moved. The muscles just above and below the affected joints are wasted. Sweating of the hands and feet, a feeble circulation leading to coldness of the limbs, and anæmia are common. It is in this type of arthritis above all that infection plays a large part in causing the condition, and if the infection can be traced and dealt with before changes in the joints have gone too far for the joints to regain their proper positions and power of movement, there is every chance of a complete cure. It has already been mentioned that the teeth, the tonsils and the air sinuses connected with the nose are sources of this infection. The infection is caused by germs which manufacture poisons which circulate in the blood and act on the tissues of the joints. Another very important place from which infection may spread into the blood is the lower bowel, and it is rare to find a severe case of " secondary " rheumatoid arthritis in which a history of long-standing constipation is not obtained.

Treatment. This is first, removal of the infection when this is traced. Next comes the building up of the general health by means of fresh air, sunshine, and a suitable diet, which need not exclude red meat. Vaccines are sometimes of great help in clearing up the infection. Light massage to the joints and the application of heat, either dry or moist, is advisable. Where many joints are affected, baths of a certain type and of high temperature are often given. After the swelling of the joints has gone down, movement at the affected joints must be encouraged. (*See also* BATHS ; RHEU-MATISM, ACUTE ; VACCINES.)

RHINITIS. This is the medical name for inflammation of the mucous membrane of the nose such as is found in the common cold. It shows itself as catarrh. (*See also* NASAL CATARRH ; NOSE.)

RIBS are curved bones which enclose the chest cavity and serve to protect the heart and lungs from injury. There are twelve pairs of ribs, of which the upper seven are directly attached to the breast bone (or sternum) in front. These are called the true ribs. Of the remaining lower five pairs of ribs, each of the upper three is attached in front, not to the breast bone, but to the most forward part of the rib above it, the part which is called the costal cartilage, as it is not made of bone, but of a softer material, gristle. The lowermost two ribs are not attached to other ribs in front ; their most forward parts lie free, and these last two ribs are therefore called floating ribs. Behind, the ribs are all attached to the back part of the spinal column (back-bone). They are so attached by means of two joints that the ribs are able to turn on the spine, making a movement rather like that of a handle of a bucket. At some distance from the junction of the ribs with the spinal column, each rib, with the exception of the last two, has a bend in it, this bend being called the angle of the rib. The spaces between the ribs are called the intercostal spaces (inter- between, costa- a rib), and these spaces are filled in by muscles, some of which run downwards and forwards, and others of which run downwards and backwards. The muscles which run downwards and forwards raise the rib just below ; those which run downwards and backwards pull the rib above immediately downwards. Along the lower border of each rib, on its inner side, is a groove, in which run the blood-vessels and nerves which supply the muscles of the intercostal spaces. (*See* Plate XVI.)

Fracture of a rib. " A broken rib " is often taken very lightly, but if the broken piece is forced inwards instead of outwards, as unfortunately so often happens, then the injury may be very serious. A broken rib is more frequently the result of crushing of the chest, as when a vehicle runs over the body, than the result of a blow. The fracture usually occurs at the angle of the rib, and the broken pieces are displaced outwards.

Treatment, where there is outward displacement of the broken ends of the bone, is to strap the chest with strapping-plaster well above and below the broken rib, so that the plaster overlaps. As a rule, a broken rib heals very quickly and the victim of such an accident soon forgets his injury. But if the broken ends of the bone are displaced inwards, as sometimes happens when the fracture is the result of a direct blow on the chest, then there is a great danger that, unless carefully watched for, any sudden movement on the part of the patient may drive the broken ends of bone into the lung or into the covering to the lung—the pleura. If this happens, not only will the patient cough up blood from damage to the tissues of the lung, but there is also the danger of infection reaching the lung from the skin covering the chest wall if this has been torn by the blow causing the fracture.

RICKETS is a disease of growing children and infants which occurs most commonly between the ninth month and third year. It is very seldom seen in its early stage after the age of three years. The disease is due to a lack of a certain substance known as Vitamin D, either because this substance is not being supplied in sufficient amount in the diet, or because it is not being manufactured by the child in its body. Vitamin D is present to a large extent in most animal fats. It is abundant in normal human milk, but is most abundant in cod-liver oil. In the body, this vitamin is formed in the skin when certain rays of light (known as ultra-violet rays, which are found both in natural and artificial sunlight) act upon the skin. It is important to remember that the beneficial action of these rays is prevented unless they have free access to the skin ; that is to say, these rays cannot penetrate clothing or ordinary window glass.

Symptoms. The first signs to make their appearance are restlessness, sweating of the head, especially during sleep, and irritability. The child's appetite becomes poor and it is either constipated or has bouts of diarrhœa. The child is commonly fat and flabby, and the abdomen sticks out, giving a " pot-bellied " appearance. Teething is delayed. The most striking evidence of the disease is given by the changes in the bones. These are softer than normal, due to the formation of an abnormal type of bony tissue which has fewer lime salts in it than it should have. Because the bones are softer than normal, they bend more easily when any strain is put upon them, which explains why a child with rickets who is allowed to walk, or to sit with its legs tucked under it, gets deformities of the legs, such as bow-legs or knock knees. If the child rests much weight on the arms, these may also become bent. The spine may develop a hump, and the walls of the chest become flattened. Rows of enlarged softened bone appear down each side of the chest in front, forming what is called a " rickety rosary " and the skull increases in size, producing a square, broad forehead.

The muscles in rickets are flabby and the whole appearance of the child is one of fatness and limpness. Owing to the bending of the bones of the legs, walking is difficult and will be late. Apart from the deformities associated with the changes in the bones, children with rickets are in danger of suffering from chest troubles. Convulsions are also a source of danger, though they are not often fatal in themselves. A peculiar spasm of the throat which almost chokes the child may occur in rickets. This is known as laryngismus stridulus and is a frightening sight to watch. The child catches its breath, and makes a crowing sound, which is particularly noticeable when the child cries. Just as it goes blue in the face, it will breathe out, and the spasm will relax. A hot bath is the first-aid treatment for this condition, and also for the general convulsions which may occur during the course of the disease.

Treatment. *This may be summed up in one word : Prevention. No child should ever be allowed to get rickets.* In breast-fed children there is little chance of the condition developing if the child is weaned at the proper time, but in artificially-fed children it is wise to give cod-liver oil or halibut oil from the third month. Amounts of 5 drops should be given twice daily to start with and the dose should be gradually increased, so that by the ninth month the child is receiving two teaspoonsful daily. In addition, the child should have as much natural sunlight as possible, and the minimum of clothes which will keep the infant warm should be put on. If the disease has already developed, large doses of cod-liver oil, or better still, calciferol or one of the new preparations of Vitamin D should be given, and the child should be exposed to artificial ultra-violet light. It should not be allowed to walk or crawl until the bones are strong enough to bear its weight, and to prevent its doing so it may be advisable to attach long, light splints to either side of the body and to the limbs. Gentle massage is useful for toning up the flabby muscles. Great patience is needed to overcome such deformities as knock-knees, bow-legs or humped back if these have been allowed to develop. As a general rule, with correct treatment by diet and Vitamin D, these deformities disappear ; but in some instances it may be necessary to call in the aid of surgery. (*See also* VITAMINS ; DEFICIENCY DISEASES.)

RIGOR is a sudden severe shivering fit which occurs in certain fevers, particularly in malaria, and may occur at the commencement of an attack of pneumonia or septicæmia. It is essential that during the rigor the patient should be kept warm.

RIGOR MORTIS is a stiffening of the muscles which occurs after death and is due to chemical changes in the composition of the muscles when blood ceases to flow through them.

RINGWORM. Ringworm is a skin disease caused by a fungus. It attacks any part of the skin, and its manifestations vary greatly in different areas.

Ringworm of the *scalp*. In the adult this is exceedingly rare ; most of the cases occurring between 5 and 12, and, even if untreated, tend to die out at puberty. One or more rounded spots, partially bald, are seen, in which the remaining hairs are short, dull, and twisted. The diseased spots are scaly, and often outlined with a reddish ring. The fungus can be seen in the hairs (and skin scrapings) under the microscope.

Ringworm of the *beard* appears in two forms : (1) As ringworm of the body ; (2) resembling barber's itch. The affected parts are swollen, painful, and nodular.

Ringworm of the *body*. Here the " rings " to which the disease owes its name are chiefly seen. The patches are red and scaly. These cases spread rapidly, especially in the armpits and the groins, where heat and moisture are present.

Ringworm of the *palms*, *soles*, and *nails*. This is far from uncommon. On the palms are found two forms : (1) The acute, which resembles an acute dermatitis ; (2) the chronic, where the palm is dry, scaly, and slightly reddened. So little inconvenience is caused that the patient may go on for years without treatment. The soles may be similarly affected, but in the commonest form the skin between the toes is white and sodden, peels off in large flakes, and leaves an oozing red surface. Cracks at the base of the toes are common, and itching is troublesome. The nails have a dirty, yellowish, " eaten-away " appearance which is very suggestive. All these cases are very difficult to diagnose unless scrapings from the skin are examined microscopically.

The *outlook* in ringworm depends on various factors. If ringworm of the scalp is untreated, it lasts till the child reaches puberty. Otherwise, 8 months at least is considered necessary for a cure. Ringworm of the nails requires very persevering treatment, and the time taken to cure it on the palms and soles varies with its thoroughness. Ringworm of the beard takes 6–8 weeks to cure, and that of the non-hairy skin 6–10 days.

Treatment is far from easy. It is simple enough to destroy the ringworm fungus itself ; the difficulty in practice is to destroy the fungus without affecting the patient.

Ringworm of the *scalp* is treated by shaving the head, washing daily, and thorough rubbing in of an antiseptic ointment. Care is taken in using brushes, towels, caps, etc., and the affected child must sleep alone. Other children should always be carefully examined for traces of the disease. X-ray, in expert hands, is one of the best and quickest methods, thousands of cases being treated successfully every year. The method is to expose the scalp to carefully estimated " doses " of the rays. After 2–3 weeks, the hair comes out entirely. Then the scalp is treated regularly with antiseptic ointment until clear. New hair appears in 6–8 weeks, and is fully grown in 3–4 months.

Ringworm of the *beard* is treated by removing the hairs with forceps and thoroughly rubbing in an antiseptic ointment.

Ringworm of the *body* is easily cured by antiseptic ointment. If the groins and armpits are affected, soothing remedies, such as boric ointment, are applied as preliminary treatment.

Ringworm of the *palms* and *soles* is treated by antiseptics ; a good plan is to have a daily 10 minutes' soak with dilute Condy's fluid, and then apply antiseptic ointment.

Ringworm of the *nails* is by far the most obstinate of all forms. If untreated it remains for life. The best method is to apply a solution which softens the nails, such as Fehling's solution, so that they can be removed without pain. Antiseptic treatment is then applied to the nail-bed until no trace of the fungus remains.

RODENT ULCER (Latin *rodens*, gnawing) is a surface cancer of the skin where the ulceration is the chief feature. It commences in the ordinary way as a small hard nodule in the skin, and, as it grows, stretches the skin over it until a raised, " mother-of-pearl," shiny area appears. It is very constant to certain situations, 95 per cent. occurring on the face, and of these about 46 per cent. on the side of the nose where it joins the cheek, a little higher than the middle, and about 24 per cent. at the outer corner of the eye. Only very rarely does it occur on other parts of the body.

No pain is felt, though the patient may complain of itching ; pain, indeed, is rarely felt even in bad cases, though the itching increases with the growth of the ulcer. When it begins to grow, the sides extend and the centre sinks, " it is like a lake surrounded on all sides by hills." Soon the centre breaks down and ulcerates, but the discharge is generally very small ; the ulcer also spreads towards the margins, and may heal by scarring at the centre. Finally the whole of the surface sloughs or comes away, except the rolled edge, and the typical *rodent ulcer*, as it is usually first seen by the doctor, has formed.

If untreated, or, worse still, if treated by quack medicines, the disease attacks and destroys every structure with which it comes in contact, such as the eyelids, the walls of the nose, and the bones of the face, leading to the most hideous deformities, and finally to the death of the patient from haemorrhage, erysipelas, meningitis (inflammation of the coverings of the brain), or exhaustion.

Treatment. The outlook for untreated or maltreated cases, as already stated, is almost hopeless, but if patients are seen early and correctly treated, it is safe to say that in 100 per cent. of the cases a cure is certain. Treatment varies a little with the stage at which the patient is first seen. In the early stages, it is possible to remove the growth completely. A scab forms, which remains on for about a fortnight, and when it comes away the wound underneath is generally entirely healed.

Caustics, such as salicylic acid, chromic acid, pyrogallol, resorcin, and arsenious acid, the last being the best, are also frequently used. These mentioned have what is called a " selective action," that is, they cause more destruction to the tissues of the rodent ulcer than to the healthy skin around. This caustic method is very satisfactory in skilled hands, but is at first very painful. One of the newer methods, which seems to be giving good results, especially in early cases, is the painting once weekly with a 10 per cent. solution of potassium bichromate in water. It appears to act as a slow caustic. In this and the more severe methods a scab is formed, and, when this falls off, a healthy healing surface is seen.

The most satisfactory method, however, especially in the early stages, is radium. X-rays are next in value, especially in neglected and widespread cases. Several applications may be required of both radium and X-rays.

ROMBERGISM. This is a term applied to the inability to stand without falling over, when the eyes are shut. It is found as a symptom in some diseases of the nervous system, especially in locomotor ataxia.

ROUND LIGAMENT. A flat cord-like ligament that attaches the womb to the groin on each side of the body is called the round ligament. This term is also applied to a ligament of the liver, which is in reality a closed blood-vessel. It is the umbilical vein which before birth carries blood from the mother to the child. (*See also* CORD.)

RUPTURE. Rupture, or hernia, usually refers to the protrusion of part of the intestine or abdominal contents through the abdominal wall. The weak places where ruptures are liable to occur are at the naval or in its immediate neighbourhood (umbilical rupture), or in the groin (inguinal or femoral rupture). The chief surgical authorities assert that a rupture is always due to a congenital weakness in the wall of the abdomen, and that exertion or accident never play a really important part in the production of a rupture.

The weak places are, however, stretched as a result of manual labour, such as the lifting of heavy weights, constant straining due to a stricture, chronic constipation, or repeated pregnancies. A rupture may occur at the site of an operation where the fibrous tissues are subjected to more strain than they can stand without stretching.

A hernia will be felt as a bulge in the abdominal wall, which is more noticeable when the patient strains in any way, as in coughing. If the swelling can be pushed back into the abdominal cavity, the hernia is said to be reducible ; if the mass will not return, the hernia is irreducible, and if the circulation in the contents of the hernia becomes interfered with, it becomes strangulated. If a strangulated hernia cannot be reduced, immediate operation is necessary in order to prevent that portion of the bowel from becoming dead or gangrenous. The symptoms are acute pain, violent vomiting, and intestinal obstruction.

In children, the commonest form of hernia is the umbilical. It is due rather to a retarded development than to a definite weakness, and it is treated by a truss such as can be conveniently prepared at home. A flat disc, such as a penny, is strapped over the swelling and kept there night and day, with replacements only for the sake of cleanliness, until the muscles have fully developed and the weak area has disappeared.

Inguinal hernia (rupture in the groin) is rather more common in boys ; it is usually easily reducible by placing the child on its back and pressing gently on the swelling, at the same time supporting the edges of the opening with the other hand. If the protrusion keeps returning, operative treatment must be considered, or a properly fitting truss must be worn all the time. (*See also* ABDOMINAL BELT ; HERNIA.)

SACCHARIN. Saccharin is an intensely sweet crystalline powder derived from toluol (methyl-benzol). It is chiefly employed as a sweetening substance, especially in cases of diabetes and obesity when sugar cannot be taken.

SACRUM. The lower part of the spinal column is composed of five vertebræ which join together to form a massive bone known as the sacrum, or sacred bone. This bone lies between the two haunch-bones, and it forms the back wall of the pelvis, and in consequence, is slightly wider in women than in men. (*See also* PELVIS.)

ST. ANTHONY'S FIRE. *See* ERYSIPELAS.

ST. VITUS'S DANCE is a disease chiefly of children between the ages of five and fifteen years, and it occurs more often in girls than in boys. If only one attack of St. Vitus's dance occurs, it is likely, to say the least of it, that the heart will be damaged unless extreme care and caution are taken to give the child the necessary rest ; but if more than one attack is suffered, then the heart will almost certainly become diseased. This is because St. Vitus's dance, or to give it its medical name, *Chorea,* is one of the more severe forms of that scourge of childhood, rheumatism. Every child who has had even a slight attack of chorea is a candidate for rheumatic heart disease unless every precaution is taken against it.

The name " St. Vitus's dance " was given to the condition chorea because of the curious movements which the children who suffer from it make. These movements are spasmlike, quite outside the control of the will and very irregular.

In a considerable number of cases, the most obvious sign to the parents is a weakness or apparent paralysis of one arm or leg. The other important symptom of chorea is the mental change. A child with chorea becomes nervous, rather inclined to cry easily, and often silent.

Treatment. From what has already been said it will be realized that the main fear in chorea is that the rheumatic agent, whatever it may be, will attack the heart. Rest in bed, alone in a room, or at least behind a screen, is the only treatment that matters. The child must be kept in bed until all movements have ceased for at least a week, and until the doctor is satisfied that no further damage can be done to the heart by the attack the child has passed through. The diet must be light but very nourishing, and for a time it may be necessary to give a liquid diet if the child has difficulty in swallowing ordinary food. An unbreakable feeding-cup is sometimes better when the movements of the jaws and face are very bad. Milk and cod-liver oil are good for these children, and may be given in large quantities.

When sleeplessness is very pronounced it may be necessary to give drugs to induce sleep. For the disease itself many different drugs are prescribed, of which arsenic and iron and aspirin are the most in favour.

Chorea may show itself in its most severe form either at the beginning of adolescence or during pregnancy. During these times of stress, the movements may be exceedingly violent and the mental changes may be so severe as to lead to the necessity for temporary institutional care. But with the recovery from the attack of chorea, the mind regains its normal state.

One variety of St. Vitus's dance occurs in the aged. It has no real relation to the ordinary rheumatic chorea such as has been described, but the movements somewhat resemble those of that disorder, so it has been named **Huntingdon's Chorea,** after the discoverer. It is due to a degeneration of the nerve cells in a particular part of the brain. (*See also* DELIRIUM ; DEMENTIA.)

SALICYLATE. The salicylates are much used in the treatment of rheumatism both internally and externally.

SALICLYIC ACID is a colourless crystalline acid which is found in Nature in wintergreen and in the sweet birch tree, but it is now more cheaply prepared from carbolic acid, a product of coal tar. Salicylic acid has many uses in medicine as it has the property of reducing fever and is also an antiseptic, prohibiting the growth of germs. It is given internally in acute rheumatism and rheumatic fever, and also in sciatica and certain forms of neuralgia. For its antiseptic properties it is used in skin diseases, and because it assists in dissolving off the outermost thickened layers of the skin it forms the chief ingredient in many corn cures. (*See also* RHEUMATISM.)

SALIVA or spittle is a somewhat sticky, cloudy liquid and consists mainly of the products of the activity of the salivary glands in the mouth, but may also contain mucus, and cells which are shed by the lining of the mouth.

SALIVARY GLANDS are those glands which produce the saliva. There are three pairs of these glands : the parotid, which lies in the cheek, just in front of, and below the ear ; the submaxillary, which is placed just below the body of the lower jaw ; and the sublingual, which lies in the floor of the mouth, underneath the front part of the tongue. There are several disorders of the salivary glands, of which the most uncomfortable for the patient is the formation of small stones in the glands. This happens usually in the submaxillary and sublingual glands, and the pain caused by the movement of the stones along the passages or ducts of the glands leading into the mouth is often very distressing, being noticed most particularly when food is taken into the mouth, as the glands then attempt to discharge the saliva along the ducts which are blocked by the stones. Removal of these stones is a simple operation ; but their formation may persist, unless the infection of the teeth and gums which is always present is attended to. The parotid gland shares in the general enlargement of the glands due to mumps, and is nearly always the first symptom of that disorder. (*See also* MUMPS ; PAROTID GLAND.)

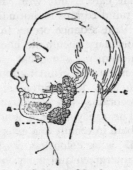

Salivary Glands
A. Sublingual; B. Submaxillary; C. Parotid

SALPINGITIS is an inflammation of the tubes which lead from the ovaries to the womb (Fallopian Tubes). It occurs after infection of the womb in childbirth or after an abortion, and is also one of the chief complications of gonorrhœa in women. (For the symptoms of the condition *see also* PERIMETRITIS ; GENITAL SYSTEM ; GONORRHŒA.)

SALTS mean in popular language saline purgatives. They include Glauber's salt, which is sodium sulphate ; Epsom salt, which is magnesium sulphate ; Rochelle salt, which is potassium and sodium tartrate ; " fruit salts," and others.

SALVARSAN, which is also known as " 606," arsenobillon, arsphenamine, arsenobenzol, is a valuable drug which is used in the treatment of syphilis, and in other diseases which are caused by similar coiled germs called spirochætes. It was discovered by Ehrlich early this century, and owes its name " 606 " to the fact that it was the six hundred and sixth experiment which gave Ehrlich the chemical composition of the drug for which he had been seeking, that is, one which would kill the spirochætes in the living body without being poisonous to the tissues of the body.

SAL VOLATILE is ammonium carbonate, or aromatic spirit of ammonia, and it is a favourite remedy for faintness. About fifteen drops drunk in half a wineglassful of water usually serves the purpose. (*See also* AMMONIA.)

SANTONIN is chiefly used in children to cure round-worms. The drug must be given on an empty stomach and a suitable purgative such as calomel must be given at the same time or just after the santonin. (*See also* WORMS.)

SAPRÆMIA is a condition in which the poisons or toxins manufactured by germs in some local hiding-place in the body escape into the blood and circulate throughout the body. This condition occurs most commonly in connection with childbirth or a miscarriage, if all the afterbirth or blood clot is not expelled from the womb. The symptoms of sapræmia are those of a mild septicæmia. The treatment is that of the source of the infection and once this has been traced and removed, the outlook for complete recovery is good. (*See also* SEPTICÆMIA ; TOXÆMIA.)

SCAB is a crust which is formed over an ulcer or wound. It is composed mainly of blood-clot, clotted lymph, or pus. It is difficult for healing to occur under a scab, and usually this has to be removed in order to allow healing to take place. Scabs may be softened and removed by soaking the part with a hot solution of bicarbonate of soda, or by means of a poultice composed of boracic acid or starch.

SCABIES. (*See* THE ITCH.)

SCALD is inflammation or damage to tissues by the action of hot liquids or gases. It resembles a burn in every way except how it is caused, and the treatment is that of a burn. (*See also* BURN.)

SCALE is a tiny flake of dead skin which is thrown off by the skin. Many such scales may be thrown off in the late stages of an attack of scarlet fever, when the process is called desquamation. (*See also* DESQUAMATION.)

SCALP consists of the three outermost layers of the covering to the top of the skull, or cranium. Actually there are five layers covering the bone, these being the skin, the fatty layer, a specialized portion of muscle called an aponeurosis, a loose connective tissue layer, and a thick membrane called the epicranium.

Scales are often shed by the scalp, and these are described as dandruff. Cysts are fairly common on the scalp, caused by blocking up in the sebaceous glands of the products of their activity. These cysts are called wens. (*See also* DANDRUFF ; WEN.)

SCAPULA is commonly known as the shoulder blade. It is a broad, triangular bone which lies on the upper part of the back of the chest, to which it is firmly attached by strong muscles. If these muscles are paralysed that part of the scapula facing the spine will be so turned that its edge can be seen when the arm is pushed forwards. This condition is called winged scapula. As the bone is triangular, it has three angles. The bottom one is called the inferior angle of the other two angles, the superior one is that facing the spine, whilst the external angle is replaced by a thickened mass of bone in which there is a cup-like cavity in which the head of the arm bone, the humerus, rests. From the front of this thickened

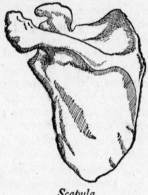

Scapula

mass of bone runs a beak-like piece of bone, the coracoid process, which serves as an attachment for the important biceps muscle. On the back of the scapula there is another thickening of bone, called the spine of the scapula, which runs in an upward and outward direction, at its outer edge being much thickened to form a

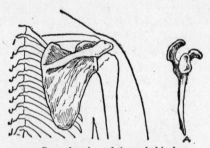

Scapula viewed from behind

A. showing glenoid fossa at upper end, where the humerus articulates

process, called the acromion, to which the collar-bone is attached by means of a joint. Injuries of the scapula are not very common as it is well protected by muscles.

SCAR is the natural result of healing of tissue which has been damaged or destroyed by injury or disease. (*See also* GRANULATION TISSUE ; KELOID.)

SCARLET FEVER is an acute infectious disease caused by a certain variety of the germ known as the streptococcus, which enters the body through the nose and throat, and first produces its effects in a localized sore throat. Afterwards, when general spread of the infection occurs, constitutional symptoms and a characteristic rash appear, the results of spread of the poisons produced by the germ in the throat and nose.

Scarlet fever is a disease of childhood, especially of the ages between five and ten years. But it is much more fatal in children up to the age of three years than in older children. The onset of the illness is usually abrupt : the incubation period is commonly two to three days, but may be anything from one to seven days. Sore throat, vomiting, headache, shivering fits, and a rise of temperature up to 102° to 103° F. and a quick pulse are the usual symptoms. The throat is very red and the tonsils also appear intensely red. The tongue is furred at the onset of the illness. The surface is covered with a creamy white fur through which bright red spots project. Later, the fur strips off from the edges inwards, leaving a perfectly clean, bright red tongue, to which the name of " red strawberry tongue " has been applied. On the second day the rash appears. This is seen first on the neck, then it spreads down gradually over the body and limbs, but rarely appears on the face. The forehead and cheeks are flushed, and there is a pale area round the mouth which forms a striking contrast. The rash is composed of tiny red spots, each being surrounded by a paler pink area. These spots are so closely packed together as to give the appearance of intense redness to the skin. The rash fades in the same order in which it appeared, and this is followed by peeling of the skin which was affected by the rash. Peeling goes on for at least two to three weeks, and the skin peels off in fine flakes—which are infectious. Even in a case of simple scarlet fever, without any complications, there is often some enlargement of the glands of the neck, but in the co-called septic type of the disease, this enlargement is marked, there is much discharge of pus from the nose and septicæmia may end the disease fatally. In rare cases, the poisons produced by the germs are so powerful that the body is unable to cope with the invasion and death takes place after only a few days' illness, during which there is high fever, continued vomiting and delirium. (*See also* SEPTICÆMIA.)

Complications of Scarlet Fever. The most common of all the complications is middle ear disease. Young children, especially those with enlarged adenoids and tonsils, are most liable to this complication. Rupture of the drum of the ear and the discharge of pus—which may continue for months or even years—is the usual sequel, unless the drum is cut at the most suitable point by the ear surgeon, when the condition in favourable cases clears up rapidly. Infection may travel backward from the middle ear and cause disease of the mastoid air cells, in which case an operation on the mastoid (simple mastoid operation) would be necessary.

Another serious complication of scarlet fever which occurs in the second or third week of the illness is inflammation of the kidneys. The amount of urine passed is greatly diminished and contains albumen and blood. Swelling of the feet, legs, and face accompanies this complication, which may become chronic and leave the victim with permanently damaged kidneys. In order to recognize the complication at the earliest possible moment, the urine should be examined at frequent intervals during the course of the illness.

Inflammation may occur in the joints, the picture then resembling that of acute rheumatism, and sometimes the heart may be involved also. Cases of scarlet fever are very liable at any stage in the illness to catch diphtheria, possibly owing to the damage already done to the tissues of the throat.

Treatment of Scarlet Fever. Until quite recently the treatment of scarlet fever was simply that of an infectious disease, and of the condition of fever ; but, since the discovery that the germ causing the disease produces a poison or toxin, like the germ which causes diphtheria, it has been possible to make an anti-toxin in the same way that diphtheria anti-toxin is prepared, and this is given in suitable doses, depending on the severity of the case. In most cases, one or two injections are given into the muscles ; in a severe case, the injection is given into a vein. The effects are commonly produced within twelve hours ; the temperature and pulse rate fall, the general symptoms of germ poisoning are lessened or may even disappear and the rash fades. There is ample evidence that the injection of scarlet fever anti-toxin reduces the liability to complications and shortens convalescence.

It is very important to prevent the spread of the germs causing the disease. Close contact with a person suffering from it is usually the way it is conveyed, but clothes from the patient, or things handled by the patient may also spread infection. Epidemics have been known to have been caused by infected milk. Patients who are convalescent may yet carry the germs of the disease in their throats and so infect others. That is why isolation of patients is insisted upon for at least four weeks. As long as there is any discharge from the nose, the patient can infect others by " droplet " infection.

Treatment by the sulphanilamide drugs, such as prontosil, is advised, but is not yet so successful as in some other infections.

SCIATICA is an inflammation of the supporting tissues of the sciatic nerve. The symptoms of true sciatica are very characteristic and consist in pain along the course of the nerve from the buttock to the ankle. The nerve itself is tender to the touch and much pain is produced on stretching the nerve by bending the extending leg at the hip joint. The cause of sciatica is unknown, but frequently it has been noticed that an attack follows an injury to the leg, or exposure to cold. Sciatica is a disease of early and middle adult life and it is most common in men.

In the very acute stages of the attack, when pain is intense, rest in bed is essential. The leg should be steadied by means of sandbags or in a light splint if this can be borne. Hot applications to the limb sometimes give relief. It may be necessary in the most painful stage to give drugs to ease the pain. After the severe pain has passed, the injection of oxygen into the back of the thigh near the nerve may be considered, or if the attack shows no signs of clearing up within a reasonable time, the injection of a salt solution into the sheath of the nerve may be undertaken. After such an injection massage and movements of the limb are useful. In these chronic cases it is sometimes found that they are being kept up by poisons —from bad teeth or loaded bowels—which are circulating in the blood.

SCIATIC NERVE is the largest nerve in the body, being about the thickness of the little finger. It supplies all the muscles at the back of the thigh, the calf and the foot and in addition, it contains many fibres which convey sensation from the skin of the back of the leg and foot. Thus the sciatic nerve has a very wide distribution. At the back of the knee-joint the nerve divides into two branches, the internal and external popliteal nerves. The external popliteal nerve lies very near the surface at the lower part of the back of the knee-joint and may, in a thin person, actually be felt. Inflammation of the sheath of the sciatic nerve is called sciatica.

The small sciatic nerve is a nerve which only contains fibres conveying sensation from the skin. It supplies the skin of the buttock, the back of the thigh and the upper half of the skin of the calf. (*See also* SCIATICA.)

SCIRRHUS is a particular type of cancer which is characterized by its hardness and firmness. A scirrhus cancer is especially common in the breast and in the prostate. (*See also* CANCER.)

SCLERODERMA (Hidebound Skin). This disease is characterized by a hardening of the skin, and is found in two forms, the diffuse and the circumscribed. The latter is often called morphœa.

Diffuse scleroderma usually affects a special region of the body such as an arm, or one side of the face and neck. It prefers the upper parts of the body, occurs more often in women, and usually begins in the thirties.

Morphœa appears as rounded patches, " old ivory " in colour, which have the appearance as if a piece of leather had been inserted into the skin. The patches are usually surrounded by a pinkish-violet ring. On the limbs, morphœa appears in " ribbon " form.

The treatment consists chiefly in building up the general health and in *time.* Many medicines have been suggested, thyroid substance being the most useful.

SCLEROSIS means hardening and is used to indicate certain changes in tissues, which as the result of disease, become firmer than normal. Hardening of the arteries, or arterio-sclerosis is due to a thickening of the middle and inner coats of their walls with the deposition in them of lime salts.

SCROFULA is the old name for tuberculosis of the lymphatic glands and bones. (*See also* TUBERCULOSIS.)

SCROFULODERMIA is a skin infection which is due to tuberculosis.

SCROTUM is the pouch which contains the testicles. It consists of two pocket-like compartments, lying side by side, the division between them being marked by a seam on the surface. The left compartment is the larger and hangs lower down. Underneath the skin of the scrotum, which is thin, and brown in colour, is a layer called the dartos, which contains many muscle fibres. When these fibres contract the skin of the scrotum is thrown into folds. Swelling of the scrotum may be due to an enlargement of the testicle itself, or to a hernia (q.v.), or to a collection of fluid, which is called a hydrocele, or to enlarged and congested veins, which condition is called a varicocele.

SCURVY is due to an error in diet which is now known to be due to lack of a vitamin, vitamin C.

Scurvy is rare in adults ; in children, however, the condition is not uncommon in those who are fed only on boiled or preserved milk or unsuitable patent foods.

Scurvy in children is often called Barlow's Disease, after the English physician who first described it. In children the disease commonly arises about the end of the first year of life. The child looks pale and anæmic, its gums bleed readily and any teeth present may drop out. The characteristic feature of scurvy in children is the pain and tenderness of the bones, especially near the joints. This tenderness is so great that the child does not wait to scream until the limb is touched ; it yells as soon as anyone approaches and appears to be going to touch it. The cause of this painful tenderness is bleeding under the external covering of the bones, which is not only very painful, but also causes swelling of the limbs. The child lies quite still, afraid to move because of the pain, and this may give the impression that the child is paralysed.

Treatment. Treatment of both the adult and infantile forms of scurvy consists in giving a diet which contains sufficient vitamin C. This vitamin is found in fresh fruit of all kinds, but particularly in the lemon and orange. All green vegetables contain vitamin C, but some contain it in greater amount than others. Tomatoes are the best vegetables for use in the treatment of scurvy, and it is a curious fact that when they are tinned they still retain their vitamin content. Therefore, in the winter, when fresh vegetables are scarce and expensive, tinned tomatoes should be taken frequently. In children who are the victims of scurvy, the sweetened juice of two or three lemons should be given daily as well as fresh tomato juice. Recovery is the rule in scurvy, except if there has been such an occurrence as bleeding into the brain which, fortunately, very rarely happens. (*See also* INFANTILE PARALYSIS.)

SEASICKNESS. Here are a few suggestions to assist those who are not experienced enough to have made their own individual rules :

On the day before the voyage, take an aperient.

An hour or so before going on board, take a little light food and a cup of strong coffee (this upsets some people but may suit most.)

Secure a good position on the boat, away from the sides ; a deck chair ; have a rug over your knees, close your eyes, sleep if possible, if not, think pleasant thoughts.

If, after all precautions, sickness does come on, a hot drink (not alcoholic) from a thermos flask may help, or a saline effervescent drink. Chloretone in 5-grain capsules, one every hour, should be taken during the crossing if necessary.

SEBORRHŒA (Greasy Skin). This term means excessive activity of the sebaceous glands of the skin, so that the skin and scalp tend to be oily.

Treatment. The head should be washed daily with soap spirit, or, if this is irritant, with a milder soap. Slight cases will be cured by this means alone, but as a rule seborrhœa of the scalp is very obstinate to treatment, and other measures will be required. A sulphur and salicylic ointment is the best, or a lotion may be used. For treatment of cases where a true dermatitis occurs, *see* DERMATITIS. Seborrhœa of the face is treated in the same way as acne vulgaris.

SEDATIVE is a remedy which lessens excitement and reduces excessive activity. Many drugs are general sedatives. Of these, opium and the bromides are the best known. Hot baths, especially if taken for a fairly long time, are excellent as a general sedative ; whilst the application of dry or moist heat to the skin locally also can be regarded as having a sedative effect.

SEMEN. Semen is the fluid of the male which is secreted by the testicles and contains spermatozoa, the male generative element. It is referred to as the seminal fluid. (*See also* TESTICLE ; SPERMA-TOZOA.)

SENILE DECAY is the result of age upon the various organs of the body.

SENNA is one of the most popular of all purgatives.

SEPSIS is poisoning by the products of decomposition of tissues and is caused by the agency of germs. A wound invaded by germs which produce pus is called a septic wound and takes much longer to heal than one in which no such germs are present.

SEPTICÆMIA is a condition in which germs gain entrance to the general blood-stream from some part of the body and continue to live there. Although in many infectious diseases, such as typhoid or pneumonia, the germs causing these conditions may get into the general blood-stream, they are soon killed off by the resistance which the patient develops, and the disease process then remains only in certain organs of the body. In true septicæmia on the other hand, once certain germs have got a hold it may be in some quite small and insignificant spot such as a finger prick, or a small wound in the skin, they are able to break through the barriers which separate them from the general blood-stream and are constantly passing into it, so that though they may not actually grow and multiply in the blood stream, the germs are constantly entering into the blood and the outlook for the patient is a poor one. There are two kinds of germs which commonly produce this condition of septicæmia. One kind forms long or short chains and is called the streptococcal group. The other kind, when grown outside the body, produces forms which resemble bunches of grapes. This kind is called the staphylococcal group.

Streptococcal Septicæmia is a particularly important form because it causes the death of thousands of mothers yearly. After an apparently easy confinement it is found that the womb has somehow become infected with germs of the streptococcal group and the onset of shivering attacks or rigors, associated with an irregular fever, diarrhœa and anæmia means that yet another life has to be sacrificed to septicæmia. Even more often does strepto-coccal septicæmia follow abortion, where often less care is taken to prevent germs from gaining admittance to the womb.

Treatment. One treatment is by means of what are called anti-streptococcal sera, which contain certain substances that should normally be produced by the human body, to kill the germs. Sulphanilamide drugs, such as prontosil, are often successfully prescribed. The only other measures to be taken are those designed to make the patient more comfortable. Tepid sponging if the fever is high; large quantities of fluid to drink; and a transfusion of blood to retain his strength must all be employed.

Staphylococcal Septicæmia is usually the result of an infection of the skin, such as the common boil. It occurs only in those patients whose resistance to disease is very low. The onset of septicæmia is marked by shivering fits and a high temperature ; but, unlike the streptococcal type of septicæmia, in this form abscesses accompany the septicæmia state and these may occur in any part of the body, such as the kidneys, the lungs and the bones.

SERUM. When blood is taken from an animal and allowed to stand quietly in a clean vessel it clots. This process consists first in the formation of a very fine net of fibrin crystals throughout the blood. After a time this net-work of fibrin shrinks and in doing so retains all the undissolved parts of the blood within its meshes, but squeezes out the remaining fluid. This is a clear, yellowish liquid called blood-serum, or more shortly serum. Should the blood happen to contain substances which are poisonous to micro-organisms, or germs (so-called anti-bacteriological bodies), or substances which can neutralize non-living poisons, or toxins (so-called anti-toxins), then these will be present in the serum. Since the use of whole blood for the purpose of administering these antibodies is impractical, serums are used in medical treatment.

Serums and Anti-Toxins used in Medicine. In those diseases where powerful sera or anti-toxins are available they constitute the very best method of treating the disease, for it is the natural way by which the body normally conquers its enemy. Diphtheria treated adequately on the first day of infection is practically non-fatal ; on the sixth it kills about one in four persons. Furthermore, the use of these substances is also of the greatest value in preventing the onset of disease. (*See also* DIPHTHERIA.)

SEX HYGIENE. The education of children in sex has been much argued, but it is possible to make too much of teaching " the facts of life." Children who keep rabbits or a cat soon learn a good deal about the facts of life, and the prospective arrival of kittens, their birth, and their early feeding teach a child more, and in a far better way, than any lecture in the schoolroom. Puberty is the time for preliminary instruction. No girl should be allowed to have the

shock of a first menstruation without some knowledge of what it
means. It is a mistake to treat menstruation as a disease and put
a girl to bed because of it, and girls should be allowed to lead their
ordinary routine of life and play games regardless of menstruation.
In the same way emissions of semen at night in boys should be
looked upon in the proper perspective. Seminal emissions are quite
normal in boys at puberty, and any suggestion of " lost vitality "
is simply nonsense. If they become too frequent consult a doctor.

In the case of youths in early manhood sex may become an urgent
problem. The best way to deal with the problem at this time is to
push it into the background, or " sublimate " it, by emphasizing
games and other interests and ambitions, or by a healthy interest
in someone of the opposite sex. Young women are said to feel the
urgency of this problem less than do young men, and those who do
feel it are often looked upon as abnormal, but this is an unfair view.
The modern young woman has her sex problems almost as much
as the young man does, and her remedies are the same as his, which
are mentioned above. Healthy companionship of the two sexes in
work and play is the best safeguard against sex difficulties.

In early married life other sex problems arise. Every family
doctor has known cases of young people who have not consummated
their marriage simply because their knowledge of how the sexual
act should be performed was inexact.

Nowadays, however, there are plenty of authoritative text books
that will serve as counsellor and guide to young people.

Birth Control. The human race has been kept within reasonable limits in the past by famine, pestilence and war. With the
gradual disappearance of two of these—one would hope of all—
other methods of birth control raise their heads. Even celibacy is
essentially a method of birth control. In this country the Ministry
of Health issued in 1930 a memorandum (153 M.C.W.) allowing
local authorities to give instruction in birth control to expectant
and nursing mothers attending maternity child welfare centres, and
who need it on medical grounds. This was extended by Circular
1408 M.C.W., 1934, allowing local authorities to provide advice for
all married women requiring it, on medical grounds, at an appropriate clinic. The Family Planning Association (formerly the
National Birth Control Association), 69 Eccleston Square, London,
S.W.1, under the presidency of Lord Horder, has been formed to
organize the different societies and groups interested in birth control
in this country. The Birth Control Investigation Committee (now
incorporated with the Family Planning Association), under the late
Sir Humphry Rolleston, subsidized research work on the subject
at the universities of Oxford, Cambridge and Edinburgh. The

Constructive Birth Control Society, 108 Whitfield Street, London, W.1, runs a clinic and travelling caravans to give free instruction in birth control to poor persons. There are other societies and clinics in different parts of the country, and more and more family doctors are becoming interested in the subject. One of the chief drawbacks, however, is that up to the present there has not been discovered a 100 per cent safe single method of birth control, though when more than one method is used at the same time, recommended by doctors and in authoritative text books, this is successful in a very large percentage of cases.

SHINGLES (Herpes Zoster). These names were originally applied to that form of the disease in which herpes started about the middle of the back, and crept round towards the front in girdle form. They are, however, rather misleading, as the disease may affect any part of the body.

Symptoms. The two main symptoms are pain, followed on the third or fourth day by crops of little blisters on a certain area. The cause is an acute inflammation of a nerve centre, together with degeneration of the nerve fibres passing through it. Hence only that area of skin supplied by the affected fibres suffers. Second attacks are almost unknown.

Treatment. The only local treatment required is to prevent breaking and infection of the blisters, as by an antiseptic dusting-powder, cotton-wool, and a bandage. The pain is treated by aspirin, phenacetin, etc., or in severe cases by morphia. A course of tonics, and especially a change of air, are valuable in convalescence.

SHOCK. The sudden severe lowering of the vitality of the body, due to injuries, operations, or profound emotion. The essential feature in shock is a lowering of the blood-pressure, due to paralysis of the brain centre that controls the contracting of the blood-vessels.

Treatment. The patient is kept at rest, the foot of the bed is raised so that blood flows back into the brain, and hot-water bottles are put all round the patient (care being taken not to touch the patient with the hot bottle, as it may cause a severe burn) so that the blood is drawn back to the surface. Hot coffee, tea or other drinks may be given; alcohol is not good, as a depressing effect follows the preliminary stimulating effect. Injection of saline solutions, with glucose, and various drugs are useful, but must be left to the doctor.

SHORTNESS OF BREATH. This condition may be a symptom in many different disorders, or, on the other hand, it may only occur after exercise and be unimportant. Shortness of breath is also known as dyspnœa or breathlessness. (*See also* BREATHLESS-NESS.)

SHOULDER is the part of the body where the arm joins on to the trunk, formed by the meeting of the humerus (bone of the upper arm) with the scapula (shoulder-blade) and clavicle (collar-bone), and the muscles associated with them.

SICK HEADACHE. (*See* MIGRAINE.)

SIGHT, ERRORS IN, or ASTHENOPIA. In general use the word is only used to mean want of power to use the eyes for any sustained effort of vision. A person who is asthenopic is unable to enjoy full use of his eyes, because any attempt to gaze fixedly at anything is accompanied by more or less wobbling or dimness of the sight.

Treatment. The treatment of asthenopia is to treat the cause. Glasses should be prescribed if they are found necessary ; alcohol, tobacco, tea, and coffee may have to be forbidden ; the general health should be regulated with tonics, if necessary.

The headache so often complained of generally disappears with the above treatment. If, however, it persists, showing that it is really a nervous headache, electric treatment may be tried, and eye-drops obtained from the doctor.

Astigmatism. This is a common error of eyesight due to the cornea (the clear membrane in front of the eye) being unequally curved in different directions, so that rays of light in different meridians cannot be brought to focus on the retina except by continued and irregular strain of the muscle. The condition causes objects to seem distorted and out of place.

Astigmatism may be remedied by suitable spectacles. (*See also* EYE.)

Short Sight (Myopia). In this condition, the distance from the lens to the retina is too great, so that distant objects are focussed in front of the retina and seem blurred. Near objects, however, can be seen more clearly and easily than with normal eyes. (*See also* EYES ; SQUINT.)

SIGMOID FLEXURE. The S-shaped bend in the colon or large bowel is sometimes referred to as the sigmoid flexure. (*See also* INTESTINE.)

SILICOSIS. This disease is a form of fibrosis of the lungs and is due to the inhalation of particles of dust. (*See also* ANTHRACOSIS ; FIBROSIS.)

SINUS. A sinus is a hollow or cavity, and the term is applied medically to a suppurating tract that has not healed up (such as a sinus leading from an abscess to the skin), but also to large channels containing blood (especially the venous sinuses of the brain, such as the lateral sinus), and to cavities within a bone (such as the maxillary and frontal accessory sinuses of the nose). *Sinus disease* is a term which is popularly applied to infection of one or more of the accessory sinuses of the nose (maxillary sinus or antrum, frontal sinus, ethmoid sinuses, and sphenoid sinus), which are situated in the bones adjacent to the nose and communicate with it, containing air. The condition commonly follows influenza, though maxillary sinus infection may sometimes be caused by a tooth abscess. The treatment is usually surgical, though recently a successful medical treatment called " displacement " has been introduced by an American specialist, Proetz, by which antiseptic oils or other liquid are introduced into the sinuses by a suction apparatus which draws out the air in them, to be " displaced " by the antiseptic fluid.

" SIX-O-SIX." *See* SALVARSAN.

SKELETON is the bony framework that supports the soft parts of the body.

SKIN. The skin is made up of two layers, the epidermis, which covers the surface, and the dermis or " true skin " underneath. Below the true skin is the subcutaneous or " under-skin " layer, which is a loose tissue containing fat, blood-vessels, and nerves, and serves to protect the deeper structures underneath, and to give roundness to the body. (*See also* DERMATITIS *and* SKIN, DISEASES OF.)

SKIN, DISEASES OF. Inflammation of the skin (*dermatitis*) attacks every part of the body, and it is possible, though not probable, to find the different forms on every part at different times. Certain forms, however, have a fondness for certain regions, and these are discussed under separate headings. (*See also* ACNE-ROSACEA ; CHEI-LITIS ; DERMATITIS ; ECZEMA ; FROST-BITE ; HEAD LOUSE ; INTERTRIGO ; LUPUS ; PAGET'S DISEASE ; PELLAGRA ; PSORIASIS ; RINGWORM ; SCABIES ; SEBORRHŒA ; SUMMER PRURIGO ; XERO-DERMA.)

SKULL. The skull is the bony framework of the head, and is divided into two parts—the cranium and the face. The cranium encloses the brain and is made up of the occipital, frontal, two parietal, two temporal, and ethmoid and splenoid bones. The bones of the face comprise the two upper jaw-bones (superior maxillæ) and one lower jaw-bone (inferior maxilla), two malar, two nasal, two lachrymal, two turbinal, two palate bones, and the vomer.

SLEEPING SICKNESS. This disease is also known as try-panosomiasis, and it is caused by the bite of the tsetse fly. It occurs amongst the natives of Africa, and it is often described as African lethargy or negro lethargy.

Symptoms. Some people begin to show symptoms two or three weeks from the time of being bitten, while others again do not show any sign of the disease for several months. The small puncture in the skin made by the bite may or may not feel irritable, and unless some redness shows the patient may overlook the affair. The first stage commences with fever, and the temperature in the evening is usually higher than in the morning. The fever may come and go during the first few weeks, but gradually it becomes more pronounced, and in time the patient becomes weakened and anæmic. The glands of the neck and other parts of the body become swollen, and there may be a rash of pink ring-shaped patches over certain areas of the skin. The next stage in the condition is

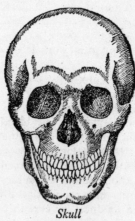

Skull

where the symptoms of sleeping sickness begin to show themselves. The patient becomes careless in his work and in his habits, his walk becomes a slouch, and he tends to fall asleep on all occasions. There are tremors of the tongue and hands and he may complain of dull headache in his wakeful moments. He will eat food if it is brought to him, but very often the effort of raising food to the mouth is too much for the patient. Gradually he becomes very thin and wasted in appearance, and he may die of sheer exhaustion unless carried off earlier by some other condition.

Treatment. The best form of treatment is the new drug known as Bayer 205, and in the earlier stages of the disease it is sometimes possible to effect a cure. Among other substances which have been used with favourable results are atoxyl, soamin, arsacetin, salvarsan and tartar emetic.

SLEEPLESSNESS. Insomnia is another term for sleeplessness. (*See also* INSOMNIA.)

SLEEPY SICKNESS. This condition is in no way related to the disease known as *sleeping sickness* ; the medical term for sleepy sickness is *encephalitis lethargica*. (*See also* ENCEPHALITIS.)

SLING. A bandage for the support of a limb is known as a sling. (*See also* BANDAGE.)

SMALLPOX. Smallpox, or variola as it is also called, is an infectious disease, the chief symptoms of which are fever and an eruption of the skin. The cause of the disease is believed to be due to a very tiny germ, but what is definitely known is that smallpox is one of the most contagious of all diseases. The infection is spread by the breath of the patient and by contact with him or his personal belongings. The infection can also be carried by the clothes of third persons not themselves infected, and it is believed that the germs can be carried through the air for some considerable distance.

Symptoms. About twelve days after the infection, the disease begins with an attack of shivering, headache, pains in the back, and vomiting. In children there may be convulsions. On the third day, the fever declines a little and a rash, somewhat resembling that of scarlet fever, makes its appearance. It commences on the face and head, spreads to the arms and trunk, and lastly appears on the legs. The distribution of the rash is important and it is one of the points of value to the doctor when he is making his diagnosis. During the period between the third and sixth day the rash undergoes a change in appearance, the raised " pocks " become filled with a clear fluid and in the centre there is a slight depression. On about the eighth day these vesicles or blebs become larger in size and the fluid inside them changes into pus or yellow matter. The skin surrounding each " pustule " is inflamed and swollen, and as the eruption is more thickly spread on the features they become very disfigured indeed.

The eruption is present on the mucous membranes as well, particularly in the mouth and throat, and the inflammation and swelling which takes place is often a serious matter to the patient, as there is great danger of obstruction of the air passages. The fever which had somewhat declined after the first two days now makes its appearance again (secondary or suppurative fever), and the patient is extremely restless from the irritation caused by the rash. On the eleventh or twelfth day the pustules either break or dry up and blackish crusts form. The temperature usually drops at this stage, but there is great itching of the skin where a scab has formed over each pustule. The scabs gradually fall off leaving a scar or " pit " which is one of the characteristic marks of smallpox.

In some outbreaks the type of the disease is much more severe. In the type of the disease known as *confluent smallpox* the symptoms are much more severe from the very onset, and the rash, instead of showing itself in isolated spots, appears in large patches, and the pocks are so numerous that they run into one another. An even more severe type of the disease is the *hæmorrhagic* type in which bleeding takes place into the pocks after they are formed. *Discrete smallpox* is the term used to describe mild cases, and *varioloid* cases are those in which the symptoms are very slight.

Treatment. The general treatment of smallpox is conducted along the same lines as for any other infectious disease. The patient is removed to hospital, which is usually situated some distance from a town. All those who have been in contact with the patient are vaccinated, and the public health authorities keep a very strict watch in order to check any spread of the infection. The house and clothing must be thoroughly disinfected. The patient should lie in a well-ventilated room, and one form of treatment allows only red light to be admitted to the room in order to protect the skin from the chemical rays of light, and thereby lessen the subsequent facial disfigurement from pitting. Skilled nursing is of vast importance in this disease and the patient must be kept strictly isolated until the skin is thoroughly healed. The length of time in hospital is usually about eight weeks. (*See also* INFECTIOUS DISEASES.)

SMOKING. *See* TOBACCO.

SNEEZING. Any irritation in the nose may cause a fit of sneezing as this is Nature's way of getting rid of the irritation and infection. (*See also* CATARRH, NASAL ; HAY FEVER ; INFLUENZA.)

SNOW BLINDNESS. A condition of the eyes in which the conjunctiva becomes inflamed, through continuous gazing at large tracts of snow under a dazzling sun, is known as snow blindness. (*See also* BLINDNESS ; CONJUNCTIVITIS.)

SOFTENING OF THE BRAIN is a term commonly applied to syphilis affecting the brain, or to suppuration of the brain due to brain abscess. It may signify interference with the nourishment of the brain through its blood supply. When a part of the brain is suddenly deprived of blood it ceases to be able to do its work properly, and in the case of a large area of the brain this means that serious consequences follow to health, if not to life. If a blood-vessel in the brain bursts, giving rise to hæmorrhage, it is unlikely that the patient will survive ; if he does, some severe form of paralysis is almost certain to result. But a blood-vessel may become so narrowed by disease—such as arterio-sclerosis—that it closes up, again depriving the part of the brain supplied by that vessel of its proper nourishment, and in such a case, although serious paralysis may follow, especially a hemiplegia in many cases, yet the danger to life is not so great. Another cause of " softening of the brain " is destruction of the brain by a tumour. This condition is usually fatal, unless the tumour is in such a situation and of such a nature that it is removable by operation. (*See also* ARTERIO-SCLEROSIS ; HEMIPLEGIA ; PARALYSIS.)

SOFT PALATE. The soft palate is the roof of the mouth at the back of the throat which is a muscular continuation of the bony arch forming the hard palate ; it ends at the uvula. (*See also* PALATE.)

SOFT SORE. Soft sore, or soft chancre, is a venereal ulceration which forms in the region of the groins. It is non-syphilitic, but it is often mistaken for the syphilitic hard chancre. (*See also* SYPHILIS.)

SOMNAMBULISM. This is another name for sleep-walking.

SOPORIFIC. Any drug which tends to induce sleep is known as a soporific. (*See also* HYPNOTIC ; NARCOTIC.)

SORE. This is a popular term for ulcer. (*See also* ULCER.)

SORE THROAT. (*See* CLERGYMAN'S SORE THROAT ; DIPHTHERIA ; LARYNGITIS ; PHARYNGITIS ; TONSILLITIS.)

SPEAKER'S THROAT. *See* CLERGYMAN'S SORE THROAT.

SPERMATIC CORD. This structure is made up of arteries, veins, nerves, etc., which are associated with the testicle. Twisting of this cord causes strangulation of the blood-vessels, and, if immediate treatment is not carried out, gangrene usually sets in and the testicle and cord may have to be removed by operation. The veins of the spermatic cord may become varicose and the condition is called a varicocele.

SPERMATORRHŒA. This term is applied to the involuntary discharge of semen from the urethra in the male without any sexual excitement. The condition is normal if the discharges are not too frequent, otherwise a doctor should be consulted, who will probably prescribe a sedative mixture. The most common causes are due to such conditions as constipation, irritation of the sexual organs by walking or riding, varicose veins, a long foreskin, intestinal worms, or reading exciting or pornographical literature before retiring to bed.

Treatment consists in removing the cause once it has been discovered. Cold baths, suitable exercise, and often a change of surroundings or companions will help considerably. A soothing mixture containing bromide taken before going to bed will often give a night free from symptoms.

SPERMATOZOON. The human male germ which is able to fertilize the female ovum, or egg, is known as a spermatozoon. It is microscopical in size but consists of a head, a neck, a body and a tail. The tail is by far the longest part and acts as a powerful propeller which makes the tiny cell capable of active movement.

These cells are able to live for quite a few days if kept at body temperature, but they soon die if exposed to the cold. (*See also* SEMEN.)

SPHENOID BONE. This bone lies at the base of the skull and in shape it bears a close resemblance to a bird. It consists of a hollow central part or body from which arises thin structures on either side known as

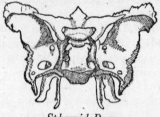

Sphenoid Bone

the great wings. The hollow in the central part communicates with the nose and is called the sphenoidal sinus. (*See also* BONE.)

SPINA BIFIDA. This term means literally a cleft spine and it aptly describes the condition. In the early days of growth, the spinal cord is represented by a groove along the back of the child while it is still in the mother's womb. The borders of this groove grow together and form a tube which is the central canal of the spinal cord. It is easy to see that if this tube fails to develop, the child will be born with the spinal cord open to the surface of the back. In such a case the child will probably be stillborn. Sometimes the neural tube has closed and the spinal cord is more or less perfectly formed but the outer covering of tissue may have failed to grow and enclose it, and the child is said to be born with split spine, or spina bifida. The usual appearance in this condition is a swelling in the lower part of the spine which contains cerebro-spinal fluid. The treatment of the condition is surgical and many cases have been successfully operated upon. (*See also* SPINAL CORD.)

Spinal Column showing Vertebræ

SPINAL COLUMN. The spinal column is also known as the spine, the backbone, or the vertebral column and it forms a very important part of the skeleton. (*See also* BACKBONE.)

SPINAL CORD is a part of the nervous system which is directly continuous above with the medulla (q.v.) and extends downwards as far as the lower part of the loins.   It is contained in a bony canal—the spinal canal, which is enclosed by the vertebral column. It gives off the spinal nerves, which pass out through spaces in the vertebral column to form the nerves to the limbs, trunk and internal organs.   (*See also* BRAIN ; NERVOUS SYSTEM ; REFLEX ACTION.)

SPINAL CURVATURE.   Deformity of the backbone consists of an exaggeration of its normal curves, or a new curve may form in a lateral or sideways direction.   *Kyphosis*, commonly known as round shoulders, is described under its own heading, and *lordosis*, which is an increase of the forward curve in the small of the back, is also described under its own heading.   *Scoliosis*, which is the name

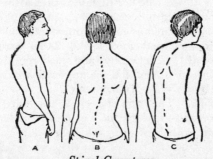

Spinal Curvatures
A. Kyphosis and Lordosis; B. Scoliosis; C. Spondylitis Deformans

given to a sideways curve of the spine, may be due to rickets in early childhood, to tuberculosis of the hip, or to great muscular weakness.   In young growing children the habit of standing badly is very liable to lead to curvature of the spine.   Diseases of the chest, such as pleurisy, in which the chest becomes collapsed, are also liable to cause an alteration in the shape of the spine.   The treatment of these conditions consists in keeping the general health in as good condition as possible by means of fresh air, suitable exercise, good food, and tonics if necessary.   Special exercises should be practised daily, and any habit of standing or sitting badly should be avoided.   Growing children should never be allowed to carry heavy weights.   It is only in extremely marked cases that special mechanical supports are necessary, but massage is good as it helps to strengthen the muscles of the back.

Angular curvature of the spine, which is also known as *Pott's disease*, is a much more serious condition, and it is almost always caused by tuberculosis.   The deformity in this condition is due to caries or rotting of the vertebræ, and, as the bone is destroyed, the spine gives way at the site of the disease, thus causing a sharp curve forward. A similar condition may occur as the result of a fall in the case of a young child, or a severe blow upon the back of an older person. Deformity of the spine does not begin to appear until quite late in the disease. The first symptom is dull, aching and constant pain in the back which is increased by sudden movement or by jarring of the spine. In order to avoid pain, the back is held very stiff and rigid and this attitude is one of the characteristics of the disease. On being requested to bend down it is found that the spine tends to move as a whole, and a child will crouch down, bending his knees while still maintaining the rigid straightness of the spine. X-ray examination should be carried out as early as possible to see whether disease is present or not whenever there is constant pain in the back.

Treatment is the same as for any other tuberculous condition : that is, rest, fresh air and good food. Early treatment may be successful in preventing deformity, and good results are often obtained by sunlight treatment and the application of suitable plaster casts. (*See also* BACKBONE ; TUBERCULOSIS.)

SPIROCHÆTE. The term spirochæte is applied to a group of tiny germs or organisms which have a spiral structure like a corkscrew. They are capable of wriggling their way through the blood or tissues, and it has been proved that they are the cause of several important diseases in human beings, especially syphilis and Vincent's angina. (*See also* GERMS.)

SPITTING OF BLOOD. (*See* BLOOD SPITTING, *also* HÆMO-PTYSIS.)

SPLEEN. The spleen is an organ of the body, about 5 in. long, situated behind the stomach in the upper left corner of the abdomen, which is connected with the rest of the body only by its nerves, lymphatics, and comparatively large blood-vessels.

SPLEEN, Diseases of. *Enlargement of the Spleen* is an important sign in a number of diseases, especially malaria and typhoid fever ; other diseases in which it may be enlarged are streptococcal septicæmia, syphilis, tuberculosis, rickets, pernicious anæmia, leukæmia, splenic anæmia, and the tropical disease kala-azar.

Rupture of the Spleen is a not uncommon result of an accident, especially when a vehicle has passed over the abdomen. The injured person has severe abdominal pain and shows signs (pallor, faintness) of internal hæmorrhage. A surgical operation is necessary to save life.

Splenic anæmia (Banti's disease) is a primary disease, but the cause is unknown ; it is probably due to an infection. It occurs chiefly in young men, and is characterised by anæmia, bleeding from the nose, stomach or bowel, and enlargement of the spleen ; it usually requires an expert physician to recognize the disease. If untreated, it is always fatal, but surgical removal of the spleen, if done early in the course of the disease, gives good results.

SPLINTS. Splints are used for keeping the ends of a fractured bone at rest and for maintaining the shape of a limb. In an emergency splints may be made out of walking-sticks, broom-handles, branches, thick newspaper, and in fact anything of suitable length and stiffness. (*See* FRACTURES.)

SPONDYLITIS DEFORMANS. This condition has in the past been classed with infective or atrophic arthritis (chronic rheumatism), but is now believed to be a separate disease, of a metabolic type (i.e. due to a chemical upset of the body). It begins in the back, affecting the vertebræ and the cartilaginous discs between them, and spreads to the large joints—hips, shoulders and jaw. It is treated by over-extending the spine, moving the chest, hips and shoulders and rotating the head, if possible, by underwater manipulation, as is done at Bath. (*See also* RHEUMATOID ARTHRITIS.)

SPOTTED FEVER. *See* CEREBRO-SPINAL FEVER.

SPRAINS AND STRAINS. A sprain is a wrenching of a joint producing a stretching or tearing of the ligaments. A strain is the wrenching of muscles or tendons. In a sprain, one or more of the ligaments of a joint are torn so that there is bleeding and weakness of the joint. The blood is usually seen under the skin in the form of a bruise. The membrane which forms the lining of the joint becomes inflamed and pours out a certain amount of fluid so that the joint swells and becomes stiff and painful to move. If possible, a firm bandage should be applied immediately so as to prevent the swelling becoming too large and also to prevent bleeding. It is the absorption of blood from the tissues which makes the cure of a sprain such a lengthy business. The parts surrounding the sprain should be gently massaged so as to keep the blood circulating at its best, and a suitable support such as adhesive strapping may be used to rest the part. The patient should be encouraged to exercise the joint gently as soon as he is able, otherwise adhesions may form. An X-ray examination is desirable in order to make sure that no damage has been done to any of the surrounding nerves.

SPRING CATARRH. A form of conjunctivitis or inflammation of the eye which occurs chiefly in children and is worst in the spring and summer months. No method of treatment is more than palliative, though radium and X-rays are now said to give promising results. Astringent lotions and smoked glasses may be helpful,

E.F.D. 17

and the patient is advised to keep as cool as possible, and to avoid any exposure to bright sun and wind.

SQUINT (Strabismus). Squint or strabismus is caused by a number of conditions : (1) By an error in development ; (2) By injury to one of the muscles which move the eye ; (3) By injury, disease, or over-stimulation of one of the nerves supplying these muscles, which causes paralysis and lengthening, or over-contraction and shortening, of the muscles ; (4) By the presence of some defect in the eye, such as long- or short-sight. This is called *concomitant*, since it is (almost) equal whether the eyes be looking to right or left. *Divergent* squint occurs when one or both eyes turns outwards ; *convergent* when one or both turns inwards. The former is sometimes found when there is constant excessive strain in short-sight, the latter in long-sight. The *treatment* of " muscular " squint is, first, that of the injury or disease which has caused the trouble. Prismatic lenses may have to be used to correct the double vision that sometimes occurs. If all treatment fails, and only then, operative measures are attempted. The treatment of concomitant squint, in both long- and short-sight, is to wear suitable spectacles, which in most cases relieves the condition. Exercises, prescribed by an ophthalmic specialist, are proving successful treatment nowadays.

STAPHYLOCOCCUS. This is the name given to a particular type of germ which is responsible for various pus-forming diseases in man. (*See also* GERM.)

STATUS LYMPHATICUS. A condition in which all the lymphatic tissues, the thymus, the spleen, and the bone marrow, etc., are markedly overgrown, is known as status lymphaticus or lymphatism. It occurs most commonly in young children, usually of the plump and flabby type. The condition may never be suspected by the parents as the child always appears to be in good health, but death may occur quite suddenly from a slight shock, and a large percentage of patients who die while under an anæsthetic suffer from status lymphaticus.

STETHOSCOPE. An instrument used for listening to the sounds produced anywhere within the body. (*See also* AUSCULTATION.)

STICKING-PLASTER. *See* ADHESIVE PLASTER.

STIFF NECK. The commonest cause of stiff neck is muscular rheumatism or fibrositis, usually the result of more or less prolonged exposure to cold, damp, or a draught. (*See also* FIBROSITIS ; RHEUMATISM.)

STILL-BIRTH. A child which measures over thirteen inches in length and which shows no sign of life after it has been born, is termed a still-born child. According to English law, every infant born alive must be notified to the medical officer of health within thirty-six hours of birth, and with regard to still-births, the registrar of births and deaths must be notified as well. (*See also* ABORTION ; CHILD-BIRTH ; LABOUR.)

STILL'S DISEASE. This is a rare form of arthritis, called after the London children's specialist who described it. It occurs in young children. (*See also* ARTHRITIS.)

STIMULANT. Any drug or other agent which is capable of increasing the activity of the body is described as a stimulant. Alcohol in small doses acts as a stimulant, but in larger quantities it depresses the brain centres. Ammonia administered as smelling-salts. Strong coffee or tea also act as stimulants. The application of heat will stimulate the action of the skin and cause increased sweating to take place. (*See also* ALCOHOL ; AMMONIA ; CAFFEINE.)

STING. *See* BITES AND STINGS.

STITCH. A sudden spasm of pain in the side usually due to cramp in the muscles is popularly referred to as stitch. The pain may go as suddenly as it comes, and rubbing may give some relief if the part still feels tender. (*See also* CRAMP.)

STOMACH. The stomach is a large, more or less pear-shaped dilatation of the digestive canal, about one foot in length and four or five inches in breadth, holding normally about two or three pints of fluid ; it communicates at its upper end with the gullet

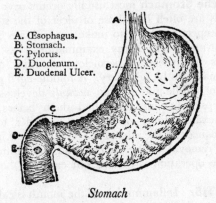

A. Œsophagus.
B. Stomach.
C. Pylorus.
D. Duodenum.
E. Duodenal Ulcer.

Stomach

(œsophagus) and at its lower end with the first part of the small intestine (duodenum) through a valve-like opening called the pylorus. It is situated in the upper part of the left side of the abdomen.

The walls of the stomach contract in rhythmic waves, which take about half a minute each to pass along the whole length of the stomach. The food is received by the stomach, masticated and mixed with saliva and mucus, and the business of the stomach is to continue the process of digestion that has been begun. The stomach wall has four layers, an outer layer of peritoneum, next a muscular layer, then a sub-mucous layer, and last an internal layer of mucous membrane, in the folds of which are innumerable microscopic glands, some of which secrete mucus and some the gastric (digestive) juice. This juice contains two ferments, (1) pepsin, which softens and dissolves the fibrous part of meat ; and (2) rennin, which digests and coagulates milk. It also contains hydrochloric acid, which keeps the digestive action of the pepsin and also helps to prevent putrefaction of the food in the stomach.

This is not absorbed in the stomach—alcohol is an exception in being absorbed straight from the stomach, even water is sent on to the intestine—but is mixed thoroughly there and converted into a milky semi-fluid substance called " chyme," and then squirted gradually through the small pyloric opening into the duodenum, where more important processes of digestion take place ; absorption into the body takes place in the small intestine.

STOMACH, DISEASES OF. With the exception of cancer of the stomach—which follows herewith—the diseases of the stomach are dealt with under separate headings. (*See also* DYSPEPSIA ; GASTRIC ULCER ; GASTRITIS.)

Cancer of the Stomach most usually occurs over the age of 40. The symptoms are often like those of ulcer of the stomach, and it will need an expert specialist to make an accurate diagnosis, with the aid of test-meals and X-ray examinations ; as the symptoms are sometimes like those of pernicious anæmia (q.v.), a blood examination may also be necessary. A middle-aged person (especially about the middle fifties) who *suddenly* develops symptoms of chronic dyspepsia, having never had them before, should have these expert examinations carried out in order to exclude the possibility of cancer of the stomach. The *treatment* is obviously an operation for removal of the cancer, and the ultimate outlook is bad unless the operation is carried out early in the course of the disease.

STOMATITIS. Inflammation of the mouth is called stomatitis. It is treated by alkaline mouth-washes, such as warm bicarbonate of soda solution or glycothymoline, and attention to the teeth or other cause.

STONE. *See* CALCULUS ; GALL-STONES.

STOOLS. Fæces is the term applied to discharges from the bowel, but the terms stools or motions are more commonly used. Normal fæces are brown in colour and the quantity discharged in one day by an adult should be approximately six ounces. This brown colour is due to substances in the bile, the chief of which is a pigment called *stercobilin*. Certain articles of food may change the colour of the fæces ; for example, if the diet consists largely of meat, the discharges from the bowel will be darker in colour, while milk and starchy foods tend to make them a light yellow colour. Too much fat in the diet may produce stools of an almost milky whiteness, or this may be the result of some disease of the pancreas in which fat is not being properly digested. Pale, clay-coloured stools usually indicate that the normal amount of bile is not entering into the intestines. This usually occurs in jaundice and the odour of the stools may be particularly offensive. The motions of children suffering from diarrhœa are, most commonly, bright green in colour. This is thought to be due to bacterial decomposition.

Bright red blood mixed with the fæces may come from a hæmorrhage round about the anus or rectum, such as from piles or some other affection of that region. When the stools are tarry-looking this is termed melæna, and this condition is caused by the presence of blood which has altered in appearance in its passage through the intestines. This condition indicates that there is a hæmorrhage high up in the bowel or in the stomach, usually from a gastric or duodenal ulcer. The colour of the stools may vary as a result of taking certain drugs. For example, drugs such as iron or bismuth may cause them to turn black ; while rhubarb and senna may give them a bright colour. Incontinence of the bowel, or inability to hold the stools, is a symptom of certain diseases of the nervous system, or it may be due to laxness of the muscles surrounding the anus. Pain at stool is a very characteristic symptom of a fissure or it may be due to inflamed piles. (*See also* CONSTIPATION ; DIARRHŒA.)

STOUTNESS. *See* article on OBESITY.

STRANGURY. This term is used to describe the condition in which there is a desire to pass urine, but the discharge is very slow and painful and only a few drops may come away.

Treatment of the condition naturally depends upon the cause, but hot baths and large quantities of bland fluids will help to relieve the immediate pain. (*See also* URINE.)

STREPTOCOCCUS. A special variety of germs which, when seen under the microscope, have the appearance of a string of beads. They are responsible for a very wide range of diseases, including tonsillitis, scarlet fever, and erysipelas. (*See also* GERMS.)

STRICTURE. The narrowing of any of the natural passages of the body, such as the urethra, the bowel or the gullet, is known as stricture. Most cases are caused by inflammation or as a result of scarring of the tissues, but it may be due to the growth of a tumour or to pressure caused by such a growth in a neighbouring organ.

STROKE. A stroke is a sudden and severe attack of apoplexy or of paralysis, or it may be used to describe sunstroke. (*See also* APOPLEXY ; PARALYSIS ; SUNSTROKE.)

STRYCHNINE. Strychnine is an alkaloid drug which is prepared from the seeds of an Eastern plant known as nux vomica. Tincture of nux vomica is often given as a tonic in convalescence or in indigestion.

Strychnine is capable of increasing the tone of the muscles, and because of its stimulating effect it is included in many nerve tonics ; as a hypodermic injection it is a powerful heart stimulant.

Poisoning by strychnine. Large doses are very poisonous indeed and may have fatal consequences. It causes the muscles all over the body to contract violently with the result that the patient is unable to breathe. The convulsion lasts a minute or two, then the muscles relax, and the patient feels exhausted and sweats all over. The convulsions soon come on again and increase in severity. The slightest noise or even a bright light will bring on the convulsions, and unless treatment is given the patient may die from exhaustion and asphyxia. The symptoms of strychnine poisoning are similar to tetanus.

Treatment. The patient should at once be put under chloroform or ether. The stomach should be washed out with a solution of permanganate of potash and large doses of chloral hydrate or bromide should be injected into the rectum. Apply artificial respiration if necessary. Rectal injections of a new drug, known as avertin, are also recommended. (*See* POISONS.)

STYE (Hordeolum). This consists in the formation of a boil in the " socket " of an eyelash. It may occur on either the upper or the lower lid ; and styes often appear in crops, now on one lid, now on the other. It is often very painful, and the conjunctiva covering the eyeball may swell, causing much distress and alarm to the patient. A single stye may be caused by local infection ; repeated styes, however, always indicate a poor condition of general health, or point to the need of glasses. Local treatment consists in removal of the eyelash, either by forceps or an incision, squeezing out the pus, and applying a warm boric acid fomentation (this is cleaner and easier to apply than a poultice). To prevent recurrence, the eyes should be bathed with warm boric lotion several times daily, and the lids then massaged with " golden ointment." If styes persist in spite of local treatment, tonics, or glasses, chloride or sulphide of calcium internally helps to check their occurrence.

STYPTICS. Styptics are substances which check bleeding either by making the blood-vessels contract or by causing the blood to clot. Cold water or ice is often valuable for this purpose, or sometimes very hot water applied directly on the bleeding surface will cause it to stop. Drugs which are capable of arresting bleeding include adrenaline, ergot, hydrogen peroxide, perchloride of iron, nitrate of silver, tannic acid, and alum. (*See also* HÆMORRHAGE.)

SUFFOCATION. The sensation of choking is also described as suffocation or asphyxia. (*See also* ASPHYXIA.)

SULPHANILAMIDE. A chemical compound used under various trade names (e.g., prontosil, proseptasine, rubiazol, etc.) for the treatment especially of streptococcal infections, such as cellulitis, erysipelas, tonsillitis, ear inflammation, puerperal fever, septicæmia, in which it has proved very successful.

SULPHAPYRIDINE. Known also by the trade name of M. & B. 693, a chemical compound used successfully in the treatment of gonorrhœa, meningitis, pneumonia, and other serious infections.

SULPHONAMIDE. The name given to a group of chemical drugs which includes sulphanilamide (prontosil, etc.) and sulphapyridine (M. & B. 693, etc.).

SULPHUR. Sulphur, a yellow non-metallic element, is used in medicine in two forms, the sublimated sulphur, or flowers of sulphur, and precipitated sulphur, also known as milk of sulphur. Sulphur ointment rubbed into the skin is one of the best treatments for the itch, or scabies. Mild sulphur preparations, especially a lotion made of the milk of sulphur, may be used for acne. Sulphur is a very good laxative, especially for children, and it is very commonly mixed with liquorice powder.

SUMMER DIARRHŒA. This form of diarrhœa is common in young children, usually from contaminated milk, and may be a serious condition. (*See also* DIARRHŒA.)

SUNSTROKE. Sunstroke, or heatstroke, are the terms applied to the conditions produced by exposure to the strong rays of the sun or to overheated air. The symptoms may vary in severity from a headache to severe collapse, high fever and delirium. Mild cases may occur in this country, especially at the beginning of a holiday unless due precautions are taken to cover the head, neck and spine.

Treatment. The patient should be kept in a darkened room and given plenty of cool drinks. Sponging the body with cold or tepid water at frequent intervals is very soothing and beneficial. In severe cases strong stimulants for the heart may be necessary.

SUPPOSITORY. Suppositories are usually made of cacao butter or oil of theobroma, and they are a convenient method of introducing drugs into the rectum, urethra, or vagina.

SUPPURATION. This term is used to indicate the formation of pus or matter. (*See also* ABSCESS; INFLAMMATION; PUS.)

SUSPENSORY BANDAGE. A support for the scrotum or testicle is known as a suspensory belt. It consists of a waist-band from which a bag is suspended. This form of support is necessary in diseases of the scrotum or testicle. (*See also* ABDOMINAL BELT.)

SWEATING, DISAGREEABLE. *Bromidrosis* is the term given to a condition in which the sweat becomes evil-smelling, and may be general or local. It occurs in some diseases in their acute stage, and may then, to the trained nose, be an almost certain guide to the diagnosis, each of the diseases having their characteristic odour. They are, chiefly, rheumatic fever, diphtheria, small-pox, cholera, typhoid, syphilis, tuberculosis, uræmia, anæmia and scurvy. In some people not only the breath, but the perspiration, becomes odorous after taking such substances as onions, garlic, sulphur, musk, and various others. Bromidrosis under the arms and on the soles of the feet is due to the decomposition of the sweat and of the softened upper layer of the skin by various bacterial organisms, and is equally irksome for the sufferer and for those near him.

Treatment. For the armpits frequent bathing with very hot water may suffice ; together with the use of a dusting powder composed of boric acid, orris root and talc in equal parts (starch powders should *not* be used, as the starch forms a happy breeding-ground for the organisms). The use of dress-shields may aggravate the condition by damming back the sweat, and so helping on both the disagreeable decomposition and the softening of the skin ; a form of eczema may follow. For the feet there are many varieties of treatment, but all physicians are agreed that great attention to cleanliness is the chief thing, not only as regards the feet themselves, but also the stockings and shoes. The feet must be washed morning and evening, and, if necessary, during the day, after which an astringent lotion such as Eau-de-Cologne, or boric acid, $\frac{1}{2}$ oz. to 1 pint water, should be used, followed by the powder mentioned above. Salicylic acid, grs. 20–48, to talc 1 oz., may be used as a powder ; this helps to absorb the perspiration. A fresh pair of *boiled* stockings should be worn daily, or, if there is much perspiration, as often as the feet are washed. The shoes should be easy-fitting ; if possible, new ones should be bought, and changed as often as the stockings, each pair being well aired when not in use.

SYNCOPE. This is another name for fainting. (*See also* FAINTING.)

SYPHILIS is a serious chronic disease which may be either " acquired " or " inherited." It is due to the entrance into the body of a special kind of germ, shaped like a corkscrew and having from ten to twenty-five spirals in its length. This germ was only discovered in the early part of this century, although the disease which it causes has been known since the Middle Ages. The germ is conveyed from one person to another most commonly through sexual intercourse, although it may (but exceptionally) enter the body if a person comes into accidental contact with such articles as towels or cups which have been used by someone suffering from the active disease, who has deposited material containing the germs upon them. In congenital syphilis the children are infected before birth by the mother, and therefore syphilis is not—strictly speaking —an *inherited* disease, as it is acquired by the unborn child whilst in the mother's womb.

Symptoms. It is usual to describe the results of syphilitic infection in three stages. In the first stage, after infection has taken place about a month, a small hard, painless sore appears at the place where the germ gained entry to the body. The bottom of the sore is very hard and the surrounding parts feel hard also. A slight colourless discharge accompanies the sore, in which the germ can be found. The glands in the neighbourhood of this sore enlarge, though this enlargement may not be noticed by the patient as it is completely painless. If no treatment is carried out during the period when the sore is present, it gradually decreases in size, until at about the end of two months only a small scar remains. But during this time the germs have got into the blood and have been carried to all parts of the body. As soon as they are able to become active in the various organs of the body, the secondary stage of the disease may be said to have been reached. This usually happens in between two to three months from the time of infection.

In the secondary stage, symptoms of a general nature appear. There is nearly always severe headache, usually worse at night; slight fever; pains in joints and bones or there may be severe anæmia. But the chief and most obvious feature of the secondary stage of syphilis is a rash. This rash may imitate nearly every known skin disease, and without certain tests it may be very difficult to tell if the rash is due to syphilis or not. During the secondary stage of the disease the germs get into the nervous system and, although at this time there may be no symptoms of any disease of the nervous system, examination of the fluid which surrounds the spinal cord, the cerebro-spinal fluid (q.v.) will show whether or not the particular person in the secondary stage is likely to suffer later from either of the two severe diseases of the nervous system caused by syphilis, namely, general paralysis of the insane (q.v.) or locomotor ataxia (q.v.). In this stage too, the germs invade the heart and walls of the blood-vessels, so that later on diseases of these important organs may occur, due to the effect of the activity of these germs. It is hardly necessary to stress, in view of what has been said of the

17*

later results of syphilis (which are responsible for a greater number of deaths and lives of chronic invalidism than the mildness of the disease in its early stages would suggest), that no one should allow the secondary, or if possible the first, stage of the disease to go untreated. But if left untreated, the secondary stage appears to clear up, and there is a period of freedom from symptoms which may last from two to twenty years ; but, sooner or later, other symptoms arise and these form what is termed the tertiary or third stage of the disorder. During this period of freedom from symptoms the resistance of the body prevents further activity on the part of the germs which are, however, lying hidden away in all the organs of the body. Many of these germs die out in the course of years, but some remain alive, and at any time they may re-awaken to activity.

There is no organ which may not be attacked in the third, or tertiary, stage of syphilis. Generally speaking, the disease in this stage takes the form of the production of tumour-like masses which become soft in the middle and then become ulcers. These tumour-like masses are called gummas, and they vary in size from a pin-head to an orange. The ulcers which replace them are slow to heal unless properly treated. The skin, the bones and joints, the liver, the palate, the tongue, the mouth, are all common places where this ulceration occurs. The ulceration of the tongue is particularly dangerous as it is apt to be followed by cancer of the tongue. The end of the third stage of syphilis is often accompanied by disease of the large blood-vessel, the aorta (q.v.), whilst later still the germs which have been allowed to remain undestroyed in the brain and spinal cord, where they settled down during the secondary stage, become active and give rise to obvious symptoms of disease of the nervous system.

Treatment of Syphilis in Adults. The importance of early treatment of the disease has already been stressed. But before treatment can be started, accurate recognition of the condition in its earliest stage is essential, and it should be the duty of everyone who notices a sore after exposure to infection to be examined by a doctor. If treatment is commenced early in the disease, by means of salvarsan (q.v.) or similar preparations of arsenic, before the germs have had time to get into the blood and spread themselves throughout the body, there is every reason to suppose that the disease may be really cured. But once the secondary stage has been reached and germs have managed to get hidden away in the various organs, there is always a danger that however energetic treatment may be, many germs may not be reached, and later on they may resume their activity. Fortunately there is a certain test, the Wassermann reaction, which can be carried out, which not only shows the doctor whether or not syphilis is present in a particular patient, but also tells him how the treatment is affecting the course of the disease. If no treatment has been given until the third stage of the disease has been reached, then salvarsan is of little value, and the older remedies of mercury and potassium iodide are the ones employed. The question of marriage is often a problem to the patient who has suffered from syphilis. It can be stated that during the first and secondary stages the disease is highly infectious, and an individual who married, even whilst undergoing treatment, in either of these stages would be committing a crime against the human race. In the tertiary stage the chances of infection are less, but they are still probable. It is impossible to lay down any fixed period after infection when it would be absolutely safe for an individual who has suffered from untreated syphilis to marry. With regard to patients who have been energetically treated, the doctor who has treated them is the one who is best able to judge when the disease has been stamped out ; the earlier treatment is begun, the more likely is the chance of complete cure.

Congenital Syphilis. The children born of parents suffering from syphilis are liable to show the symptoms of the later stages of the disease. In the children the disease is always generalized, and any part of the body may suffer. The bones, the skin, the joints, and the liver are commonly affected. The eyes may be attacked if the children survive the infant period, whilst a particularly complete form of deafness may occur in the early teens. The nervous system also may share in the general involvement of the body, and general paralysis of the insane is not uncommon in the victims of congenital syphilis, coming on from about the eleventh or twelfth year onwards.

Treatment of Congenital Syphilis. The treatment of congenital syphilis really begins with the treatment of the mother whilst she is pregnant. If such treatment is vigorously carried out, there is every chance that a healthy child will be born. Once the child is born, the treatment follows the same lines as those of adults. Salvarsan or other arsenic compounds are well tolerated by children, and rubbing with mercury is also valuable ; but the disease is so generalized in the victims of congenital syphilis that it is rare for a real cure to occur.

SYRINGE. Syringes are used for injecting fluids into the body or into its passages and cavities. A very useful form of syringe is that known as Higginson's syringe, and it is chiefly used for giving enemas or for using as a vaginal douche, though it is also useful for douching the nose or the ear. Hypodermic syringes are made in many sizes, and they are used for injecting drugs directly into the body under the skin or into a vein.

TABES. Means *tabes dorsalis* or *locomotor ataxia*, a nervous disorder caused by an old syphilitic infection of the spinal cord and brain. (*See also* LOCOMOTOR ATAXIA ; SYPHILIS.)

TACHYCARDIA. Rapid action of the heart-beat in the absence of any obvious cause is described as tachycardia. (*See also* HEART ; PULSE.)

TANNIN. Tannic acid, or tannin, is obtained from oak-galls and it is also present in several varieties of plants. When brought in touch with any tissue or mucous membrane, tannic acid draws it together and dries it up, and because of this action tannin is used in the treatment of ulcers, sores, and various moist eruptions. A solution of tannic acid sprayed over a burn will act as a protective covering. (*See also* GALL.)

TAPEWORM. *See* WORMS.

TARTAR. The deposit which collects round the necks and adjoining parts of the teeth is described as dental tartar. It is hard, firmly adherent, light brown in colour, and is derived from stagnating saliva or mucus on parts of the teeth not generally subject to friction. As it presses on the gum, it sets up inflammation, favouring the growth of germs and helping to produce pyorrhœa. Tartar should be regularly removed by scaling of the teeth.

TARTARIC ACID. Either in the form of free acid or of acid tartrate of potassium, tartaric acid is widely distributed in the vegetable kingdom, the most abundant source being the grape.

TEETH. A tooth is made up of a crown, a neck and one or more roots or fangs. The greater part of the tooth is composed of dentine, or ivory, and over the crown there is a hard, brittle, white shell called enamel. The dentine surrounds a cavity containing the pulp. This consists of fine blood-vessels, nerves and connective tissue. On the top of the crown are two or more elevations or cups which aid the chewing of the food. The teeth are fixed in sockets in the upper and lower jaw-bones, and between the root of the tooth and the wall of the socket is a substance called the cement or crusta petrosa. The gum covers the borders of the jaw-bones, embraces the teeth at their necks and occupies the space between the teeth.

In a grown-up person there are thirty-two teeth, eight on each side above and below. These are called the second or permanent teeth. The upper row consists of four incisors in the centre, sharp and chisel-shaped ; on each side of the incisors is one pointed canine ; next to the canines are two premolars ; then there are three molars on each side. The bottom row is placed in the same way, each upper tooth having a similar one opposite to it. The incisors and canines are for cutting purposes, the pre-molars and molars, with their broad ridged tops, are for grinding the food. The so-called wisdom teeth are the last molars and they do not erupt till about the twenty-first year. Occasionally, they do not appear at all.

The first or milk teeth are cut gradually, the first to appear being the lower central incisors about the sixth month. Then follow the upper central and lateral incisors, and, in this order, the first molars in the twelfth month, the canines in the eighteenth, and the second molars in the twenty-fourth month. There is some degree of variation of the times of eruption even in normal children, but

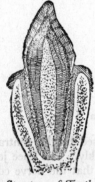

Structure of Tooth.

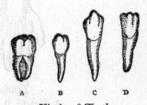

Kinds of Teeth

A. Molar. C. Canine.
B. Pre-molar. D. Incisor.

in rickety children, dentition is very much delayed. The second dentition begins to appear about the sixth year with the appearance of the first permanent molars and each year after this the other permanent teeth are cut ; the central incisors, the laternal incisors, the first pre-molar, the second pre-molar, the canines, and the second molars.

TEMPORAL BONE. This bone takes part in the formation of the temple, but is more important as having the internal ear placed deeply in it, protected by the mastoid air cells.

TENDON. The white fibrous structure which connects a muscle to the bone is termed a tendon. Its fibres are tough and strong and do not give much. Tendons vary in their shape ; they may be rounded like cords—long and slender as in the limbs, while others may be flat and sheet-like as in the case of the abdominal (belly) muscle. Where it passes over a bone, a tendon usually runs in a fibrous sheath lined with a smooth moist membrane.

Small bones may develop in the tendon (sesamoid bones), the knee-cap being an example of this.

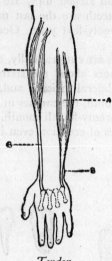

Tendon
A. Muscle; B. Tendon

TENDON JERK is the response caused by the contraction of a muscle when the tendon is tapped briskly. The knee jerk is an example of this and its presence denotes that the nerve continuity to and from the spinal cord is intact.

TENESMUS. Painful, spasmodic, frequent straining to empty the bowel, usually ineffectual, is termed tenesmus. Sometimes a little blood or mucus is passed. It may arise when the bowel is loaded with hard masses of fæces, or it may be provoked by a fissure of the anus or a growth in the rectum. Tenesmus is quite frequently caused by diarrhœa, particularly the diarrhœa associated with dysentery. In young children it may be produced by worms in the bowel or it may be caused by intussusception. In this latter condition the infant has fits of screaming and blood and slime are passed. A similar condition may arise in the bladder, known also as stranguary or dysuria, due to a very acid urine, gravel or inflammation.

TERTIAN FEVER. A variety of the tropical fever called Malaria. (*See also* MALARIA.)

TESTICLE. The testicle is the male sex gland and corresponds to the ovary in the female. There are two, a right and a left, each occupying a compartment in the scrotum, a purse-like bag. The testicles develop originally in the cavity of the abdomen (belly), and just before or after birth reach the scrotum. The testicle has a complicated journey to make before it finally arrives at the scrotum and it carries with it a tube-like process of the lining of the abdomen (the peritoneum) which becomes closed at its upper end and which covers the testicles in front and at the sides. This lining is called the *tunica vaginalis* and, being smooth, it diminishes any friction that might arise from the movements of the testicles. Sometimes fluid collects in the bag, a condition called *hydrocele*.

The testicle produces sperm cells or spermatozoa. These are the male seeds which, when they fertilize the female eggs, produce a new individual. The sperms are contained in small tubes and make their way along a number of small ducts to reach the main duct of the testicle, called the vas deferens. This leads to the seminal vesicle (reservoir), from which the sperms are discharged during sexual intercourse. In addition to this function, however, the testicle has yet another equally important function. Certain cells (interstitial cells) in the gland produce a secretion which is passed directly into the blood-stream, called an " internal secretion," and it is this secretion which is responsible for the development of the mature sex characters. Absence of the secretion, which may arise after castration (removal of testicles), causes the individual to remain boyish in figure ; the skin is smooth and hairless, penis small, voice high-pitched, and there is a tendency to fatness. Such a person is described as a eunuch. (*See also* EPIDIDYMIS ; HYDROCELE ; SCROTUM ; SPERMATIC CORD ; VARICOCELE.)

TETANUS. Tetanus, which is more commonly known as lockjaw, is due to a germ which enters the body and sets up a condition of contraction in the muscles, usually commencing in the jaw and neck, but gradually affecting the rest of the body. The germ is found in soil, and as it is extremely resistant to the effects of heat and cold it may go on living for years. It is even resistant to the effects of ordinary antiseptics, so it is easy to understand that such powers of resistance make the wiping out of tetanus a difficult problem. The germ lives in the intestines of horses and cattle, and any manured soil is liable to become infected. For the development of tetanus it is necessary that there should be some opening in the skin through which the germ can gain entrance to the body and the wound must come in touch with the germ through soil.

Symptoms. Symptoms usually begin to appear seven or eight days after infection of the wound, but the longer the symptoms take to appear, the better the chances are of recovery. The first signs of the disease are stiffness of the throat muscles, with difficulty **in**

swallowing. The patient has difficulty in opening the mouth, and gradually the neighbouring muscles begin to contract, giving the face a peculiar expression. The spasm extends to the muscles of the back, chest, abdomen and limbs, and the patient has frequently recurring seizures which are terrible to watch. The skin is moist or sweating, but the patient never loses consciousness and is unhappily aware of his serious condition. In *local tetanus*, the contractions are limited to the muscles surrounding the wound but such cases never become severe. *Tetanus neonatorum* may occur in newborn infants, the symptoms showing themselves within a week or so of birth. Infection usually takes place through the severed umbilical cord and convulsions may be the first sign of the disease.

Treatment. The early administration of anti-tetanic serum should be carried out in any case of a wound which may have been contaminated by soil. Once the symptoms of tetanus appear much larger doses are given, and they should be injected into the spinal canal or into the skull cavity. Various drugs are given to relieve the spasms and to allow the patient to take nourishment. Only liquid food is given and a feeding-tube may be used if necessary. The patient must be kept absolutely quiet in a darkened room as the slightest disturbance is liable to cause a spasm. When the spasms are very severe, relief may be given with inhalations of chloroform. (*See also* SERUM.)

TETANY. This is an affection in which there arise spasms of certain muscles. It is due to over-excitability of the nervous system. The muscles most often affected are those of the arms and hands. The elbows and wrist are bent, and the fingers squeezed together. Sometimes the lower limbs are similarly affected, and occasionally the face. In children, rickets is the chief cause, especially if it is associated with some derangement of digestion. In adults the condition arises also in connection with dilatation or sagging of the stomach and it follows removal of the parathyroid glands, tiny structures situated in the thyroid gland in the neck. The actual disorder is believed to be due to some disturbance of the calcium (lime) salts in the blood. The spasms may occur spontaneously or may be brought about by slight irritation of the nerves from pressure or any other cause.

Treatment of tetany in the child calls for the remedying of the co-existing rickets. Sunshine, ultra-violet rays, cod-liver oil and nourishing food generally are indicated. Large doses of calcium chloride also help. Occasionally, it may be necessary to prescribe small doses of a nerve sedative such as chloral hydrate. In adults, attention to the digestive system by dieting and relief of constipation are essential to cure the condition. Extract of parathyroid gland with calcium is also given for this affection. (*See also* RICKETS.)

THERAPEUTICS. This word signifies the branch of medicine which deals with the treatment and cure of the sick in all aspects.

.THERMOMETER. This is an instrument for recording and measuring temperature.

In Great Britain we use the Fahrenheit scale, the freezing point being fixed at 32° and boiling point at 212°. On the Continent the Centigrade and Réaumur scales are used ; in the first the freezing point is 0, or zero, and the boiling point 100° ; in the second the freezing point is also 0, but the boiling point is fixed at 80°.

To convert the Fahrenheit scale to Centigrade, subtract 32, divide by 9 and multiply by 5 ; to convert Centigrade to Fahrenheit, divide by 5, multiply by 9 and add 32.

Normal body temperature, 98·4° F, is generally marked with an arrow on the clinical thermometer.

THIGH. That part of the lower limb from the hip to the knee is described as the thigh. The large bone of this region is called the femur and it is clothed with large and powerful muscles. In front are the quadriceps which straighten the leg at the knee, behind are the hamstrings which bend the knee, and on the inner side are the adductor muscles passing from the haunch bone to the femur and serving to adduct or bring the thigh towards its fellow. All the muscles are enclosed in a strong fibrous sheath from which partitions arise and pass between the different muscles. In men, the outlines of the various muscles are visible to the eye ; but in women the greater amount of fat under the skin obscures them. There are two other very important structures in the thigh, the femoral artery and the sciatic nerve. The main artery enters about the middle of the groin, where it can be compressed against the bone in an emergency, and runs down to the inner side of the knee where it passes behind into the space behind the knee. The sciatic nerve, the largest in the body, runs down the middle of the back of the thigh and in the lower part divides into two branches. Painful conditions of this nerve are called sciatica ; frequently this affection is of rheumatic origin, but it may, though less frequently, arise from some pressure within the pelvis.

THORACIC DUCT. This is the main lymphatic channel of the body. It is a tube about 18 in. long, commencing in the upper part of the abdominal cavity and passing upwards through the diaphragm, thence through the thorax or chest cavity to reach the root of the neck where it joins the junction of the two large veins, the left internal jugular and the left subclavian veins.

THORAX. The bony cage forming the skeleton of the upper

part of the trunk is called, in anatomy, the thorax. It is bounded in front by the sternum or breast-bone, behind by the vertebral column and at the sides by the ribs. Separating it from the abdomen is the diaphragm muscle. (*See also* CHEST ; LUNG ; PLEURA.)

THREAD-WORM. *See* WORM.

THROAT. This region is limited in medicine to the upper part of the digestive canal, from the tonsils to the beginning of the œsophagus or gullet. It is described as the pharynx, and is dealt with under that heading ; the larynx, or voice-box, is under its own heading.

THROBBING. *See* PALPITATION.

THROMBOSIS. This term refers to the clotting of blood within the heart or blood-vessels during life and the clot is itself described as a thrombus. Healthy blood does not clot in healthy vessels, but if the circulation is slow or if there is any roughening in the vessel walls, or if there are certain blood changes, clots readily form and tend to grow and extend to where the blocked vessel joins a larger one.

Symptoms. These depend upon the stopping of the blood supply. In some cases, thrombosis is beneficial, as in aneurysm where there is a dilatation of an artery and the walls are consequently weakened. In this condition the clot tends to strengthen the arterial wall and prevent its rupture. In general, however, the effects of thrombosis are harmful. If it occurs in the leg, pain, swelling and disablement arise. Vein thrombosis in the leg sometimes occurs after child-birth or during typhoid fever. In the brain, thrombosis leads to some degree of paralysis which tends to become more extensive, while in the heart thrombosis may cause sudden death.

Sometimes a clot may soften and there is a danger that a small piece may be washed off and carried to a distant organ to block a blood-vessel. This is called embolism. Should there be any infection in the clot, the septic fragments may give rise to abscesses in various parts of the body, a grave state of affairs. In other cases, the clot may be converted into scar or fibrous tissue, obliterating completely the aperture of the blood-vessel. It is in this way that a varicose vein may be cured naturally.

Treatment naturally depends upon the cause. The immediate remedy is rest for the affected part. In the case of a limb, it should be well-padded with cotton-wool and the patient is not permitted to move the limb. Over a tender and swollen vein an ice-bag may give relief from the pain. (*See also* EMBOLISM ; PYÆMIA ; WHITE LEG.)

THRUSH. This is an inflammatory disease of the mouth and throat occurring chiefly in delicate and poorly nourished children.

It is due to an infection with a fungus, called *oidium albicans*, and it shows itself as greyish-white patches scattered over the mouth. Tenderness of the mouth, digestive disturbance, diarrhœa with green stools, and general irritability are the chief symptoms. Occasionally, the disease may spread to the stomach and intestines and it may infect the vagina. Cleanliness and the use of an antiseptic lotion, weak peroxide of hydrogen, along with a purge of castor oil, are the main methods of treatment.

THUMB. The thumb is the most movable of all the digits. There are only two segments as compared with three in the case of the fingers, but the metacarpal bone moves very freely on the wrist bones, while those of the fingers are much more restricted. Certain muscles in the forearm move the thumb, but there is also a small group of muscles forming the ball of the thumb, called the thenar muscles, which widens the range of muscular activities of the thumb. (*See also* FINGER ; HAND.)

THYMUS GLAND. This is a pear-shaped gland with the point upwards, consisting of a right and left lobe, situated in the chest immediately beneath the breast-bone. It extends upwards into the neck and its base lies upon the heart.

As with other lymphoid tissues, the thymus manufactures white blood cells ; but its other functions are a matter of doubt. There appears definitely to be some connection between the thymus and the sex glands. Removal of the sex glands causes persistence of the thymus and when the thymus is unduly enlarged (Status lymphaticus) the sex development is delayed. It would appear as if the secretion of the thymus gland restricts and controls the activities of the sex glands and prevents their precocious development. (*See also* STATUS LYMPHATICUS.)

THYROID EXTRACT. This extract is obtained from the fresh thyroid glands of sheep which are dried and reduced to a powder. The extract is standardized to contain a definite percentage of iodine and it is usually employed in tablet form. It is also available in the form of a liquor. Thyroid extract is used extensively in medical practice, particularly in the treatment of thyroid deficiency in children (cretinism) and in the same condition in adults (myxœdema). Occasionally it is taken in the treatment of obesity, but in all cases it must be used with care and under a doctor's control.

THYROID GLAND. The thyroid gland belongs to the endocrine system or " ductless " glands of internal secretion. (*See also* CRETINISM ; DUCTLESS GLANDS ; ENDOCRINE GLAND ; GOITRE ; MYXŒDEMA.)

TIBIA. This is the shin-bone and it is the larger of the two bones of the lower leg. The bone is triangular in section, ending above in two expansions which joint with the thigh-bone and below by forming the inner prominence of the ankle. The greater part of the tibia is immediately under the skin and can be felt by the finger. (*See also* FIBULA ; LEG.)

TIC is a movement which is repeated time after time without any definite cause or object, and which is due to a neurosis (q.v.). The beginning of a tic (or habit spasm, as it is often called) can often be traced to the continued performance of a movement which at one time was made with a definite and proper purpose.

The treatment of tics is difficult, especially in adults. In children, wholesome neglect of the habit, attention to the general health and mental development is sufficient to cure many cases. In adults, the habit of a tic is usually part of an obsession (q.v.) and is suitable for treatment by psychotherapy.

Tic douloureux is a spasm of the muscles of the face which must not be confused with ordinary tics, as it is due to a neuralgia of the trigeminal nerve. (*See also* NEURALGIA and TRIGEMINAL NERVE.)

TINEA. This is the common name applied to a group of vegetable parasites or fungi which cause a number of skin diseases. The fungi produce spores, and while some varieties of tinea produce disease exclusively in man, others affect both animals and man. The tinea microsporon is the cause of scalp ringworm in children. Cats and dogs are susceptible to a variety of this tinea and this infection can be communicated to human beings.

TINNITUS, or noises in the ears, is one of those complaints which is not serious in itself, but is annoying and difficult to get rid of. It usually, but not always, accompanies deafness, and in a young woman with commencing deafness is usually looked upon as one of the symptoms of otosclerosis. Tinnitus is usually treated by giving the patient a mild sedative (such as dilute hydrobromic acid) and inflating the ears ; but treatment often has to be a prolonged affair. (*See also* DEAFNESS ; OTOSCLEROSIS.)

TISSUE is a collection of the microscopic cells or elements of the body to form a distinct structure, from which the various parts and organs are built up. Some structures, such as cartilage, are formed of one tissue only with but the slightest admixture of another ; other structures are simple in form, such as the blood-vessels, which are formed of fibrous tissue, elastic fibres and muscular fibres, with an inner layer of endothelial cells ; while other structures are much more complex, such as the liver.

TOBACCO. Immoderate use of tobacco in any form is detrimental to health. Irritation of the throat, loss of appetite, sickness and diarrhœa may arise. The heart becomes irritable, palpitations are experienced, and breathlessness on the slightest exertion is produced. Heart pain may be produced from excessive smoking. Very serious is the effect of tobacco upon the sight. It commences with a dimness of vision and inability to read fine printing. The colour sense is often affected and unless the tobacco consumption is immediately cut down the condition may go on to blindness (Tobacco amblyopia). Both eyes are affected equally in this disease.

Cigarette smoking is the least harmful especially if the cigarette has a filter tip or is smoked through a holder containing a removable wad of cotton-wool. Cigar smoking and pipe smoking are more liable to produce symptoms of tobacco poisoning. Should any symptom appear, it is essential that the use of tobacco should be given up until such time as complete health is restored.

TOE. Each toe consists of three segments, or phalanges, except the great toe, which has only two. In new-born babies the great toe shows much resemblance to a thumb in its grasping power and free movement.

Diseases and deformities of the toes are exceedingly common, mainly as a result of wearing ill-fitting footwear. In consequence, the big toe is bent inwards towards the second toe and may actually be over or under it. This condition is called *hallux valgus*, and to relieve the pressure on the projecting part of the great toe a bursa or serous bag forms. This is very liable to become inflamed and is known as a bunion. Radical treatment for this condition requires the removal of part of the bone by surgical operation. Stiffness of the great toe causing immobility at the chief joint is usually associated with flatfoot. Correction of the flatfoot and the use of proper footwear is necessary in treatment, but an operation may be required in severe cases.

Hammer toe may affect any of the toes, but is most often seen in the second. In this condition there is over-extension at one joint, with marked flexion at another, with the result that the first two segments of the toe become V-shaped with the point upwards. Operation is required to relieve the deformity. Deficient blood-supply due to over-tight footwear favours the development of chilblains in the young and gangrene in the old. The poor nutrition from this cause also leads to rheumatoid changes in the joints. (*See also* CORNS ; FOOT ; HALLUX VALGUS ; HAMMER TOE.)

TONGUE. The tongue is the mobile muscular organ accompanying the floor of the mouth. Its muscle fibres go in various directions and are interlaced. Covering the surface of the tongue is a moist mucous membrane. At the back of this organ there is a V-shaped series of red spots which are called the circumvallate papillæ. In front of the V there are numerous little elevations termed the filiform papillæ, and dotted here and there are larger and redder elevations called the fungiform papillæ.

The tongue is symmetrical and has a median groove stretching from the tip to the back portion and representing the position of the librous partition which divides the tongue into lateral halves. The back part of the tongue is bound down to the floor of the mouth by structures which together constitute the root of the organ. In front the tongue is free, and its under-surface has a smooth covering which is prolonged forwards to form a fold attaching the tongue to the floor of the mouth. This fold is called the frenum and, on either side of it, open the ducts of the submaxillary salivary glands. Occasionally the frenum is too short and hampers the movements of the tongue in speaking. This condition is called tongue-tied and is easily remedied by the doctor snipping the fold with a pair of scissors.

The tongue is richly supplied with blood, large branches of the external carotid artery, called the lingual, passing into the organ on both sides. All the muscles have a special nerve supply, the hypoglossal cranial nerve. The mucous membrane is supplied by fibres from the fifth and ninth cranial nerves and some fibres from the seventh cranial nerve.

The tongue has four chief functions, concerned respectively with taste, mastication, swallowing of food and with speech. In chewing, the tongue assists by moving the food to and fro in the mouth and against the hard palate. In swallowing, the tongue pushes the food mass into the pharynx and at the same time pulls up the opening of the larynx (air passage) and so allows the food to pass directly into the gullet.

Tongue in Health and Disease. Normally, the tongue should be of a pink colour and slightly moist all over. Variations in the appearance of the surface of the tongue give valuable infor-mation as to the state of the health. If the tongue is furred it is generally an indication that the digestive system is out of order either from constipation, dyspepsia, fever or some constitutional disease. The fur consists of moulds and other germs mixed with food remains and cast-off surface cells. In certain diseases there are certain constitutional changes in the tongue. In scarlet fever a strawberry tongue is observed, from resemblance of the tongue to the fruit. In diabetes the tongue is red and beefy in appearance ; in kidney disease, it is dry and cracked ; in certain diseases of the nervous system, notably general paralysis, it is very tremulous.

Diseases of the Tongue. Sometimes the tongue is affected with ulcers. These may arise from the pressure of a jagged tooth or may simply be an evidence of poor general health. Inflammation of the tongue is called glossitis. This may be caused by excessive smoking, or the drinking of too hot and pungent liquids, or from some germ infection. There is a certain amount of swelling and pain and occasionally the inflammation may go on to an abscess formation. In inflammation of the tongue, there is sometimes a danger of extreme swelling of the organ leading to complete suffocation. If such a condition should arise prompt incision of the tongue is necessary. Treatment of the glossitis requires the removal of the irritant, if any, and the use of bland antiseptic mouth washes such as borax and glycerine.

White flaky patches may form on the surface of the tongue, a condition called leukoplakia. This disease is generally associated with syphilis and excessive smoking and drinking. The white flakes may peel off and leave a cracked and fissured surface which may become cancerous. In some cases, cancer commences as a wart on the tongue which is quite painless. Later, the wart breaks down, ulcerates and the glands under the chin become involved causing pain and swelling. Operation for removal of part of the tongue and of the glands, along with radium treatment, are the only methods of cure and if these are to be successful they must be carried out in the early stages. *Therefore, it must be emphasized that any little ulcer or hard lump in the tongue should be regarded seriously and expert advice obtained as to the real nature of the trouble.*

Simple tumours may also form in the tongue, warts, fatty overgrowths, and cysts. Underneath the tongue, a small fluid swelling may collect as a result of a dilatation of a mucous gland or duct. The condition is called the ranula and it is easily remedied by an operation. Occasionally, a black patch forms at the back of the tongue. It is due to a fungus, aspergillus niger, which leads to overgrowth of the filiform papillæ. The patch should be painted with a solution of salicylic acid in glycerine, 5 grains to the ounce. *Injuries* to the tongue are often associated with considerable bleeding. This may be arrested by stitching the wound but not infrequently it is necessary to ligate (tie) the tongue artery in the neck.

Insect stings of the tongue often lead to great swelling which may obstruct the air passage. If there is any danger of suffocation, the tongue has to be freely incised.

TONIC. Any agent which increases the tone of the body generally or of any organ or tissue is described as a tonic.

TONIC SPASM. A spasm of a muscle or group of muscles which is continuous, not intermittent, is described as tonic. Such a spasm is observed during the first stage of an epileptic fit when the whole body becomes quite rigid. This stage is followed after 20 to 30 seconds by intermittent spasms called clonic. More localized tonic spasms are seen in lockjaw (tetanus) and in strychnine poisoning. Occasionally, tonic spasms of a group of muscles may be of hysterical origin.

TONSIL. The tonsils consist of two oval masses of lymphoid tissue—the same tissue of which lymph glands are composed—about an inch in length and half an inch from before backwards, placed at the back of the mouth, facing one another on opposite sides of the upper part of the throat. The tonsils are not the only lymphoid tissue structures in this part of the body ; in addition there is a smaller mass of it on the back of the tongue, called the lingual tonsil, which is sometimes enlarged, especially in adults, and also another mass up behind the uvula, between the back of the nose and the mouth, called Lushka's tonsil or, when enlarged, adenoids.

This whole chain of separate masses of lymphoid tissue is called Waldeyer's ring. It is believed to have a protective function, though in reality very little is known about the function of the tonsils. It has been suggested that they produce an internal secretion, like the ductless glands of the body, but this has never been proved or disproved. It has also been suggested that a function of the tonsils is the production of white blood corpuscles (lymphocytes), but this function, if it is of any importance in the tonsil, is in any case shared with the numerous other lymph glands of the body. It may be taken, however, that whatever other functions the tonsils may be discovered to have, their chief function is a defensive one, either acting themselves as bulwarks against infection or stimulating the body (as some authorities have suggested) to defend itself against infection, and this function is most active in childhood.

It used to be imagined that enlarged tonsils did harm only because they obstructed the airway, and the method of treating the condition was to cut off part of the enlargement, which, indeed, often did the patient some good. It is now realized, however, that a tonsil does the real harm when it is diseased (infected by bacteria), and that while many enlarged tonsils are unhealthy, a small hidden tonsil may be more septic and may cause much more harm than an enlarged tonsil. With regard to the question of whether the tonsils should be removed or not, there is to-day rather a reaction against the wholesale removal of enlarged tonsils in children. Nowadays no doctor wants to remove tonsils merely because they are enlarged ; but when foul matter can be squeezed out of tonsils, and the glands of the neck are enlarged, and perhaps the child is of poor physique and suffers from various gastro-intestinal disorders—in other words, when the tonsils are no longer doing their job properly and are infecting the rest of the body—then undoubtedly the tonsils *ought* to be removed. Doctors to-day are rather disinclined to remove tonsils before the age of five, for it is up to that age that their protective function is most active, but even before that the tonsils should be removed if they are unhealthy and causing enlarged glands of the neck. It is not nowadays considered so certain as it was that unhealthy tonsils cause rheumatism in children ; nor will removal of the tonsils have much effect on asthma or bronchitis ; but it is doubtful if the tonsils ever fully recover from an attack of scarlet fever or diphtheria, and it is probably well to remove them when a child has fully recovered from these infectious diseases.

There is no question about the removal of adenoids ; the very term adenoids means that the lymphoid tissue behind the uvula is enlarged and unhealthy, and as this affects the breathing, causes deformity of the mouth (gothic-arched palate), and frequently causes inflammation of the ears and deafness, it is evident that adenoids should be removed whenever their presence is discovered, even if the child is only a week old. Unfortunately, up to the present nothing has been discovered to take the place of surgical removal of adenoids, though breathing exercises and simple nasal drops may be useful in preventing their development.

TONSILLITIS, or inflammation of the tonsils, may be either chronic or acute.

Chronic tonsillitis means the condition of enlarged and unhealthy tonsils, to which a great variety of ailments have been attributed, some justly, some unjustly ; but certainly in adults they appear to have an evil influence in rheumatism, certain types of heart disease, boils, certain types of kidney disease, persistent inflammation of the conjunctiva (white of the eye), dyspepsia, and certain types of deafness, to mention only a few that reliable authorities have catalogued. If the tonsils are not bad enough to be removed the best treatment is to paint them regularly with Mandl's paint (which is not a proprietary preparation but is called after the long-dead physician who invented the formula) which contains iodine in glycerine, flavoured with peppermint.

Acute tonsillitis is sometimes divided up into different headings —catarrhal tonsillitis, lacunar tonsillitis, and parenchymatous tonsillitis, but in reality all these are merely different stages of the same disease.

A common cause of tonsillitis is infection with the germ called the streptococcus. The tonsils are the favourite entrance of the streptococcus into the body, and it causes an acute reddening of the throat, sometimes a membrane on the tonsil resembling the membrane of diphtheria (a swab should always be taken by the doctor when the membrane is present, in case it may be the latter) and a sharp rise of temperature (up to 104° or 105° F., sometimes).

Treatment. The patient must be kept in bed, given two aspirin tablets every four hours, and warm gargles of hydrogen peroxide or glycerine of thymol; the throat may be painted with Mandl's paint, and the doctor, who should always be called in, as tonsillitis may mean the beginning of scarlet fever or some other serious condition, will probably prescribe a sulphanilamide, such as prontosil.

Quinsy, or tonsillar abscess, may develop after tonsillitis either inside the tonsil or in the tissues behind it. When a quinsy has definitely developed a doctor should be called in to open it, otherwise the pus in it may track down more deeply and cause severe inflammation. The tonsils should be removed after an attack of quinsy, as subsequent attacks are otherwise rather common.

TOURNIQUET. This is a French word used to denote any mechanical instrument for the arresting or prevention of bleeding.

TOXÆMIA. Any condition of blood poisoning caused by the toxins or poisons produced by disease germs within the body is described as toxæmia. It is to be distinguished from septicæmia, a condition in which the germs are present and multiply in the blood.

TOXICOLOGY. This is a section of medical science which deals with poisons, their nature and composition, their effects upon the body and the methods of their detection.

TOXIN. This word is used to denote the poisonous substances produced by germs (bacteria) either in the body or in artificial media.

TRACHEA, or windpipe, is the tube, about four inches or rather more in length, which conveys the air from the lower part of the throat down to the lungs. It begins just below the Adam's apple in the neck (i.e., below the larynx), and ends in the thorax by dividing into the right and left bronchi.

TRACHEOTOMY is an urgent operation in which the trachea or windpipe is opened from the front of the neck to allow air to get down to the lungs when the upper part of the throat is obstructed by inflammation (such as diphtheria), a foreign body, or some other cause.

TRANSFUSION OF BLOOD. If a great deal of blood is lost, as when an artery is torn in an accident, or in severe cases of anæmia, it may be necessary to replace the blood by transfusion. This operation consists of withdrawing blood from a person called the donor and transferring it to the bloodless person called the receiver. The blood may be passed directly to a vein of the receiver, but sometimes the blood is first passed into a vessel, treated with oil or sodium citrate to prevent clotting, and then allowed to run into the receiver's vein. Before the operation is carried out, it is necessary first to find out if the donor's and receiver's blood are compatible.

TREPHINE. The operation of boring a circular opening in the skull is performed by means of a special cylindrical saw called a trephine.

TREPONEMA PALLIDUM. This is the organism or germ which causes syphilis. It is a long slender organism containing six to fourteen spirals and it is actively mobile, moving in a corkscrew fashion. (*See also* SYPHILIS.)

TRICHIASIS. Inversion of the eyelashes is termed trichiasis. Normally, the eyelashes protrude outwards from the eyelids, but, as a result of inflammation of the lid margins, one or more of the eyelashes may be directed inwards so that they rub against and irritate the delicate surface of the eye. This may in time give rise to ulceration of the cornea with impairment of the vision. Treatment is simply the pulling out of the offending eyelash and the complete destruction of the root by electrolysis. (*See also* EYELIDS.)

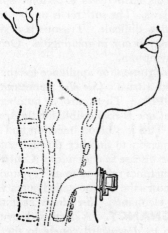

Tracheotomy Tube

TRICHINOSIS. This is a disease caused by eating pork infected with a tiny round worm called the trichina spiralis. The parasites invade the voluntary muscles setting up inflammation. The worms become encysted between the muscle fibres, remaining alive for years. No satisfactory cure is known. (*See also* WORMS.)

TRICUSPID VALVE. This is one of the heart valves. It is situated between the right auricle and the right ventricle, and is provided with three cusps. Unlike the mitral valve, it is not frequently the seat of disease. (*See also* HEART.)

TRIGEMINAL NERVE is the nerve which controls the muscles of chewing, and it also enables us to feel such sensations as pain, heat and cold, and touch, on our face and in our eyes, nose, mouth and teeth. It is the " nerve of toothache." Our sense of taste is also, to some extent, governed by the trigeminal nerve and any damage to the nerve in a particular part of its course in the skull will cause the sense of taste to be diminished or abolished on the front two-thirds of the same side of the tongue. The trigeminal nerve is connected with nearly every other nerve supplying the head and neck, and because it has all these connections it has situated on it, outside that part of the brain from which it arises, a mass of grey nervous tissue called a ganglion. This ganglion, the Gasserian ganglion, separates out, as it were, the different parts of the nerve that are going to supply different areas of the face, and these separate parts, or branches of the nerves, leave the skull through separate holes.

TRISMUS. This term refers to a tonic spasm of the muscles which clench the jaws. The sufferer is unable to separate the teeth and feeding becomes difficult. Trismus is a symptom of lockjaw (tetanus) and it may occur in meningitis. Occasionally, it occurs as an hysterical symptom.

TRUSS. An instrument or appliance for the control of a hernia or rupture is called a truss. (*See also* ABDOMINAL BELT ; HERNIA.)

TRYPANOSOMA. There are a number of trypanosomas, some harmless, but one is responsible for the tropical disease called sleeping sickness. This is a blood infection and the disease is transmitted from one person to another through an intermediate host, the tsetse fly. The disease is endemic in Central Africa and South America. It is sometimes referred to as Trypanosomiasis. A variety of trypanosoma causes the disease called surra which affects horses, dogs, camels and elephants. (*See also* SLEEPING SICKNESS.)

TUBAL PREGNANCY. A fertilized ovum arrested in the Fallopian tube on its downward course to the womb gives rise to tubal gestation or pregnancy. As this is an abnormal place for the development of the embryo, the tube usually ruptures between the sixth and twelfth week of pregnancy, a dangerous happening—for it is associated with great shock and severe internal bleeding. An immediate operation is generally necessary.

TUBERCULIN is an emulsion of dead tuberculosis germs and is used in weak dilutions in the treatment of tuberculosis. The great success once hoped for by employing tuberculin has not been realized, but it is still valuable when combined with other methods of treatment. It is also of undoubted value as a method of diagnosis of tuberculosis. (*See also* TUBERCULOSIS.)

TUBERCULOSIS. Pulmonary tuberculosis, or consumption, is the term applied to tuberculosis affecting the lungs. It starts off by the formation of " tubercles," small abnormal masses of tissue due to the presence of a germ called *Koch's bacillus*. Koch was a famous German bacteriologist (1843–1910) who first described the germ which is the cause of tuberculosis. It is contagious from one person to another, from animals to man, and from man to animals. There are three main varieties of the tubercle bacillus : the human, the bovine and the avian. Infection from human sources is probably much more frequent than from any other ; but quite a large amount of human tuberculosis is caused by germs of the bovine type, and tuberculosis may be communicated to man from infected cow's milk, and from tuberculous meat, either beef or pork.

The germ can invade any part of the human body, but it usually becomes localized in the lung passages. It may be confined to the lungs alone, to the bronchial tubes only, or to both bronchial tubes and the lungs, and may manifest itself in an acute form (galloping consumption), a less acute form (subacute), or in a chronic form (fibroid tuberculosis).

It is quite possible to have tuberculosis of the lungs without knowing it, though it may be present and active, unsuspected by the patient or his doctor, at the time of death from some other cause, and further, it may have been active and have healed up completely without any definite treatment and have given no signs of its presence during life. Once recognized, however, tuberculosis of the lungs is so far advanced that it rarely heals up completely, though it can very often be arrested and life is not shortened although some evidence of the past activity of the disease remains.

Diagnosis. It is most important that this should be early in order that the treatment may be successful. Unfortunately the onset of tuberculosis is very insidious, and the disease may be very extensively spread in the lungs without causing sufficient ill-health to make a person consider himself sufficiently ill to consult a doctor. The following symptoms are suggestive of consumption :

Symptoms. Cough and Sputum. In most cases cough with *sputum* is the earliest indication, and in a young adult persistent cough, especially when accompanied by *purulent sputum* (phlegm containing a great deal of matter), is very suspicious unless there is some obvious cause for it such as an unhealthy state of the nose and throat due to over smoking, etc. In older people chronic bronchitis is very common, and unless a marked change appears in the type of cough and the sputum, little importance can be placed on their presence.

Hæmoptysis or bleeding from the lungs. This is the first sign in roughly 18 to 20 per cent of cases. It varies from streaks of bright colour in the sputum, definitely bloodstained phlegm, to the *coughing up* of practically pure blood (hæmoptysis). Bleeding from the lungs in a young adult, with or without symptoms of ill-health in phlegm which persists may be taken as practically certain to mean consumption. It is important to remember that a brisk hæmorrhage is often absolutely the first symptom, and that there may be as much as one pint of blood lost without previous cough or presence of phlegm, and without a careful physical examination of the chest revealing any abnormalities in the lungs.

Pain. Tuberculosis of the lungs in an early stage is usually painless, but in practically every case, however, there is sooner or later an attack of pleurisy (inflammation of the lining membranes of the lung and inner surface of the chest wall) which does cause definite pain. In about 5 per cent of all cases the pleurisy is the first symptom. The history of a cold or of an influenzal attack followed by pain characteristic of inflammation of the lining membranes of the lungs should always be regarded as a most suspicious circumstance.

Difficulty in breathing; Dyspnœa. In cases where much of the lung has been attacked without symptoms, accompanied or followed by extensive healing and the formation of scar tissue, it may cause difficulty in breathing, or cause the patient to seek advice for this alone. In some cases fluid will fill up the space between the lung and the chest wall without causing any pain, though it may cause much difficulty in breathing.

Influences on the general health. This is often very slight, and is often ignored or disregarded by both the patient and by the physician. The symptoms are common to many illnesses, and may only be of use as corroborative evidence. The most important are : *Malaise :* an indefinite feeling of tiredness lasting for months. Sometimes it appears only as undue tiredness at the end of the day's work. It may show itself as a general disinclination to work or play, or as a definite feeling of exhaustion whether the patient is up and about or lying in bed. It us usually partly physical and partly mental. *Weight Loss :* If a young adult loses weight in a rapid and marked fashion it is very important. *Night-Sweating :* This is common at the beginning and usually disappears as the case settles down. The point here is that the sweats occur although the patient is not conscious of having had any fever. The perspiration may be so copious as to necessitate many changes of night attire. *Fever :* Often the temperature is raised without the patient being aware of anything unusual. The high temperature is very suggestive, though it is often missed as it is unusual for one to take one's temperature when in apparently normal health. *Anæmia :* This may be severe owing to the general poisoning of the system owing to the germ of tuberculosis. The heart muscle is weakened, and this will cause palpitation and difficulty in breathing. In women the anæmia may be sufficient to cause suppression of the periods for a time. *Digestive disturbances :* These are commonly complained of during a period of about two years before the first signs suggesting consumption appear. These disturbances are so common that they are not very important. *Ischio-rectal abscess and Fistula :* An abscess in the region of the anus is a common complication. Every case of this condition should be carefully examined, as it may be the means by which the presence of consumption is detected.

Question of Temperature. The temperature of a normal individual is 98·4° F., with possible variations of from below normal in the morning to just above in the afternoon about six o'clock. A daily swing of more than one and a half degrees is definitely abnormal. For the purpose of testing for tuberculosis the temperature should be taken night and morning (5 p.m. and 8 a.m. are good average times.)

X-ray Examination. This is a very useful aid to diagnosis, but some degree of skill is required to interpret the picture. The X-ray picture must always be regarded as definitely subsidiary to the other points mentioned above, and the diagnosis as a whole depends entirely on the collection and weighing up of various items of evidence for and against.

Types of Acute Tuberculosis of the Lungs. *Miliary :* So-called because there are numerous lesions the size of a millet-seed. This only occurs in the lungs when it is part of a general infection all over the body.

Broncho-pneumonic Tuberculosis. (" Galloping Consumption ") : This is a rapidly progressive condition and is usually fatal within six months. The lining membrane of the smaller bronchial tubes are infected most and there is a great deal of destruction of tissue. *Pneumonic :* This is not very common. Large areas of lung become solid and the patient usually dies within a few months ; but some cases manage to survive the acute stage and become chronic. Large areas of tissues are destroyed and *cavities* are thus produced.

Types of Chronic Tuberculosis of the Lung. These are more common than the acute types. The route by which the germ reaches the lung is not definitely known, but it is most probably by the germs being breathed in when they are present in the air in dust, etc. In some cases the germs may be swallowed in food, as in the case of infected milk, and may travel by means of the blood or lymph streams to the lungs. Once there the germ produces a small *tubercle* or lump which gradually grows bigger. The centre portion is cut off from its blood supply and breaks down, a process known as *caseation*. The natural defence of the body is to grow fibrous tissue round the outside of the tubercle. Sometimes this is successful, and the result is a small fibrous nodule only. Lime salts are often laid down in the centre portion of the tubercle, a process known as *calcification*. If nature's attempt at healing is not successful the area of disease increases and the original tubercle joins up with others which have formed near it. The enlargement is very irregular, and the disease may be advancing in one direction while healing by fibrosis is occurring in another. Finally, one of the walls of the smaller bronchial tubes becomes ulcerated through, and the broken-down portion inside is emptied into the air passages which, in their turn, are so irritated that they try to get rid of this dead matter by coughing. In this way the germ of tuberculosis will appear in the phlegm.

Treatment. The treatment is long and troublesome and may have to be carried on throughout life. Endless steadfastness, courage, self-discipline and self-denial are required, and the final result depends more on the presence or absence of these qualities than on anything else. Financial and home conditions are also of importance, as the treatment may last for a year or two and must be adapted to suit the environment.

Some patients do not come to be treated until the chance of cure is passed ; but it must be realized that treatment, if successful, will result in the patient being able to lead a happy and useful life, though it is likely to change for the worse should a proper mode of life not be persisted in. The chief aim and object of *sanatorium treatment* is to teach the sufferer this mode of life, and is not expected to cure the patient completely. The treatment can, of course, be carried out at home, but there are many arguments in favour of institutional *versus* home treatment. The groundwork of all treatment is a monotonous disciplined daily routine, so much so that it is very difficult for the patient to carry it out alone. The treatment will completely upset the usual routine of a home, and it is not uncommon to find that the rest of the family cannot put up with it.

Another important point is that the condition of the patient may alter from day to day, and that such alterations should be met by slight deviation of treatment ; these details are very important in the long run, and mean that daily supervision is necessary. The family doctor can rarely afford to devote so much time to one patient, nor in many cases can the patient afford the expense.

Fresh Air and Sunlight. As many hours as possible should be spent in the open air, and when indoors the windows must be widely opened, or taken out of their sashes.

Routine and discipline, and education. The essentials of sanatorium treatment must be followed for the rest of the patient's life, and this must become automatic, as otherwise the worry of attention to detail would be a burden both to the patient and to those around him. The strict routine of a sanatorium produces this atmosphere and, like other forms of physical training, takes some months to do its work, and then only if persisted in day by day for several months, without relaxation.

Food. Special diet is not necessary : three good meals a day should be taken and the food thoroughly masticated and digested. Teeth must be put right so that the food can be properly chewed. The normal weight in health for each individual patient should be the aim to which he must strive to return.

Preventive Hygiene. People who live in the same house as the consumptive should not sleep in the same room. They must try to avoid infection when the patient coughs, and should wash their hands frequently, especially before meals. They should also wash after touching anything belonging to the patient, e.g. eating and drinking utensils, and these should be boiled after use. *Marriage :* Any active tuberculous disease in a girl is a definite contra-indication to marriage, or more particularly to pregnancy. Often the tuberculous disease seems to be arrested during pregnancy, only to flare up after the birth of the child, and the result is frequently fatal. An abortion may be necessary in the mother's interest, though even when procured early in the pregnancy there is always some risk that the tuberculous disease may be aggravated. *Lactation :* The feeding of an infant at the breast by a woman who has active consumption should not be permitted both in the interests of the mother and of the child. In the mother's case, nursing is a drain which she can ill afford to undergo, and which will accelerate the disease ; in the case of the infant, infection from the mother is a real danger, and it must be remembered that the earlier the age at which the infant is infected the worse is the outlook.

No child has ever been born suffering from tuberculosis when the mother is afflicted, but many catch it at an early age. A child born of a consumptive parent should, in its own interest, be separated from the parent affected and brought up in the country. It should exchange the town life for a country life ; indoor for outdoor life ; warm baths for outdoor bathing ; mental activity for physical exercise : to sum up, it should live a natural life. At a later stage the child should attend an open-air school.

Tuberculosis is not transmitted as a hereditary disease, but there is a greater tendency to develop the complaint in children born of infected parents or parent.

Tuberculosis of joints is most common in childhood and early youth, but it may occur at any age and is not uncommon in old people. It is a chronic condition and comes on insidiously, and when established there is swelling of the joint (" white swelling "), pain on movement, and the limb is often drawn up (by the pull of the muscles) ; at a later stage there is destruction of the joint, and deformity results. General signs of tuberculosis, such as evening rise of temperature, night sweats, and wasting, are also present. When the diagnosis is made early by the doctor and time not wasted by people considering the condition " rheumatism " or " growing pains," the outlook is favourable, though treatment is always prolonged.

Treatment. The joint is usually fixed in a useful position by means of a carefully moulded plaster of Paris splint or other apparatus and kept absolutely immobile for at least six months after the active disease has settled down, and may take up to two or three years. Open air and sunlight are essentials in treatment.

TUMOUR. In a popular sense, a tumour refers to any abnormal swelling in the body, but pathologically it refers to an abnormal growth of cells and is sometimes also termed a neoplasm or new growth.

Any tissue of the body can develop a tumour, and tumours are classified according to the type of tissue involved. Broadly, there are two main classes : the connective tissue tumours and the epithelial tumours. These, in turn, can be each divided into malignant and benign (harmless) tumours, according to whether they are a menace to life or not. Tumours are also named according to the name of the actual tissue affected. Thus, there are *lipomas* —fatty tumours ; *fibromas*—fibrous tumours ; *angiomas*—blood-vessel tumours ; *neuromas*, nerve tumours, and so on. Sarcomas are so called because to the eye their substance resembles a fleshy mass. Carcinoma is a cancer, and is so called because processes grow out from the parent tumour like the claws of a crab.

The actual causation of tumours is unknown and it is probable that a variety of causes are operative. Some form of irritation, chemical or bacterial, is certainly very often a precursor of cancer.

This is most noticeable in chimney-sweeps' and paraffin-workers' cancer. Also, cancers can be produced artificially in animals by the application to the skin of irritant tars. Some tumours are probably of embryonic origin, i.e. groups of cells get misplaced during development within the womb and in later life they commence to grow in an uncontrolled manner. Teratomata probably arise in this way.

Many tumours are quite harmless and only produce symptoms when their bulk interferes with the work of an organ. Others, however, grow very rapidly, infiltrating the organ in which they originate and spreading to other parts of the body by the transit of tumour cells in the blood stream or in the lymphatic channels. Secondary growths are set up and tissues and organs are destroyed by these new growths. Cancers and sarcomas are tumours of this type and are consequently destructive to life. Innocent or benign tumours grow very slowly, while the reverse is the case with the malignant variety.

The appearance of a tumour need not be a cause for alarm but it is always advisable to seek medical advice immediately. In a majority of cases, the person concerned will be reassured that the tumour is harmless ; but should the verdict be otherwise the chances of cure are very much greater in the early stages of a malignant tumour as compared with the later stages. Pain does not necessarily accompany a tumour, but that in itself is not evidence that the tumour is harmless. The early stages of cancer are nearly always painless. Simple tumours are only removed if they are disfiguring or are pressing on some organ. With malignant tumours early removal by surgical operation, along with radium treatment, are essential as soon as they are detected.

TYMPANITES. This term is used to denote distension of the abdomen (belly) as a result of the presence of gas, or air, in the intestines or peritoneal cavity. Normally, there is a certain amount of gas in the intestines, but under certain conditions it becomes excessive in amount. Tympanites is especially liable to arise when the bowel muscle is weakened or paralysed through the absorption of poisons. This occurs in general peritonitis and notably in typhoid fever. It may also arise after an abdominal operation, as a result of shock, and in association with intestinal obstruction. Occasionally it occurs as an hysterical symptom.

Treatment. An enema of soap and water with a dessert-spoonful of turpentine may be given or poultices may be applied to the abdomen. Sal volatile or oil of peppermint by the mouth may be helpful in some cases.

TYMPANUM. This is the middle ear, an air-filled cavity in the temporal bone of the skull. It lies just behind the ear-drum or tympanic membrane and contains a chain of three small bones, the malleus, the incus and the stapes, which lead from the drum to the internal ear and probably have a protective function. It also contains two tiny muscles which act upon the ossicles. The tympanum communicates with the throat by a small canal called the Eustachian tube, and is also connected with the air-cells in the mastoid process of the temporal bone. (*See also* EAR.)

TYPHOID FEVER. This is an acute disease characterized by a special ulceration of the small intestine, with the eruption of rose-coloured spots, and a typical course of temperature.

Symptoms. After infection, there is an incubation period of from one to about two weeks. Then the disease shows itself rather insidiously by headache, feeling of tiredness, nose bleeding and abdominal pain. Fever appears and the temperature steadily rises during the first week, each night the temperature being higher than the preceding night (Staircase temperature.) The pulse is slow, tongue white and coated, and constipation is more common than diarrhœa. The rash makes its appearance at the end of the first week and consists of isolated rose-red spots, slightly raised but disappearing on pressure. They appear first on the abdomen and may spread to the chest and limbs. During the first week the glands in the small intestine (Peyer's patches) are becoming inflamed and by the second week they have become ulcerated. Then the patient begins to look seriously ill and exhausted. The face is very pale with flushed cheeks. The tongue is dry, the sufferer dull and listless. Diarrhœa sets in and the motions are pea-soup-like with an unpleasant odour and often containing blood. The abdomen becomes distended and tender, the temperature continues high, the pulse rapid and sometimes weak.

During the third week the symptoms depend upon the severity of the ulceration. In a severe case the abdominal signs become more marked and the patient becomes prostrated and emaciated. Disturbance of the nervous system is shown by delirium, muscle tremors, drowsiness, and, in extreme cases, coma or unconsciousness. It is at this stage that there is a grave danger of perforation of the bowel and of intestinal hæmorrhage or bleeding. Should this arise, the outlook is very bad.

In a favourable case, towards the end of the third week the temperature begins to fall gradually, and the other symptoms subside. The diarrhœa passes off, the tongue becomes clean, and the convalescent stage is reached by the end of the fourth week. During this period great care has to be taken with the diet, as an injudicious meal may readily induce a relapse.

The diagnosis of typhoid fever in the early stages is by no means easy as it may be mistaken for pneumonia, generalized tuberculosis or even appendicitis. Fortunately, if typhoid is suspected it is possible to confirm the diagnosis by means of a laboratory test, as the blood of typhoid patients gives a special reaction within ten days of the onset of the disease (Widal test). Also, it may be possible even earlier to cultivate the typhoid bacilli from a sample of the suspected person's blood.

Complications. It has already been noted that perforation of the bowel and hæmorrhage may arise during the third week of the disease. These are revealed in the case of the first, by abdominal pain and collapse, and in the case of the second by the temperature falling to subnormal, the patient becoming collapsed, and sometimes blood being passed by the bowel. Other complications include gall-bladder inflammation, pneumonia, pleurisy, meningitis, abscesses in the bones or joints, and a painful condition of the spine (typhoid spine) due to an inflammation of the cartilage discs between the vertebræ. Thrombosis (clotting of blood) may also arise in the femoral vein of the leg during convalescence.

Paratyphoid fevers. These are illnesses which closely resemble the less severe forms of typhoid. They are caused by two different organisms or germs, paratyphoid A and paratyphoid B, and infection is acquired in much the same way as in true typhoid. The diagnosis is dependent upon bacteriological examination in the laboratory.

Treatment. It is usually advisable for a typhoid patient to be nursed in a special hospital. This is particularly advisable, as complications may arise which necessitate immediate attention on the part of the physician or surgeon. Special care is essential in the management of typhoid patients to disinfect all the body discharges and soiled clothing to prevent spread of infection. As there is an inflammation of the bowel, only a minimum of food should be given. Two to three ounces of peptonized milk should be given every two or three hours, but this should vary according to the digestive powers of the patient. Water can be freely given, and, to break the monotony of the milk diet, small quantities of beef tea and chicken broth. Attention to the skin is important, a cold antiseptic lotion being used frequently, and care should be taken, especially in prolonged cases, to prevent bed-sores. If the temperature is high, cold spraying or even cold baths are very beneficial. There are no specific drugs of value in the treatment of typhoid, though intestinal antiseptics such as beta-naphthol and oil of cinnamon may be given. Distension of the abdomen (tympanites) can be treated by giving oil of cinnamon by the mouth in 2–5 minim doses and by applying turpentine fomentations to the abdomen. Any constipation during the course of the disease should be treated by enemata and not purgatives, as these may irritate the bowel and lead to perforation. Stimulants may be necessary, but these are to be given with great discrimination. During convalescence, diet must be carefully supervised, and all solid food strictly avoided.

TYPHUS FEVER. This infectious disease, once very prevalent in this country, is now fortunately very rare. It has been all but conquered by cleanliness and sound sanitation. Essentially, it is a disease of dirt, overcrowding, starvation and fatigue.

Treatment. Strict isolation is essential in cases of typhus fever. Good nursing is vital.

ULCER. An ulcer may be described as an open sore resulting from inflammation on the surface of the skin, or on the surface of the membrane lining any cavity within the body. Death occurs in the tissues of the infected area, and because of this loss the ulcer is usually depressed below the surface of the healthy tissue. Any irritation to the skin may cause an ulcer to form, but the commonest cause of all is the presence of disease germs. Other factors which often encourage the development of ulcers are poorness of the blood, a general state of bad health, or poor circulation which leads to varicose conditions of the veins. Constant pressure or friction is liable to cause ulceration of the skin, for example, bedsores. Any malignant growth, cancer or sarcoma, is liable to break down and ulcerate. Rodent ulcer is the chief amongst these malignant ulcers and usually is situated on the face.

Varieties. Ordinary simple inflammatory ulcers are usually rounded, depressed areas consisting of a " floor " or surface covered with greyish-yellow material, from which there is a discharge. The surrounding parts are red and swollen, and there is a blue line which marks the edge of the healthy tissue. When the destructive process has ceased, the ulcer becomes cleaner and the floor is more or less covered with red granulation tissue. The parts surrounding the ulcer then become less angry-looking and the discharge is more watery in appearance.

When healing the new tissue contracts, giving a puckered appearance to the scar and the edges show the blue line of advancing healthy skin. Ulcers may be described as *local* when they occur at one spot only, and *constitutional* when there are several of them on different parts of the body. Constitutional ulcers are generally the result of some disease such as syphilis, tuberculosis, anthrax, Oriental sore, and yaws, and they are known as *infective ulcers*. Local ulcers include many varieties according to their symptoms and appearance. *Callous* or *indolent ulcer* is the commonest type and it occurs chiefly on the legs of women in middle life. They are often of considerable size and the edges are thick, hard, and raised above the surface. There are few granulations, and the discharge is thin and small in amount, but is often offensive and irritating. *Irritable ulcer* is one which is very painful, especially at night, and they appear to be commonest about the ankle. *Weak ulcers* are met with in weakly people, especially those suffering from dropsy. In this type the ulcer is soft, bleeds easily, and the granulations project above the surface forming what is popularly known as proud-flesh. *Varicose ulcers* are met with on the legs of patients who suffer with bad varicose veins, and there is danger of the vein rupturing and severe bleeding occurring. The ulcer itself may belong to any of the above mentioned types but it has a tendency

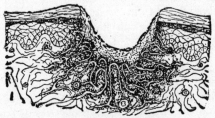

Cross Section of Ulcer

to develop into a callous ulcer. *Internal ulcers* tend specially to develop in the mouth, stomach and intestines. *Gastric ulcer* is fully described under GASTRIC or STOMACH ULCER and ulcer of the upper part of the intestine will be found under DUODENAL ULCER.

Treatment. For ordinary inflammatory ulcers the treatment consists of rendering the part clean with moist, warm, antiseptic applications, such as acriflavine, carbolic lotion, or perchloride of mercury solution, and the dressing covered with oiled-silk. As soon as the ulcer is rendered clean, these antiseptics must be stopped, as they interfere with the healing processes. The importance of complete rest cannot be too strongly emphasized and the patient should be given good nourishing food and tonics. *Weak ulcers,* or any ulcer in which the granulations are too prominent and above the level of the surrounding skin, may be treated with blue stone (copper sulphate), silver salts, or other substances which have a reducing effect upon the proudflesh. Once an ulcer has reached the healing stage, all that is necessary is to keep the surface clean and free from irritation and as much rest as possible must be given to the part. The ulcer may be kept covered with a piece of lint spread over with boracic ointment, or an elastic plaster bandage may keep a zinc gelatin dressing on the leg. The usual interval allowed to elapse between dressings is two days, but if there is any discharge or if the ulcer is not clean, the dressing must be changed oftener. The lint must be thoroughly soaked before removal, and never pulled away roughly. The healing of a large ulcer, after it has been rendered clean, may often be hastened by grafting its surface with skin from another part of the body. (*See also* DUODENAL ULCER ; GASTRIC ULCER ; GRANULATION TISSUE ; LUPUS ; PROUD-FLESH.)

ULITIS. This term is applied to inflammation of the gums. (*See also* GINGIVITIS ; GUMS, DISEASES OF.)

ULNA. The inner of the two bones which form the skeleton of the forearm is known as the ulna, and when the palm of the hand is turned upwards it can be traced with the finger from the point of the elbow down to the wrist. At the lower end of the ulna is a small rounded knob which stands out prominently, especially in thin people. (*See also* BONES ; FRACTURES ; ARM ; ELBOW.)

ULNAR. The *ulnar artery* is one of the branches of the brachial artery which supplies the upper arm. It commences at the elbow, passes down the forearm and eventually joins the arteries which supply the palm and fingers. The *ulnar nerve* lies very close to the ulnar artery and the two structures travel together down the forearm into the palm. This nerve supplies sensation to the palm and back of the hand and to the little finger and ring finger. (*See also* ARM ; ELBOW ; FINGERS.)

ULTRA-VIOLET RAYS. The invisible rays of light given off at the higher (violet) end of the spectrum are described as ultra-violet rays. They have a powerful action upon all forms of life, and nowadays are greatly used in the treatment of many diseases and conditions. (*See also* LIGHT TREATMENT.)

UMBILICUS. More commonly referred to as the navel, the umbilicus is the little depressed button-like scar lying somewhat below the middle line of the abdomen. (*See also* HERNIA ; RUPTURE.)

UNDULANT FEVER. This disease is more commonly known as Malta fever, Mediterranean fever, or Rock fever, but is now recognized to be not uncommon in this country where slight long-continued infections are much commoner than was formerly realized. It is due to infection of milk by a germ, *Brucella abortus*, and it is calculated that 60 per cent of the herds of cows in England are infected to a greater or less extent. It can be prevented by thorough pasteurization of the milk. Treatment of the fever is by a vaccine or by arsenic preparations. *See* MALTA FEVER.

URACHUS. A fibrous cord which passes from the bladder to the umbilicus is known as the urachus. It represents the remains of the canal which, in the unborn child, joins the bladder with the allantois, one of the fœtal membranes. (*See also* EMBRYO ; FŒTUS ; LABOUR and CHILDBIRTH.)

URÆMIA. This is a poisonous condition of the blood which arises in diseases of the kidney. The poisonous materials which normally should be passed in the urine are retained in the blood, and many serious symptoms are produced in consequence. Uræmia is one of the most serious results of chronic Bright's disease (nephritis) but it may occur in other diseases of the kidney, such as stone in the kidney or tuberculous disease, or in some cases where there is suppression of the urine, or, when the kidneys are sound, from an enlarged prostate or other cause of retention of urine. (*See also* NEPHRITIS.)

UREA. Urea is a compound which is always present in the urine and sweat ; but in disease, especially disease of the kidney, it may be greatly increased. One of the uses of this compound is to stimulate the functions of the kidney, and it is sometimes given for this purpose in cases of dropsy of the heart or in kidney disease. The hypnotic drugs known as veronal, dial, medinal and luminal are very closely allied to urea. (*See also* HYPNOTICS.)

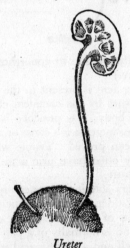

Ureter

Showing connection between Ureter and Bladder

URETER. The ureters are two in number, and they are the tubes which convey the urine from the kidneys to the urinary bladder. Each ureter measures from ten to twelve inches in length

18*

and they are lined by a delicate mucous membrane. Obstruction of the ureter may be a serious condition ; it is usually caused by a stone from the kidney, giving rise to very intense pain. Twisting of the ureter may cause sharp attacks of abdominal pain, with nausea, and perhaps vomiting. (*See also* BLADDER ; URINE.)

URETHRA. In the male, the urethra is the tube inside the penis which extends from the neck of the bladder to the exterior. It measures from seven to eight inches in length and is the passage for both urine and seminal fluid. The female urethra is a narrow canal about one and a half inches long and it lies embedded in the wall of the vagina. Inflammation of the urethra is known as urethri-

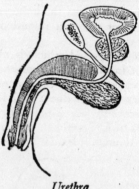

Urethra

tis, and it is nearly always due to gonorrhœa. (*See also* GLEET ; GONORRHŒA ; KIDNEY.)

URIC ACID. Uric acid is present in the urine and blood and it is formed in the tissues by the chemical changes which protein foods undergo in the body. Its presence is greatly increased in disease, but whether this increase is a cause or a result of a particular disease has not yet been proved. People who suffer from rheumatism and gout very often have uric acid crystals deposited in the urine. (*See also* GOUT.)

URINE is the watery solution excreted by the kidneys by way of the ureters to the bladder, which is emptied periodically through the urethra. It consists of waste substances which result from the activity of the body, and is normally of a pale yellow colour with a distinctly aromatic smell and a slightly acid reaction. The amount of urine excreted by a normal adult in 24 hours is 50 ounces, about 38 ounces by day and 12 ounces by night.

The colour of urine may vary in different diseases and also after taking various drugs. Over-secretion of urine may be due to such diseases as diabetes or chronic Bright's disease (of the kidneys), but it may also be due to such comparatively trivial causes as nervousness or drinking too much tea or beer.

Under-secretion of urine is due to inflammation of the kidney, to such an operation as passing a catheter, or to various fevers, or it may be due only to sweating or violent exercise.

Urine, Retention of. *Retention* of the urine is the term applied to the involuntary holding back of the urine in the bladder on account of something preventing urination, although the urine is secreted by the kidneys ; *suppression* of urine is an even more serious condition, as it is due to the failure of the kidneys to produce the urine, usually from acute inflammation of the kidneys or an acute fever. Retention of the urine, on the other hand, is usually due to an obstruction of the passage through which it should be passed, from a stricture, or a stone, or enlargement of the prostate gland at the neck of the bladder (common in old men), or to the shock of an operation or childbirth. Sometimes a warm bath will relieve the condition, but it is usually relieved by the passage of a sterilized catheter—which may have to be repeated frequently—or an operation. (*See also* CATHETER.)

URTICARIA. This is popularly known as nettle-rash and it is characterized by weals on the skin. Any alkaline application will be found soothing and baths containing bicarbonate of soda will relieve the itching. There is a form of the disease known as *giant urticaria*, or *angio-neurotic œdema*, in which sudden swellings may occur in the eyes, lips, mouth and throat. The eyes may be completely closed, or similar swellings may develop in the tongue or larynx causing very distressing symptoms. An injection of adrenaline should be given ; but in swelling of the larynx intubation of the larynx may have to be carried out in order to save the patient's life. The condition known as *lichen urticatus* is a disease similar to urticaria, and the legs and trunk seem to be the chief sites of the eruption. Children, particularly, are affected with this condition and the rash sometimes resembles the blisters of chickenpox. The diet must be carefully gone into and the regularity of the bowels should be maintained. The affected parts should be sponged with bicarbonate of soda dissolved in warm water. (*See also* ALLERGY ; ANAPHYLAXIS ; LICHEN.)

UTERUS, or womb, is the hollow organ in which the development of the fœtus from the ovum takes place. (*See also* WOMB.)

UVULA is the small muscular mass that hangs down from the middle of the soft palate between the pillars of the fauces. In relaxed conditions of the throat it may be enlarged or elongated, usually due to unhealthy tonsils or an unhealthy condition of the nose, and when one or other of these is put right the uvula becomes normal again.

VACCINATION. Vaccination is simply the introduction into the human body of the virus of cowpox, a modified form of small-pox ; with the object of producing a mild attack of the disease and stimulating the natural resistance of the body to gain an immunity to smallpox. (*See also* SMALLPOX.)

VAGINA. This is the passage between the womb and the vulva or external genital organs in the female. It lies between the urinary bladder in front and the rectum behind, the urethra being embedded in the lower half of the front wall. The lower opening of the vagina is partially closed by the hymen in the virgin. Inflammation, or vaginitis, may be caused by gonococcal infection or by the presence of a foreign body such as a pessary or tampon. It may occur as a complication of measles, scarlet or other infectious fevers. There is generally a certain amount of discharge, and the passage may become painful and tender, according to the severity of the in-flammation. Leucorrhœa, or " whites," is the term applied to a discharge from the vagina. (*See also* DOUCHE ; LEUCORRHŒA ; REPRODUCTIVE ORGANS.)

VAGINISMUS is a condition of hypersensitiveness of the vulva and vagina which leads to painful spasms of the muscles at the entrance to the genital canal whenever any attempt at sexual inter-course is made. It may be caused by excessive smallness of the open-ing, rigidity of the hymen, or some painful inflammatory disorder of the parts. The treatment naturally depends upon the cause ; sexual intercourse should be avoided until the condition clears up.

VALVE. In the heart, veins, and lymphatics of the human body there are flaps of tissue which permit of the blood or lymph flowing only in one direction. Should the fluid attempt to flow backwards, the flaps are floated outwards and so block the passage. Such flaps are termed valves, and they are an essential part of the mechanism of the heart and veins.

VARICOCELE. This is a dilated and twisted condition of the veins of the spermatic cord. These veins drain the testicle and its coverings, and the condition shows itself as a slight swelling in the scrotum which disappears when the patient lies down. It feels like a bag of worms, and the condition occurs most often in the left side. Varicocele occurs in young adults and its production is favoured by constipation. Very often no symptoms are produced, but sometimes there is experienced a feeling of weight and dis-comfort—the latter occasionally amounting to a neuralgic pain. The discomfort is generally worse during vigorous exercise and during hot weather.

In mild cases, the best treatment for a varicocele is to ignore it ; in more severe cases a suspensory bandage may be worn. The affection can often be relieved by cold baths, which have a bracing effect generally, and by attention to the bowels. If the condition is causing anxiety, an operation can be performed by means of which a portion of the venous network is removed, or it may be obliterated by injection, like varicose veins. (*See also* SPERMATIC CORD ; TESTICLE.)

VARICOSE VEIN. A vein is called varicose when it is dilated, twisted and knotty in appearance. Actually, the twisting is due to the elongation of the vein. Many veins in different parts of the body can be so affected, but the commonest situation is the leg. Most often it is the saphenous vein which passes up the inner side of the leg and thigh which becomes varicose.

The fundamental cause of varicose veins of the leg is a hereditary weakness of the walls of the veins and of the valves. These valves are unable to withstand any extra call upon the blood circulation, so that they become incompetent and do not help to support the long column of blood. The result is that there is a certain amount of sluggishness of the venous return of blood—and sometimes a back flow so that the veins become dilated, lengthened and finally twisted. There are certain contributory factors which tend to produce varicose veins. Anything constricting the limb, such as tight garters, leads to this affection while the strain of standing for prolonged periods is a common precipitating cause. This explains the frequency of the condition in shop assistants and policemen. In women, the pregnant womb by pressing on the great veins in the pelvis may lead to varicose veins and similarly any abdominal tumour or even an overloaded bowel, as in constipation, may have the same adverse effect.

The earliest symptom is a feeling of weight and fullness in the limb after standing or a long walk. On examination, the veins will be seen to be prominent and, as the condition develops, the veins bulge out and are seen to be twisted and knotted under the skin. The feeling of weight increases and there is a marked weariness of the limbs after even a short period of standing. Nearly always there is a certain amount of swelling of the ankles, for the obstruction of the venous flow causes a local dropsy. This leads to impairment of the nutrition of the skin and blood pigment is deposited which is irritating. Any friction on the part is then apt to lead to dermatitis which may ultimately cause a breakdown of the tissues, or, in other words, a varicose ulcer.

Treatment. Once the condition is established, it is difficult to cure except by the modern method of injecting chemical substances which lead to obliteration of the veins, or by operation. In some cases, the varicose veins can be controlled by the wearing of an elastic bandage. This should be put on first thing in the morning *in bed*, and should not be taken off again until the person is again in bed at night. The object sought after is to prevent a large column of blood from collecting in the veins and so further dilating them. Massage or gentle rubbing in an upward direction is also beneficial, but it must be carefully carried out so as to avoid injury to the veins. Should redness and pigmentation of the skin in the lower part of the leg develop, the part affected should be freely dusted with a zinc oxide and fine boracic powder. For the treatment of eczema and ulceration *see* under respective headings.

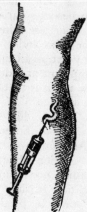

Injection treatment of Varicose Vein

The most recent treatment for varicose veins is by the local injection into the veins of a solution of salicylate of soda or a quinine salt or soda morrhuate which produces a firm clot within the veins. This clot ultimately becomes hard and fibrous and so obliterates the venous channel. This treatment may take some time, but it does not necessitate the patient lying up and it prevents the need of a more extensive surgical operation. Some people might imagine that the formation of a clot in the vein might be dangerous but this is not so, as there is no sepsis involved, and thousands of cases have been done in this country without fatality. (*See also* VEIN.)

VASA VASORUM. These are the tiny microscopic blood-vessels which supply the walls of the arteries and veins. Like all other tissues, the large blood-vessels require a constant supply of nutriment.

VAS DEFERENS. This is one of the two main ducts of the

testicle along which the secretion of that organ is conveyed to its temporary storehouse in the seminal vesicles.

VEIN. The tubes which carry the blood to the heart are called veins. They are similar in structure to the arteries, and possess three coats—an inner elastic lining, a middle muscular coat, and an outer covering of fibrous connective tissue. In contrast with an artery, the middle muscle-coat of a vein is much less developed, so that the vein collapses when empty while the artery retains its tubular form. The veins are provided with valves which permit the blood to flow in one direction only, the valves being floated back to close the vein if there is any backward flow of blood.

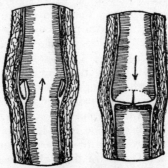

Vein: showing closure of valve

The blood in the veins is dark purplish in colour, for much of its oxygen has been lost to the tissues. There is one exception to this in the case of the pulmonary veins which take the pure oxygenated blood from the lungs to the heart. The veins more or less follow the course of the arteries and are named after the arteries they accompany.

Diseases and injuries of veins. An injury to a vein is generally a much less serious affair than an injury to an artery, as the blood flows slowly and the flow can easily be controlled by pressure. Bleeding from a large vein, however, such as a ruptured varicose vein in the leg, may be dangerous as also a wound of one of the large veins in the neck or armpit. In the latter case, there is the added risk of air being sucked into the vein, causing an air-embolus, and this may lead to death. Veins which have become dilated, twisted and knotty are termed *varicose*. (*See* Varicose Veins). Clotting of blood in a vein is termed *thrombosis*; it causes stoppage of the flow of blood; the vein swells and the function of the part involved is handicapped. This condition arises during the course of prolonged illnesses when the blood is in a septic state as in typhoid fever.

Inflammation of a vein is called *phlebitis*. (*See also* CIRCULATION OF BLOOD ; THROMBOSIS ; WHITE LEG.)

VENA CAVA. The two great veins which collect all the blood from the whole of the body and pass it into the right auricle of the heart are called the superior and the inferior vena cava. (*See also* VEIN.)

VENEREAL DISEASE. A disease acquired through the act of sexual intercourse is termed a venereal disease. Into this category come *syphilis, gonorrhœa* and *soft chancre* or sore. All these diseases are dependent upon micro-organisms or germs, and they may in a few cases be acquired other than venereally, e.g. by contact with infected towels in the case of gonorrhœa or drinking vessels in the case of syphilis. The occurrence of venereal diseases is one of the greatest of all social problems, yet they are essentially preventable diseases provided reasonable sanitary precautions are taken. (*See also* GONORRHŒA ; CHANCRE ; SYPHILIS.)

VENTRICLE. The literal meaning of this word is " little stomach," and it is used to describe two of the muscular chambers of the heart, the spaces in the brain filled with cerebro-spinal fluid, and to certain spaces in the larynx or voice box.

VERTEBRA. The back bone is made up of a number of segments each superimposed upon the other and the individual bones are called vertebra. There are thirty-three vertebræ, varying in size and shape, but they are all constructed on a similar plan.

There is a rounded or oval body from which two portions are directed backwards to form an arch which ends in a spine-like process. The body is composed of spongy bone, and between the bodies of the vertebræ are disks of fibro-cartilage, thus making a solid yet flexible column. Projecting from either side of the arch is a bony outgrowth called the transverse process, and in the neck region this is perforated for the transmission of the vertebral artery. On the arch there are also articular processes by which the arch of one vertebra joints with that of another. The superimposed arches with their ligaments form the spinal canal in which is placed the delicate spinal cord. There are seven cervical, twelve dorsal, five lumbar, five sacral and four coccygeal vertebræ. The neck vertebræ are small and permit of free movement. The first cervical vertebra is called the atlas and it joints with the occipital bone of the skull. The second cervical vertebra is called the axis. To the dorsal vertebræ are attached the ribs. The lumbar vertebræ are very strong, while the five sacral vertebræ are fused together in early life to form a solid triangular bone. The coccygeal vertebræ are very small and insignificant and are often fused together.

The vertebral column may be affected by tuberculosis as in

Pott's Disease, and it is sometimes the site of secondary cancer following cancer of the breast. Rheumatoid arthritis of the spinal column may also occur, converting the flexible column into a rigid, unbending mass. (*See also* POTT'S DISEASE ; SPINAL CORD.)

VESICAL. This is an adjective used to denote anything referring to the urinary bladder. Thus the blood vessels supplying the bladder are called vesical arteries and veins, and a stone in the bladder is called a vesical calculus.

VILLUS. This is a small finger-like process which is found in the lining membrane of the small intestine. Villi are present in great numbers and give the interior of the intestine the appearance of a velvet pile. Each villus contains blood-vessels and one or more lacteals, small tubes which carry off the fat absorbed from the intestine. By means of villi the absorptive capacity of the bowel is greatly increased.

The term villi is also given to the small processes on the outer surface of the chorion, which is one of the membranes of the developing embryo in the womb. On one part the chorionic villi are greatly developed and form the placenta, by means of which nourishment is conveyed from the mother to the child.

VINCENT'S ANGINA. *See* ANGINA.

VIRUS. This is the term which signifies the morbid poisonous material produced in the course of an infective disease, by which the disease can be reproduced when it is inoculated into another person. The virus may contain germs visible through the microscope, but in some cases these cannot be demonstrated though they are presumed to exist. Certain types of virus such as those of smallpox, rabies, and foot-and-mouth disease, are able to pass through a fine porcelain filter and they are described as filterable viruses. (*See also* BACTERIA.)

VISCERA. This is the term applied collectively to the internal organs of the body. A single organ is described as a *viseus*.

VISCEROPTOSIS. Sagging of the abdominal organs is termed visceroptosis. The condition is also known by the name Glenard's disease or abdominal ptosis. It is a fairly common complaint, being much more frequently observed in women than in men. The commonest age period is from 25 to 30 years.

Symptoms. The severity of the symptoms does not correspond to the degree of the visceroptosis. Those who do suffer complain of a feeling of weight and dragging pain in the abdomen and loins, aggravated by the erect posture and by exertion, and eased by lying down. It is believed that these sensations are produced by dragging on the nerves contained in the peritoneal attachments of the organs. There are usually some dyspeptic symptoms, and, owing to the development of bands which tend to kink the intestines, symptoms of intestinal self-poisoning arise. In many of these cases, there develops a neurasthenic element which is a difficult factor to deal with in treatment.

If this condition of visceroptosis is suspected, on examination, the lower part of the abdomen will be found to be unduly prominent, especially in the erect posture, and it may be possible to detect the actual organ which is displaced by palpation. Should there be any doubt, an X-ray investigation after a bismuth meal will yield evidence of the existence of this affection.

Treatment. If it is commenced sufficiently early, much can be done by toning up the abdominal muscles by massage and suitable graduated exercises. A belt or bandage may be worn. It is imperative to keep the bowels well open, and to this end a roughage-containing diet should be eaten. The neurasthenic factor must also be treated by psychological methods. In some cases, the Weir-Mitchell treatment has proved very beneficial. Should these simple methods fail, the possibility of a surgical operation must be considered. The unduly movable organs can be fixed to the back wall of the abdominal cavity. These operations are not always successful, however, and any relief which is afforded may not be permanent. (*See also* ABDOMEN ; BELT ; INTESTINE.)

VITAMINS. These are substances present in various food-stuffs of a very complex composition which are essential for the maintenance of health. Up to the present five vitamins have been recognized, A, B, C, D and E, with a possible sixth, K. It is only recently that the separate identity of A and D has been established, and six elements have been recognised in the original B, of which two, B_1 and B_2 (the latter sometimes called G) appear to be important. Further research will probably reveal the presence of further vitamins.

Vitamin A (the fat-soluble vitamin) is derived from the green chlorophyll in plants and so is present in milk and butter, animal fats and fish livers. The deficiency diseases directly due to lack of this vitamin are rare, but deficiency of it is responsible for a lowering of resistance to infection. Vitamin B (the water-soluble vitamin) has two main elements, B_1 (the lack of which causes beri-beri) and B_2 (the lack of which causes pellagra). These diseases are rare, but deficiency of this vitamin causes such disorders as constipation and anæmia, and pregnant and nursing mothers appear to require it especially. It is found in the germ or outer covering of wheat and other seeds, in yeast, oranges, tomatoes and lean meat. Vitamin C, the scurvy preventing vitamin, is present in oranges, lemons, potatoes, green vegetables, lean meat and slightly in un-cooked milk. Vitamin D is present in most of the foodstuffs in which vitamin A is present (except green vegetables, carrots and tomatoes) which explains why at first they were not recognized as separate substances. Vitamin D prevents rickets and almost all living cells contain a substance (ergosterol) which when irradiated by ultra-violet rays becomes anti-rachitic. The chief source of vitamin D is cod-liver oil. Vitamin E is related to reproductive capacity, and wheat germs are the chief source of it. Vitamin K, which has been isolated in America from the alfalfa plant, is said to slow up the clotting of the blood. Any ordinary good mixed diet, with fresh fruit or vegetables, lean meat and milk, will contain a sufficiency of the vitamins for good health. (*See also* DEFICIENCY DISEASES.)

VOCAL CORDS. These are two cords consisting of tense elastic bands which stretch from back to front of the larynx. Each is controlled by small muscles supplied by nerves under the control of the will. It is through the vibration of these cords that speech is chiefly produced. During swallowing, the vocal cords approximate and so prevent food from passing into the larynx on its way to the gullet. Above the " true " vocal cords are the false vocal cords, which are simply folds of tissue which take no part in phonation. (*See also* LARYNX.)

VOLVULUS. The twisting of a length of bowel upon itself so as to obstruct the passage of the bowel contents is called volvulus. The portion most usually affected is the sigmoid colon, and the affection is associated with chronic constipation. (*See also* INTESTINE: OBSTRUCTION.)

VOMITING. The violent and forcible expulsion of the stomach contents through the mouth is called vomiting. This act is generally preceded and accompanied by a feeling of sickness or nausea and by a free flow of saliva.

The causes of vomiting are exceedingly numerous and many are not related to the digestive organs. The commonest cause, however, is irritation of the stomach from the eating of unsuitable foods, the drinking of excessive amounts of alcohol, or from the swallowing of irritant chemical poisons. Vomiting is a symptom of gastric catarrh, acute or chronic, and of other organic diseases of the stomach such as ulcer and dilatation of that organ. In the case of gastric ulcer, vomiting usually takes place immediately after a meal. In dilatation of the stomach there is vomiting of large quantities of fluid at considerable intervals of time. After very severe vomiting from any cause, the vomit may be streaked with blood, and this is merely due to the effects of straining upon the membranes of the stomach. In cancer of the stomach, the vomit may be " coffee-ground " in appearance; this is due to the gastric secretion altering blood which has oozed from the cancer.

Vomiting may arise from reflex causes, i.e. from irritation in some distant organ. Thus it may arise from tickling of the throat, from coughing, in colic, appendicitis, worms in the intestines, gall-stones, gall-bladder inflammation, liver and pancreatic disorders, and strangulated hernias. It may also occur in nervous and mental disorders, in hysteria, migraine, locomotor ataxia, brain tumour and abscesses, concussion and compression of the brain and meningitis. Any disagreeable smells or unpleasant sights may invoke vomiting in sensitive persons. The motion of a boat at sea is a common cause of vomiting. In children, periodic attacks of vomiting may arise, cyclical vomiting, which is associated with a diminution of the alkalinity of the blood (acidosis). In the early months of pregnancy, sickness, sometimes amounting to actual vomiting, is a common symptom. Finally, vomiting can be caused by direct irritation of the vomiting centre in the brain through the action of an emetic drug such as apomorphine or from the circulation in the blood of the poisons of certain infectious fevers.

Treatment. It should be remembered that vomiting is in itself merely a symptom, and it is the fundamental cause which requires treatment. If it is due to irritant foods or drinks, the vomiting will rid the stomach of the cause of the trouble, and in such cases the vomiting is to be encouraged. Plenty of warm water should be drunk as this helps to wash out the stomach and also relieves the distress and discomfort of the vomiting. In gastritis or gastric catarrh, regulation of the diet is all important. For some days the diet should be limited to fluids, milk, egg and albumen water and, when all vomiting has ceased, semi-solid foods can then be taken. Distressing vomiting from any cause may be relieved by sipping hot water or iced soda water, or by the application of a mustard plaster to the abdomen. In children who suffer from cyclical vomiting, large doses of alkali (sodium bicarbonate) and of glucose will cut short the attacks. Alcoholic cases will benefit by a saline purge every morning. A great many drugs are used in the treatment of vomiting, tincture of opium, chloretone, dilute hydrocyanic acid, and others ; but an effective remedy is to use a drop of tincture of iodine in a tablespoonful of tepid water and repeat the dose four or five times at fifteen-minute intervals. (*See also* DYSPEPSIA ; EMETIC ; GASTRITIS ; SEA SICKNESS.)

VULVA. This is the name given to the external genital organs of the female. They consist of two pairs of lips or double folds of skin which surround and conceal the vaginal opening. These lips are called the labia majora and the labia minora. The front ends of the labia minora surround the clitoris, which is a sensitive erectile structure similar to the penis in the male sex.

Inflammation of the vulva, or vulvitis, may arise from lack of cleanliness of the parts or from the irritation of threadworms (especially in the case of children), but is commonly caused by gonorrhœa. The symptoms include a feeling of itching and burning with intense discomfort and the presence of a purulent discharge. The vulva become red and swollen. Treatment necessitates rest in bed with frequent bathing and douching, with the use of a mild antiseptic ointment. Gonorrhœal vulvitis requires special treatment under the direction of a doctor. (*See also* GENITAL SYSTEM.)

WARTS. Warts are small harmless tumours of the skin. They may appear on any part, and are thought to be due to an infection. They are certainly contagious. There are four varieties : (1) the common raised wart found on the hands ; (2) the flat wart found on the hands and face, and most commonly in children ; (3) the corn-like warts found on the soles, rarely on the palms, at sites of pressure ; (4) " cauliflower " or venereal warts, found chiefly about the genitals and anus. Warts may also occur on a skin affected with seborrhœa, and on a senile skin. These may become cancerous.

Treatment. The simplest method is to freeze the warts with ethyl chloride and snip them off with scissors ; or they may be destroyed by freezing with carbon dioxide snow. Caustic, such as salicylic or acetic acids, are efficient but slow, and the pain naturally lasts over a longer period. Venereal warts owe their size to the heat and moisture of the parts, and when treated with a simple drying powder containing 5 per cent. salicylic acid readily shrivel up. Seborrhœic and senile warts are treated by curetting and cauterizing. Accompanying seborrhœa, and the itching so often found with senile warts, are treated under their individual headings.

The effect of X-rays on warts is, in careful hands, remarkable, large crops often disappearing in a very short time. On the other hand, in some cases this treatment may fail entirely.

Internally, arsenic in small doses, Epsom salts, or green iodide of mercury will sometimes produce a cure ; and the injection of salvarsan (an arsenical preparation) is successful in some cases.

WASSERMANN REACTION. This is a test introduced by Wassermann in 1906 for the detection of syphilitic infection. It is a very complicated reaction and requires to be carried out by a skilled pathologist. (*See also* SYPHILIS.)

WATER-BRASH. This is the regurgitation into the mouth of a hot, bitter fluid from the stomach. Very often it is accompanied by heartburn. Water-brash is a symptom of acid dyspepsia. (*See also* HEARTBURN.)

WATER-HAMMER PULSE. In severe disease of the aortic valve of the heart, in which there is regurgitation of blood, the pulse has a characteristic up and down movement. There is a strong impulse at the pulse which falls away very rapidly. This thumping pulse is called the water-hammer or Corrigan's pulse. (*See also* HEART.)

WEIL'S DISEASE. This is a febrile disorder associated with jaundice and bleedings and occurring in epidemic form. (*See also* JAUNDICE.)

WEN. This is the popular term for a sebaceous cyst. It forms in the skin, most often of the scalp, face or back, and results from the blocking of a duct of a sebaceous gland. Normally, the oily secretion of these glands is poured out on the skin, but should

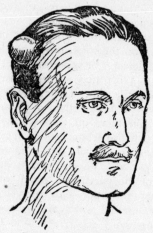

Wen or Sebaceous Cyst

the duct of the gland be obstructed from any cause, the secretion accumulates and a soft swelling forms which gradually enlarges to considerable dimensions if untreated. The skin over the wen in time becomes thin and red and may become inflamed if irritated. Suppuration may then arise, and the wen ruptures with the discharge of offensive pus. Apart from this complication, wens are disfiguring, and they should be removed when of quite moderate size. The operation is very simple and is carried out under a local anæsthetic. It consists of opening the cyst, evacuating its contents, and then removing the whole of the cyst wall.

WHITE LEG. This is the popular expression used to describe a swelling of the leg which sometimes complicates the puerperium, i.e., the first 2 or 3 weeks after childbirth. The condition is due to an inflammation of the lymph vessels of the leg which partially obstructs the channels and leads to a white swelling of the limb.

The infection probably enters the lymphatic system through injury of the tissues at the neck of the womb. Most often the left leg is involved.

The swelling is first noticed in the thigh and gradually extends to the whole leg. It is dead white in colour and the swelling is hard and unyielding. There is usually a certain amount of fever which persists for a few days. Treatment necessitates absolute rest in bed with elevation of the limb by means of pillows. Pain is relieved by a glycerine and belladonna mixture applied locally, and the bowels are kept freely open. Within a few weeks, the condition subsides and recovery is complete, although in a few cases the swelling of the leg may reappear on exertion. Massage is useful in such cases. Swelling of the lower limbs may also arise from clotting of the blood in deep veins during the course of infective fevers such as typhoid or pneumonia. (*See also* LYMPHATIC SYSTEM ; PHLEBITIS ; THROMBOSIS.)

WHITES. The name " whites " is popularly used for a thick white or yellow vaginal discharge due to an unhealthy condition of the vagina and cervix. It is described under its medical name of LEUCORRHŒA.

WHITLOW. This is a painful septic inflammation occurring usually in one of the fingers or thumb. It is most often caused by the prick of a dirty pin or some such sharp object.

A superficial whitlow commences as a red tender spot which becomes a blister filled with pus. If the inflammation spreads more

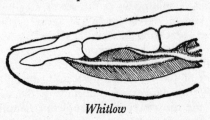

Whitlow

deeply, pain and tenderness become very marked, and there is also throbbing. The whole finger commences to swell, the glands in the elbow and armpit become tender and the pain gets progressively worse in the finger and may be so severe as to prevent sleep. There is often a certain amount of fever and constitutional disturbance according to the degree of the inflammation.

Suppuration in a tendon sheath may extend into the palm, and this is almost certain to cause subsequent disability in the use of the hand. If the tendon of the thumb or little finger is involved, the inflammation may spread to the wrist and forearm and abscess formation may take place. In the most severe cases there may be sloughing of the tendons and the bone may be affected, causing its destruction. In such a case, it may become necessary to sacrifice the hand by amputation to prevent further spread of the suppuration, and there is always a danger of a serious blood infection or septicæmia arising as a further complication and not infrequently proving fatal.

It is therefore clear that a whitlow is a potentially dangerous condition and should always be regarded seriously. If the whitlow does not immediately respond to home methods of treatment, there should be no delay in seeking expert treatment from the doctor. It is nearly always in cases where the sufferer has continued to attempt self-treatment that the grave complications mentioned arise.

With a superficial whitlow, the best immediate treatment is to open the blister with a sterile needle or pair of scissors, allow the contents to escape, remove any loose skin, and then apply a boracic fomentation and continue fomenting until all pain and redness disappear. Deeper types of whitlow require free incision deeply into the skin in order to allow any pus to drain away. This should be performed by the doctor. Subsequently hot boracic fomentations are applied at frequent intervals until the condition clears up. Meanwhile the arm should be supported by a sling with the hand well raised. (*See also* ABSCESS.)

WHOOPING COUGH. An acute infectious fever characterized by peculiar spasmodic outbursts of coughing ; whooping cough is also known by the technical term pertussis. It is an epidemic disease, occurring in childhood and generally before the age of ten. Infection is conveyed by droplets of discharged fluid laden with germs, but the risks of infection diminish after the early stages of the fever are past, and, during the spasmodic coughing stage, the danger of transmitting the disease is slight. One attack of the disease confers complete immunity for the rest of life.

The incubation period is from one to two weeks and the fever is conveniently divided into three stages. Firstly, lasting from 7 to 10 days, there are symptoms suggesting a severe cold in the head with a certain amount of feverishness. There is some degree of bronchitis with a hard cough, and then in the second stage there develops the typical spasmodic cough. This consists of a series of short expiratory coughs without any air entering the lungs, the sufferer becoming black in the face at times. Then follows a long crowing expiration, producing the characteristic " whoop." A number of attacks usually follow on each other and, as a rule, relief does not arise until either vomiting occurs, or a considerable quantity of sticky mucous secretion is brought up. The paroxysms most often come on at night-time before sleeping, and sometimes after meals. They are liable to be induced by a fright or by hearing someone else cough.

During the attacks the eyes bulge and may become bloodshot and bleeding may occur into the conjunctiva. The child holds on to the bed or an adult and is in great fear. Bleeding from the nose not infrequently arises, and very occasionally bleeding into the brain may result. Convulsions may also be induced in very young children. Interference with the child's sleep and the inability to take proper nourishment and the vomiting may produce considerable exhaustion and wasting.

In the third stage, the whooping cough gets gradually less and within three or four weeks the child should be practically well. In some debilitated children an occasional whoop may persist for some months. The complication most to be feared in whooping cough is catarrhal pneumonia, and for the prevention of this everything depends upon careful nursing and treatment of the child. Persistent bronchitis and emphysema may also be sequels to severe attacks. There is also a danger that the weakened resources of the child may render it a prey to tubercular infection. As whooping cough is very infectious in the early stages, complete isolation of the child is essential in the interests of other children. Six weeks is generally reckoned as an adequate time ; and children who have been in contact with a known case of the disease should be isolated for three weeks as a precautionary measure. During an epidemic of whooping cough, a child who develops an acute cold in the head with bronchitis should be carefully watched and preferably isolated until the real nature of the illness is manifest.

Treatment. In the case of strong children there may be no need to put them to bed, especially in the summer. They should have as much fresh air as possible and should be kept warm and given nutritious food. With more delicate children—and in winter —they should be kept in bed exclusively in one room until the temperature has subsided and the symptoms have considerably abated. The air of the room may be impregnated with cresoline or similar drugs. If there is much vomiting, the diet should be restricted to milk, beaten eggs and custard. Drugs such as bromide and chloral may be prescribed to control the paroxysms, and there is now available a vaccine which is preventive in the earliest stages and mitigates the disease if it develops. Recently injections of adrenaline have been employed with considerable success. Injections of ether deeply into the muscles have also been advised.

During a paroxysm, someone should always be present to comfort and reassure the child, as the mental strain to a young child so induced is very great. Care should be taken to disinfect and destroy any sputum from the child, especially in the early stages. (*See also* BRONCHO-PNEUMONIA ; DISINFECTION ; INFECTIOUS DISEASE.)

WOMB. The uterus, or womb, is a pear-shaped organ freely movable in the pelvis and situated between the bladder and the rectum. It measures $3\frac{1}{2}$ inches long, 2 inches wide by 1 inch thick ; its narrow end or neck projects into the vagina, while its upper expanded end, or fundus, has the Fallopian tubes springing from its sides. These pass outwards to be loosely attached to the ovaries and they convey microscopic ova (eggs) from the ovaries to the womb.

The womb consists of an outer or serous coat, a middle or muscular coat, and an inner or mucous coat. The mucous membrane is of peculiar structure and is constantly undergoing changes. During the child-bearing period it periodically becomes engorged with blood, culminating in menstruation. The membrane is reconstructed every month unless pregnancy takes place, when it undergoes another complete change. After birth, it slowly returns to its normal condition and remains quiescent until lactation has ceased.

Owing to its movability, the womb is constantly being affected by its neighbouring organs, especially the bladder, the varying size of which necessitates accommodating movements of the womb. In close association with the Fallopian tubes are two muscular cords, the round ligaments, which extend upwards and pass to the external genital organs (labia majora) and help to support the womb. There are six other supporting ligaments which are composed of folds of peritoneum, the lining membrane of the abdominal cavity. Inside the uterus there is a triangular cavity into which the Fallopian tubes open above, and which is prolonged downwards into the cavity of the neck of the womb as the cervical canal. This opens into the vagina, the opening being termed the external os (to distinguish it from the internal os), which is the place where the cervical canal joins the cavity of the body of the womb.

Displacement of the Womb. Normally the womb is bent forwards upon itself at the junction of the neck with the body, this position being described as *anteflexion*. It is also bent forward in the pelvic cavity and this is termed *anteversion*. When it is bent backwards this is called *retroflexion*, and when it is tilted right back on itself this is called *retroversion*. One of the commonest forms of womb trouble is one or other of the displacements to which the organ is subject. It may be displaced in various directions by pressure exerted by tumours or swellings in the abdomen, or by adhesions to other organs which drag upon it, or by its own weight, especially if there is a co-existing weakness of the supporting ligaments and muscular floor of the pelvis.

Prolapse, or "falling of the womb," is a downwards displacement. It is most common in elderly women whose muscles have lost tone or who have become thinner, and so have lost the support of the internal pads of fat which help to maintain the womb in position. It may also arise following a confinement in which the birth passages have been injured and torn and the tissues have not firmed up adequately. Frequent straining as a result of chronic constipation or a chronic cough, also tends to downward displacement especially if there is any weakness of the ligaments and the pelvic floor.

The first symptom is generally a feeling of inward heaviness, with backache and a sensation of always being tired. There is also frequent desire to pass water and to empty the bowels, while menstruation is often excessive and more prolonged than usual. At this stage the patient should consult a doctor, for much can be done by exercises, general tonic treatment, fresh air, correct dieting and the relief of constipation to prevent further trouble and avoid the need for an operation. Once a displacement is definitely established a pessary or womb support will be required or an operation resorted to. In an otherwise healthy woman the latter is preferable, as a pessary is only palliative, and unless correctly fitted is of no value. In very severe cases, the womb may appear outside the body and then it is apt to become ulcerated and bleed. Part of the bladder and bowel may also protrude (cystocele and recticele) and cause discomfort. In such cases an operation is desirable.

Inflammation of the womb mucous membrane is termed endometritis, of the muscle—metritis, and of the tissues surrounding the womb—perimetritis. It is treated usually by hot douches ; but an operation (curettage) may sometimes be necessary. (*See also.* Genital System ; Menstruation ; Pessary ; Visceroptosis.)

WORM. Various types of worm are parasitic in the human body and are productive of disease. There are two main groups, the flatworms which consist of the tapeworms and flukes, and the roundworms. These parasites gain entrance to the body through the eating of infected food, drinking infected water or directly through the skin.

The roundworms most often infecting man are the thread or pinworm, the ascaris lumbricoides—or intestinal roundworm, and the whipworm or tricocephalus dispar. There is one other variety, the ankylostoma, but this worm is rarely met with in this country. The *ascaris lumbricoides* resembles the ordinary earthworm ; it has

a pinkish colour, tapers at each end, and the mouth is surrounded
by three projections armed with fine teeth. In length it varies
from 4 to 12 inches. It is probable that the mouse or rat is the intermediate host by swallowing the eggs. These develop into larvæ
and are deposited on human food, and the infection so conveyed
to man. The worms live in the small intestine and may make their
way into the bile ducts, stomach, gullet and thence to the air
passages. They are expelled by the bowel or they may be vomited.
As a rule only two or three worms are present, but occasionally
there are large numbers.

If only a few are present, there may be no symptoms and the
condition is only discovered when a worm is detected in the motion.
On the other hand, there may be a capricious appetite, with itching
of the nose, sickness and vomiting, and sometimes blood in the
motions. In children convulsions may arise. If a worm enters the
bile duct, jaundice may be caused and, if a large number of worms
are present, they may lead to obstruction of the bowel. The best
treatment is the correct administration of the drug santonin or oil
of chenopodium. A light diet precedes the use of the former drug,
which is given in doses from 1 to 5 grains along with 2 grains of
calomel at bed-time. In the morning a saline purge is taken. Santonin must be administered with care as it sometimes upsets the
patient, producing yellow vision amongst other unpleasant symptoms, and two nights should elapse before the dose is repeated.

The **threadworm** or *oxyuris vermicularis* is an exceedingly common
infection in children. This worm is about ¼- to ¾-inch in length,
the female being 2 to 3 times larger than the male. The worm
gets into the body by the swallowing of the eggs which hatch out
in the intestine where the worms mature. Their habitat is the large
intestine from the cæcum to the anus, and the impregnated female
discharges her eggs in the rectum, from which they are voided in
the stools.

The worms often wriggle out of the anus, causing intense itching,
especially at night. In females, they may enter the vagina, causing
irritation and discharge. Children are apt to scratch these parts
and convey the eggs to the mouth and so infect themselves. Children
so infected are peevish, irritable, complain of colicky pain and
exhibit reflex symptoms such as grinding of the teeth at night, night
terrors, and occasionally convulsions. The appetite may be voracious.
The condition is easily detected by finding the worms in the motions.
They resemble small wriggling pieces of white thread.

To rid the bowel of the worms, frequent enemata of infusions
of quassia are necessary. The young child should be given an
injection into the bowel of about 6 ounces and older children up

to $\frac{3}{4}$-pint. Salt and water or lime water are also used for this purpose, but are not so effective as infusion of quassia. Internally, small doses of santonin are beneficial, but this drug should be given only under medical supervision. On rising in the morning the child's anus should be washed after the bowels move, and a weak mercurial ointment applied fairly liberally to the part. Regular action of the bowels is essential, and if the child scratches at night a close pair of knickers should be worn. Every precaution should be taken to prevent the child re-infecting itself.

In all forms of tapeworm, when infected meat is eaten, the cyst is dissolved in the stomach, the head is set free and fixes itself to the mucous membrane of the intestine and develops segments. The symptoms are variable and the infection may only be discovered by finding segments of worms in the expelled motions. Colic may be complained of or the appetite may be unusual. Occasionally, there is headache, depression and irritability, these nervous symptoms being due to poisons liberated by the worm. Tapeworms may live for years in the human body, and there may be several present at the same time.

Treatment. The most usual remedy is oil of male fern. This is administered with some carminative such as peppermint or cinnamon first thing in the morning before breakfast and after a fast which has commenced at 6 p.m. the night before. Two hours afterwards a saline purge is taken, or four hours later a dose of castor oil, and the motions are passed into warm water. It is essential that the head be sought for, otherwise, unless it be passed, the segments will grow again. Should the head not be passed, it will be three months before more segments are passed, and it is therefore advisable to wait until that time before recommencing treatment. *It is important* that the castor-oil should never be taken at the same time as the male fern, as it dissolves a harmful substance in the latter. Other remedies used to kill tapeworm are oil of turpentine, and decoction of pomegranate bark. (*See also* BILHARZIASIS ; FILARIASIS ; HYDATID DISEASE ; MALE FERN ; SANTONIN.)

WRIST. The region between the hand and the forearm is popularly described as the wrist. It may be conveniently taken as that part of the upper limb comprised by the lower ends of the radius and ulna, the eight carpal or wrist bones, and the adjacent parts of the metacarpal bones. The eight small bones are arranged in two rows of four, the upper four joining with the radius to form the radio-carpal joint, or the wrist joint proper. There is a considerable range of movement at the wrist, flexion (forward bending), extension (backward bending), adduction (bending to little finger side) and abduction (bending to thumb side). Forward and backward movements are also combined with side movements so that the wrist is exceedingly flexible. Consequently, dislocation is an infrequent injury, though sprains are comparatively common.

The wrist region is devoid of muscles, but there are numerous tendons by which the hand and fingers are moved and these strengthen the part considerably. (*See also* FOREARM ; GANGLION ; RADIUS ; SPRAIN.)

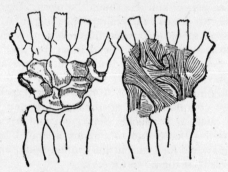

Bones and Ligaments of Wrist

X-RAYS. Known also as the Rontgen rays, after their inventor, the X-rays are a form of radiant energy, originally derived from the sun. A vast number of radiations are given off by the sun which travel through the ether in waves of different length and vibration. There are the obvious luminous rays, but there are many more invisible rays, the ultra-violet rays, wireless telegraphy rays, X-rays and certain rays of radium.

To-day, the X-ray examination adds greatly to the accuracy of diagnosis of a great many diseases. There is the obvious value of X-rays in detecting fractures, dislocations, and in locating needles, bullets and other metallic objects in the tissues ; but the X-rays are equally valuable in investigating the deeper organs. The condition of the heart, great vessels and lungs can be determined by X-ray examination of the chest ; the alimentary canal can be photographed by giving the patient a meal containing bismuth and barium, which are opaque to the X-rays, and much information obtained as to their state of functioning. It is even possible to bring such organs as the brain, kidneys and gall bladder within the scope of accurate X-ray diagnosis by the injection into these organs of opaque substances.

A recent and very important development of X-ray diagnosis is in the detection of dental disease. It is impossible to tell the condition of the roots of teeth other than by the use of X-rays. The X-rays have shown that abscesses may exist without any pain or other symptom, yet these abscesses are dangerous to health, by poisoning the blood stream. X-ray films give well-defined pictures of the teeth and reveal clearly any existing infection at the roots.

X-rays as Curative Agent. Radio-therapy, or treatment of disease by means of X-rays, has made rapid strides in recent years. In the treatment of cancer the value of X-rays is considerable. In some cases, the growth may be completely destroyed, and in others it is so reduced that it can be removed by operation. In inoperable cancers, X-rays treatment enables the sufferer to live for a longer period and in greater comfort than would otherwise be the case. The term "deep therapy" is applied to X-radiation designed to reach organs affected with malignant disease deeply situated within the body and inaccessible to the surgeon. In the treatment of skin diseases, X-rays are of established value. In ringworm of the scalp, the hair can be caused to fall out and later it will return in a healthy state. Chronic eczema, pruritis, or itching, and lupus, (tuberculosis of the skin) can also be benefited. The X-rays in small doses benefit the skin, but in large doses will produce redness which may go on to actual destruction of the tissue—a so-called X-ray burn.

YAWS. This is a tropical disease, variously known as framboesia, purru, parangia and coko, and it is seldom met with in European countries. Yaws is a very contagious disease and is caused by a micro-organism called the treponema pertenue, which is somewhat similar to the organism which causes syphilis, the treponema pallidum. The disease is thought to be carried from one person to another by insects which have become infected from the sores of a sufferer. It may also be spread through direct contact with infected persons or their belongings, and insanitary and unhygienic conditions generally tend to increase its incidence. Infection can only take place through an abrasion or wound of the skin.

YELLOW FEVER. This is an acute specific tropical fever, now restricted mainly to West Africa and South America, and characterized by jaundice, bleeding, gastro-intestinal disturbance, and sometimes suppression of urine. The disease affects white people much more than coloured people ; it is most prevalent in swampy, low-lying country and in insanitary overcrowded towns.

Yellow fever is caused by a micro-organism which is carried by a special variety of mosquito, called the stegomyia fasciata.

In treatment, a special serum invented by Noguchi, if injected during the first day or two of the disease, is likely to be beneficial and lead to recovery, but after the third day this serum is comparatively ineffective. Otherwise the usual methods for the management of fever are adopted. The occurrence of yellow fever has been greatly diminished by the destruction of mosquitoes and by preventing their breeding, and by draining swamps. Persons suffering from the disease should be carefully screened to prevent being bitten by mosquitoes and so spreading the infection. A vaccine is now available in preventing this deadly disease. (*See also* MOSQUITO ; TROPICAL HYGIENE.)

ZOSTER. Herpes Zoster is the medical name for a form of shingles, and the condition is described under the heading SHINGLES.

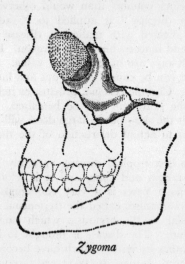

Zygoma

ZYGOMA. This is the name applied to a bridge of bone which joins the temporal bone with the malar bone. (*See also* BONE ; TEMPORAL BONE.)